# IFMBE Proceedings 103

The IFMBE Proceedings Book Series is an official publication of *the International Federation for Medical and Biological Engineering* (IFMBE). The series gathers the proceedings of various international conferences, which are either organized or endorsed by the Federation. Books published in this series report on cutting-edge findings and provide an informative survey on the most challenging topics and advances in the fields of medicine, biology, clinical engineering, and biophysics.

The series aims at disseminating high quality scientific information, encouraging both basic and applied research, and promoting world-wide collaboration between researchers and practitioners in the field of Medical and Biological Engineering.

Topics include, but are not limited to:

- Diagnostic Imaging, Image Processing, Biomedical Signal Processing
- Modeling and Simulation, Biomechanics
- Biomaterials, Cellular and Tissue Engineering
- Information and Communication in Medicine, Telemedicine and e-Health
- Instrumentation and Clinical Engineering
- Surgery, Minimal Invasive Interventions, Endoscopy and Image Guided Therapy
- Audiology, Ophthalmology, Emergency and Dental Medicine Applications
- Radiology, Radiation Oncology and Biological Effects of Radiation
- Drug Delivery and Pharmaceutical Engineering
- Neuroengineering, and Artificial Intelligence in Healthcare

IFMBE proceedings are indexed by SCOPUS, EI Compendex, Japanese Science and Technology Agency (JST), SCImago. They are also submitted for consideration by WoS.

Proposals can be submitted by contacting the Springer responsible editor shown on the series webpage (see "Contacts"), or by getting in touch with the series editor Ratko Magjarevic.

Guangzhi Wang · Dezhong Yao · Zhongze Gu ·
Yi Peng · Shanbao Tong · Chengyu Liu
Editors

# 12th Asian-Pacific Conference on Medical and Biological Engineering

## Proceedings of APCMBE 2023
## May 18–21, 2023
## Suzhou, China—Volume 1: Biomedical Signal Processing, Imaging and Rehabilitation Engineering

Springer

*Editors*
Guangzhi Wang
Department of Biomedical Engineering
School of Medicine
Tsinghua University
Beijing, China

Dezhong Yao
School of Life Science and Technology
University of Electronic Science and Technology
Chengdu, China

Zhongze Gu
State Key Laboratory of Bioelectronics
School of Biological Science and Medical Engineering
Southeast University
Nanjing, China

Yi Peng
Institute of Basic Medical Sciences
Chinese Academy of Medical Sciences and School of Basic Medicine Peking Union Medical College
Beijing, China

Shanbao Tong
School of Biomedical Engineering
Shanghai Jiao Tong University
Shanghai, China

Chengyu Liu
State Key Laboratory of Bioelectronics
School of Instrument Science and Engineering
Southeast University
Nanjing, China

ISSN 1680-0737 ISSN 1433-9277 (electronic)
IFMBE Proceedings
ISBN 978-3-031-51454-8 ISBN 978-3-031-51455-5 (eBook)
https://doi.org/10.1007/978-3-031-51455-5



This Springer imprint is published by the registered company Springer Nature Switzerland AG
The registered company address is: Gewerbestrasse 11, 6330 Cham, Switzerland

Paper in this product is recyclable.

# Preface

The 12th IFMBE Asian-Pacific Conference on Medical and Biological Engineering (APCMBE 2023) was held in Suzhou, China, from 18–21 May 2023. The conference was organized by the Chinese Society of Biomedical Engineering (CSBME) and was endorsed by the International Federation for Medical and Biological Engineering (IFMBE).

Aimed to gather talents in the fields of medicine, enterprise, research, and education, APCMBE 2023 focused on key fields and key technologies of biomedical engineering and promoted the integration of multiple disciplines. Special attention was paid to the frontiers of biomedical engineering, including medical artificial intelligence, neural engineering, medical imaging, computer-aided surgery, biosensors, rehabilitation engineering, medical informatics, biomechanics, and other hot topics and key issues. The progress of biomedical engineering has provided strong support for the realization of translational medicine and personalized medicine based on interdisciplinary cooperation and information sharing. Improving medical standards and ensuring people's health are a long journey and a highly challenging undertaking. We need to maintain an open, innovative, and cooperative spirit, jointly address the challenges, and promote the continuous progress and transformation of technology in biomedical engineering.

In total, we received 363 contributions, out of which 181 contributions were full-length scientific papers, and the rest were short abstract submissions. In total, 100 papers met the standards for publication in the Proceedings of APCMBE 2023.

We, the local organizers, would like to thank IFMBE for its support in organizing APCMBE 2023. Our thanks go to the members of the International Organizing Committee for their contribution. We extend our thanks to the organizers of topical sessions and the reviewers. They made the creation of these proceedings possible by devoting their time and expertise to reviewing the received manuscripts, and thus allowed us to maintain a high standard in selecting the papers for the Proceedings. And last, but certainly not least, we would like to thank Springer Nature publishing company for the support and assistance in publishing this Proceedings.

| | |
|---|---|
| Beijing, China | Guangzhi Wang |
| Chengdu, China | Dezhong Yao |
| Nanjing, China | Zhongze Gu |
| Beijing, China | Yi Peng |
| Shanghai, China | Shanbao Tong |
| Nanjing, China | Chengyu Liu |

# APCMBE 2023 Committees

## Presidium

### President

| | |
|---|---|
| Xuetao Cao | Chinese Academy of Medical Sciences |

### Executive President

| | |
|---|---|
| Shengshou Hu | Fuwai Hospital, Chinese Academy of Medical Sciences |

### Vice Presidents

| | |
|---|---|
| Jing Cheng | Tsinghua University |
| Hui Chi | Medical Information Research Institute, Chinese Academy of Medical Sciences |
| Xiaosong Gu | Nantong University |
| Jinxiang Han | Shandong First Medical University |
| Deyu Li | Beihang University |
| Suiren Wan | Southeast University |
| Guangzhi Wang | Tsinghua University |
| Guosheng Wang | Henan Tuoren Medical Device Co., Ltd |
| Dezhong Yao | University of Electronic Science and Technology of China |
| Yiwu Zhao | Naton Medical Group |
| Hairong Zheng | Shenzhen Institutes of Advanced Technology, Chinese Academy of Sciences |

### Secretary General

| | |
|---|---|
| Hui Chi | Medical Information Research Institute, Chinese Academy of Medical Sciences |

## Scientific Committee

### Director

| | |
|---|---|
| Guangzhi Wang | Tsinghua University |

### Deputy Directors

| | |
|---|---|
| Luming Li | Tsinghua University |
| Xuemin Xu | Shanghai Jiao Tong University |
| Hairong Zheng | Shenzhen Institutes of Advanced Technology, Chinese Academy of Sciences |

### Members

| | |
|---|---|
| Yilin Cao | The Ninth People's Hospital Affiliated to Shanghai Jiao Tong University School of Medicine |
| Zhengtao Cao | Air Force Specialty Medical Center |
| Jin Chang | Tianjin University |
| Jianghua Chen | The First Affiliated Hospital, Zhejiang University School of Medicine |
| Weiyi Chen | Taiyuan University of Technology |
| Wenjuan Chen | Huawei Technologies Co., Ltd |
| Hui Chi | Medical Information Research Institute, Chinese Academy of Medical Sciences |
| Yazhou Cui | Shandong Pharmaceutical Biotechnology Research Center |
| Jianrong Dai | Cancer Hospital, Chinese Academy of Medical Sciences |
| Yubo Fan | Beihang University |
| Jinxiang Han | Shandong First Medical University |
| Feilong Hei | Beijing Anzhen Hospital, Capital Medical University |
| Xiaotong Hou | Beijing Anzhen Hospital, Capital Medical University |
| Jingbo Kang | The Sixth Medical Center of PLA General Hospital |
| Deling Kong | Nankai University |
| Deyu Li | Beihang University |
| Jinsong Li | Zhejiang University |
| Zongjin Li | Nankai University |

| | |
|---|---|
| Hongen Liao | Tsinghua University |
| Kangping Lin | Chung Yuan Christian University |
| Chengyu Liu | Southeast University |
| Hongbing Lu | Air Force Medical University |
| Changsheng Ma | Beijing Anzhen Hospital, Capital Medical University |
| Dong Ming | Tianjin University |
| Hongwei Ouyang | Zhejiang University |
| Yingxin Qi | Shanghai Jiao Tong University |
| Qizhu Tang | Wuhan University |
| Jie Tian | Key Laboratory of Molecular Imaging, Chinese Academy of Sciences |
| Suiren Wan | Southeast University |
| Tao Wan | The Second Military Medical University |
| Shulin Wu | Guangdong Provincial People's Hospital |
| Yifei Wang | Jinan University |
| Zhibiao Wang | Chongqing Medical University |
| Mengyu Wei | University of Macau |
| Xunbin Wei | Peking University |
| Huayuan Yang | Shanghai University of Traditional Chinese Medicine |
| Dezhong Yao | University of Electronic Science and Technology of China |
| Ming Zhang | The Hong Kong Polytechnic University |
| Yiwu Zhao | Naton Medical Group |
| Changren Zhou | Jinan University |

## Organizing Committee

### Director

| | |
|---|---|
| Qingming Luo | Hainan University |

### Deputy Directors

| | |
|---|---|
| Zhongze Gu | Southeast University |
| Xueqing Yu | Guangdong Provincial People's Hospital |
| Qiang Zhang | Shanghai United Imaging Healthcare Co., Ltd |
| Hairong Zheng | Shenzhen Institutes of Advanced Technology, Chinese Academy of Sciences |

**Local Organizing Committee Members**

| | |
|---|---|
| Xin Chen | Shenzhen University |
| Xun Chen | University of Science and Technology of China |
| Xiang Dong | Naton Medical Group |
| Jianzeng Dong | Beijing Anzhen Hospital, Capital Medical University |
| Qianjin Feng | Southern Medical University |
| Feng Fu | Air Force Medical University |
| Xingming Guo | Chongqing University |
| Gang Huang | Shanghai University of Medicine and Health Sciences |
| Baohua Ji | Zhejiang University |
| Linhong Ji | Tsinghua University |
| Hua Jiang | Zhejiang University |
| Xieyuan Jiang | Beijing Jishuitan Hospital |
| Xinquan Jiang | The Ninth People's Affiliated Hospital of Shanghai Jiao Tong University School of Medicine |
| Yan Kang | Shenzhen Technology University |
| Xixiong Kang | Beijing Tiantan Hospital, Capital Medical University |
| Bin Li | Shanghai Sixth People's Hospital Affiliated to Shanghai Jiaotong University |
| Changying Li | Beijing Aeonmed Co., Ltd. |
| Tao Li | Tianjin Third Central Hospital |
| Pengcheng Li | Huazhong University of Science and Technology |
| Jun Liang | The Second Affiliated Hospital of the Air Force Military Medical University |
| Peixue Ling | National Glycoengineering Research Center |
| Gang Liu | Xiamen University |
| Hui Liu | Chinese Academy of Medical Sciences |
| Lihua Liu | The Fourth Hospital of Hebei Medical University |
| Yajun Liu | Beijing Jishuitan Hospital of Capital Medical University |
| Zhicheng Liu | Capital Medical University |
| Aili Lu | Tsinghua University |
| Jiaxin Liu | Chinese Academy of Medical Sciences |
| Ling Lv | The Fourth School of Clinical Medicine of Nanjing Medical University |
| Zhenhe Ma | Northeast University |
| Chenxi Ouyang | Fuwai Hospital, Chinese Academy of Medical Sciences |

**International Organizing Committee Members**

# Contents

## Biomedical Signal Processing

## Neural Engineering



## Rehabilitation Engineering

# Biomedical Signal Processing

# A Risk Probability Prediction Model for Sudden Cardiac Death Based on Heart Rate Variability Metrics

Supeng Yan[1], Xin Song[1], Liang Wei[1], Yushun Gong[1], Houyuan Hu[2], and Yongqin Li[1](✉)

[1] Department of Biomedical Engineering and Imaging Medicine, Army Medical University, Chongqing, China
18719808855@139.com

[2] Department of Cardiology, Southwest Hospital, Army Medical University, Chongqing, China

**Abstract.** The estimated annual number of sudden cardiac death (SCD) is approximately 4 million cases worldwide and approximately 50% of SCDs are unexpected first manifestations of cardiac disease. The identification of subjects at high risk for SCD is of great importance as the prevention of SCD events would be possible with the implantable cardioverter defibrillator (ICD). However, there is no reliable method to estimate individualized SCD risk for prevention. In this paper, we introduced a novel approach to predict individualized SCD risk probability based on heart rate variability metrics (HRV). First, we selected 11 commonly used HRV metrics. The heart rate (HR) corrected HRV metrics ($HRV_C$) and ventricular beat rate (VBR) from 1 h electrocardiogram(ECG) segments were extract as candidate features. Then, the feature dimension was reduced by recursive feature elimination. Finally, training set of normal control and SCD victims was employed to build multi-layer perceptron (MLP) model. To evaluate the model's predictive ability, best cut-off threshold of high and low SCD risk was determined using Youden index. The SCD risk probability based on 1 h $HRV_C$ was $0.00 \pm 0.01$ for normal control and $0.99 \pm 0.01$ for SCD victims. The near-perfect results were achieved for discriminating SCD from normal control. Our method not only estimated individualized SCD risk probability reliably, but also had higher prediction accuracy than the existing methods.

**Keywords:** Sudden cardiac death · Risk probability · Heart rate variability

## 1 Introduction

Sudden cardiac death (SCD) is an unexpected sudden death due to a heart condition, that occurs within one hour of symptoms onset [1]. It is a leading cause of mortality and responsible for approximately half of all deaths from cardiovascular disease [2]. The estimated annual number of SCDs is approximately 4 million cases worldwide and approximately 50% of SCDs are unexpected first manifestations of cardiac disease [3]. It emphasizes the importance of prevention, in which implantable cardioverter defibrillator(ICD) is the most effective approach to primary prevention, leading to substantial


G. Wang et al. (Eds.): APCMBE 2023, IFMBE Proceedings 103, pp. 3–10, 2024.
https://doi.org/10.1007/978-3-031-51455-5_1

reductions in all-cause mortality among appropriately selected patients [4]. Therefore, the identification of subjects at high risk for SCD is of great importance.

The early identification of risk factors for SCD is the philosopher's stone of cardiology, for which researchers worldwide have explored a number of different markers in the past few decades [5]. Among these, heart rate variability (HRV) is probably the most analyzed non-invasive index and has shown potential for predicting SCD. However, all related research of SCD prediction based on HRV were multi-classification models that could not quantitatively provide individualized absolute risk estimation of SCD. In present study, we developed a SCD risk probability ($P_{SCD\text{-}risk}$) prediction model based on heart rate variability metrics to estimate and identify risk of SCD. Figure 1 illustrated the block diagram of the proposed method.

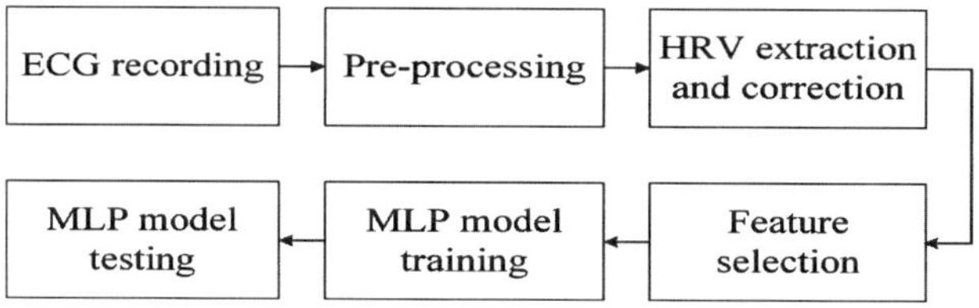


**Fig. 1.** Flowchart of proposed method

## 2 Material and Method

### *A. Study Population*

This study was approved by Ethics Committee of Southwest hospital of the Army Medical University (approval number: KY2020148). Healthy adults with Holter ECG recordings (>10 h) were recruited between May 2017 and November 2019 from Southwest hospital and served as low risk group. SCD victims were obtained from Sudden Cardiac Death Holter Database (SDDB), American Heart Association ECG databases(AHADB) and served as high risk group. Each of SCD victims had a ECG recording before onset of SCD events with data length greater than 1 h. The detailed information of subjects were described in Table 1.

**Table 1.** Summary of subjects used in this study

| Groups | Data source | N | Age, year | Sex (M, F) | ECG duration, h |
|---|---|---|---|---|---|
| Normal control | Southwest hospital | 124 | 48.67 ± 16.52 | 71, 53 | 22.30 ± 2.60 |
| SCD | SDDB, AHADB | 22 | 61.06 ± 19.33 (6 NA) | 10, 8 (4 NA) | 9.80 ± 7.39 |

*N*: Number of Subjects; *M*: Male; *F*: Female; *NA*: Not Available

*B. ECG Pre-Processing*

All the ECG recordings were sampled at 250 Hz. First of all, noise reduction in ECG recordings was done. All ECG recordings were band-pass filtered (0.05–100 Hz) using a fourth-order Butterworth filter. Baseline wander was removed with median filter and power-line frequency was removed with notch filter. Then, the Pan-Tompkins algorithm was used to detect the QRS-complexes in the ECG recordings. The rhythm of beat was revised manually to ensure correct beat classification. Finally, all artifacts and ectopic beats were removed and the resultant missing data were replaced by cubic spline interpolation from the nearest valid data.

*C. Training Set and Testing Set*

To train $P_{SCD\text{-}risk}$ prediction model, 1 h ECG segments were extracted from normal control at 2 h interval and SCD at 10 min interval. The data sets of HRV features extracted from these ECG segments were then randomly partitioned into training set and testing set at a ratio of 8:2. The data set was split cross-subject wise, hence this ensured that subjects in the training set were exclusively different from that in the testing set. Before training the model, training sets were provided with $P_{SCD\text{-}risk}$ as labels. For data in normal control, $P_{SCD\text{-}risk}$ was set to 0 for no SCD occurrence. For data in SCD victims, $P_{SCD\text{-}risk}$ depended on the data collection time, the longer the time between data collection and onset of SCD, the lower the $P_{SCD\text{-}risk}$ would be, with a 0.006 decreasing rate per hour. $P_{SCD\text{-}risk}$ immediately before onset of SCD had a maximum value as 1. The details of data set split can been seen from Table 2.

**Table 2.** Data set split

| Data set | Percentage (%) | ECG segments number |
|---|---|---|
| Training set | 80 | Normal control:1099; SCD: 928 |
| Testing set | 20 | Normal control: 282; SCD: 234 |

*D. Feature Extraction*

The following 11 commonly used HRV metrics were calculated according to published literatures [6]: (1) SDNN: the standard deviation of normally conducted RR intervals(RRI); (2) RMSSD: the root mean square of successive differences in normally conducted RRIs; (3) TINN:triangular interpolation of RRI histogram; (4) HRVTI: HRV triangular index; (5) TP: total power with frequency $< 0.4$ Hz; (6) LF: power in low frequency range (0.04–0.15 Hz); (7) nLF: relative power of the low frequency range in normalized units; (8) SD1: Poincaré plot standard deviation perpendicular the line of identity; (9) SD1/SD2: ratio of SD1 to Poincaré plot standard deviation along the line of identity (SD2); (10) SampEn: sample entropy; (11) DC: deceleration capacity of heart rate.

The heart rate (HR) corrected HRV metric ($HRV_C$) was then calculated as follows. A long-term ECG recording could be divided to several overlapping 5 min ECG segments.

The original HRV metric ($HRV_O$) and mean heart rate ($HR_m$) were obtained by the method described above for all 5 min ECG segments. Then the exponential function was used to quantify the relationship between $HRV_O$ metrics and $HR_m$ using the following Eq. (1), where α was constant, β was fitted exponential power coefficient:

$$HRV_O = \alpha \cdot e^{-\beta \cdot HR_m} \tag{1}$$

Lastly, $HRV_C$ was calculated based on the Eq. (2):

$$HRV_C = \frac{HRV_O}{e^{-\beta \cdot HR_m}} \cdot e^{-\beta \cdot HR_t} \tag{2}$$

where $HR_t$ was the target HR for correction.

In addition to 11 $HRV_C$ metrics, ventricular beat rate(VBR) was also entered in candidate features. It was because ventricular arrhythmia was common cause of SCD in patients with structural heart disease, especially under cardiac stress [7]. To avoid overfitting and minimize computational cost, the recursive feature elimination(RFE) and 10-fold crossover validation was used to select optimal feature combination that contributed the most to prediction results.

*E. Model Development*

As shown in Fig. 2, the optimal features were given to a multilayer perceptron model (MLP) with 3 hidden layers for $P_{SCD\text{-}risk}$ prediction. The number of neurons in the first hidden layer equals the number of optimal features selected in the previous step. Following, the model had 8 neurons and 1 neurons in the second and third hidden layer respectively. Sigmoid activation function was applied on the learned feature map to obtain a probability map. The batch size was 64, the loss function was MSELoss, the optimization function was Adam and learning rate was 0.001. The training was terminated when the MSELoss did not improve for more than 100 consecutive epochs.

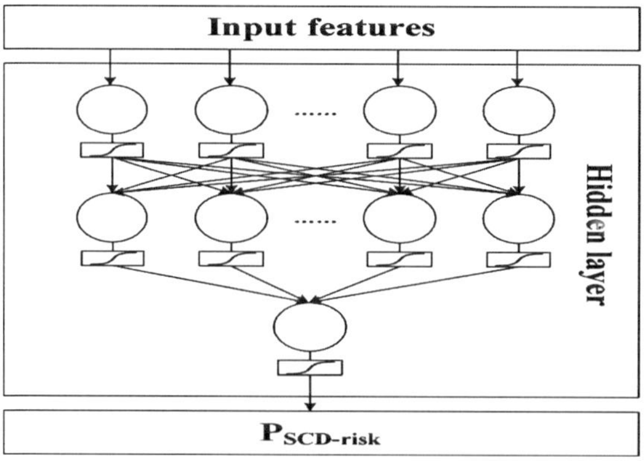


**Fig. 2.** Model structure

The high and low SCD risk cut-off thresholds were determined using Youden index. Model performances were evaluated based on accuracy, sensitivity, specificity.

*F. Statistical Analysis*

Continuous data were expressed as the mean ± standard deviation (SD) and analyzed by t-test or one-way analysis of variance. Categorical data were expressed as numbers (proportions, %) and analyzed by $\chi^2$ test. Multiple pairwise comparisons for continuous variables among the groups were made by post hoc tests (Bonferroni correction). Two-sided P values 0.05 were considered statistically significant and all analyses were performed with the use of SPSS (version 22; IBM Corp, Armonk, NY, USA).

## 3 Result and Discussion

*G. Optimal Feature Selection*

Figure 3 showed the error score results using various feature combinations. As result, we obtained an optimal combination of 7 features from all 12 features. This best subset included VBR, $TINN_C$, $HRVTI_C$, $TP_C$, $LF_C$, $nLF_C$, $SD1/SD2_C$. These 7 metrics were subsequently used for model training and evaluation. To investigate the effects of $HRV_C$ metrics on SCD risk prediction, the same procedure was also performed for these $HRV_O$ metrics as contrast.

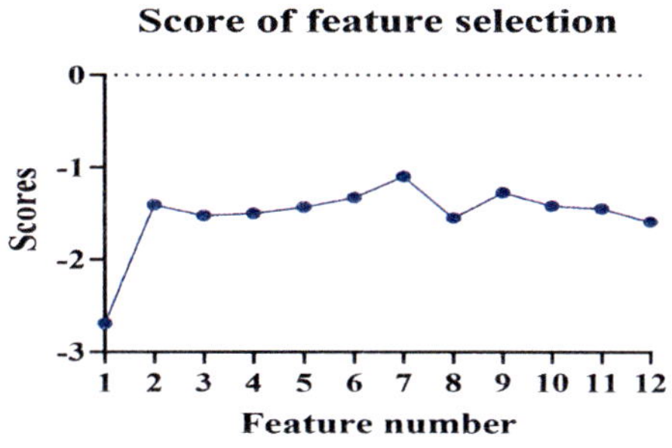


**Fig. 3.** Feature selection

*H. Comparison Between HRVC and HRVO*

Figure 4 and Table 3 showed the result of testing set. Mean $P_{SCD\text{-}risk}$ of normal control and SCD based on 1 h $HRV_O$ was 0.18 ± 0.12 and 0.80 ± 0.16; while mean $P_{SCD\text{-}risk}$ of normal control and SCD based on 1 h $HRV_C$ was 0.00 ± 0.01 and 0.99 ± 0.01. All comparisons were significant with $P < 0.05$. The $P_{SCD\text{-}risk}$ from $HRV_C$ with a lower SD was more stable and concentrated than from $HRV_O$. As shown in Table 3, the model with $HRV_C$ produced superior classification performance than the model with $HRV_O$. These results attested to the robustness of the proposed model with $HRV_C$.

Monfred et al. proved that there was a universal exponential decay-like relationship between HRV and HR [8]. $HRV_C$ was obtained from HR correction method to eliminate the effect of HR on $HRV_O$. Results were more stable and accurate after correction for

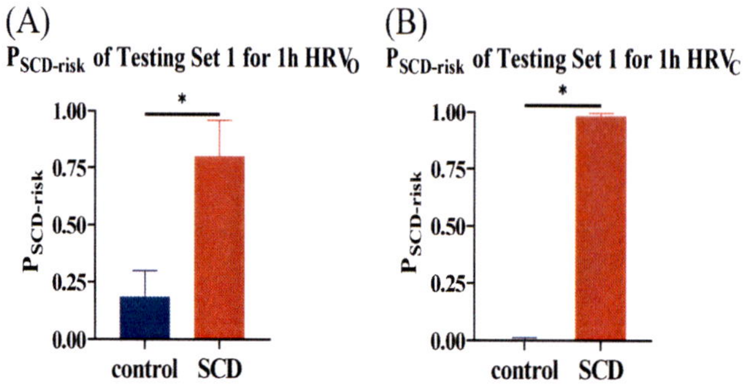


**Fig. 4.** $P_{SCD\text{-risk}}$ of testing set 1for 1 h HRV

**Table 3.** Classification performance of testing set

| Model with | Accuracy (%) | Sensitivity (%) | Specificity (%) |
|---|---|---|---|
| $HRV_O$ | 96.90 | 97.86 | 96.10 |
| $HRV_C$ | 100.00 | 100.00 | 100.00 |
| P value | 0.000 | 0.072 | 0.001 |

confounding factor of HR. Variation of individualized $P_{SCD\text{-risk}}$ from 1 h $HRV_O$ and $HRV_C$ in 24 h of 2 subjects is shown in Fig. 5. Figure 5b presents a more stable and accurate result.

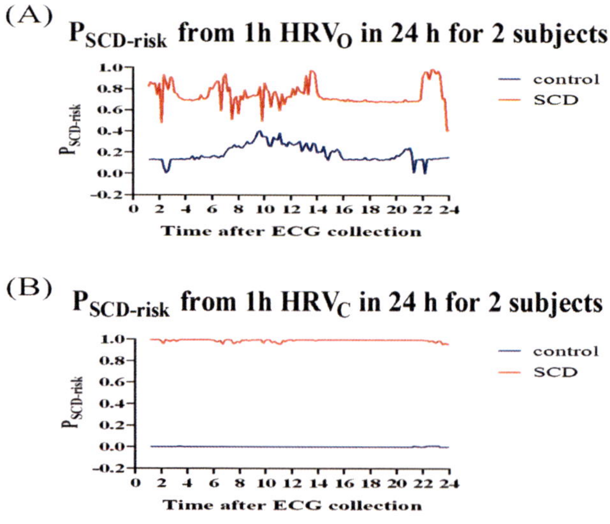


**Fig. 5.** $P_{SCD\text{-risk}}$ from 1h HRV in 24h of 3 subjects

*I. Comparison with Previous Studies*

Recent studies with top performance in this field have been summarized in Table 4. Our method outperformed the previously top-performing methods. To separate SCD from normal individuals, our best model based on $HRV_C$ metrics achieved maximum accuracy of 100% in testing set. In addition, our model showed great clinical value in predicting SCD risk as far as 24 h before the SCD event occurred. Earlier studies usually predicted SCD event several minutes to 1 h ahead of onset. If there is no medical assistance around, our method will leave more time for person who are at high risk of SCD to visit the hospital.

**Table 4.** Previous similar studies with best performance

| Autor (year) | Prediction period | Features | Compared class | Accuracy |
|---|---|---|---|---|
| Nguyen (2019) [9] | 8 s before | Raw ECG | Normal control | 99.26% |
| Rohila (2020) [10] | 1 h before | HRV, S-transform | Normal control, CAD, and CHF | 91.67% |
| Present study | 24 h before | Corrected HRV | Normal control | 100.00% |

*CAD*: Coronary Artery Disease; *CHF*: Congestive Heart Failure

## 4 Conclusion

We proposed a reliable and stable approach for predicting individualized SCD risk probability based on HRV in normal and abnormal heart conditions. The near-perfect results were achieved for discriminating SCD from normal control. Our method not only estimated individualized SCD risk probability reliably, but also had higher prediction accuracy than the existing methods. In the future, we plan to extend this work to deal with other cardiac disease and include new features of HRV. Prospective studies on its clinical usefulness may help develop an non-invasive diagnosis method for SCD.

## References

1. Kumar, A., Avishay, D.M., Jones, C.R., Shaikh, J.D., Kaur, R., Aljadah, M. et al.: Sudden cardiac death: epidemiology, pathogenesis and management. Rev. Cardiovasc. Med. **22**(1), 147–158 (2021). https://doi.org/10.31083/j.rcm.2021.01.207
2. Wong, C.X., Brown, A., Lau, D.H., Chugh, S.S., Albert, C.M., Kalman, J.M. et al.: Epidemiology of sudden cardiac death: global and regional perspectives. Heart Lung Circ. **28**(1), 6–14 (2019). https://doi.org/10.1016/j.hlc.2018.08.026
3. Obrova, J., Sovova, E., Kocianova, E., Taborsky, M.: Sudden cardiac death—a known unknown? Biomed. Pap. Med. Fac. Univ. Palacky Olomouc Czech Repub. **166**(3), 258–266 (2022). https://doi.org/10.5507/bp.2021.065

4. Stecker, E.C., Nazer, B.: The shadows of sudden cardiac death. J. Am. Coll. Cardiol. **77**(19), 2363–2365 (2021). https://doi.org/10.1016/j.jacc.2021.03.321
5. Sessa, F., Anna, V., Messina, G., Cibelli, G., Monda, V., Marsala, G. et al.: Heart rate variability as predictive factor for sudden cardiac death. Aging (Albany NY) **10**(2), 166–177 (2018). https://doi.org/10.18632/aging.101386
6. Task Force Report: Heart rate variability. Standards of measurement, physiological interpretation, and clinical use. Task Force of the European Society of Cardiology and the North American Society of Pacing and Electrophysiology. Eur. Heart J. **17**(3), 354–381 (1996)
7. Feng, Y., Cheng, J., Wei, B., Wang, Y.: CaMKII inhibition reduces isoproterenol-induced ischemia and arrhythmias in hypertrophic mice. Oncotarget **8**(11), 17504–17509 (2017). https://doi.org/10.18632/oncotarget.15099
8. Monfredi, O., Lyashkov, A.E., Johnsen, A., Inada, S., Schneider, H., Wang, R. et al.: Biophysical characterization of the underappreciated and important relationship between heart rate variability and heart rate. Hypertension **64**(6) (2014)
9. Nguyen, M.T., Nguyen, B.V., Kim, K.: Deep feature learning for sudden cardiac arrest detection in automated external defibrillators. Sci. Rep. **8**(1), 17196 (2018). https://doi.org/10.1038/s41598-018-33424-9
10. Rohila, A., Sharma, A.: Detection of sudden cardiac death by a comparative study of heart rate variability in normal and abnormal heart conditions. Biocybern. Biomed. Eng. **40**(3), 1140–1154 (2020). https://doi.org/10.1016/j.bbe.2020.06.003

# A Faster Single-Channel SSVEP-Based Speller Using Peak Filter Extended Canonical Correlation Analysis

Xietian Wang[1], Heng Cui[1], Aiping Liu[1], and Xun Chen[1,2](✉)

[1] School of Information Science and Technology, University of Science and Technology of China, Hefei, China
xunchen@ustc.edu.cn
[2] Institute of Dataspace, Hefei Comprehensive National Science Center, Hefei, China

**Abstract.** Steady-state visual evoked potential (SSVEP) based brain-computer interface (BCI) can provide an effective speller for disabled people. With the attempts in building user-friendly BCIs, training-based systems using a single electroencephalogram (EEG) channel attract attention increasingly. One important step for training-based BCIs performance improvement is to construct clean templates. However, since band-pass filters can not precisely extract the fundamental and harmonic frequency components, there remains much noise in the templates extracted by existing methods. A novel peak filter extended canonical correlation analysis (PF-eCCA) was proposed in this work. Firstly, a peak filter strategy was developed to construct templates, which can emphasize the specific frequencies and suppress unrelated components. Then, eCCA was employed for classification. This method is evaluated on the Benchmark dataset and achieved the highest information transfer rate (ITR) of 138.7 bits/min, which significantly outperformed the state-of-the-art method. The proposed peak filter strategy can also be used to improve several other existing methods with low additional computation costs.

**Keywords:** Brain-computer Interface · Electroencephalogram (EEG) · Single-channel Detection · Steady-state Visual Evoked Potential (SSVEP)

## 1 Introduction

Brain-computer interfaces (BCIs) have the potential of helping people in communicating. The steady-state visual evoked potential (SSVEP) is the most widely adopted paradigm [1] because of its high information transfer rate (ITR). The users need to stare at a flickering target, then the sinusoidal response which is correlated to the focused flash frequency can be observed by electroencephalogram (EEG).

The earliest SSVEP detection methods are training-free. The most widely adopted methods are power spectrum density analysis (PSDA) [2], canonical correlation analysis (CCA) [3] and filter bank CCA (FBCCA) [4].


G. Wang et al. (Eds.): APCMBE 2023, IFMBE Proceedings 103, pp. 11–17, 2024.
https://doi.org/10.1007/978-3-031-51455-5_2

Unlike the training-free method, the training-based method takes into account user variability and can use phase information to obtain a higher ITR. One of the first attempts is the extended-CCA (eCCA), which significantly improves the performance [5]. Task-related component analysis (TRCA) directly uses the correlation between training and test data for classification [6]. However, this method can only be used for multi-channel conditions.

Multi-channel EEG can benefit SSVEP classification by using the combination of channels to provide higher SNR [7]. However, multi-channel devices need a complicated setup for each electrode. Thus, single-channel recorded SSVEP detection is more capable of BCI applications [8, 9]. The representative methods are individual template CCA (ITCCA) [10] and transfer template CCA (ttCCA) [11]. One of the state-of-the-art (SOTA) methods uses the fast Fourier transform based convolutional neural network (FFT-CNN) [12]. However, FFT-CNN needs 20 training trials for each target, which will cause fatigue and reduce comfort [13].

This study aims to achieve a single-channel SSVEP-based BCI speller with high ITR. Based on the assumption that SSVEP consists of fundamental and harmonic frequency components, this study proposed the peak filter (PF) strategy, which can precisely extract the stimulus-related frequency components and eliminated the noise. To verify the ability of the PF strategy to benefit target identification, we proposed peak filter eCCA (PF-eCCA) and tested using a 40-target Benchmark dataset [14]. This study also combined the PF strategy with other competitive methods and compared the performance in the same condition.

The rest of this paper is organized as follows. Section 2 introduces the proposed strategy. Section 3 presents the data acquisition and compares the performance of different methods. Finally, Sects. 4 and 5 report the discussion and conclusion.

## 2 Method and Data Acquisition

A. *Preliminaries*

Standard CCA applies weight vectors to maximize the correlation coefficient between two random signals [3]. Given two variables $\boldsymbol{X}$ and $\boldsymbol{Y}$, CCA finds the weight vector $\boldsymbol{W_X}$ and $\boldsymbol{W_Y}$ by solving the following problem

$$\max_{\boldsymbol{W_X},\boldsymbol{W_Y}} \rho\left(\boldsymbol{X}^T\boldsymbol{W_X}, \boldsymbol{Y}^T\boldsymbol{W_Y}\right) = \frac{E\left[\boldsymbol{W_X}^T\boldsymbol{X}\boldsymbol{Y}^T\boldsymbol{W_Y}\right]}{\sqrt{E\left[\boldsymbol{W_X}^T\boldsymbol{X}\boldsymbol{X}^T\boldsymbol{W_X}\right]E\left[\boldsymbol{W_Y}^T\boldsymbol{Y}\boldsymbol{Y}^T\boldsymbol{W_Y}\right]}}. \tag{1}$$

In a standard multi-channel recorded SSVEP condition, $\boldsymbol{X}$ is an $N_c \times N_s$ EEG data matrix which is sampled using sampling rate $f_s$. $N_c$ is the number of channels, $N_s$ is the number of samples. $\boldsymbol{Y}$ is defined as

$$\boldsymbol{Y}_{f_k} = \begin{bmatrix} \sin(2\pi f_k n) \\ \cos(2\pi f_k n) \\ \vdots \\ \sin(2\pi N_h f_k n) \\ \cos(2\pi N_h f_k n) \end{bmatrix}, n = \frac{1}{f_s}, \frac{2}{f_s}, \ldots, \frac{N_s}{f_s}. \tag{2}$$

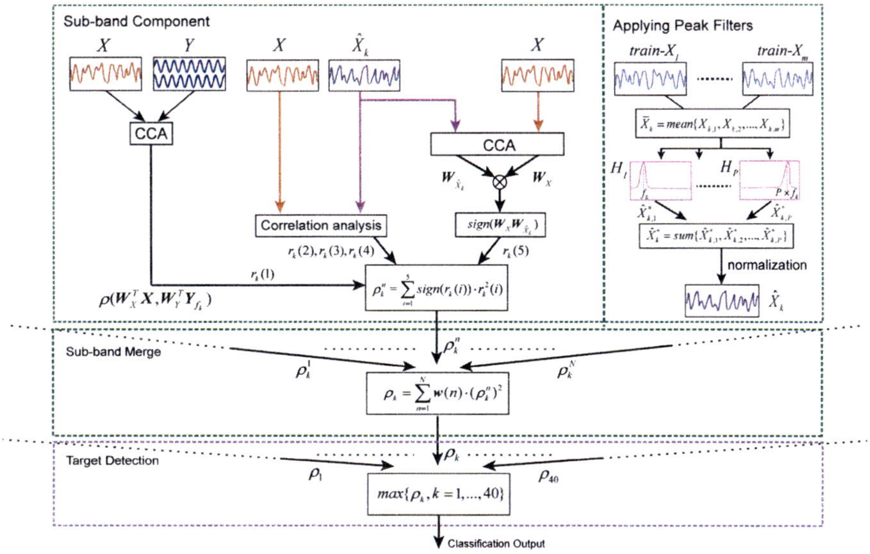


**Fig. 1.** Flowchart of peak filter strategy. $\boldsymbol{X}$ denotes the test signal, $\boldsymbol{Y}$ denotes the sine-cosine reference signal, $\boldsymbol{X}_{k,l}$ is the $l$ th signal in the training data of target $k$. $l$ ranges from 1 to $m$, $m$ is the number of training data. $\widehat{\boldsymbol{X}}^{*}_{k,p}$ is the signal obtained after the $p$ th peak filter. $p$ ranges from $l$ to $P$. $H_1$ to $H_p$ are several PFs at fundamental and harmonic frequencies

$f_k$ is the frequency of the $k$ th stimulus target, and $N_h$ is the number of harmonics.

Filter bank CCA [4] decomposes signals using band pass filters and uses CCA to calculate the correlation coefficient $\rho_k^n$ in the $n$ th sub-band. The final correlation value is

$$\rho_k = \sum_{n=1}^{N} w(n) \cdot \left(\rho_k^n\right)^2, \; w(n) = n^{-a} + b, n \in [1, N]. \tag{3}$$

$a$ and $b$ are hyperparameters. $N$ is the number of sub-bands.

Extended-CCA (eCCA) combines FBCCA with individual template. The correlation coefficient in the $k$ th sub-band is calculated as

$$\boldsymbol{r}_k = \begin{bmatrix} r_k(1) \\ r_k(2) \\ r_k(3) \\ r_k(4) \\ r_k(5) \end{bmatrix} = \begin{bmatrix} \rho\left(\boldsymbol{X}^T \boldsymbol{W}_X\left(\boldsymbol{X}, \boldsymbol{Y}_{f_k}\right), \boldsymbol{Y}_k^T \boldsymbol{W}_Y\left(\boldsymbol{X}, \boldsymbol{Y}_{f_k}\right)\right) \\ \rho\left(\boldsymbol{X}^T \boldsymbol{W}_X\left(\boldsymbol{X}, \widehat{\boldsymbol{X}}_k\right), \widehat{\boldsymbol{X}}_k^T \boldsymbol{W}_X\left(\boldsymbol{X}, \widehat{\boldsymbol{X}}_k\right)\right) \\ \rho\left(\boldsymbol{X}^T \boldsymbol{W}_X\left(\boldsymbol{X}, \boldsymbol{Y}_{f_k}\right), \widehat{\boldsymbol{X}}_k^T \boldsymbol{W}_Y\left(\boldsymbol{X}, \boldsymbol{Y}_{f_k}\right)\right) \\ \rho\left(\boldsymbol{X}^T \boldsymbol{W}_X\left(\widehat{\boldsymbol{X}}_k, \boldsymbol{Y}_{f_k}\right), \widehat{\boldsymbol{X}}_k^T \boldsymbol{W}_Y\left(\widehat{\boldsymbol{X}}_k, \boldsymbol{Y}_{f_k}\right)\right) \\ \rho\left(\widehat{\boldsymbol{X}}_k^T \boldsymbol{W}_X\left(\boldsymbol{X}, \widehat{\boldsymbol{X}}_k\right), \widehat{\boldsymbol{X}}_k^T \boldsymbol{W}_{\widehat{\boldsymbol{X}}_k}\left(\boldsymbol{X}, \widehat{\boldsymbol{X}}_k\right)\right) \end{bmatrix}. \tag{4}$$

Template $\widehat{\boldsymbol{X}}_k$ is the average of all training data at frequency $f_k$. $\boldsymbol{X}$ and $\widehat{\boldsymbol{X}}_k$ have the same dimension of $N_c \times N_s$. Denotes that $\boldsymbol{W}_{\boldsymbol{A}}(\boldsymbol{A}, \boldsymbol{B})$ is the weight of the matrix $\boldsymbol{A}$ that maximizes the correlation coefficient between $\boldsymbol{A}$ and $\boldsymbol{B}$ by CCA, and $\boldsymbol{W_B}(\boldsymbol{A}, \boldsymbol{B})$ is the weight of the matrix $\boldsymbol{B}$. The correlation values are obtained in the same way as FBCCA. The target $k$ that generates the maximum $\rho_k$ is considered as the classification output.

B. Peak Filter eCCA (PF-eCCA)

1. Peak Filter Strategy

The component of the SSVEP response of target $k$ is considered as Eq. (5). $\boldsymbol{X}_k(t)$ denotes the acquired single-channel EEG data and $n(t)$ is the noise of zero means. $s_k(t)$ is the response signal containing several harmonics of the stimulus frequency $f_k$. In different trials, each user has the equivalent amplitude and phase combination individually.

$$\boldsymbol{X}_k(t) = s_k(t) + n(t). \tag{5}$$

By averaging all training data for a single target, the output template can approach $s_k(t)$. We are usually unable to get enough data to build a model without noise, which reduces the accuracy. The peak filters can be used to extract signals at a specified frequency with a more accurate frequency selection. We used a set of infinite impulse response (IIR) peak filters to construct the templates. After averaging the data of all trials, $\overline{\boldsymbol{X}}_k(t)$ was produced and then filtered by several peak filters. A power normalization by unifying the maximum amplitude was applied later. The model construction of $\widehat{\boldsymbol{X}}_{\boldsymbol{k}}$ could be written as

$$\widehat{\boldsymbol{X}}_k^*(t) = \sum_{p=1}^{P} \mathit{peak\,filter}_{k_p}\left(\overline{\boldsymbol{X}}_k(t)\right), \tag{6}$$

while the $\mathit{peak\,filter}_{k_p}()$ has the peak-frequency of $p \times f_k$, $P$ is the number of PFs. With a series of PFs, the output $\widehat{\boldsymbol{X}}_{\boldsymbol{k}}$ would only contain $s_k(t)$ and noise in frequency $f_h$.

2. Peak Filter eCCA

We used the PF strategy in eCCA and set the quality factor of peak filter to 9. The diagram of PF-eCCA is shown in Fig. 1. PF strategy only changes the generation method of individual template $\widehat{\boldsymbol{X}}_{\boldsymbol{k}}$ in eCCA and it is readily pluggable.

First, $\overline{\boldsymbol{X}}$ was calculated by averaging all training data of target $k$. Then, the averaged data was filtered by several PFs separately. The output of all PFs was cumulated to $\widehat{\boldsymbol{X}}_k^*$. Normalization makes $\widehat{\boldsymbol{X}}_{\boldsymbol{k}}$ and $\overline{\boldsymbol{X}}_k$ had the same maximum amplitude.

Since the data has only one channel, the rank of signal $\boldsymbol{X}$ and $\widehat{\boldsymbol{X}}$ is 1, thus the weight vector $W_X\left(\boldsymbol{X}, \widehat{\boldsymbol{X}}_{\boldsymbol{k}}\right)$, $W_X\left(\boldsymbol{X}, \boldsymbol{Y}_{f_K}\right)$, $W_X\left(\widehat{\boldsymbol{X}}_{\boldsymbol{k}}, \boldsymbol{Y}_{f_K}\right)$ are scalars. Without loss of generality, we set these weights to 1. Thus, $r_k(2)$, $r_k(3)$, and $r_k(4)$ are the correlation coefficient between $\boldsymbol{X}$ and $\widehat{\boldsymbol{X}}$. $r_k(5)$ is

$$r_k(5) = \begin{cases} +1, \mathit{sign}\left(\boldsymbol{W_X W_{\widehat{X}_k}}\right) = 1 \\ -1, \mathit{sign}\left(\boldsymbol{W_X W_{\widehat{X}_k}}\right) = -1 \end{cases}. \tag{7}$$

C. *Data Acquisition*

To make our validation process more convincing, we used a 40-target open access Benchmark dataset [14] to evaluate all methods. Total of 40 targets arranged in a 5 × 8 stimulus matrix are modulated using frequency ranges from 8.0 to 15.8 Hz with an interval of 0.2 Hz. We used channel Oz as the single-channel data resource. Each volunteer participates in 6 blocks and each block contains 40 trials. Data in the first 0.1 s after stimulus onset was discarded to avoid visual latency. The 0.1 s was taken into account when estimating ITR.

## 3 Results

In this section, we compared the performance of several methods before and after applying the PF strategy. We calculated the ITR using

$$ITR = \left(\log_2 N_f + P\log_2 P + (1-P)\log_2\left[\frac{1-P}{N_f - 1}\right]\right) \cdot \left(\frac{60}{T}\right). \tag{8}$$

$P$ is the classification accuracy, $N_f$ is the number of targets, $T$ (in second) is the length of time window.

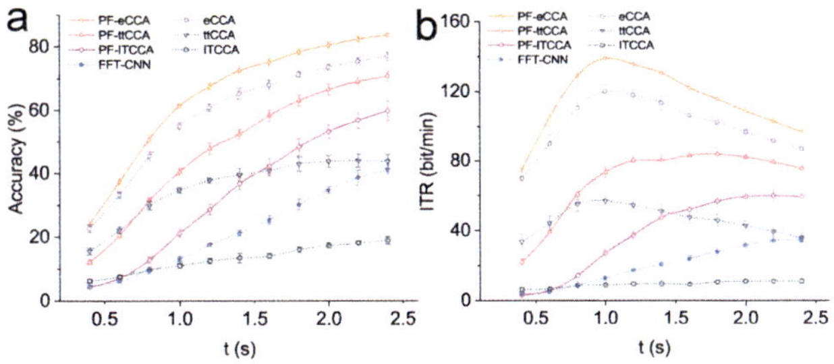


**Fig. 2.** The averaged classification accuracy (**a**) and ITR (**b**) using data lengths from 0.4 to 2.4 s. Error bars indicate the standard errors

We used leave-one-block-out cross-validation. The 6 blocks of data were divided into 5 training blocks and 1 test block. Each block was used once as test data. Figure 2 illustrates the accuracy and ITR comparison between different methods. We used 5 sub-bands and 3 harmonics of the target frequency. The proposed method PF-eCCA gets the highest ITR of 138.7 bits/min. Compared with the original eCCA method, the paired t-tests indicates the significant improvement in accuracy (76.9 ± 1.4% vs. 83.5 ± 0.7%, $p = 1.30 \times 10^{-5}$) and the maximum ITR (119.8 ± 3.9 bits/min vs. 138.7 ± 2.2 bits/min, $p = 8.47 \times 10^{-6}$). For the maximum ITR of other compared methods using PF strategy, the significance is observed with (1) ttCCA (56.9 ± 2.5 bits/min vs. 83.3 ± 3.6 bits/min), $p = 2.42 \times 10^{-6}$ (2) ITCCA (11.0 ± 1.3 bits/min vs. 59.5 ± 3.9 bits/min), $p = 5.13 \times 10^{-7}$. Comparing PF-eCCA with FFT-CNN, the significance is $p = 1.03 \times 10^{-9}$.

All comparisons show significant improvement after applying the PF strategy. The resultant ITR in this study is 138.7 bits/min. To our knowledge, this is the highest ITR reported in single-channel SSVEP-based systems (i.e., 76.5 bits/min [15], 57.9 bits/min [16] and 15.4 bits/min [17]).

## 4 Discussion

It is worth mentioning that most performance improvement strategies increase the operation time of the decision while our strategy was only applied to the template data. This strategy is readily pluggable and pushed the training-based CCA method to a stronger one.

Since the SSVEP component consists of the fundamental and harmonic frequencies of the stimulus, we implemented the PF strategy to extract the frequency information precisely. The modification of the template is shown in Fig. 3. Only the signal parts are retained, and the other frequency components are eliminated.

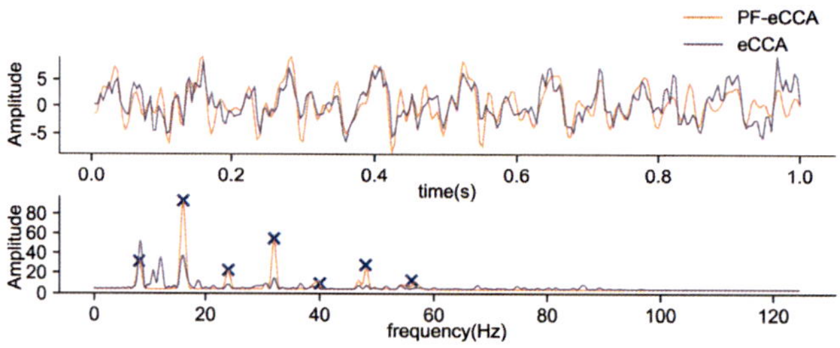


**Fig. 3.** The template waveform and frequency spectrum at stimulus frequency 8 Hz in the first sub-band. The purple line is the average of all training data, the orange line is the model produced by PF strategy. The blue "×" indicates the location of 8 Hz and its harmonics

We observed the influence of sub-band merge parameters $(a; b)$ is (1.25, 0.00) according to the grid search approach. The optimization brings little accuracy gain compared to the suggested value (1.00, 0.00) in the conventional eCCA (i.e. 62.43% vs. 62.07%, $t = 1.0s$).

In our proposed method, the number of PFs determines the number of harmonic components in detection. The highest accuracy was achieved when using three PFs. It is possible that using fewer harmonics can not make well use of the SSVEP components, while high harmonics are easily affected by noise and result in low accuracy.

## 5 Conclusion

This study developed the PF strategy considering that SSVEP only contains fundamental and harmonic frequency components. Several peak filters were designed to filter the individual templates. With low computation cost and high performance enhancement, this strategy can be generalized in training-based methods and improve performance. Since single-channel systems require little effort in data acquisition, this research can further expand the application scenario of SSVEP-based BCIs.

## References


1. Li, M., He, D., Qi, C.: Brain-computer interface speller based on steady-state visual evoked potential: a review focusing on the stimulus paradigm and performance. Brain Sci. **11**, 450 (2021)
2. Kawala-Sterniuk, A., Browarska, N., Al-Bakri, A., et al.: Summary of over fifty years with brain-computer interfaces–a review. Brain Sci. **11**, 43 (2021)
3. Lin, Z., Zhang, C., Wu, W., et al.: Frequency recognition based on canonical correlation analysis for SSVEP-based BCIs. IEEE Trans. Biomed. Eng. **54**, 1172–1176 (2007)
4. Chen, X., Wang, Y., Gao, X., et al.: Filter bank canonical correlation analysis for implementing a high-speed SSVEP-based brain–computer interface. J. Neural Eng. **12**, 046008 (2015)
5. Nakanashi, M., Wang, Y., Wang, Y.-T., et al.: A comparison study of canonical correlation analysis based methods for detecting steady-state visual evoked potentials. PLoS ONE **10**, e0140703 (2015)
6. Nakanashi, M., Wang, Y., Chen, X., et al.: Enhancing detection of SSVEPs for a high-speed brain speller using task-related component analysis. IEEE Trans. Biomed. Eng. **65**, 104–112 (2018)
7. Haider, A.: A brief review of signal processing for EEG-based BCI: approaches and opportunities. In: IEEE International Conference on Electronics and Information Technology, Mt. Pleasant, America, pp. 384–394 (2021)
8. Karunasena, S., Sanduni, P., Ariyarathna, D., et al.: Single-channel EEG SSVEP-based BCI for robot arm control. IEEE Sensors Appl Symp Sundsvall, Sweden **2021**, 1–6 (2021)
9. Arpaia, P., De Benedetto, E., Donato, N., et al.: A wearable SSVEP BCI for AR-based, real-time monitoring applications. IEEE International Symposium on Med. Meas. & Appl. Neuchâtel, Switzerland **2021**, 1–6 (2021)
10. Nwachukwu, S., Sandra, E., Shi, M. et al.: An SSVEP recognition method by combining individual template with CCA. In: Proceedings of the 2019 3rd International Conference on Innovation in Artificial Intelligence, Suzhou, China 2019, pp. 6–10 (2019)
11. Yuan, P., Chen, X., Wang, Y., et al.: Enhancing performances of SSVEP-based brain–computer interfaces via exploiting inter-subject information. J. Neural Eng. **12**, 046006 (2015)
12. Nguyen, T.-H., Chung, W.-Y.: A single-channel SSVEP-based BCI speller using deep learning. IEEE Access **7**, 1752–1763 (2018)
13. Zerafa, R., Camilleri, T., Falzon, O., et al.: To train or not to train? A survey on training of feature extraction methods for SSVEP-based BCIs. J. Neural Eng. **15**, 051001 (2018)
14. Wang, Y., Chen, X., Gao, X., et al.: A benchmark dataset for SSVEP-based brain-computer interfaces. IEEE Trans. Neural Syst. Rehabil. Eng. **25**, 1746–1752 (2017)
15. Sözer, A.T.: Enhanced single channel SSVEP detection method on benchmark dataset. In: 15th International Conference on Elect. Eng., Comput. Sci. & Autom. Control, Mexico City, Mexico, 2018, pp. 1–4 (2018)
16. Ojha, M., Mukul, M.K.: Detection of target frequency from SSVEP signal using empirical mode decomposition for SSVEP based BCI inference system. Wirel. Pers. Commun. **116**, 777–789 (2021)
17. Acampora, G., Trinchese, P., Vitiello, A.: Applying logistic regression for classification in single-channel SSVEP-based BCIs. In: IEEE International Conference on System, Man and Cybernetics, Bari, Italy, 2019, pp. 33–38 (2019)

# Respiratory Function Monitor Based on Surface Diaphragm Electromyography

X. Song[1], Y. C. Li[1], W. G. Zhang[2], S. P. Yan[1], and Y. Q. Li[1](✉)

[1] Department of Biomedical Engineering and Imaging Medicine, Army Medical University, Chongqing, China
sphere_song@163.com

[2] Department of Critical Care Medicine, Army Medical University, Chongqing, China

**Abstract.** To design a respiratory function monitoring system with surface diaphragm electromyography that can be used to monitor respiratory function in the home or with medical agents. Based on the STM32F411VET6 microcontroller system, two electrodes were used to detect the surface EMG signals. Additional two circular disposable Ag/AgCl electrodes were applied for the output of high-frequency excitation and the input of ECG and bio-impedance signals. The hardware system included a diaphragm EMG detection circuit, ECG detection circuit, bio-impedance detection circuit, constant current source excitation circuit, and microcontroller. The analog signals were digitalized by the A/D mode of the MCU, and the digitalized signals were stored in a secure digital memory card through the secure digital input and output protocol. After the system design, the system was validated by acquiring signals from 10 patients with mechanical ventilation due to respiratory dysfunction and 10 healthy adults. Fifteen respiratory function-related parameters were calculated and compared between groups. The signal-to-noise ratio of the signal collected by the system was > 10 dB, the common mode rejection ratio was > 80 dB. Compared with healthy adults, inhalation time, exhalation time, tidal volume, peak-to-peak value of the bio-impedance signal, variation of bio-impedance signal in one second, diaphragmatic EMG low-band power (LF, 20–40 Hz), diaphragmatic EMG high-band power (HF, 150–250 Hz), the ratio between high-band power and low-band power., diaphragmatic electromyography area, diaphragmatic electromyography peak-to-peak, and cardiopulmonary coupling coefficient were significantly lower *($P < 0.05$)*, but heart rate was significantly higher in mechanically ventilated patients ($P < 0.05$). In addition, there were no significant differences in respiratory rate, diaphragmatic electromyography time, and inhalation and exhalation ratio between the two groups. The designed respiratory function monitoring system was demonstrated to be reliable. It can be used for continuously and non-invasively monitoring respiratory function in real time.

**Keywords:** Surface diaphragm electromyography · Electrocardiography · Bio-impedance · Respiratory function monitoring


G. Wang et al. (Eds.): APCMBE 2023, IFMBE Proceedings 103, pp. 18–28, 2024.
https://doi.org/10.1007/978-3-031-51455-5_3

## 1 Introduction

Breathing is the most basic life activity of the human body, its main function is to inhale oxygen and excrete carbon dioxide, maintain acid-base balance, and normal metabolism in the body. Respiratory diseases are one of the most common diseases in China, according to the data of the China Health Statistics Yearbook 2020, respiratory diseases ranked fourth in the mortality rate of major diseases among urban and rural residents in 2019 [1]. In modern medical monitoring technology, human respiratory function monitoring is increasingly becoming an essential part of routine monitoring. Respiratory function monitoring helps diagnose respiratory illness. Itis useful in assessing disease status and is useful in guiding mechanical ventilation therapy [2]. The ideal monitoring system should have the characteristics of monitoring results to guide treatment, high sensitivity and specificity, and be simple and portable.

Currently, clinicians evaluate respiratory function by evaluating physical examinations such as skin color, nasal flap, accessory respiratory muscle exertion, and abnormal breath sounds (wheezing, stridor) [2]. This method is simple and easy to implement, and it is widely used clinically, but it is only a rough understanding of the patient's respiratory function, so it is not accurate enough. To accurately assess respiratory function, it is necessary to use a pulmonary function test instrument with high sensitivity and specificity, and pay attention to changes in the subject's lung ventilation function, dynamic lung volume, and residual gas volume [3]. The results of pulmonary function tests are more convincing than clinicians' physical examinations. However, subjects need to do blowing experiments, and it is difficult to meet the experimental requirements for critically ill patients. Respiratory mechanics monitoring is an effective tool for respiratory function evaluation, treatment effect evaluation, and optimization of ventilator applications, but the prevalence of mechanical monitoring and non-invasive respiratory mechanical monitoring methods are not perfect, so it has not been routinely used in clinical work [4].

Each of these respiratory monitoring methods has shortcomings. The respiratory function monitoring system based on body surface diaphragm myoelectric can make up for the shortcomings of the above monitoring methods, and has the advantages of continuous non-invasive monitoring, simple and portable, and a wide range of applications. The diaphragm is the most important inspiratory muscle, and continuous monitoring of diaphragmatic electrical signals can truly reflect the respiratory needs of the respiratory center and visually assess whether the respiratory function is abnormal [5]. In this study, two pairs of Ag/AgCl electrodes were used as signal detection electrodes to realize synchronous signal acquisition and storage. Based on retrospective analysis of signals, non-invasive, continuous, and qualitative monitoring of respiratory function is realized.

## 2 Methods and Materials

The respiratory function monitoring system mainly includes a hardware system and a software system. The hardware system is divided into hardware circuit design and embedded program design, which mainly completes the synchronous acquisition and data storage of diaphragmatic electromyography, ECG, and thoracic impedance signals.

The software system mainly completes the retrospective analysis of data. The system design schematic is shown in Fig. 1. The power module provides 3.3 V DC for digital circuits and ±5 V DC for analog circuits; the analog circuit is mainly composed of three parts: diaphragmatic electromyography detection circuit, ECG detection circuit, and thoracic impedance detection circuit; The digital circuit consists of a single-chip microcomputer STM32F411 and basic peripheral circuits. The analog signal is converted to digital by the ADC of the STM32F411, and the data is stored in the SD card through the SDIO interface. The stored data can be uploaded to the PC host through the Type-C interface, and the signal characteristic parameters can be obtained through the software analysis system.

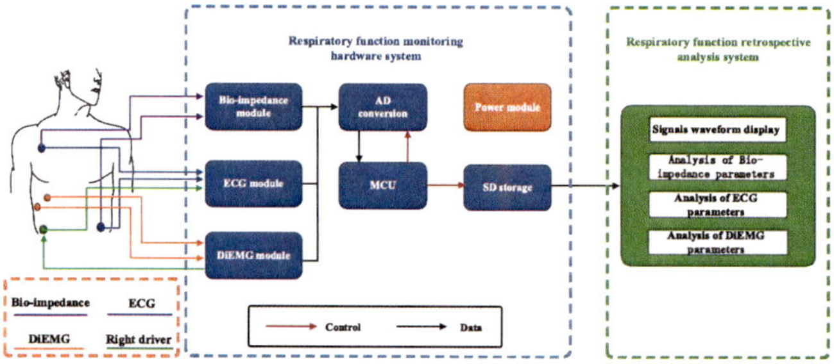


**Fig. 1.** The system design schematic

*A. Hardware and program design*

1. Power supply

This system requires ±5 V and 3.3 V dc. The power module is powered by a DC12 V rechargeable lithium battery, which provides ±5 V for analog circuits and 3.3 V for digital circuits through the DC-DC voltage isolation conversion module (DW5-12D05A1) and LDO regulator chip (H7650-33GR).

2. Diaphragmatic EMG signal detection circuit

It is mainly composed of a pre-amplification circuit, a high-pass filter, a low-pass filter, a 50 Hz notch, and a post-amplification circuit. The preamplifier circuit uses OPA2277UA and AD620 to form a dual op-amp integrated instrument amplifier circuit to improve input impedance and common-mode rejection ratio. Adding the right leg drive to the front circuit can effectively suppress the power frequency interference signal. To preserve the diaphragmatic EMG signal component as much as possible, the second-order high-pass filter cutoff frequency is 8 Hz; the second-order low-pass filter cutoff frequency is 194 Hz; The circuit includes three stages of amplification, 100x preamplification, 20x second amplification, and 4x third amplification, with a total gain of 12500x. The 50 Hz notch uses a dual-T dual-follow notch circuit with better performance that can independently adjust the figure of merit [6]. The AD620 integrated instrumentation op-amp is selected for the post-amplification circuit.

3. ECG signal detection circuit

It is mainly composed of a pre-amplification circuit, a filter circuit, and a post-amplification circuit. The preamplifier input is connected in parallel with the bidirectional transient suppression diode P6KE20CA to avoid circuit breakdown caused by positive and negative transient high-voltage pulses. The ECG electrode is used as an input electrode of the excitation constant current source, and the input of the pre-op amp is connected to a first-order passive low-pass filter to initially filter out the interference of high-frequency excitation signals. The AD620 constitutes an ECG preamplification circuit, and a second-order active high-pass filter filters out baseline drift caused by respiratory movement with a cutoff frequency of 0.5 Hz; Second-order active low-pass filtering filters out high-frequency interference with a cutoff frequency of 159 Hz; 50 Hz notch filters out power frequency interference; The ECG signal amplification circuit is divided into three stages, 10 times in the pre-amplification, 13 times in the second stage, and 4 times in the third stage, and the total gain of the circuit is 1000 times.

4. Transthoracic impedance signal detection circuit

It is mainly composed of a constant current source excitation circuit, pre-amplification circuit, demodulation circuit, filter circuit, and post-amplification circuit. In this study, the MAX038CPP integrated chip from MAXIM was used to generate high-quality high-frequency sine wave signals. A precision V-I conversion circuit through the AD620 generates a constant current source signal of 50 kHz/0.5 mA [7]. The preamplifier circuit uses AD620 to form a differential op amp circuit, and the circuit is amplified by 10 times; The AD637 RMS converter demodulates the breathing signal from the carrier with a 9x amplification in the second stage, a bandpass filter with a cutoff frequency of 0.15–25 Hz to filter out DC impedance and high-frequency interference, and a third stage amplified by 28x, with a total gain of 5000x.

5. Digital circuit and embedded program

The digital circuit adopts the STM32F411 single-chip microcomputer, which mainly includes the minimum system and basic peripheral circuit of the single-chip microcomputer to complete the tasks of system control, data sampling and storage, storage progress display, and so on. The analog-to-digital conversion mode is DMA synchronous acquisition. According to the Nyquist sampling theorem, the sampling frequency is set to 500 Hz using the timer Timer2. Write and debug single-chip microcomputer programs in the MDK Keil V5.0 software environment. The program design mainly completes clock initialization, ADC initialization, SD card storage initialization, ink screen initialization, system control, etc.

*B. System technical parameters test*

The respiratory function monitoring system was tested with parameters such as magnification, input impedance, signal-to-noise ratio, common-mode rejection ratio, and bandwidth. The test method of parameters is carried out according to YY0885-2013 and YYT1095-2015 standards. The test results of technical parameters are shown in the Table 1.

**Table 1.** Technology parameters test results

| Parameters | DiEMG | ECG | Bio-impedance |
|---|---|---|---|
| Theoretical gain | 12500 | 1000 | 5000 |
| Actual gain | 12800 | 973 | 4873 |
| Input impedance /MΩ | 5.0 | 10.4 | 5.5 |
| SNR/dB | 10.4 | 14.7 | 11.2 |
| CMRR/dB | 110 | 90 | 85 |
| Bandwidth/Hz | 20–185 | 0.5–100 | 0.15–25 |

*C. Acquisition and processing*

1. Volunteer enrollment

There were 10 patients with mechanical ventilation in the Department of Intensive Care Medicine (mean ± standard deviation: age 55.50 ± 1.69 years, height 166.50 ± 2.22 cm, weight 67.30 ± 2.65 kg, male: 7, female: 3). In addition, 10 healthy volunteers (mean ± standard deviation: age 48.60 ± 3.18 years, height 163.80 ± 1.51 cm, weight 64.30 ± 2.28 kg, male: 4, female: 6). There were no statistical differences in age, height, weight, and sex between the two groups ($P > 0.05$). The experimental protocol was approved by the Medical Ethics Committee of the First Affiliated Hospital of the Army Medical University of the Chinese People's Liberation Army (approval number: KY2020148) and the written informed consent of the subjects.

2. Measurement protocol

The electrodes of ECG and thoracic impedance detection are located in the second intercostal space at the right edge of the sternum and the junction of the left fifth intercostal and midaxillary lines. The diaphragmatic electrode is located in the sixth and eighth intercostal spaces between the midline of the right clavicle and the anterior axillary line. The exact location is shown in Fig. 1. Connect to the monitoring system, wait for subjects to lie resting on their backs for 5 min, and start the test, each subject records 3 min. After the data acquisition is completed, run the application compiled on the MATLAB R2020a (version R2020a, MathWorks, Natick, Massachusetts, USA) platform to read, preprocess, and calculate the characteristics of the stored data.

3. Signal processing

(a) Diaphragmatic EMG Signal Processing

To facilitate the extraction of signal features, it is necessary to filter out the electrical interference of the body surface diaphragm EMG center. The specific signal processing process is as follows

(1) The steady-state wavelet transform is used to filter out ECG interference in the diaphragmatic EMG signal

(2) The RMS value was calculated one by one for the filtered diaphragmatic EMG signals one by one, and the envelope curve with the same density as the diaphragm EMG signal before calculation was obtained
(3) According to the envelope curve, the diaphragm discharge time, the peak-to-peak of the diaphragmatic electrical signal, the diaphragm discharge area, and other parameters were obtained; According to the diaphragmatic EMG signal after filtering out ECG interference, the diaphragmatic EMG high-frequency power, diaphragmatic EMG low-frequency power, HF/LF and other parameters are calculated. Schematic diagram of diaphragmatic electromyography pre-processing is shown in Fig. 2.

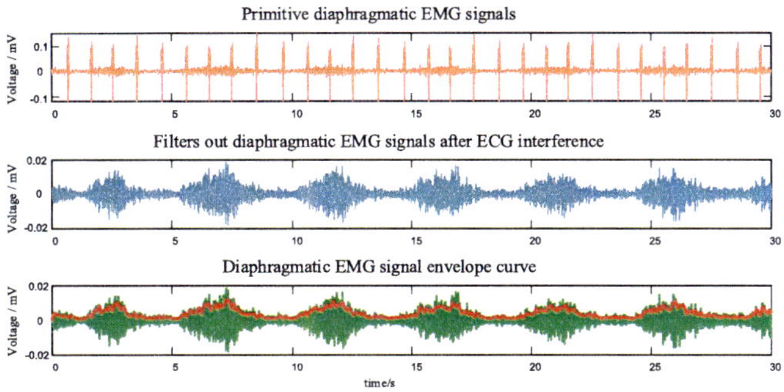


**Fig. 2.** Schematic diagram of diaphragmatic electromyography pre-processing

(b) ECG signal processing

Studies have shown that there is a certain relationship between the amplitude change of the R wave of the ECG signal and the human respiratory movement, and the respiratory signal derived from the ECG has a high consistency with the measured respiratory signal. The cardiopulmonary coupling coefficient comprehensively analyzes the ECG signal and respiratory signal, which can well reflect the influence of the body's autonomic nervous system on cardiovascular and respiratory function. The specific signal processing process is as follows

(1) Identify the QRS complex, and calculate the R wave occurrence time, amplitude, and other relevant parameters
(2) The ECG will produce certain changes with the occurrence of respiratory movement, so the respiratory signal can be obtained from the method of extracting the respiratory signal from the ECG
(3) The abnormal conditions (such as premature beats) in the signal sequence of the NN interval were eliminated to obtain the normal sinus NN interval sequence and EDR signal
(4) After adjusting the sampling frequency, and resampling the two signals obtained in (3), the mutual power spectrum and coherence of the NN interval sequence signal and the EDR signal were calculated for each window based on the fast Fourier transform, and the product of the square and coherence of the mutual power spectrum value was used as the cardiopulmonary coupling coefficient.

(c) bio-impedance signal processing

There is ECG interference in the chest impedance signal, and the specific processing process of the signal is as follows: (1) 400-point smooth filtering is used to denoise the chest impedance signal; (2) The dynamic differential threshold method was used to detect the peak and trough position of the breathing wave; (3) Calculate the respiration-related parameters, and the difference between adjacent peaks and troughs is the peak-to-peak of chest impedance signal; The sampling frequency of this system is 500 Hz, the time interval between each sampling point is 0.02 s, and the acquisition of 500 points is 1 s, so the wave peak is 500 points after 1 s is the impedance value after 1 s, and the difference with the wave peak is the change of chest impedance of 1 s. The number of peaks detected in one minute is the respiration rate. Schematic diagram of bio-impedance signal characteristic parameters as shown in the Fig. 3.

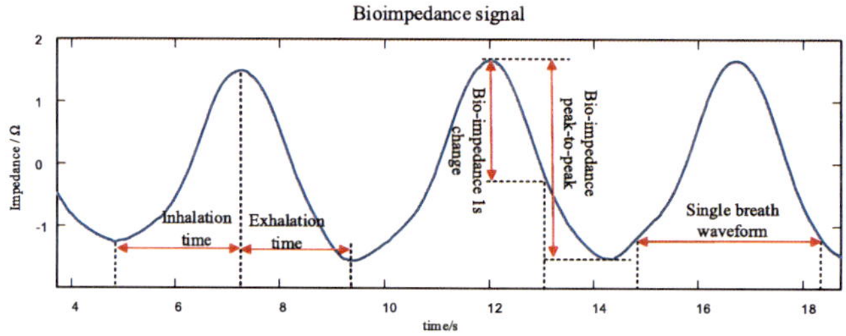


**Fig. 3.** Schematic diagram of bio-impedance signal characteristic parameters

The specific meaning of the feature parameters is shown in the Table 2.

4. Statistical Analysis

SPSS23.0 software is used for statistical analysis, first check whether the data follow the normal distribution, the standard deviation of the mean is used for obedience, and the data that does not follow the normal distribution is represented by M(Q1, Q3). If the data follow a normal distribution and the variance is homogeneous, the t-test is used for two independent samples, otherwise the Wilcoxon rank sum test is used. When $P < 0.05$, the difference between the two groups was statistically significant.

## 3 Results

*A. Hardware*

The signal acquisition composition is shown in the Fig. 4 shown. In this study, the signals of mechanically ventilated patients and healthy adults were collected, and then the data was exported from the Type-C interface to a local PC, and the original signal waveform drawn by the Matlab application was shown in the Fig. 5 shown.

*B. Comparison of variances in parameters*

The inspiratory time, expiratory time, tidal volume, peak-to-peak of thoracic impedance signal, 1s change of thoracic impedance signal, diaphragmatic discharge area,

**Table 2.** The specific meaning of the feature parameters

| Parameters abbreviation | Unit | Description |
|---|---|---|
| RR | f/min | Respiration rate per minute |
| Inspi time | s | Inhalation time |
| Expi time | s | Exhalation time |
| It:Et | | Suction ratio |
| VT | L | Tidal volume |
| Imped P-P | Ω | Bio-impedance peak-to-peak |
| Imped Vari | Ω | Bio-impedance 1s change |
| DiEMG LF | | Diaphragmatic EMG low-band power (20–40 Hz) |
| DiEMG HF | | Diaphragmatic EMG high-band power (150–250 Hz) |
| HF/LF | | Ratio between high-band power and low-band power |
| DiEMG Area | μV*s | Diaphragmatic electromyography area |
| DiEMG time | s | Diaphragmatic electromyography time |
| DiEMG P-P | μV | Diaphragmatic electromyography peak-to-peak |
| HR | f/min | Number of heart beats per minute |
| CPC | | Cardiopulmonary coupling coefficient |

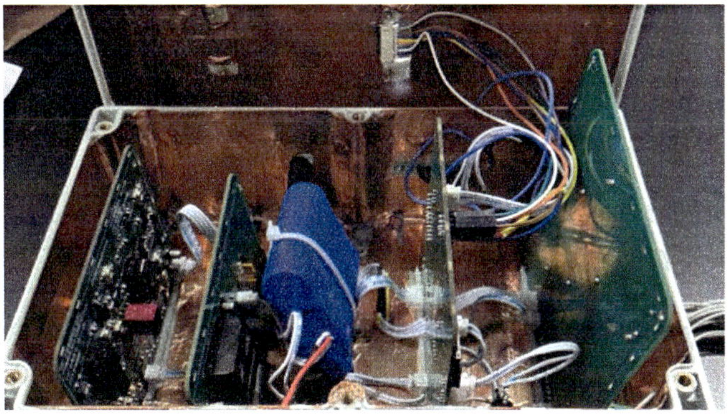

**Fig. 4.** The signal acquisition composition

low-frequency power of diaphragmatic EMG, high-frequency ratio and low-frequency of diaphragmatic EMG signal, peak-to-peak of diaphragmatic EMG signal and cardiopulmonary coupling coefficient were significantly lower than those of healthy adults ($P < 0.05$). Heart rate was significantly higher in mechanically ventilated patients than in healthy adults ($P < 0.05$). There were no significant differences in respiration rate, aspiration ratio, and diaphragm discharge time between the two groups ($P > 0.05$). The

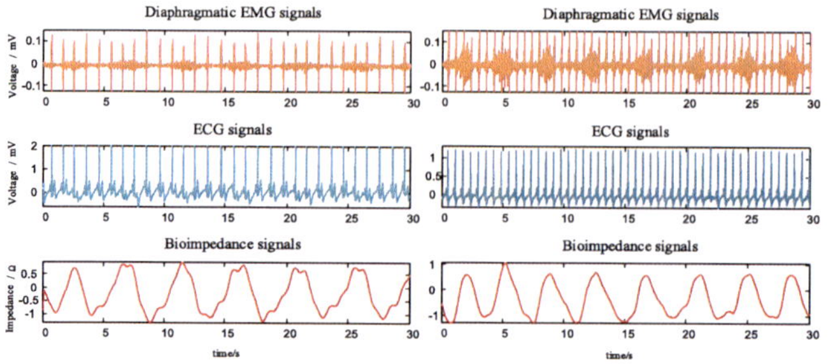


a) The healthy b) The patient

**Fig. 5.** The original signal waveform

**Table 3.** The analysis of respiratory-related parameters of patients and healthy adults

| Parameters | Patients (n = 10) | Healthy volunteers (n = 10) | *P* |
|---|---|---|---|
| RR (f/min) | 15.900 ± 2.359 | 12.400 ± 0.267 | 0.529 |
| Inspi time(s) | 1.199 ± 0.182 | 1.947 ± 0.088 | 0.003 |
| Expiry time (s) | 1.344 ± 0.158 | 2.176 ± 0.124 | 0.001 |
| It:Et | 0.920 ± 0.102 | 0.933 ± 0.085 | 0.928 |
| VT(L) | 0.493 ± 0.066 | 0.913 ± 0.119 | 0.007 |
| Imped P-P (Ω) | 1.165 ± 0.177 | 6.086 ± 0.886 | 0.000 |
| Imped Vari (Ω) | 1.209 ± 0.238 | 4.074 ± 0.679 | 0.002 |
| DiEMG LF | 6.201 ± 2.318 | 19.442 ± 4.336 | 0.011 |
| DiEMG HF | 0.488 ± 0.208 | 14.957 ± 5.394 | 0.000 |
| HF/LF | 0.189 ± 0.095 | 0.772 ± 0.265 | 0.002 |
| DiEMG area (μV*s) | 67.525 ± 17.634 | 155.692 ± 27.601 | 0.007 |
| DiEMG time (s) | 2.163 ± 0.288 | 2.704 ± 0.130 | 0.105 |
| DiEMG P-P(μV) | 30.077 ± 6.186 | 57.515 ± 9.856 | 0.029 |
| HR (f/min) | 92.000 ± 5.217 | 69.300 ± 4.224 | 0.003 |
| CPC | 0.397 ± 0.068 | 0.590 ± 0.028 | 0.043 |

analysis of respiratory-related parameters of patients and healthy adults is shown in the Table 3.

## 4 Conclusion

In this study, the design of a respiratory function monitoring system based on body surface diaphragm myoelectric was completed, and the synchronous acquisition and storage of diaphragmatic myoelectric, ECGand thoracic impedance were realized. After clinical experiments, the system works stably and can collect physiological signals with a high signal-to-noise ratio in complex electromagnetic field environments, providing clinical data for respiratory function research.

The excitatory signal of the respiratory center is transmitted to the diaphragm through the phrenic nerve, causing diaphragm excitation, which is contracted by the excitation-contraction coupling mechanism, thereby producing diaphragmatic EMG. Human respiratory activity is closely related to respiratory muscle activity, and the middle diaphragm of respiratory muscle is particularly important, providing 60–80% ventilation power for normal inhalation in adults. Therefore, monitoring the respiratory function of subjects by diaphragmatic electromyography is theoretically the most reliable and accurate. The results showed that the peak-to-peak and diaphragmatic discharge area of diaphragmatic electrical signals in mechanically ventilated patients were lower than those in healthy adults ($P < 0.05$). This is because the respiratory rate of patients with respiratory dysfunction is accelerated, resulting in a significant reduction in the single contraction of the diaphragm. Patients with respiratory dysfunction rely on ventilators to assist ventilation, and the activity of the diaphragm is weakened, so the high and low band power of diaphragm EMG is lower than that of healthy adults ($P < 0.05$). Prolonged mechanical ventilation can cause increased diaphragmatic fatigue. When diaphragm fatigue, the low-frequency component of diaphragm discharge increases and the high-frequency component decreases, so HF/LF is significantly lower in mechanically ventilated patients than in healthy adults ($P < 0.05$).

During breathing exercises, the shape of the human thoracic cavity will change accordingly, the ECG axis will be deflected, and the amplitude of the ECG signal R fluctuation will change. This varies by increasing the amplitude of the R wave with exhalation and decreasing the amplitude of the R wave on inhalation. The cardiopulmonary coupling coefficient was calculated using the ECG NN interval sequence signal and the derived respiratory signal was significantly lower in patients than in healthy adults ($P < 0.05$). The cardiopulmonary coupling coefficient reflects a decrease in cardiopulmonary coordination and decreased cardiopulmonary function.

The respiratory movement will cause the rhythmic expansion and contraction of the thoracic cage due to the contraction and relaxation of the respiratory muscles, and the distribution resistance of the thoracic surface will also change, and by detecting the change in impedance, it is possible to judge the human respiratory activity, observe the speed and amplitude of breathing. Comparing whether there is a difference in chest impedance signal parameters with healthy adults can determine whether the subject's respiratory function is abnormal. The results showed that the changes in inspiratory time, expiratory time, peak-to-peak of thoracic impedance, and intra-1 s chest impedance in patients with abnormal respiratory function were significantly lower than those in healthy adults ($P < 0.05$). Because patients generally breathe shallow and fast, each inhalation is small, but the frequency is fast; Healthy subjects generally breathe deeply and slowly, with relatively large and slower inhalations per inhalation.

Studies have shown that the monitoring system can collect diaphragmatic EMG, ECG, and thoracic impedance signals in real-time, and can work continuously for a long time with good stability. There were significant differences in respiratory function-related parameters between the two groups, indicating that the system was able to assess the respiratory function of the monitored person. However, there are still some shortcomings in this system: the monitoring system is still relatively large, and the portability needs to be improved; The sample size of the initial clinical experiment is small and insufficient to fully verify the working performance of the system. In the future, we will continue to improve the circuit design and collect more clinical samples in response to the above shortcomings.

**Acknowledgments.** This work was supported by the national key research and development plan (2021YFC0122404).

## References

1. Zhang, X.G.: China Health Statistical Yearbook 2020, vol. 4. China Union Medical College, Beijing (2020)
2. Liu, C.W., Xu, S.X.: Critical Care Organ Support and Care, pp. 33–34. People's Health Publishing House, Beijing (2001)
3. Pulmonary function of respiratory branch of Chinese medical association. Guidelines for pulmonary function examination (Part I)—overview and general requirements. Chin. J. Tubercul. Resp. Med. **37**(6), 402–405 (2014)
4. Li, L.C., Luo, H., Zhang, H., et al.: Clinical significance of mechanical ventilation with respiratory mechanics monitor. Int. J. Resp. **37**(17), 1320–1323 (2017)
5. Liu, H.G., Wu, A.P., Yang, Y., et al.: Monitoring and application of diaphragmatic electrical activity. Chin. J. Resp. Crit. Care **9**(04), 447–450 (2010)
6. Wang, T.: Design of Electrostatic Sensor Amplification Filter Circuit and Its Electromagnetic Compatibility Research. Xi'an University of Technology (2018)
7. Zhuo, C.N.: Development of a Miniature Cardiac Function Monitoring Device with Two Electrodes. Chongqing University (2015)

# Aortic Pressure Waveform Estimation Based on Variational Mode Decomposition and Gated Recurrent Unit

Shuo Du[1], Jinzhong Yang[1], Guozhe Sun[2], Hongming Sun[1], Lisheng Xu[1](✉), and Dingchang Zheng[3]

[1] College of Medicine and Biological Information Engineering, Northeastern University, Shenyang, China
xuls@bmie.neu.edu.cn

[2] Department of Cardiology, China Medical University, Shenyang, China

[3] Research Centre of Intelligent Healthcare, Coventry University, Coventry, UK

**Abstract.** Objective: Aortic pressure waveform (APW) can provide vital indices for the diagnosis of cardiovascular diseases. Although various APW estimation methods have been reported to avoid the risks of direct invasive measurement, more accurate and practical estimation models still need to be developed to promote the application of APW in routine monitoring. To solve this problem, a hybrid model based on variational mode decomposition (VMD) and gated recurrent unit (GRU) named VMD-GRU was proposed to estimate the APW from the brachial pressure waveform (BPW). Methods: Invasive APWs and BPWs from 34 subjects were used to validate the proposed hybrid model. Initially, new samples were obtained from these measured APWs and BPWs using data augmentation technology. Subsequently, VMD was employed to decompose the augmented BPWs into multiple intrinsic mode functions (IMFs). Next, the GRU network was utilized to learn the complex relationship between the IMFs and augmented APWs. The trained GRU network can be used to estimate the APWs with the IMFs obtained from the BPWs and VMD approach. The root-mean-square-error of total waveform and mean absolute errors of commonly adopted hemodynamic indices in clinic including systolic and diastolic blood pressures and pulse pressure were used to evaluate the proposed hybrid model. The performance of the proposed hybrid model was obtained from leave-one-subject-out cross validation. Results: The proposed hybrid model achieved smaller errors of total waveform (3.33 vs. 3.50 mmHg, $P < 0.05$) and pulse pressure (3.02 vs. 3.64 mmHg, $0.05 < P < 0.10$) compared to the GRU. Conclusion: The proposed hybrid model can provide more accurate APW in comparison to the GRU network.

**Keywords:** Variational mode decomposition · Gated recurrent unit · Aortic pressure waveform · Brachial pressure waveform


G. Wang et al. (Eds.): APCMBE 2023, IFMBE Proceedings 103, pp. 29–38, 2024.
https://doi.org/10.1007/978-3-031-51455-5_4

# 1 Introduction

Numerous studies have shown that aortic pressure waveform (APW) provides more physiological and pathological information for the diagnosis and treatment of cardiovascular diseases than peripheral pressure waveforms [1]. Direct invasive measurement with a pressure catheter, as the gold standard means of obtaining the APW, carries significant drawbacks of high invasion and expensive cost [2]. These drawbacks limit the clinical application of APW in routine monitoring. On the contrary, peripheral pressure waveforms can be measured less invasively using a catheter [3] or non-invasively using an applanation tonometry [4]. Hence, various indirect APW estimation methods using the peripheral waveforms were proposed to avoid the drawbacks of invasive measurement.

An approximation using carotid pressure waveform is the earliest method in clinical practice owing to its simple operation although it gives unsatisfactory performance [5]. At present, the commercial devices based on generalized transfer function (GTF) are widely adopted to obtain APW from one-channel peripheral pressure waveform [6–8]. However, the GTF method can lead to a serious low precision problem owing to its limited ability to simulate the characteristics of pulse transmission in the complex and nonlinear cardiovascular system. To improve the precision, Windkessel [9], tube-load [10], T-tube [11] and one-dimensional [12] models have been introduced to the estimation of APW. Unfortunately, these physical-model-based methods usually rely on simultaneous collection of multiple-channel signals, which leads to an intractable practical problem. Recently, nonlinear neural network has shown excellent performance in APW reconstruction task owing to its powerful feature extraction ability [13]. Moreover, similarly to the GTF, the neural network only utilizes one-channel peripheral pressure waveform, which can facilitate the application of this method in clinical practice. In this paper, a hybrid model based on variational mode decomposition (VMD) and gated recurrent unit (GRU) named VMD-GRU was proposed to reconstruct the APW from the brachial pressure waveform (BPW) for a higher estimation accuracy in comparison to the neural network only based on GRU.

# 2 Methods

As shown in Fig. 1, new samples were obtained from the measured BPWs and APWs with data augmentation technology during training process firstly. Next, intrinsic mode functions (IMFs) of the augmented BPWs were obtained using the VMD approach. Subsequently, a GRU network was trained with these IMFs and augmented APWs. During the estimation process, the VMD approach was performed to obtain IMFs from the measured BPWs. Then, these IMFs were input to the trained GRU network to estimate APWs.

*A. Data collection*

The proposed method was validated with invasive APWs and BPWs from 34 patients who underwent cardiac catheterization at the First Hospital of China Medical University. The APWs and BPWs were measured simultaneously by pressure wires (RadiAnalyzer Xpress, St. Jude Medical, Minnesota, USA). Sampling frequency was 100 Hz. This

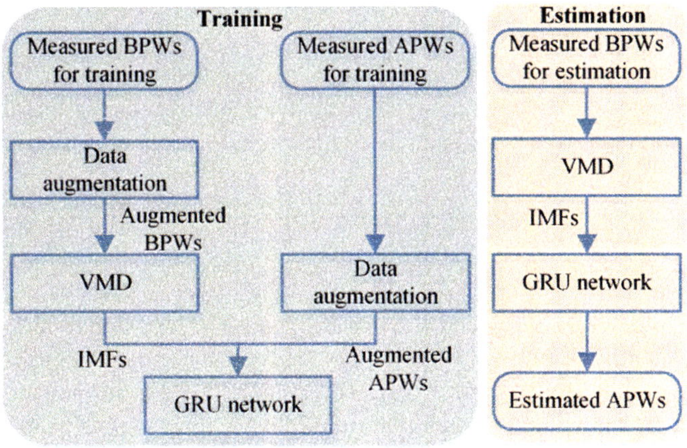


**Fig. 1.** Procedures of the modeling of the VMD-GRU.

study was approved by the Ethics Committees of College of Medicine and Biological Information Engineering, Northeastern University (EC-2020B016). All subjects gave their informed and signed consents. Table 1 summarizes some information of the patients and corresponding data.

**Table 1.** Patient and data characteristics.

| Characteristics | Mean ± SD or number |
|---|---|
| Male | 14 |
| Age (y) | 56 ± 14 |
| Height (cm) | 165 ± 8 |
| Weight (kg) | 68 ± 12 |
| SBP (mmHg) | 150 ± 23 |
| DBP (mmHg) | 79 ± 13 |

SBP and DBP denote brachial systolic blood pressure and diastolic blood pressure, respectively.

*B. Data augmentation*

Over-fitting phenomenon often occurs when complex neural networks are employed in small datasets. Hence, the data augmentation technology of window slicing was performed to increase the number of samples in the training set [14]. The data of each subject were cut into 300 segments to form multiple new samples.

*C. Variational mode decomposition*

VMD is an adaptive and quasi-orthogonal signal decomposition method, which can non-recursively decompose the original signal $f(t)$ into $K$ IMFs which are compact around a center pulsation [15]. The VMD can be written as a constrained variational problem:

$$\begin{cases} \min_{\{u_k\},\{\omega_k\}} \left\{ \sum_k \left\| \partial_t \left[ \left( \delta(t) + \frac{j}{\pi t} \right) * u_k(t) \right] e^{-j\omega_k t} \right\|_2^2 \right\} \\ s.t. \sum_k u_k = f(t) \end{cases} \tag{1}$$

where $\{u_k\} = \{u_1, u_2, \cdots, u_K\}$ and $\{\omega_k\} = \{\omega_1, \omega_2, \cdots, \omega_K\}$ denote the sets of IMFs and their corresponding central accuracies, respectively. $\delta(t)$ and $j$ are the Dirac function and imaginary number unit, respectively. The constrained variational problem can be addressed with an augmented Lagrangian function:

$$\begin{aligned} L(\{u_k\}, \{\omega_k\}, \lambda) = {} & \alpha \sum_k \left\| \partial_t \left[ \left( \delta(t) + \frac{j}{\pi t} \right) * u_k(t) \right] e^{-j\omega_k t} \right\|_2^2 + \left\| f(t) - \sum_k u_k(t) \right\|_2^2 \\ & + \left\langle \lambda(t), f(t) - \sum_k u_k(t) \right\rangle \end{aligned} \tag{2}$$

where $\alpha$ and $\lambda(t)$ are the penalty parameter and Lagrangian multiplier, respectively. The alternate direction method of multipliers is adopted to obtain the solutions of the Eq. (2). All the IMFs gained from the solutions in spectral domain are expressed as:

$$\hat{u}_k(\omega) = \frac{\hat{f}(\omega) - \sum_{i \neq k} \hat{u}_i(\omega) + \frac{\hat{\lambda}(\omega)}{2}}{1 + 2\alpha(\omega - \omega_k)^2} \tag{3}$$

where $\hat{u}_k(\omega)$, $\hat{f}(\omega)$, $\hat{u}(\omega)$ and $\hat{\lambda}(\omega)$ are the Fourier transforms of $\hat{u}_k(t)$, $\hat{f}(t)$, $\hat{u}(t)$ and $\hat{\lambda}(t)$, respectively.

As reported by Li, the value of $K$ is equal to the level of empirical mode decomposition on the same signal [16]. Hence, this study set $K$ to 6 according to the mode of level of empirical mode decomposition on the adopted BPWs. As shown in Fig. 2, IMFs were obtained from the BPW using the VMD algorithm.

*D. Gated recurrent unit*

GRU, as a time recurrent neural network, can extract the nonlinear features in time series [17]. It is a simpler alternative to the long short-term memory and has been proved to be suitable for small datasets [18]. As shown in Fig. 3, a GRU cell contains an update gate outputting $z_t$ and a reset gate outputting $r_t$. The update and reset gates decide how to get the current hidden state $h_t$ from the current input $x_t$ previous hidden state $h_{t-1}$.

$$\begin{cases} z_t = \sigma\left( \boldsymbol{W_z}[h_{t-1}, x_t] + \boldsymbol{b_z} \right) \\ r_t = \sigma\left( \boldsymbol{W_r}[h_{t-1}, x_t] + \boldsymbol{b_r} \right) \\ \tilde{h}_t = \tanh\left( \boldsymbol{W_h}[r_t h_{t-1}, x_t] + \boldsymbol{b}_h \right) \\ h_t = (1 - z_t) h_{t-1} + \tilde{h}_t \end{cases} \tag{4}$$

where $\boldsymbol{W_*}$ and $\boldsymbol{b_*}$ denote weight matrix and bias vector, respectively; $\sigma(\cdot)$ and $\tanh(\cdot)$ are the sigmoid and tanh functions, respectively.

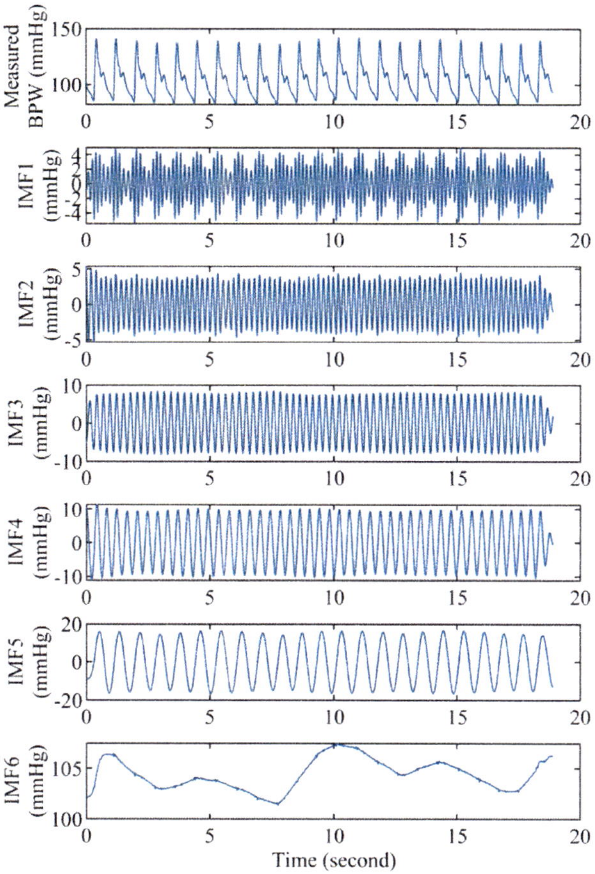


**Fig. 2.** Measured BPW and the IMFs obtained from VMD.

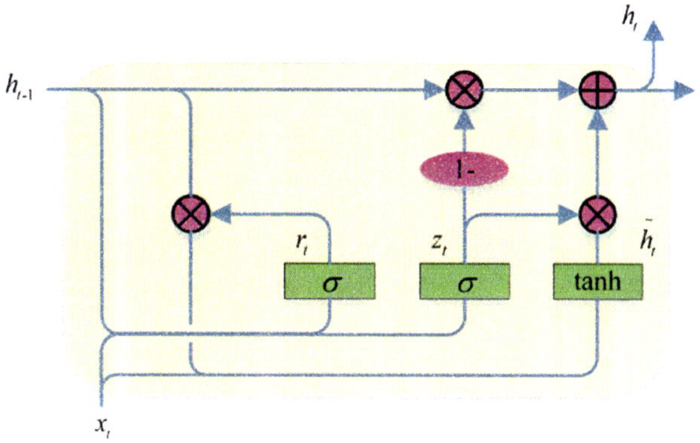


**Fig. 3.** The structure of a GRU cell.

In this study, the IMFs derived from the VMD are input into the two layers of GRU network with 200 GRU cells. The number of epochs and the batch size were set to 30 and 100, respectively. Adma optimizer and mean squared error loss function were adopted in the GRU network and the learning rate was set to 0.0001.

*E. Performance evaluation*

Root-mean-square-error of total waveform (TW), mean absolute errors of systolic blood pressure, diastolic blood pressure and pulse pressure (SBP, DBP and PP, respectively) were used to evaluate the proposed method. Leave-one-subject-out cross-validation was adopted. The performance of the proposed hybrid model was compared to that of the GRU using paired *t*-test.

## 3 Results

Figure 4 compares the measured APW, from a representative subject (ID 2), with those derived from the GRU and the proposed hybrid method. It is obvious that the estimated APW from the proposed hybrid model is closer to the measured one in comparison to the GRU alone.

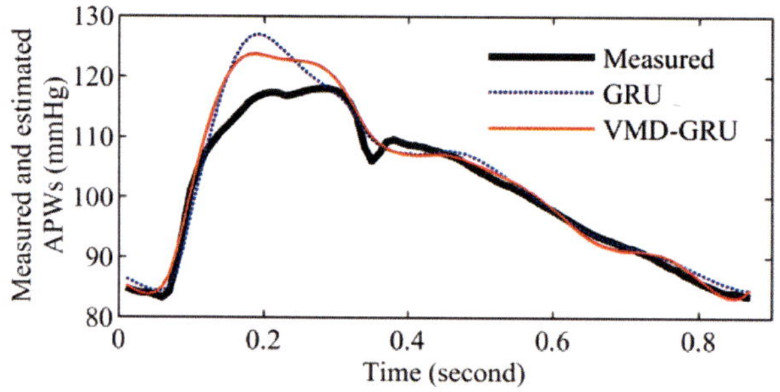


**Fig. 4.** Comparison of the measured (black thick solid line) and estimated APWs from subject # 2 using the VMD-GRU (red solid line) and GRU (blue dashed line).

Figure 5 shows the Bland-Altman analysis results of the GRU and VMD-GRU. The VMD-GRU obtained not only lower bias (−0.39 vs. 0.47 mmHg, −0.38 vs. 1.40 mmHg, 0.33 vs. 0.76 mmHg and −0.71 vs. 2.16 mmHg, respectively) but also more narrow limits (14.08 vs. 14.68 mmHg, 15.49 vs. 16.12 mmHg, 8.22 vs. 8.65 mmHg, and 14.61 vs. 15.57 mmHg, respectively) of TW, SBP, DBP and PP compared to the GRU.

Table 2 lists the performance comparison in error measures of the GRU and VMD-GRU. The VMD-GRU achieved lower errors of TW (3.33 vs. 3.50 mmHg, $P < 0.05$) and PP (3.02 vs. 3.64 mmHg, $0.05 < P < 0.10$) and similar errors of SBP and DBP (3.10 vs. 3.29 mmHg and 3.02 vs. 3.64 mmHg, respectively, both $P > 0.10$) compared to the GRU.

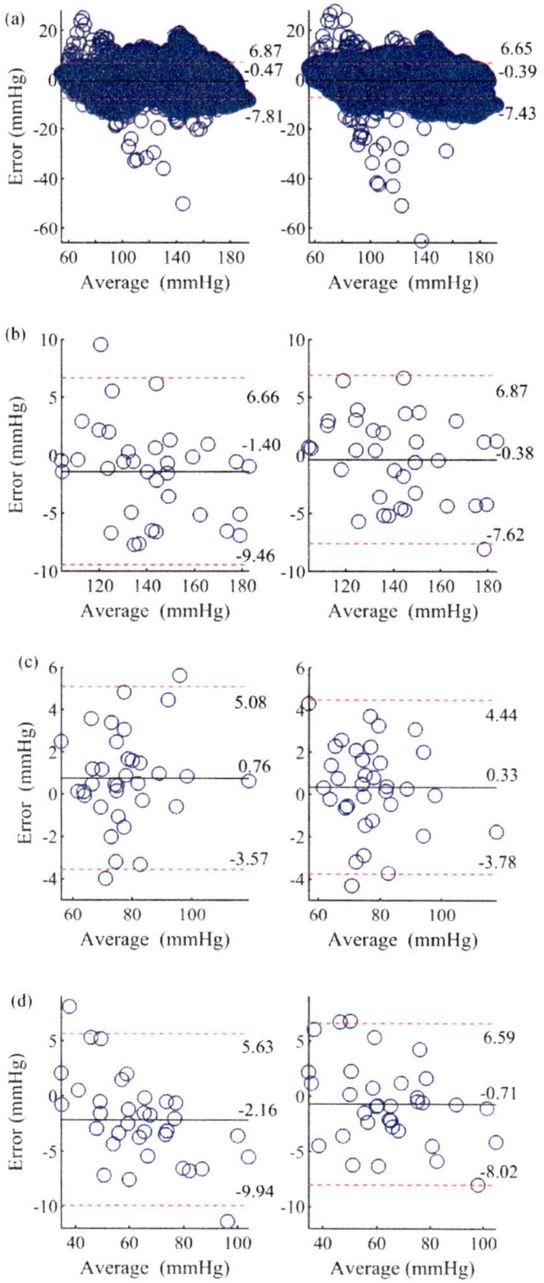


**Fig. 5.** Bland-Altman analysis results of the GRU (left) and VMD-GRU (right) for the **a** TW, **b** SBP, **c** DBP and **d** PP.

**Table 2.** Performance comparison of GRU and VMD-GRU.

| | TW (mmHg) | SBP (mmHg) | DBP (mmHg) | PP (mmHg) |
|---|---|---|---|---|
| GRU | $3.50 \pm 1.18$ | $3.29 \pm 2.79$ | $1.76 \pm 1.51$ | $3.64 \pm 2.64$ |
| VMD-GRU | $3.33 \pm 1.12$* | $3.10 \pm 1.98$ | $1.70 \pm 1.25$ | $3.02 \pm 2.25^{\#}$ |

* and # denote $P < 0.05$ and $0.05 < P < 0.10$, respectively.

## 4 Discussion

The transmission process of pressure waveform is essentially nonlinear [19]. Hence, this study proposed two nonlinear APW reconstruction methods including the GRU and the hybrid model VMD-GRU. Comparison experiments have showed that the hybrid model is more accurate than the GRU. The pressure waveform contains multiple components caused by complex physiological activities including cardiac pulsation, respiration [20] and neural regulation [21]. The VMD can decompose the BPW into multiple IMFs, which may be beneficial for the GRU to extract the features corresponding to the above physiological activities from the BPW for reconstructing the APW. The current analysis was based on the subjects with cardiovascular diseases. Further research is required to extend the proposed method to a wider range of subjects. This study adopted invasive data to validate the proposed method, while a non-invasive peripheral pressure waveform is more suitable for routine monitoring than an invasive one. Hence, it is necessary to estimate the APW with non-invasive peripheral pressure waveforms.

## 5 Conclusion

Estimation of the APW from the measurements of peripheral pressure waveform is a low-risk approach compared with direct invasive measurement. This study validated the effectiveness of the hybrid model based on VMD and GRU for obtaining such estimations by measuring BPW. Experimental results have shown that the proposed method is more accurate than the neural network only based on GRU and provides a step towards the development of an improved and clinically useful non-invasive approach for estimating the APW.

**Acknowledgments.** This work was supported by the National Natural Science Foundation of China (No. 62273082, and No. 61773110), the Natural Science Foundation of Liaoning Province (No. 20170540312, and No. 2021-YGJC-14), the Basic Scientific Research Project (Key Project) of Liaoning Provincial Department of Education (LJKZ00042021), Fundamental Research Funds for the Central Universities (No. N2119008), the Shenyang Science and Technology Plan Fund (No. 21-104-1-24, No. 20-201-4-10, and No. 201375).

## References


1. Williams, B., et al.: 2018 ESC/ESH Guidelines for the management of arterial hypertension. Eur. Heart J. **39**, 3021–3104 (2018)
2. Mceniery, C.M., Cockcroft, J.R., Roman, M.J., Franklin, S.S., Wilkinson, I.B.: Central blood pressure: current evidence and clinical importance. Eur. Heart **35**, 1719–1725 (2014)
3. Imholz, B.P.M., Wieling, W., Van Montfrans, G.A., Wesseling, K.H.: Fifteen years experience with finger arterial pressure monitoring: assessment of the technology. Cardiovasc. Res. **38**, 605–616 (1998)
4. Harju, J., et al.: Comparison of non-invasive blood pressure monitoring using modified arterial applanation tonometry with intra-arterial measurement. J. Clin. Monit. Comput. **32**, 13–22 (2018)
5. Mitchell, G.F., et al.: Arterial stiffness and cardiovascular events: the Framingham heart study. Circulation **121**, 505–511 (2010)
6. Ott, C., Haetinger, S., Schneider, M.P., Pauschinger, M., Schmieder, R.E.: Comparison of two noninvasive devices for measurement of central systolic blood pressure with invasive measurement during cardiac catheterization. J. Clin. Hypertens. **14**, 575–579 (2012)
7. McEniery, C.M., Wilkinson, I.B., Hickson, S.S., McDonnell, B.J., Maki-Petaja, K.M., Richardson, C.J.: Comparison of estimates of central systolic blood pressure and peripheral augmentation index obtained from the Omron HEM-9000AI and SphygmoCor systems. Artery Res. **3**, 24–31 (2009)
8. Climie, R.E., Schultz, M.G., Nikolic, S.B., Ahuja, K.D., Fell, J.W., Sharman, J.E.: Validity and reliability of central blood pressure estimated by upper arm oscillometric cuff pressure. Am. J. Hypertens. **25**, 414–420 (2012)
9. Sooriamoorthy, D., Shanmugam, S.A., Juman, M.A.: A novel electrical impedance function to estimate central aortic blood pressure waveforms. Biomed. Signal Proces. **68**, 102649 (2021)
10. Gao, M., Rose, W.C., Fetics, B., Kass, D.A., Chen, C.H., Mukkamala, R.: A simple adaptive transfer function for deriving the central blood pressure waveform from a radial blood pressure waveform. Sci. Rep. **6**, 33230 (2016)
11. Liu, W., et al.: Noninvasive estimation of aortic pressure waveform based on simplified Kalman filter and dual peripheral artery pressure waveforms. Comput. Meth. Programs Biomed. **219**, 106760 (2022)
12. Khalife, M., Decoene, A., Caetano, F., de Rochefort, L., Durand, E., Rodriguez, D.: Estimating absolute aortic pressure using MRI and a one-dimensional model. J. Biomech. **47**, 3390–3399 (2014)
13. Xiao, H., Liu, C., Zhang, B.: Reconstruction of central arterial pressure waveform based on CNN-BILSTM. Biomed. Signal Proces. **74**, 103513 (2022)
14. Meng, T., Shi, H., Wang, C., Wu, B.: Application of principal component analysis in measurement of flow fluctuation. Measurement **173**, 108503 (2021)
15. Dragomiretskiy, K., Zosso, D.: Variational mode decomposition. IEEE Trans. Signal Proces. **62**, 531–544 (2014)
16. Li, Y., Li, Y., Chen, X., Yu, J.: Research on ship-radiated noise denoising using secondary variational mode decomposition and correlation coefficient. Sensors (Basel) **18**, 1 (2017)
17. Chen, J., Jing, H., Chang, Y., Liu, Q.: Gated recurrent unit based recurrent neural network for remaining useful life prediction of nonlinear deterioration process. Reliab. Eng. Syst. Safe **185**, 372–382 (2019)
18. Gruber, N., Jockisch, A.: Are GRU cells more specific and LSTM cells more sensitive in motive classification of text? Front. Artif. Intell. **3**, 40 (2020)
19. Patel, A.M., Li, J.K.: Validation of a novel nonlinear black box Wiener System model for arterial pulse transmission. Comput. Biol. Med. **88**, 11–17 (2017)

20. Baselli, G., et al.: Model for the assessment of heart period and arterial pressure variability interactions and of respiration influences. Med. Biol. Eng. Comput. **32**, 143–152 (1994)
21. Furlan, R., et al.: Continuous 24-hour assessment of the neural regulation of systemic arterial pressure and RR variabilities in ambulant subjects. Circulation **81**, 537–547 (1990)

# Research on Intelligent Calibration Test Fault Diagnosis Model of Automatic Chemiluminescence Immunoassay Analyzer

Xinqi Pan[1,2], Xiao Sun[1,2(✉)], and Lifeng Sha[3]

[1] School of Biological Sciences and Medical Engineering, Southeast University, Nanjing, China
xsun@seu.edu.cn
[2] Southeast University-Monash University Joint Graduate School, Southeast University, Suzhou, China
[3] Jiangsu Avatarget Biotechnology Co. Ltd., Suzhou, China

**Abstract.** In this study, three fault diagnosis models for the calibration test of the automated chemiluminescent immunoassay analyzer (ACLIA) are developed. The models are trained, validated and tested with a large amount of historical calibration testing data. We compare the performance of three machine learning methods of Random Forest (RFC),Extreme Gradient Boosting (XGB) and Light Gradient Boosting Machine (LGBM). The results on independent test datasets show that the RFC model performs the best, with accuracy, F1, and AUC metrics of 0.979, 0.982, and 0.930, respectively; the XGB model performs similarly to the RFC model, with accuracy, F1, and AUC metrics of 0.964, 0.974, and 0.910, respectively; the LGBM model has the AUC metric of 0.900. In summary, the RFC,XGB and LGBM models trained in this study can effectively diagnose the calibration fault categories of ACLIA, which can help medical instrument manufacturers reduce the losses caused by the calibration testing process, reduce the cost of reagents, and improve the production efficiency.

**Keywords:** Fault diagnosis · Machine learning · Automated chemiluminescence immunoassay analyzer (ACLIA)

## 1 Introduction

Automated chemiluminescence immunoassay analyzer (ACLIA) is an important in vitro diagnostic product which is indispensable for clinical diagnosis in modern medical institutions. It is a new technique that combines chemiluminescence analysis and immunoassay to detect trace antigens or antibodies, using the absorption of light to analyze the analyse qualitatively or quantitatively [1]. The principle is a direct chemical immunoassay using acridine esters for labeling. The luminescence intensity is obtained by recording the photon energy generated per unit time, and the concentration of the substance to be measured can be indirectly determined by the luminescence intensity detected by the instrument according to the linear relationship between the concentration of the substance to be measured and the luminescence [2].


G. Wang et al. (Eds.): APCMBE 2023, IFMBE Proceedings 103, pp. 39–46, 2024.
https://doi.org/10.1007/978-3-031-51455-5_5

The same batch of reagents can be customized with six different concentrations at the factory, and then the corresponding luminescence values of the six different concentrations can be detected on the testing instrument. The points indicated by coordinates S0-S5 in Fig. 1 are called standard points, and the curve fitted by the algorithm for the six standard points is called the master curve.

Calibration testis the most important step before biochemical analysis by ACLIA. Differences between the instrument and the environment in which it is used may lead to different results for the same concentration of reagents, which in turn may lead to inaccuracies in the detection of the instrument. It is an important step in eliminating this variability. Calibration test process is as follows. Firstly, the luminescence values corresponding to two different concentrations of reagents will be detected on the working instrument. The points composed of concentration and luminescence values are called calibration points, which are represented by C1 and C2 in Fig. 1. Then, the mathematical linearity of the luminescence value difference conversion is calculated by the two calibration points and the points corresponding to the concentration in the main curve, and the luminescence value corresponding to the standard point is converted and calibrated to obtain the correction point, which is represented by S0′-S5′ in Fig. 1. The six correction points are refitted by the algorithm to calculate the curve called the working curve of the instrument. Calibration quality control (QC) test is a further verification of the calibration testing to measure the strength of the instrument's working curve. The process of calibration QC test is as follows. Firstly, the reagents are equipped with two known concentration range of the QC product on the instrument to obtain the corresponding luminescence value, and then obtain the concentration value corresponding to the luminescence value through the working curve, if the concentration value is within the reference range set by the QC product, it means the calibration test is successful, otherwise it means fails. The calibration test and calibration QC test flow is shown in Fig. 1.

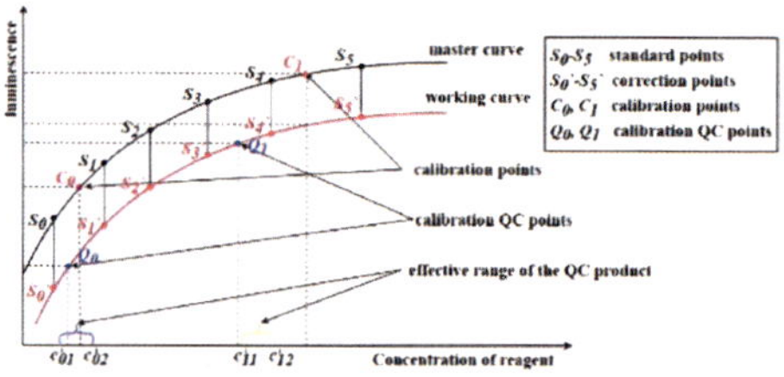


**Fig. 1.** Schematic diagram of calibration test and calibration QC test

In the traditional calibration test fault diagnosis process, calibration test fault is diagnosed by means of consuming calibration QC products. In this study we used machine learning algorithms to build calibration test fault diagnosis models, which analyze and learn from a large amount of historical testing data to explore the relationship between calibration test data and calibration results, and then to perform intelligent diagnosis and classification. Intelligent fault diagnosis model can reduce the consumption of additional calibrated quality control products during the Calibration QC testing phase, which can effectively reduce the cost of using quality control reagents, and further simplify the process and improve the efficiency of instrument use. The model construction process in this study is shown in Fig. 2.

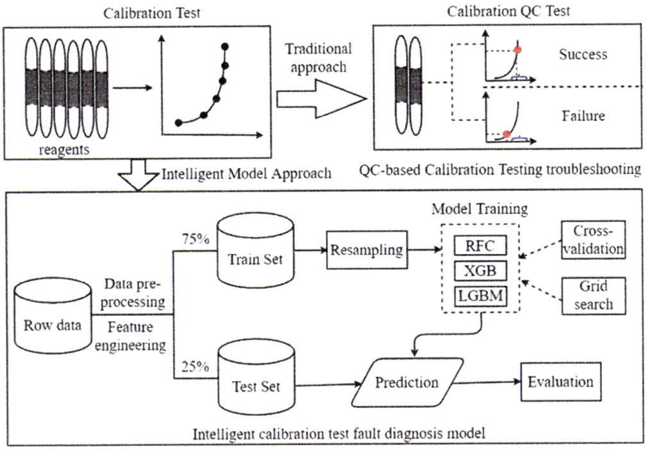


**Fig. 2.** Flowchart of intelligent calibration test diagnosis

## 2 Materials and Methods

*A. Dataset and data processing*

The data used in this study were obtained from historical calibration test data of the same model of ACLIA collected from 15 regional hospitals by a medical device manufacturer, including two types of record data: calibration test fault records and calibration test normal records. There were 6157 original calibration test records. After data cleaning, missing value processing, outlier processing, data conversion and data normalization, 5650 valid calibration test records were obtained as the original data set of this study. Among them, the calibration test fault records are 311, the calibration test normal records are 5339.

*Feature selection*: Feature selection is the core step in feature engineering and an important step in the pre-construction of the model. Based on the research problem and expert domain knowledge, the feature terms relevant to this study were extracted for the training of the fault diagnosis models, and the specific feature descriptions are shown in Table 1.

*Data resampling*: Due to the large proportion of positive and negative samples in the dataset, further data processing is required to better train the model. For the processing of unbalanced data, the main idea is to process the unbalanced sample data in binary classification by changing the distribution of the two categories so that the unbalanced data are converted to balanced data, and then classified by the classification algorithm after a series of conversions. GhoshRoy applied the SMOTE technique to the male fertility prediction model, effectively improving the performance of the classification

**Table 1.** Data feature item description

| Number | Feature coding | Feature description |
|---|---|---|
| 1 | RLU_StandardPoint0–5 | The luminous values corresponding to the six standard points S0-S5<br>The concentration values |
| 2 | Conc_StandardPoint0–5 | corresponding to the six standard points S0-S5 |
| 3 | RLU_StandardPoint05_Corrected | Corresponding luminous value of operating point S0′-S5′ after correction |
| 4 | Conc_StandardPoint05_Corrected | Concentration values corresponding to working points S0′-S5′ after calibration |
| 5 | RLU_Calibrator1 | Luminous value of fixed point 1 |
| 6 | Conc_Calibrator1 | Concentration value of calibration point 1 |
| 7 | RLU_Calibrator2 | Luminous value of fixed point 2 |
| 8 | Conc_Calibrator2 | Concentration value of calibration point 2 |
| 9 | ChemUID | Reagent type |

model [3]. The SMOTE sampling method was used in this study to resample the training set samples, which not only effectively changes the class distribution of the samples, but also helps to differentiate the samples of the boundary minority classes and more effectively improves the class imbalance of the data sample set.

*Dataset partitioning*: The original dataset was split into a training set and an independent test set according to the reagent types, where the original dataset contained a total of thirty reagent types, and the corresponding division ratio of positive and negative samples for each type of reagent was 4:1. The training set in the final division result had a total of 4521 data, including 4271 positive samples with normal calibration test and 250 negative samples with faulty calibration test; the selected independent test set had a total of 1129 data, including 1068 positive samples with normal calibration test and 61 negative samples with faulty calibration test.

*B. Machine learning methods*

*Model selection*: This study tested various machine learning models based on random forest, and finally selected the random forest classification (RFC), extreme gradient boosting (XGB) model and light gradient boosting machine (LGBM) with better evaluation indexes. RFC is a supervised machine learning method based on ensemble learning, which can balance errors and maintain high accuracy for unbalanced data sets [4]. XGB is an algorithm based on gradient lifting decision tree, which has excellent performance in parallel computing efficiency, control overfitting and prediction generalization ability [5]. LGBM is also a gradient lifting decision tree machine learning algorithm based on Histogram. Compared with the XGB model, it can solve the problems of poor computational efficiency and low scalability of XGB under the condition of multidimensional large data sets [6]. For each of the above models, a grid-based search is used for model hyperparameter optimization.

*Model evaluation*: Model evaluation is an important inaccessible step in the field of machine learning and an important indicator to assess the generalization ability of a model. Choosing the appropriate evaluation metrics for the target problem is crucial to whether the actual problem can be better solved, and the following three evaluation metrics were used in this study as reference indicators for the merits of the target classification model, among which, the AUC (area under the curve) and F1 metrics can meet the evaluation requirements in a highly unbalanced classification sample [7].

AUC indicates the size of the area under the ROC curve. The larger area under the curve represented by AUC indicates the better model evaluation index of the model classifier and the better model classification effect.

F1 is an index used to measure the accuracy of the binary model. It takes into account the accuracy rate and recall rate of classification model at the same time, which is a kind of weighted average of the former two metrics, and the larger the value, the better the model [8].

## 3 Results and Discussion

A ten-fold cross-validation approach was used to select and tune the model parameters on the training set, and finally determine the optimal parameter settings for the RFC, XGB and LGBM models on the training set. In this study, ACC, F1 and ROC_AUC were designated as the comprehensive evaluation indicators of the ten-fold cross-validation model. The ten-fold cross-validation was performed for each group of hyperparameter combinations and the average values of the corresponding evaluation indicators were obtained for ten test sets, and the model with the optimal combination was finally selected, and the average values of each evaluation indicator of the optimal model are shown in Table 2.

**Table 2.** Performance of each model on the training set

| Test Set RFC | XGB | LGBM |
|---|---|---|
| ACC 0.934 | 0.928 | 0.877 |
| F1 0.959 | 0.956 | 0.928 |
| AUC 0.927 | 0.920 | 0.904 |

The optimal results of 10-fold cross-validation show that the RFC model has the best performance, and the accuracy and F1 and AUC indexes reach 0.934, 0.959 and 0.927, respectively. The performance of XGB model is comparable to that of RFC model, and the accuracy ratio, F1 index and AUC index reach 0.928, 0.956 and 0.920 respectively. The performance of LGBM model was relatively poor. The above results show that the performance of three models on the training set is feasible.

The performance results of the above models in the independent test set show that the LGBM model performed relatively poorly on the independent test set, with accuracy and F1 and AUC metrics reaching 0.954, 0.974, and 0.900, respectively. The RFC and XGB models performed relatively well, with the RFC model having the best AUC metric of 0.930, while the F1 metric also outperformed the LGBM and XGB, reaching 0.982. The results of each model on the independent test set are shown in Table 3 and the ROC curve of each model is shown in Fig. 3.

**Table 3.** Performance of each model on the independent test set

| Independent test Set RFC | XGB | LGBM |
|---|---|---|
| ACC 0.979 | 0.964 | 0.954 |
| F1 0.982 | 0.974 | 0.974 |
| AUC 0.930 | 0.910 | 0.900 |

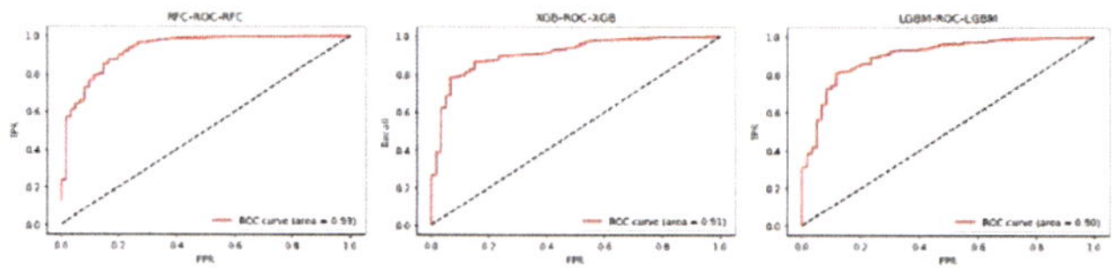


**Fig. 3.** ROC curve corresponding to models for the independent data set

In addition, in order to verify the performance of the model on individual hospital datasets, validation tests were conducted on 12 hospital datasets, and all models performed relatively well on individual hospital datasets, with the XGB model having the best performance in each index, with accuracy, F1 and AUC indexes averaging 0.990, 0.992 and 0.980 for each hospital, respectively. The RFC and XGB model accuracy and F1 indicator averages were also above 0.960 and 0.980, achieving good prediction results. The results of XGB performance indicators in each hospital dataset are shown in Table 4, and the corresponding ROC curves are shown in Fig. 4. The above results show that the models obtained by tenfold cross-validation of the training set can still perform well on the independent test set and can be applied into practical calibration fault diagnosis of ACLIA.

## 4 Conclusions

In this study, we used machine learning method establish intelligent fault diagnosis models of instrument calibration test. The models have strong applicability. By replacing the calibration quality control process with our intelligent diagnosis models, the consumption of quality control liquid reagents in the quality control test stage can be completely avoided. Another advantage of this fault diagnosis method based on machine learning is that more and more excellent model performance can be obtained through the training of a large amount of historical data, which further improves the accuracy of calibration fault diagnosis.

**Table 4.** Performance of XGB model in various hospital datasets

| Hospital Set | ACC | F1 | AUC |
|---|---|---|---|
| H1 | 0.974 | 0.982 | 0.98 |
| H2 | 1.000 | 1.000 | 1.00 |
| H3 | 1.000 | 1.000 | 1.00 |
| H4 | 0.989 | 0.994 | 1.00 |
| H5 | 0.988 | 0.994 | 0.96 |
| H6 | 0.986 | 0.993 | 0.93 |
| H7 | 0.988 | 0.994 | 1.00 |
| H8 | 0.987 | 0.980 | 0.99 |
| H9 | 0.991 | 0.987 | 0.99 |
| H10 | 0.983 | 0.992 | 0.97 |
| H11 | 0.996 | 0.997 | 0.98 |
| H12 | 0.993 | 0.996 | 1.00 |
| Average | 0.990 | 0.992 | 0.98 |

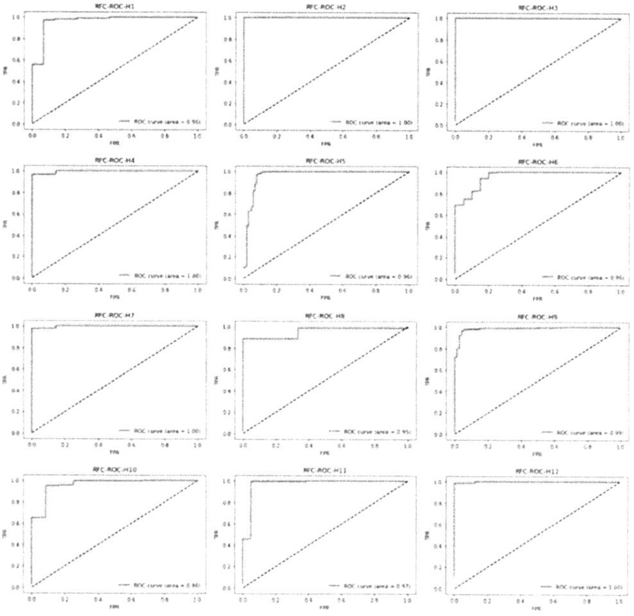

**Fig. 4.** The performance of XGB model in each hospital corresponds to ROC curve

## References


1. Boylan, B., McDermott, O., Kinahan, N.T.: Manufacturing control system development for an in vitro diagnostic product platform. Processes **9**(6), 975 (2021)
2. Zhen, Y.X., Qing, Z.L., Hao, M., Shan, C.Q., Xiao, N.Y.: Chemiluminescence Immunoassay Analyzer Control System Based on S3C2410A. Appl. Mech. Mater. (2011)
3. Debasmita, G.R., Ahmad, A.P., Santosh, K.C.: Explainable AI to Predict Male Fertility Using Extreme Gradient Boosting Algorithm with SMOTE. Electronics (2022)
4. Lisein, J., Fayolle, A., Legrain, A., Prévot, C., Claessens, H.: Prediction of forest nutrient and moisture regimes from understory vegetation with random forest classification models. Ecol. Indicat. (2022)
5. Kurse, S.: Fault detection of bearing using XGBoost algorithm and data visualization using t-distributed stochastic neighbor embedding (t-SNE) Method (2021)
6. Hartini, S., Rustam, Z., Hidayat, R.: Designing hybrid CNN-SVM model for COVID19 classification based on X-ray images using LGBM feature selection. Int. J. Adv. Sci. Eng. Inf. Technol. (2022)
7. Yuzhe, L., Haichun, Y., Zuhayr, A., Zheyu, Z., Tianyuan, Y., Jiachen, X., Yuankai, H.: Holistic fine-grained global glomerulosclerosis characterization: from detection to unbalanced classification. J. Med. Imag. (Bellingham, Wash.) (1) (2022). https://doi.org/10.1117/1.JMI.9.1.014005
8. Hossin, M., Sulaiman, M.N.: A review on evaluation metrics for data classification evaluations. Int. J. Data Min. Knowl. Manage. Process (2) (2015). https://doi.org/10.5121/ijdkp.2015.5201

# Evaluation of Cerebral Autoregulation Function Based on TCD Signal

Chenghuan Shi[1], Jiahao Ye[1], Jiading Li[1], Xingqun Zhao[1](✉), and Zhengtao Yu[1,2]

[1] School of Biological Science and Medical Engineering, Southeast University, Nanjing, China
ndt@seu.edu.cn

[2] Nanjing Osteotech Biotechnology Co., Ltd., Nanjing, China

**Abstract.** Transcranial Doppler (TCD) ultrasound is a commonly used clinical method to evaluate cerebral vascular function. The cerebral autoregulation (CA) function is a mechanism to keep the cerebral blood flow constant when the blood pressure fluctuates. Certain cardio-cerebrovascular diseases may undermine the function to some extent. However, there is no gold standard to evaluate whether the function is normal or not. The most widely used TFA method and ARI index only give a qualitative rule. Therefore, it is necessary to find a reliable evaluation method to identify people with impaired CA function. Based on the TCD signals of normal group and diabetes patient group in the physionet dataset, this paper first uses the features and indicators extracted by the above two methods to classify the subjects. Secondly, a one-dimensional convolution network structure is designed, and its classification accuracy is better than that of machine learning method, reaching 85.33%. Finally, the structure of siamese neural network is used and a new loss function is designed to further improve the accuracy to 92.00%. The method proposed in this paper has preliminarily verified the feasibility of assessing whether the CA function of different groups is damaged, but more clinical patient data is necessary to improve the accuracy and reliability of the method.

**Keywords:** Transcranial doppler · Cerebral autoregulation · Machine learning · 1D-CNN · Siamese network

## 1 Introduction

Transcranial Doppler (TCD) ultrasound is a convenient, non-invasive and real-time detection method for cerebrovascular diseases, providing important evidence for the timely warning and diagnosis of various cerebrovascular diseases [1].

Cerebral autoregulation (CA) is a regulatory mechanism that maintains the constant cerebral blood flow within a certain range of blood pressure fluctuations [2]. Many studies have shown that this regulatory function is damaged to a certain extent among patients with cerebrovascular diseases [3, 4]. However, at present, there is no gold standard to evaluate whether the CA function is normal or not.

The transfer function analysis method (TFA) is based on the linear system hypothesis and evaluates CA by obtaining the gain, phase and consistency between blood pressure


G. Wang et al. (Eds.): APCMBE 2023, IFMBE Proceedings 103, pp. 47–54, 2024.
https://doi.org/10.1007/978-3-031-51455-5_6

and blood flow velocity signals in different frequency bands. The international Cerebral Autoregulation Research Network (CARNet) further standardized the TFA calculation [5]. However, only a qualitative rule is given, that is, the greater the gain, the smaller the phase, the greater the degree of CA damage. Tiecks gives the autoregulation index (ARI) of 1–9 [6] by establishing the blood flow velocity response model after blood pressure mutation. The smaller the index, the greater the degree of CA damage.

Since it is essentially a dichotomous problem, many researchers have proposed machine learning methods based on the physiological features of TCD signals including time and frequency parameters, multi-scale entropy, and morphological characteristics [7]. However, these large number of features have problems such as low contribution to classification results and poor generalization ability. With the development of deep learning, the physiological signals can be directly input into the 1D-CNN network, and the network will automatically extract features from signals and make classification. However, deep learning depends heavily on the number of learning samples while small datasets are the pain points in medical problems, especially for TCD signals, which greatly increases the difficulty of network training.

In this paper, based on the TCD and ABP signals of normal people and diabetes patients in physionet, firstly, the indicators extracted from TFA and ARI methods are used for machine learning classification. Secondly, 1D-CNN neural network is designed to classify the signals. Finally, the siamese neural network is used to transform the direct classification process into the learning of similarity between signals. The siamese network expands the data by establishing sample pairs, and improves the accuracy of classification.

## 2 Experimental Data and Preprocess

*A. Experimental data*

The dataset is from Novak's team of Harvard Medical School, which is about the impairment of CA function in diabetes patients, and made open on physionet [8]. Research shows that diabetes can change the permeability of the blood-brain barrier, thus affecting regional metabolism, thereby damaging CA.

The data set includes 69 diabetes patients and normal people who accept continuous measurement of blood flow velocity of bilateral middle cerebral arteries, ambulatory blood pressure, end expiratory carbon dioxide partial pressure and other parameters during the process of sitting still, leaning upright and Valsalva movements, with a sampling frequency of 500 Hz. Different signal channels of the sample data segment are shown in Fig. 1.

*B. Preprocess*

For the signal obtained from the dataset, the following preprocess is necessary.

First, according to the requirements for recording duration given in the white paper [5], multiple 5-min segments are intercepted from each subject's sitting period, and finally 276 segments are obtained, including 180 in the control group and 196 in the diabetes group. The training set and test set are divided according to the ratio of 8:2.

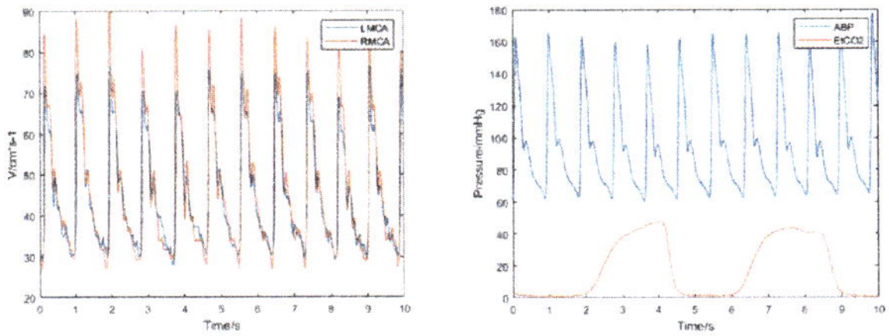


(a) (b)

**Fig. 1.** Samples of data segments. **a** Blood flow velocity of bilateral MCA. **b** Blood pressure and partial pressure of $CO_2$

Secondly, blood flow and blood pressure signals are de-sampled to 50 Hz, and Butterworth low-pass filter with cut-off frequency of 20 Hz is used.

Then, the blood flow velocity signal is normalized to obtain the percentage change, which not only eliminates the dimensional and individual differences, but also ignores the impact of the incident angle in TCD detection [5].

# 3 Methods

*C. Machine learning*

Firstly, the corresponding characteristics are obtained by using transfer function and autoregualtiont index analysis.

In the transfer function analysis method, taking blood pressure signal as input and blood flow signal as output, the transfer function is obtained by calculating their auto-correlation and cross-correlation functions, as shown in Formula (1). The gain and phase of VLF (0.02–0.07 Hz), LF (0.07–0.20 Hz) and HF (0.20–0.50 Hz) are calculated, as shown in formulas (2) and (3). The same calculation is performed on the left and right sides. Since CA regulation mainly occurs in VLF band, left and right side gain and phase are finally selected for further analysis.

$$H(f) = \frac{s_{xy}(f)}{s_{xx}(f)} = \frac{E|X(f)X^*(f)|}{E|X(f)Y^*(f)|} \tag{1}$$

$$|H(f)| = \sqrt{|H_{R(f)}|^2 + |H_{I(f)}|^2} \tag{2}$$

$$\emptyset(f) = tan^{-1}\frac{H_I(f)}{H_R(f)} \tag{3}$$

In the autoregulation index analysis method, nine (1–9) standard response models of blood flow velocity change after ABP sudden drop are constructed according to the second-order linear difference equation. The value of the standard model with the highest matching degree of the target signal, namely the minimum mean square error, is the ARI value. Finally, two ARI values on the left and right sides are obtained.

After obtaining the six characteristics which are left and right side gains, phases and ARI values, the ANOVA test is used to evaluate whether there is significant statistical difference between the characteristics of the two groups. After that, KNN, SVM, MLP, DT, RF, ADA and GBDT are used to make classification.

*D. Deep learning*

In this paper, 1D-CNN is constructed, and its structure is shown in Table 1. The input is a four-channel signal, including left and right middle cerebral artery blood flow velocity (L/RMCA), ambulatory blood pressure (ABP), and end-expiratory carbon dioxide partial pressure (EtCO2). The duration of each section of signal is 5 min, and the sampling is reduced to 10 Hz, with a total of 3000 points. Because CA occurs in the low frequency band, it needs a large receptive field to extract features, so large convolution kernels is selected at the beginning of the network, and average pooling is used. The final receptive field is 111 points, namely 0.1 Hz, which is close to VLF.

**Table 1.** Structure of 1D-CNN

| Network stuctures |
| --- |
| $3000 \times 4$(RMCA, LMCA, ABP, $CO_2$) |
| Conv ($51 \times 4 \times 128$,stride = 2) + BN + ReLU |
| AvgPool (2, strde = 2) |
| Conv ($7 \times 128 \times 32$, stride = 2) + BN + ReLU |
| AvgPoo l(2, strde = 2) |
| Conv ($5 \times 32 \times 128$, stride = 2) + BN + ReLU |
| AvgPool (2, strde = 2) |
| Conv ($3 \times 128 \times 256$, st ride = 2) + BN + ReLU |
| AvgPool (2, strde = 2) |
| Conv ($5 \times 256 \times 512$, stride = 2) + BN + ReLU |
| Conv ($5 \times 512 \times 128$, stride = 2) + BN + ReLU |
| FC-1024 |
| FC-128 |
| FC-3 |

*E. Siamese network*

Siamese neural network is a special type of neural network. Its main idea is to make a sample pair, learn the similarity between the pair through two feature extraction networks with the same structure which shares the weight, and then compare and match samples of new unknown categories according to the similarity measurement. Its structure is shown in Fig. 2, where the single network structure is the same as the 1D-CNN designed in the previous section. By constructing the original data into sample pairs, the number of samples can be expanded to a certain extent. Suppose the number of samples in the control group is N1, the number of samples in the control group is N2, the number of similar samples is N1 (N1–2)/2 + N2 (N2–2)/2, and the number of unexpected samples is N1N2.

The distance function used in the paper is Euclidean distance, The network is trained by minimizing the loss function value of a pair of samples from the same category and maximizing that from different categories. The loss function is shown in Formula (4), where Y = 1 represents the same category and Y = 0 represents different categories, $X_1$ and $X_2$ respectively represent the signal sequence, $W$ represents the weight of the network, $G_w(X_1)$ and $G_w(X_2)$ represent the eigen vectors of the signal sequence and $E_w(X_1, X_2)$ represents the Euclidean distance between the eigen vectors.

$$\begin{aligned} & L(w, (Y, G_w(X_1), G_w(X_2))) \\ & = \frac{Y}{2} E_w(X_1, X_2) + \frac{1-Y}{2} \max\{m - E_w(X_1, X_2), 0\} \end{aligned} \tag{4}$$

The threshold m is set. When the distance exceeds m, the loss function is regarded as 0, which means that the dissimilar features are far away, and the loss value should be very low. For similar features that are far away from each other, it is necessary to increase the loss value so as to continuously update the matching degree of paired samples.

In the process of inference, the signal with the smallest average Euclidean distance from other signals of the same category is selected as the template, as shown in Formula (5). The similarity between the signals in the test set and the two types of signal templates are calculated. Signals are finally divided into the type with higher similarity.

$$e = \sum Y E_w(X_1, X_2) \tag{5}$$

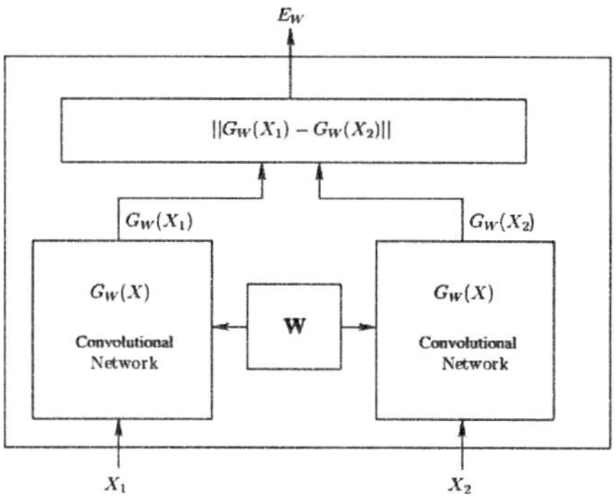


**Fig. 2.** Structure of the siamese network

## 4 Results

The features get from TFA and ARI are shown in Table 2. Before classification, the ANOVA test is used to evaluate whether there is really a statistically significant difference between these indicators in the control group and the control group.

**Table 2.** Results of ANOVA

| Features | Control Group | Diabetes Group | P |
|---|---|---|---|
| L_ARI | 5.64 ± 1.39 | 4.62 ± 1.90 | <0.01 |
| L_Gain_VLF | 0.76 ± 0.28 | 0.75 ± 0.32 | 0.86 |
| L_Phase_VLF | 50.28 ± 18.52 | 45.58 ± 19.99 | 0.06 |
| R_ARI | 5.56 ± 1.55 | 4.35 ± 1.80 | <0.01 |
| R_Gain_VLF | 0.72 ± 0.27 | 0.66 ± 0.30 | 0.21 |
| R_Phase_VLF | 46.43 ± 19.57 | 41.78 ± 21.11 | 0.09 |

**Table 3.** Results of machine learning methods

| Model | Train accuracy (%) | Test accuracy (%) |
|---|---|---|
| KNN | 61.08 | 54.67 |
| SVM | 59.26 | 53.20 |
| MLP | 64.85 | 60.33 |
| DT | 68.48 | 56.28 |
| RF | 73.12 | 60.23 |
| ADA | 67.66 | 52.67 |
| GBDT | 71.34 | 58.45 |

The classification results of each machine learning algorithm are shown in Table 3.

For the classification results of 1D-CNN, accuracy is 85.33%, precision is 85.00%, and recall is 87.18%. For the classification results of the siamese network, accuracy is 92.00%, precision is 90.24%, and recall is 94.87%.

## 5 Discussions

From the statistical results, it can be seen that there is a significant difference in the ARI index between diabetes and control groups. There was no significant difference between 2 groups in the gain and phase obtained by the TFA method. But compared with gain, the p value of phase is more than 5%, but less than 10%, which still has certain reference value. ANOVA ensures the feasibility of the subsequent classification problem.

The result of machine learning is not ideal. This may be due to the small number of cases and the expansion mode. A relatively stable segment with a duration of 5 min was selected from the original signals of 69 subjects, and 276 segments were finally obtained. Since several signal segments in the dataset come from the same subject, the intrinsic correlation of the signal fragments may be high, the generalization ability may be limited, and the performance in the testset is poor.

In the design of 1D-CNN, large convolution kernels are selected in the first few layers. This is because the autoregulation mechanism takes effect in the low frequency band. Therefore, the receptive field of the network is required to be large, so that the low frequency features can be extracted and the accuracy rate is much higher than that of the machine learning methods.

For siamese network, the relationship between m values and accuracy is shown in Table 4. In the process of reasoning, it is necessary to select the most representative template for each category. The template selection method proposed in this paper is to find the segment with the smallest average euclidean distance from other signals in the same category. The accuracy rate of the siamese neural network in the test set reached 92.00%, and the recall rate reached nearly 95%. It is verified that the siamese neural network designed based on the above 1D-CNN has solved the problem of over-fitting to a certain extent, improving the generalization ability. At the same time, the higher recall rate represents a lower false negative rate. Therefore, the TCD result lays a foundation for further diagnosis and treatment of the subjects with impaired autoregulation function.

**Table 4.** Correspondence between m-value and classification accuracy

| m | Accuracy (%) |
|---|---|
| 0 | 82.67 |
| 0.2 | 85.33 |
| 0.4 | 88.00 |
| 0.6 | 92.00 |
| 0.8 | 90.67 |
| 1.0 | 92.0 |

## 6 Conclusions

TCD signals of normal people and diabetes patients from the dataset on physionet are used to explore the method and feasibility of evaluating CA function impairment. First of all, the most widely used TFA and ARI methods are implemented, and six features including the gain, phase and ARI index of the middle cerebral arteries on both sides are extracted. The traditional machine learning method is used for classification, but the results are not ideal. After that, a one-dimensional convolution neural network is designed, and the accuracy in the test set reaches 85.33%. On this basis, the siamese neural network is used and a new loss function is designed to further improve the accuracy to 92.00%. This paper preliminarily verified the feasibility of evaluating CA function between normal and diabetes groups. However, it is still necessary to find more TCD signal data of patients with cardiovascular and cerebrovascular diseases whose CA function is impaired to verify the generalization ability of the model. At the same time, the structure design of one-dimensional convolutional neural network, the loss function and template selection of the siamese neural network can be further optimized.

## References

1. Ali, M.F.A.: Transcranial Doppler ultrasonography (uses, limitations, and potentials): a review article. Egyp. J. Neurosurg. **2021**(1)
2. Payne, S.: Cerebral autoregulation: control of blood flow in the bran. Cerebrovasc. Brain Metab. Rev. **2**(2), 161 (2016)
3. Xiong, X., Shang, et al.: Impaired cerebral autoregulation: measurement and application to stroke. Neurol. Neurosurg. Psych. **88**(6), 520–531 (2017)
4. Novak, V., et al.: Adhesion molecules, altered vasoreactivity, and brain atrophy in type 2 diabetes. Diab. Care **34**(11), 2438–2441 (2011)
5. Claassen, J.A., Meel-Van, D., Simpson, D.M., et al.: Transfer function analysis of dynamic cerebral autoregulation: a white paper from the international cerebral autoregulation research network. J. Cereb. Blood Flow Metab. **36**(4), 665 (2016)
6. Tiecks, F.P., Lam, A.M., Aaslid, R., Tiecks, F.P., Lam, A.M., Aaslid, R., Newell, D.W.: Comparison of static and dynamic cerebral autoregulation measurements. Stroke **26**(6), 1014–1019 (1995)
7. Hamilton, R., Thorpe, S., Thibeault, C., et al.: Abstract 21400: morphological analysis of transcranial doppler waveforms for large vessel occlusion diagnosis. Circulation **136**(suppl_1) (2017)
8. Novak, V., Quispe, R.: Cerebro microvascular disease in elderly with diabetes (version 1.0.0). PhysioNet (2020)

# Effect of Promoter G-quadruplex on Gene Expression and Its Interaction with Transcription Factor

Jiahuan Liu and Xiao Sun(✉)

School of Biological Science and Medical Engineering, Southeast University, Nanjing, China
xsun@seu.edu.cn

**Abstract.** G-quadruplexes (G4s) are special nucleic acid structures widely found in human genome. They are enriched in important regions such as telomeres and promoters and are involved in important biological processes including gene transcription and DNA replication. G4s are associated with many diseases. In this study, we use high-throughput sequencing data to analyze the distribution of G4s and their effects on gene expression and to explore the synergistic effects of G4s and transcription factors (TFs) on gene expression. The analysis of the interaction between G4 and TFs provides new insights into the biological functions of G4 and offers new opportunities for G4-based disease therapy.

**Keywords:** G-quadruplex · Transcription factor · Gene expression

## 1 Introduction

The basic unit of a G4 is a G-quartet, which is a planar square structure formed by the interconnection of Hoogsteen hydrogen bonds between adjacent guanine nucleotides. Within a G-quartet, a monovalent cation occupies the central vacancy, neutralizing the electrostatic repulsion of the oxygen atoms on the guanine nucleotide. Several G-quartets stacked vertically form the G-quadruplex structure (Fig. 1), which can be formed both intramolecularly and intermolecularly.

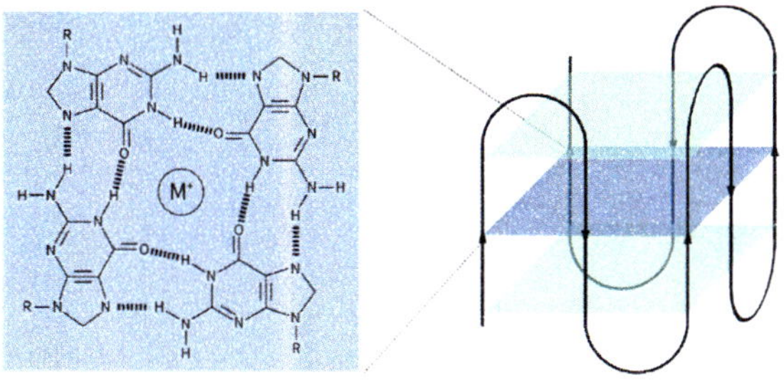

**Fig. 1.** G-quartet and G-quadruplex


G. Wang et al. (Eds.): APCMBE 2023, IFMBE Proceedings 103, pp. 55–62, 2024.
https://doi.org/10.1007/978-3-031-51455-5_7

The first high-throughput whole-genome sequencing of G4s was achieved by the G4-seq technology developed by Balasubramanian et al. [1]. The G4-seq method identified 716,310 G4s in human genome in vitro. These sequences revealed a highly non-random distribution. They were highly enriched in functional regions of the genome, especially in gene transcriptional regulatory regions.

The G4-seq technology has been improved to provide better coverage and resolution of high GC regions and was also used to build multi-species maps of G4 genomic data [2]. Comparative analysis of multi-species G4 maps revealed that in mammals such as mice, G4s were also highly enriched in promoter regions and transcription start sites.

G4s play crucial roles in various biological processes and are closely associated with numerous diseases, rendering them potential targets for drug development. For example, G4s on telomeres can disrupt the structure of the Shelterin complex, preventing telomerase from lengthening telomeric DNA properly [3]. In many tumor cells, the expression of telomerase is abnormally active, leading to extended lifespan of tumor cells. Therefore, stabilizing the G4 structure in the telomeric region could promote the apoptosis of cancer cells.

Several studies on G4s suggested that G4s enriched in the promoter region impede the binding of TFs, inhibit transcription, and need to be broken down by G4 binding proteins to promote transcription [4–6]. However, studies of the human genome have shown that G4s are enriched in regulatory regions, particularly in the promoter regions of highly expressed cancer genes [7, 8]. In a study by Spiegel et al., it was found that G4s can interact with TFs and act as a binding hub for TFs [9] instead of solely acting as transcriptional repressors. Many different TFs were recruited to the endogenous G4s with an affinity comparable to that of canonical DNA double-strand interactions. Furthermore, within a chromatin context, TFs could outcompete a G4-specific small molecule. The ability of these G4s in promoters to recruit TFs allows TFs to bind promoters more frequently, thereby facilitating the recruitment of RNA polymerase II and enhancing transcription.

This study focuses on the extensive involvement of the G4s in transcription regulation processes and their potential as valuable drug targets. It investigates the biological functions of G4s in relation to gene expression and TFs, providing new opportunities for drug design. The study demonstrates the high enrichment of G4s in promoter regions and the high correlation between G4s and up-regulation of gene expression levels, highlighting the close relationship between G4s and gene expression. By combining the sequence data of G4s and transcription factor binding sites (TFBSs) with gene expression data, this study discovers a significant enrichment of TFBSs near the G4s and proves that the interaction between G4s and TFs has a pronounced up-regulating effect on gene expression.

## 2 Materials and Methods

### 2.1 G-quadruplexes of the Human Genome

The G4 sequence data used in this study included in vitro G4-seq data [2] and in vivo G4 ChIP-seq data [9]. The in vitro G4-seq data were obtained from HEK293T cell line. The G4s were identified under both physiological $K^+$ conditions and under pyridostatin

(PDS) conditions where G4s were stabilized by PDS. In vivo G4 ChIP-seq data were obtained from K562 and HepG2 cell lines. Genome annotation information was obtained from the Gencode database [10]. TFBS data were from the ReMap database [11]. Gene expression data for K562 and HepG2 cell lines were obtained from the Cancer Cell Line Encyclopedia (CCLE) database [12], with the gene expression values reported as $\log_2(TPM+1)$.

### 2.2 Integrative Analysis of G-quadruplex, Gene Expression and Transcription Factor Binding Site

PAVIS [13] was used to analyze the number of G4s in each region and to calculate the proportion of G4s in each region. G4s sequences were shuffled 10 times across the genome to generate random sequences. For each region, the fold enrichment was calculated by dividing the actual proportion of G4s by the proportion of random sequences.

Using the genome annotation data, promoter sequences were extracted and used to identify promoter G4s. The number of G4s in the promoter of each gene was counted. The relationship between the number of promoter G4s and the gene expression was analyzed within the same cell line. Additionally, for the same gene across different cell lines, the relationship between the difference in the number of promoter G4s and the difference in the gene expression was analyzed.

The number of TFBSs at each nucleotide coordinate upstream or downstream of the G4 sequence was counted, and the statistics of TFBSs near all G4s were accumulated to obtain the relative position between G4s and TFBSs.

The sequences of genome-wide promoter TFBSs were determined, and the relationship between the number of promoter TFBSs and the gene expression was analyzed. Based on the relative position of the TFBSs with respect to G4s, the TFBSs were classified into two categories: (1) G4-relevant TFBS: TFBS sequences that overlap with G4s. (2) G4-free TFBS: TFBS that do not overlap with any G4s. The numbers of these two categories of TFBSs in promoters were analyzed in relation to the gene expression. As the gene expression data contains many genes with an expression value of zero, these genes were excluded to avoid the influence of factors like pseudogenes.

## 3 Results and Discussion

### 3.1 Distribution of G-quadruplexes Throughout the Human Genome

The analysis of the G4 sequence data from G4-seq and G4 ChIP-seq showed the distribution proportion across various regions in the genome (Table 1). The G4-seq sequences demonstrated a high proportion of distribution in introns and intergenic regions. In contrast, the G4 ChIP-seq sequences presented a higher proportion upstream of transcription start sites (1kbp) and in 5′-UTRs. In terms of experimental rationale, G4-seq as an in vitro experiment reflects less influence of intracellular environment on G4 formation than G4 ChIP-seq. The number of G4-seq sequences was much larger than G4 ChIP-seq sequences, suggesting that a substantial proportion of G4-formable sequences in vitro did not form G4 structures in vivo and that a large proportion of these sequences were present in introns and intergenic regions.

**Table 1.** Proportion of G4 sequences in different genomic regions

| Region | $K^+$ G4-seq | PDS G4-seq | HepG2 G4 ChIP-seq | K562 G4 ChIP-seq |
|---|---|---|---|---|
| Upstream of the transcription start site | 2.24% | 1.81% | 39.24% | 44.05% |
| In 5′ UTR | 0.70% | 0.71% | 11.93% | 14.71% |
| In exon | 1.10% | 1.43% | 1.50% | 2.01% |
| In intron | 41.16% | 40.87% | 25.31% | 22.01% |
| In 3′ UTR | 1.49% | 1.43% | 1.36% | 1.38% |
| Downstream of the transcription stop site | 1.08% | 1.06% | 1.09% | 1.02% |
| Other regions | 52.24% | 52.69% | 19.56% | 14.82% |

The fold enrichment results of each group of G4 sequences showed that, despite a high proportion being located in introns and intergenic regions, they exhibited minimal enrichment. However, the G4-seq sequences were more enriched upstream of transcription start sites and in 5′-UTRs (~3-fold). In both sets of G4 ChIP-seq data, the G4 sequences displayed significantly higher enrichment upstream of the transcription start sites and in 5′-UTRs to other regions (<3-fold). In K562 cell line, G4 ChIP-seq sequences were enriched 81.42-fold upstream of the transcription start sites and 68.38-fold in 5′-UTRs. In HepG2 cell line, G4 ChIP-seq sequences were enriched 69.66-fold upstream of the transcription start sites and 45.87-fold in 5′-UTRs.

The difference in the distribution patterns between G4-seq sequences and G4 ChIP-seq sequences supports the notion that G4 formation requires a relatively open chromatin environment [14]. The notable enrichment of G4s upstream of the transcription start sites and in 5′ UTRs reveals that G4s are closely associated with transcriptional regulation. Therefore, the investigation of G4s is important for understanding the regulation of gene expression.

### 3.2 Effect of Promoter G-quadruplexes on Gene Expression

The relationship between the number of promoter G4s and the gene expression was analyzed separately for the K562 and HepG2 cell lines (Fig. 2). The Spearman correlation coefficient between the number of promoter G4s and the gene expression value in K562 cell line was 0.3596522 ($P < 2.2 \times 10^{-16}$). In HepG2 cell line, the Spearman correlation coefficient was 0.2999787 ($P < 2.2 \times 10^{-16}$). The results indicate that the number of promoter G4s is positively correlated with gene expression.

The relationship between the difference in the number of promoter G4s and the difference in the gene expression for the same gene was analyzed between K562 and HepG2. The Spearman correlation coefficient between the difference in the number of promoter G4s and the difference in the gene expression was 0.3735708 ($P < 2.2 \times 10^{-16}$). These results indicate that the number of promoter G4s is positively correlated with the gene expression in both intracellular and intercellular analyses. Shen et al. used DRB and triptolide to inhibit transcription, they found that while G4 formation was not

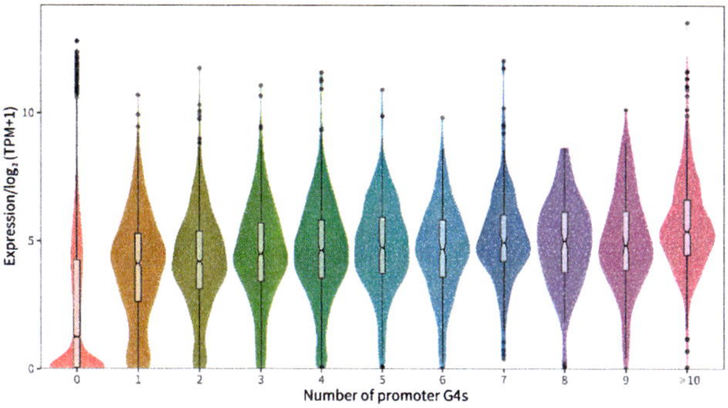


**Fig. 2.** Relationship between the number of promoter G4s and gene expression levels in K562 cell line

inhibited, chromatin compaction led to the loss of promoter G4s and RNA polymerase II [14]. This suggests that G4 formation is dependent on chromatin accessibility rather than active transcription. Additionally, G4-stabalizing ligand helped mitigate the loss of RNA polymerase II at promoters caused by chromatin compaction. These findings indicates that promoter G4s play vital role in recruit transcription elements and promote transcription.

## 3.3 Interaction of G-quadruplex and TFBS in Gene Promoter

The distribution of TFBSs around the G4-seq sequences and G4 ChIP-seq sequences was analyzed. The results (Fig. 3) revealed a peak in the center of the G4s, indicating a higher density of TFBSs on G4 sequences.

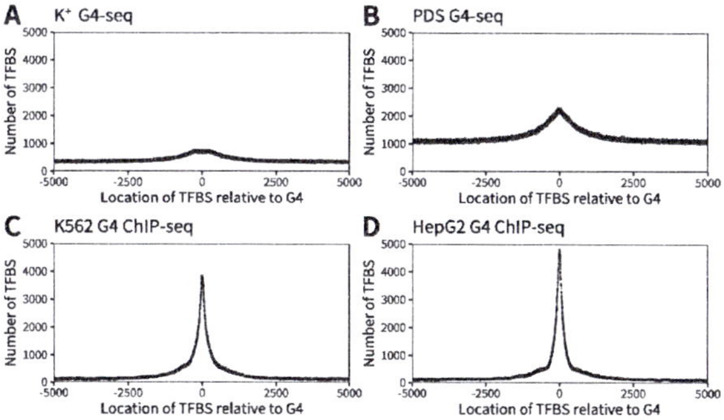


**Fig. 3.** TFBS distribution around G4s. **A** TFBS distribution around the G4-seq sequences in vitro under $K^+$ condition. **B** TFBS distribution around the G4-seq sequences in vitro under PDS condition. **C** TFBS distribution around the G4 ChIP-seq sequences in vivo in K562 cell line. **D** TFBS distribution around the G4 ChIP-seq sequences in vivo in HepG2 cell line. The x-axis indicates the position of TFBS relative to G4 and the y-axis indicates the cumulative number of TFBSs at the same position relative to G4.

PDS is a small molecule ligand that stabilizes G4s, so the overall number of G4s identified under PDS conditions is greater compared to that under $K^+$ condition, and the in vivo G4 sequences identified through G4 ChIP-seq will be less than G4-seq, resulting in a reduced count on both flanks of the distribution plots. The higher peaks in the in vivo G4 ChIP-seq results are correlated with a higher enrichment of the in vivo G4s near transcription start sites.

Further analysis in K562 cell line and HepG2 cell line revealed a positive correlation between the number of promoter TFBSs associated with G4s and the gene expression. The TFBSs were classified into G4-relevant TFBS and G4-free TFBS according to whether they overlap with G4s, and their respective relationship with gene expression was analyzed. The Spearman correlation coefficient between the number of promoter G4-relevant TFBSs (11.985%) and gene expression was 0.3761347 in the K562 cell line, and the Spearman correlation coefficient between the number of promoter G4-free TFBSs (88.015%) and gene expression was 0.3883304. In the HepG2 cell line, the Spearman correlation coefficient between the number of promoter G4-relevant TFBSs (13.830%) and gene expression was 0. 3095979 and the Spearman correlation coefficient between the number of promoter G4-free TFBSs (86.170%) and gene expression was 0. 296815.

Based on the presence or absence of G4-relevant TFBS or G4-free TFBS in the promoter, genes were classified into four categories according to the following criteria: (1) Both: genes with both G4-relevant TFBSs and G4-free TFBSs in the promoter; (2) G4-relevant TFBS only: genes with G4 relevant TFBSs and without G4-free TFBSs in the promoter; (3) G4-free TFBS only: genes without G4-relevant TFBSs and with G4-free TFBS in the promoter; (4) Neither: genes with neither G4-relevant TFBSs nor G4-free TFBSs in the promoter. Analysis of the expression of these four groups of genes (Fig. 4) revealed that in both K562 and HepG2 cell lines, the expression of the two groups with G4-relevant TFBSs in the promoter were higher compared to the two groups without G4-relevant TFBSs. Moreover, the group with both G4-relevant TFBSs and G4-free TFBSs showed the highest expression levels.

Therefore, not only does promoter G4 and promoter TFBS respectively have an activating effect on gene expression, but the interaction of these two elements leads to higher levels of gene expression.

## 4 Conclusion

This study focuses on G4, which is widely distributed in the human genome and is associated with various diseases. The objective is to explore the functions and mechanisms of G4s to provide insights for disease research and drug design. Through statistical analysis, G4s are found to be highly enriched near transcription start sites, similar to TFBSs. Additionally, a significant portion of G4s overlaps with TFBSs, and therefore their interactions and effects on gene expression were investigated. The findings reveal that the interaction between G4 and TF shows a greater expression up-regulation effect compared to TFBSs without G4 involvement. Overall, this study reveals the transcriptional activation effect of the interaction between G4 and TF, providing a new direction for the study of the biological functions of G4.

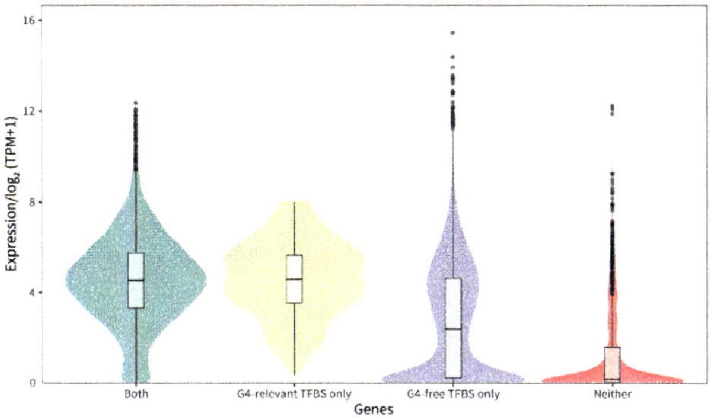


**Fig. 4.** Expression levels of different groups of genes in the K562 cell line

## References

1. Chambers, V.S., Marsico, G., Boutell, J.M., Di Antonio, M., et al.: High-throughput sequencing of DNA G-quadruplex structures in the human genome. Nat. Biotechnol. **33**, 877-+ (2015). https://doi.org/10.1038/nbt.3295
2. Marsico, G., Chambers, V.S., Sahakyan, A.B., et al.: Whole genome experimental maps of DNA G-quadruplexes in multiple species. Nucleic Acids Res. **47**, 3862–3874 (2019). https://doi.org/10.1093/nar/gkz179
3. de Lange, T.: Shelterin: the protein complex that shapes and safeguards human telomeres. Genes Dev. **19**, 2100–2110 (2005). https://doi.org/10.1101/gad.1346005
4. Thakur, R.K., Kumar, P., Halder, K., et al.: Metastases suppressor NM23-H2 interaction with G-quadruplex DNA within c-MYC promoter nuclease hypersensitive element induces c-MYC expression. Nucleic Acids Res. **37**, 172–183 (2009). https://doi.org/10.1093/nar/gkn919
5. Cogoi, S., Shchekotikhin, A.E., Xodo, L.E.: HRAS is silenced by two neighboring G-quadruplexes and activated by MAZ, a zinc-finger transcription factor with DNA unfolding property. Nucleic Acids Res. **42**, 8379-U147 (2014). https://doi.org/10.1093/nar/gku574
6. David, A.P., Pipier, A., Pascutti, F., et al.: CNBP controls transcription by unfolding DNA G-quadruplex structures. Nucleic Acids Res. **47**, 7901–7913 (2019). https://doi.org/10.1093/nar/gkz527
7. Kouzine, F., Wojtowicz, D., Baranello, L., et al.: Permanganate/S1 nuclease footprinting reveals Non-B DNA structures with regulatory potential across a mammalian genome. Cell Syst. **4**, 344–356 (2017). https://doi.org/10.1016/j.cels.2017.01.013
8. Hansel-Hertsch, R., Beraldi, D., Lensing, S.V., et al.: G-quadruplex structures mark human regulatory chromatin. Nat. Genet. **48**(10), 1267–1272 (2016). https://doi.org/10.1038/ng.3662
9. Spiegel, J., Cuesta, S.M., Adhikari, S., et al.: G-quadruplexes are transcription factor binding hubs in human chromatin. Genome Biol. **22**, 117 (2021). https://doi.org/10.1186/s13059-021-02324-z
10. Frankish, A., et al.: GENCODE reference annotation for the human and mouse genomes. Nucleic Acids Res. **47**, D766–D773 (2019). https://doi.org/10.1093/nar/gky955
11. Hammal, F., de Langen, P., et al.: ReMap 2022: a database of human, mouse, Drosophila and Arabidopsis regulatory regions from an integrative analysis of DNA-binding sequencing experiments. Nucleic Acids Res. **50**, D316–D325 (2022). https://doi.org/10.1093/nar/gkab996
12. Ghandi, M., et al.: Next-generation characterization of the cancer cell line encyclopedia. Nature **569**, 503–508 (2019). https://doi.org/10.1038/s41586-019-1186-3

13. Huang, W., Logananthara j, R., Schroeder, B., et al.: PAVIS: a tool for peak annotation and visualization. Bioinformatics **29**, 3097–3099 (2013). https://doi.org/10.1093/bioinformatics/btt520
14. Shen, J., Varshney, D., Simeone, A., et al.: Promoter G-quadruplex folding precedes transcription and is controlled by chromatin. Genome Biol. **22**, 143 (2021). https://doi.org/10.1186/s13059-021-02346-7

# Dielectric Properties for Identification of Gliomas and Normal Brain Tissues with Open-Ended Coaxial Probe

Guofang Xu[1], Xingliang Dai[2], Xuefei Yu[3], Xiang Nan[4], and Jijun Han[1](✉)

[1] Department of Medical Informatics, School of Biomedical Engineering, Anhui Medical University, Hefei, Anhui, China
hanjijun@ahmu.edu.cn

[2] Department of Neurosurgery, The First Affiliated Hospital of Anhui Medical University, Hefei, Anhui, China

[3] School of Biomedical Engineering, Southern Medical University, Guangzhou, Guangdong, China

[4] Department of Anatomy, School of Basic Medicine, Anhui Medical University, Hefei, Anhui, China

**Abstract.** The dielectric properties (DPs) of biological tissues are the crucial parameters used in discrimination between normal and malignant tissue. Open-ended coaxial probe (OCP) method has become the most common technique for measuring DPs through vector network analyzer (VNA). This technique secures its promising potential in identifying tumor for its broadband, noninvasive and easy-to-use merit. Many studies have measured the DPs of different human tissues while the technique is still hard to apply in tumor resection. One important problem is the OCP method remains unclear about the detectable tumor size. Therefore, in this work, we examine the identification size of tumor by numerical simulation from 50 MHz to 500 MHz. DPs change under tumor dimension and probe size were discussed. For probe 1 the identification size is 0.51 mm radius, for probe 2 the identification size is 0.77 mm radius, for probe 3 the identification size is 1.40 mm radius. With a better understanding of the identification limit of gliomas of the different probe, this technique is taking a step to clinical practice.

**Keywords:** Dielectric properties · Open-ended coaxial probe · Gliomas · Tumor section · Identification

## 1 Introduction

Gliomas are one of the most common malignant brain tumors [1]. According to the World Health Organization, the gliomas are classified into four grades based on their pathological and genetic properties including Grades I, II, III and IV [2, 3]. For Grades I gliomas, surgical treatment is still the most effective therapy at present, while there is currently no cure for higher-grade tumors [4]. When gliomas transform to higher grades, surgical treatment combined with chemo or radiotherapy is not effective but


G. Wang et al. (Eds.): APCMBE 2023, IFMBE Proceedings 103, pp. 63–69, 2024.
https://doi.org/10.1007/978-3-031-51455-5_8

will significantly delay progression and extend survival. To prevent gliomas undergo transformation to higher grades, the malignant tissues need to be all removed in grades I gliomas surgical resection. This requires the surgeon have a real-time knowledge of the tissue types for surgical resection. Traditional histopathological techniques have capability of a tissue identification while the routine procedure involves rapid freezing, cutting, staining and microscopic assessing by a skilled pathologist. Nevertheless, these septs for intraoperative identification are time consuming, leading to a high surgical risk.

In recent years, a technique which is promising for intraoperative real-time on-site tissue identification based on dielectric properties (DPs) was rapidly developed. The underlying theory is that the DPs exhibit significant differences between tumors and normal tissues. Therefore, the measured DPs could use to distinguish the tissue types. Open-ended coaxial probe (OCP) method is the most widely used in DPs measurement which is broadband, noninvasive and easy-to-use. In this method, vector network analyzer (VNA) transmits an incident electromagnetic signal into tissues and received a reflective signal by the open-ended coaxial probe. DPs can be retrieved with reflection coefficients according to the transmission line theory and then the obtained DPs are used for identification.

A number of studies measured different human tissue such as skin [5], colon epithelium [6], breast [7], thyroid nodules [8], prostatic [9] and so on, which proved the remarkable differences of DPs values between normal and malignant tissue. Although many investigations have measured DPs of various tissues over a wide frequency range, the DPs of gliomas are rarely reported. In the research by Lu et al., the DPs of human gliomas were measured from five patients at frequencies of 5–500 MHz and the conclusion is that the DPs of gliomas were 30% higher than the surrounding tissues [10].

Although the above studied have showed the big DPs differences between normal and malignant tissues and demonstrates the ability of intraoperative tissue identification, this method is too early to be used in a tumor resection surgery. The question is that how small the tumor could be detected and then identified. It is crucial because probes need be selected according to the estimated tumor size and the surgeons should be informed about the identifying limitation of DPs method.

In this work, the identification sizes of gliomas are investigated through numerical simulations across the range of 50–500 MHz. Three configuration probes were chosen to study the identification size and DPs change with tumor size and probe were exported. Besides, we discussed the multiple crucial parameters of identification sizes. This study focused on simulation data in order to have a controlled on the model settings and the DPs of tissues.

## 2 Material and Methods

To investigate the identification size of gliomas through OCP, we built a numerically computable gliomas dielectric model which was assigned the corresponding DPs values. Then, we calculated DPs based on the simulation data through OCP reconstruction algorithm. We examined a series of gliomas radius with three configuration probes and employ the Mann-Whitney U test to determine the minimal measurable radius, i.e., identification size.

### 2.1 Model Building

Human brain is a complex organ in structure and electromagnetic behavior. This complexity is a major challenge for establishing an accurate numerical model for simulating the interaction of electromagnetic fields with the gliomas. Therefore, a reasonable and feasible simulation model should be established for electromagnetic calculation. Here, we built the model with normal brain and gliomas as shown in Fig. 1. In the model, the normal brain tissue is simplified as a cylindrical-shaped geometry with radius of 20 mm and height of 20 mm. We simplified the gliomas as a hemisphere-shaped model, the parameter Tr in Fig. 1 determines the size of tumor which the large Tr indicates a large tumor size, and vice versa. In this work, Tr was examined from 0.1 mm to 3 mm with an interval of 0.1 mm to mimic the growth of tumor. This simplification does not compromise the accuracy of the calculation, because only the tissue closed to probe has a contribution to the measured DPs.

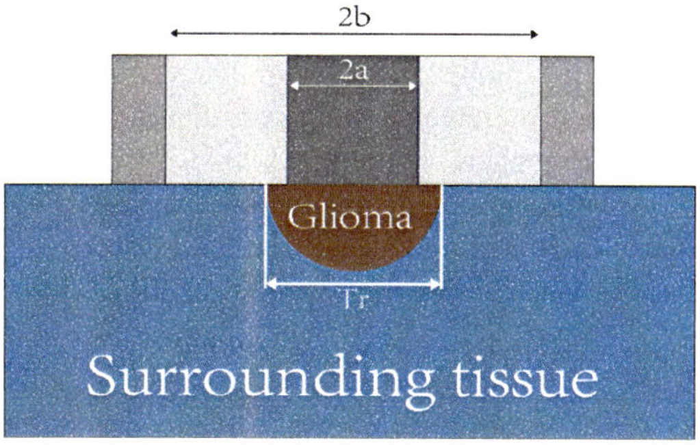


**Fig. 1.** Simulation model

To simulate the OCP measurement, the frequency-depended DPs values should be assigned to the corresponding tissue. According to the research by Lu et al., we used the interpolation method to assigned the DPs of gliomas and normal brain [10].

When taking measured in simulations, electromagnetic signals are transmitted by an open-ended coaxial probe and reflexes in the tissue which resulting reflection coefficient is received by probe. The DPs was calculated by reflection coefficient and characteristic parameters of the probe with a DPs reconstruction algorithm.

The simulations were performed within the magnetic resonance frequency band. Due to the frequency-depended property of DPs, the values of the current examined frequency are entered into the COMSOL through interpolation method.

### 2.2 Probe Setting

In this study, three configuration probes are examined as summarized in Table 1. These probes are chosen because different configuration probes have different sensing radii and sensing depths as identification size are expected to be impacted [11, 12]. We examined three commercially available probes (UT-047-M17, RG-405, RG-402) in following simulation. The open-ended port of the probe was connected to model, while another port was the feed point for providing the electromagnetic signal source.

**Table 1.** The configurations of three configuration probe

| Probe | Number | Center Conductor Diam 2a. (mm) | Insulator Outer Diam 2b. (mm) | Outer Coax Diam. (mm) |
|---|---|---|---|---|
| UT-047-M17 | Probe 1 | 0.32 | 0.94 | 1.19 |
| RG405 | Probe 2 | 0.57 | 1.68 | 2.18 |
| RG402 | Probe 3 | 1.02 | 2.99 | 3.58 |

### 2.3 OCP Reconstruction Algorithm

In simulation, the propagating mode of electromagnetic signal is transverse electromagnetic (TEM) mode which the electric field is radial and the magnetic field encircles the center conductor everywhere inside the coaxial probe except near the open tip where fringing occurs due to the abrupt change in impedance. Reflection would occur on medium/probe interface due to the impedance difference between the probe and medium. Hence, the DPs can be reconstructed by measuring reflection coefficient.

### 2.4 Data Analysis

To obtain the identification size, Mann-Whitney U test was employed to analyze data difference in this research. We programmed this test based on the rank sum test function in MATLAB with the 0.01 significance level (alpha). The inputs are the measured DPs and the literature DPs; and the p-value and h-value are outputs. The p-value of Mann-Whitney U test indicates the difference between the measured values and literature values. If the null hypothesis is rejected, the $h = 1$ is returned, while $h = 0$ means a failure to reject the null hypothesis.

Then, the DPs were exported with different tumor size at 253 MHz and the change of DPs were compared when Tr is 0.6 mm with three configuration probes.

## 3 Results

As mentioned above, it is determined that the identification size of gliomas is that the p values are both smaller than 0.01 for the measured DPs compared with gliomas. By testing the h value for each change of tumor size, the identification sizes had been determined in Table 2. If the tumor size is larger than the sizes in Table 2, then tumor could be identified through OCP.

In Fig. 2, the curves show that the DPs change with increasing tumor radius for three probes at 253 MHz.

The DPs of tumor are compared when tumor radius is 0.6 mm in Fig. 3 as follows.

**Table 2.** The identification sizes of three probes

| Shape | Probe1 | Probe2 | Probe3 |
|---|---|---|---|
| Hemisphere | R0.51 | R0.77 | R1.4 |

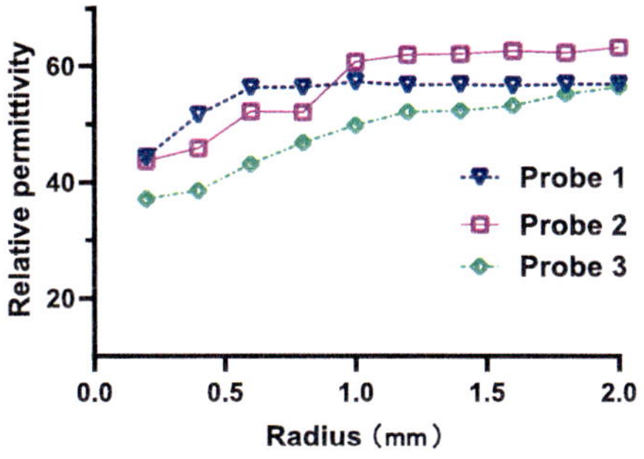


(a)

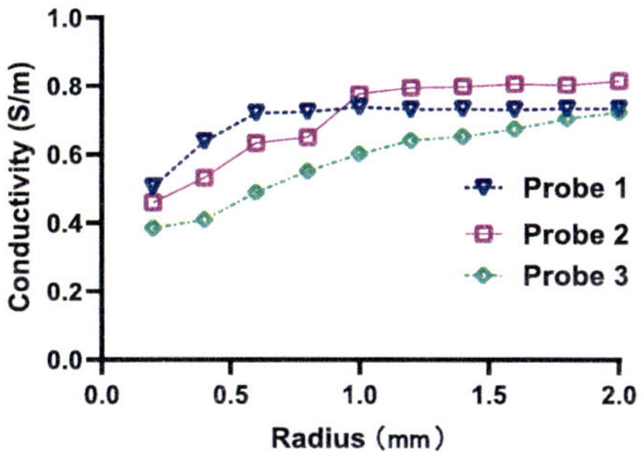


(b)

**Fig. 2.** Photographs of the: **a** relative permittivity and **b** conductivity change with tumor radius

# 4 Discussion

In this section, several factors that affect the identification size are analyzed.

From Fig. 2, we found that when tumor radius increases from 0.2 mm to 2.0 mm, the DPs increase and then gradually stabilize. It can be seen from the trend of the curve that increasing radius of cancer target contributes more to the measured DPs within a certain radius, and when the radius of cancer target reaches a certain value, the DPs have little change.

In Fig. 3, it can be seen that probe size has a greater impact on identification size. Smaller size probe of three probes has smaller identification size when detected gliomas. The conclusion is that the smaller size probe is easier to identify tumor among the three probes.

However, this study also has some limitations. The simulation model is simplified and glioma is established as a hemisphere, but the reality is more complex. At the same

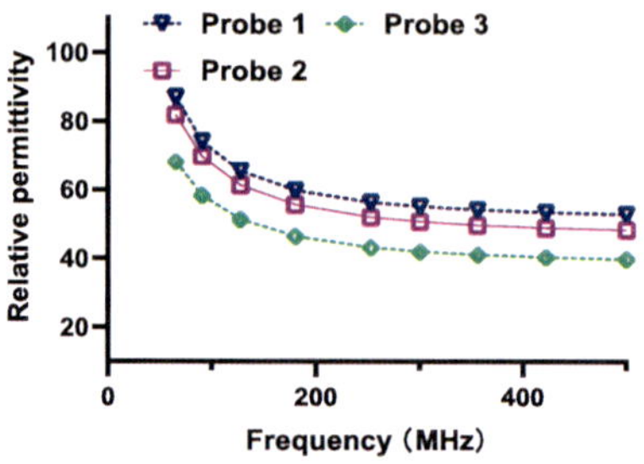


(a)

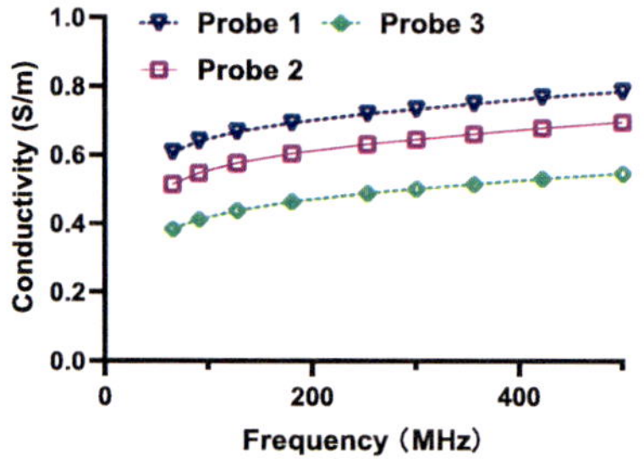


(b)

**Fig. 3.** Photographs of the: **a** relative permittivity and **b** conductivity change with probe configuration

time, to better control the size of model and assigned the DPs to corresponding tissues, we used the simulation to investigated the identification size and ignored the effect of noise which is inevitable in actual measurement.

To solve the above limitations, we will rebuild the model, making the tumor shape closer to reality through the random function and perform multiple simulation experiments. Furthermore, the database of normal tissue and gliomas would be created for deeper research through actual measurement in the hospital. With the database, we could carry out further research that is to determine how large the tissue part is malignant in the normal tissue, i.e., the volume of the tumor. Knowing the volume of the tumor will make a great progress in the treatment of cancer. This study means taking the OCP approach one step closer in tumor resection surgery.

## 5 Conclusion

In this study, we put emphasis on investigating identification size of three configuration probes. The influencing factors are also discussed. First, we conclude that the identification size of three configuration probes. For probe 1 the identification size is 0.51 mm radius, for probe 2 the identification size is 0.77 mm radius, for probe 3 the identification size is 1.40 mm radius. The crucial factors, the size of the probe and the tumor, that can affect the DPs measurements are discussed. In summary, the identification size of gliomas and crucial factors are investigated. Thus, further research would put emphasis on detecting tumor size. This work provides a discussion with how large the tumor could be identified and the influencing factors, it is crucial for quantify tumor in the detection range of the probe. We expect to contribute more useful insights in tumor resection.

## References

1. Ricard, D., Idbaih, A., Ducray, F., et al.: Primary brain tumours in adults. The Lancet **379**(9830), 1984–1996 (2012)
2. Louis, D.N., Ohgaki, H., Wiestler, O.D., et al.: The 2007 WHO classification of tumours of the central nervous system. Acta Neuropathol. **114**, 97–109 (2007)
3. Louis, D.N., Perry, A., Reifenberger, G., et al.: The 2016 World Health Organization classification of tumors of the central nervous system: a summary. Acta Neuropathol. **131**, 803–820 (2016)
4. Alis, D., Bagcilar, O., Senli, Y., et al.: The diagnostic value of quantitative texture analysis of conventional MRI sequences using artificial neural networks in grading gliomas. Clin. Radiol. **75**(5), 351–357 (2020)
5. Mayrovitz, H., Gildenberg, S., Spagna, P., et al.: Characterizing the tissue dielectric constant of skin basal cell cancer lesions. Skin Res. Technol. **24**(4), 686–691 (2018)
6. Guardiola, M., Buitrago, S., Fernández-Esparrach, G., et al.: Dielectric properties of colon polyps, cancer, and normal mucosa: Ex vivo measurements from 0.5 to 20 GHz. Med. Phys. **45**(8), 3768–3782 (2018)
7. Mayrovitz, H.N., Weingrad, D.N.: tissue dielectric constant differentials between malignant and benign breast tumors. Clin. Breast Cancer (2022)
8. Huang, S., Cai, W., Han, S., et al.: Differences in the dielectric properties of various benign and malignant thyroid nodules. Med. Phys. **48**(2), 760–769 (2021)
9. Halter R.J., Schned, A., Heaney, J., et al.: Electrical properties of prostatic tissues: I. Single frequency admittivity properties. J. Urology **182**(4), 1600–1607 (2009)
10. Lu, Y., Li, B., Xu, J., et al.: Dielectric properties of human glioma and surrounding tissue. Int. J. Hyperth. **8**(6), 755–760 (1992)
11. Meaney, P.M., Gregory, A.P., Seppälä, J., et al.: Open-ended coaxial dielectric probe effective penetration depth determination. IEEE Trans. Microwave Theory Techniq. **64**(3), 915–923 (2016)
12. Li, Z., Deng, G., Li, Z., et al.: A large-scale measurement of dielectric properties of normal and malignant colorectal tissues obtained from cancer surgeries at Larmor frequencies. Med. Phys. **43**(11), 5991–5997 (2016)

# Research on GMI Probe Performance in Biomagnetic Field Range in Unshielded Environments

Wenzhu Wu[1,2] and Mingxin Qin[1(✉)]

[1] Department of Electronic Engineering, Army Medical University, Chongqing, China
qmingxin@tmmu.edu.cn
[2] Chongqing Medical and Pharmaceutical College, Chongqing, China

**Abstract.** A gradient probe based on the Giant Magneto-Impedance (GMI) effect using the CoFeSiB glass-covered amorphous microwires. We set up a weak magnetic experiment system to test the sensitivity and linearity of the GMI probe in a magnetic field with a frequency of 1–100 Hz and an amplitude of 0–100 pT. The results show that the GMI gradient probe can detect a magnetic field signal as low as 12 pT in unshielded environments. And the GMI gradient probe has good linearity in both amplitude and frequency domain. A signal segmentation superposition process is proposed which can enhance the signal and reduce the random interference. This study is a foundation for the development of biomagnetic sensors, and provides a possibility for non-contact biomagnetic field measurement, diagnosis and analysis in unshielded environments.

**Keywords:** GMI effect · Gradient probe · Biomagnetic field · Unshielded environments

## 1 Introduction

Magnetic sensors have the advantages of being non-contact and non-destructive, and their performance is virtually unaffected by environmental factors such as dust, oil and moisture, as well as non-magnetic occlusions such as dust, skin and clothing [1]. Therefore, magnetic sensors have been used in a wide range of applications such as consumer electronics, navigation, aerospace as well as biomedical fields [2].

The detection of biomagnetic fields has always been a challenge because the amplitude of biomagnetic fields is very small, generally from tens of femrotesla ($10^{-15}$ T) to hundreds of picotesla ($10^{-12}$ T), which is much smaller than the magnetic fields in the environment [3]. For biomagnetic signal measurements, the Superconducting Quantum Interference Device (SQUID) is always the first choice as it is capable of measuring magnetic fields down to several fT ($10^{-15}$ T) [4]. However, the high cost and complexity of SQUIDs make them difficult to commercialize. On the other hand, magnetic sensors such as Optical Pump Magnetometers (OPMs) [5], fluxgate sensors [6], Giant Magneto-Resistance (GMR) sensors [7], and Giant Magneto-Impedance (GMI) sensors


G. Wang et al. (Eds.): APCMBE 2023, IFMBE Proceedings 103, pp. 70–78, 2024.
https://doi.org/10.1007/978-3-031-51455-5_9

[8, 9] are compact, highly sensitive, and can be easily integrated into the complementary metal-oxide-semiconductor (CMOS) fabrication process [10].

A GMI magnetic sensor with a magnetic field sensitivity at pT ($10^{-12}$ T) level can be used for biomagnetic field measurement, such as magnetocardiography (MCG) and magnetoencephalography (MEG) α-wave detection [11, 12]. It has the advantages of small probe size, high sensitivity, fast response time and low power consumption. In addition, GMI sensor is an AC-powered magnetic sensor, which facilitates the subsequent processing of signal modulation and demodulation, filtering, oscillation and resonance [13]. In this study, we construct a GMI gradient probe and a weak magnetic experiment system. We tested the GMI probe in a biomagnetic field range with a frequency of 1–100 Hz and an amplitude of 0–100 pT.

## 2 Theoretical Analysis of the GMI Effect

When an amorphous wire is excited with a certain frequency of alternating current, its impedance changes sensitively with a small external magnetic field, which is called the giant magneto-impedance (GMI) effect. The GMI effect in amorphous wires has been explained as the skin effect, which is characterized by the skin depth [14]:

$$\delta = \sqrt{\frac{2\rho}{\omega\mu(H_{ex})}} \tag{1}$$

where $\rho$ (130 $\mu\Omega\cdot$cm) is the resistivity of the amorphous wire, $\omega$ the angular frequency of the applied current, $\mu$ the complex magnetic permeability, $H_{ex}$ the external static magnetic field.

At a relatively high frequency ($\omega \gg 2\rho/\mu a^2$), when the penetration depth reaches the order of the thickness of the magnetic material ($\delta \ll a$), a strong skin effect occurs, the expression for the impedance Z can be expressed as [11]:

$$Z = \frac{(1+j)aR_{dc}\sqrt{\omega\mu(H_{ex})}}{2\sqrt{2\rho}} \tag{2}$$

where $R_{dc} = \frac{\rho l}{\pi a^2}$ is DC resistance of the amorphous wire, $l$ the wire length, a radius of the wire, δ the skin depth.

The sensitivity of the magneto-impedance (Z) is:

$$\frac{\partial|Z|}{\partial H_{ex}} = \frac{aR_{dc}\sqrt{\omega}}{4\rho}\cdot\frac{1}{\sqrt{\mu}}\cdot\frac{\partial\mu}{\partial H_{ex}} = A\frac{\mu^{-1/2}\partial\mu}{\partial H_{ex}} \tag{3}$$

where $A = \frac{\sqrt{\rho\omega}}{4\pi a}l$, and it suggests that the sensitivity of a GMI sensor is correlated to the value of $l/a$ and the value of $\omega$, which would affect the complex magnetic permeability ($\mu$).

# 3 GMI Probe Test

## 3.1 GMI Probe

The structure of a GMI sensor probe is shown in Fig. 1, which consists of an amorphous wire, a pick-up coil, and a drive circuit. We used a CoFeSiB glass-covered amorphous microwire with a diameter of 25 μm and a length of 10 mm, while a 500-turn enameled copper wire with a diameter of 20 μm wounding on the amorphous microwire as the pick-up coil. To induce a strong skin effect, we used the frequency of 500 kHz pulse with a voltage peak-to-peak value of 2 V as the excitation current.

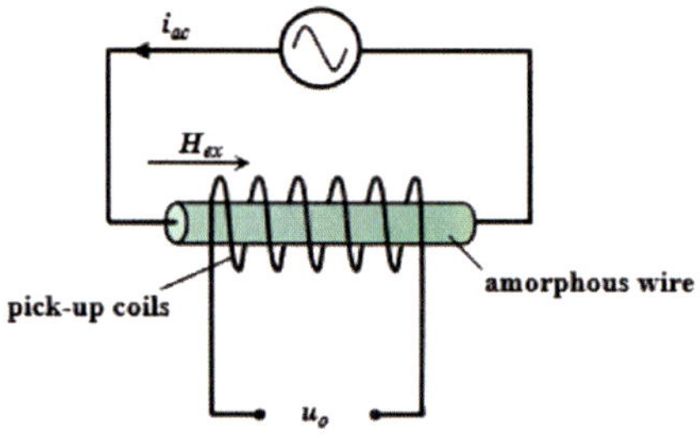


**Fig. 1.** Structure of a single GMI sensor probe

To further reduce the background noise, a gradient probe design is developed, as shown in Fig. 2. The distance between the two pick up coils is 3 cm, and the output voltage from two pick up coils is $u_O = u_{o1} - u_{o2}$.

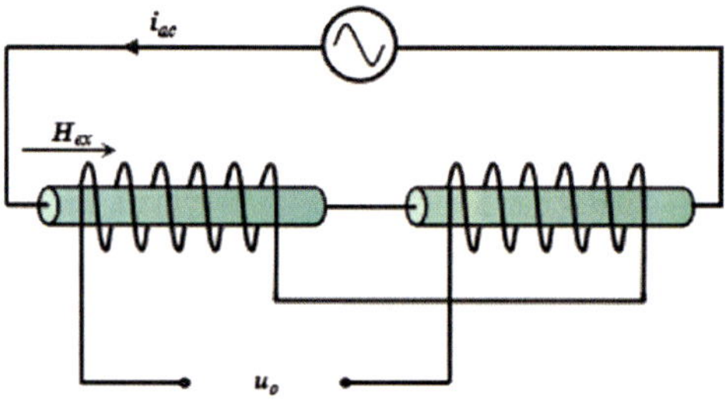


**Fig. 2.** Structure of a gradient GMI sensor probe.

## 3.2 Probe Experiments

The purpose of the experiments is to test the sensitivity and linearity of the GMI probe in a magnetic field with a frequency of 1–100 Hz and an amplitude of 0–100 pT. For biomagnetic signals such as MCG and MEG, most of their frequencies and amplitudes are in this range. We constructed a weak magnetic experimental system to test the sensitivity of the sensor probe, the schematic diagram is shown in Fig. 3a. Unit 1 acts as the sensing probe and unit 2 is the reference probe. We constructed a circuit to generate loop current that induces a weak magnetic field. The magnitude of the ambient magnetic field can be adjusted by changing the magnitude of the loop current. All experiments were conducted in an unshielded environment.

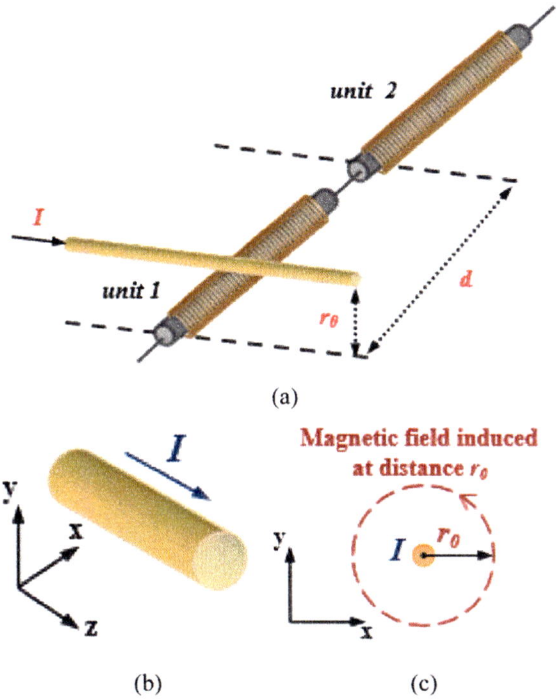


**Fig. 3.** **a** Schematic diagram of the experiment system. **b** Top/Side view and **c** front view of the direction magnetic field wrapping the wire at distance r0 from the wire.

With a current of $I$ flows in a long enough wire, it generates a magnetic field; the direction of the magnetic field induced around the wire satisfies Ampere's Law, as shown in Fig. 3b, c. The magnitude of magnetic induction intensity at distance $r_0$ is:

$$B = \frac{\mu_0 I}{2\pi r_0} \tag{4}$$

where $\mu_0 = 4\pi \times 10^{-7} \mathrm{T} \cdot \mathrm{m/A}$ is vacuum magnetic permeability, $r_0$ distance from test lead to a probe, $I$ test lead circuit current. For a gradient probe, the magnetic induction intensity between the two units is:

$$B = \frac{\mu_0 I}{2\pi r_0} - \frac{\mu_0 I}{2\pi r_1} \tag{5}$$

$$r_1 = \sqrt{{r_0}^2 + d^2} \tag{6}$$

where $d$ is the distance between two pick-up coils.

The NIcDAQ 9255, a high-precision 24-bit ADC is used as the analog-to-digital converter with a sampling rate of 500 Hz. LabVIEW is used for data acquisition, with each data acquisition lasting 20 s, and the data is further processed by filtering and time-frequency analysis in MATLAB.

### 3.3 Results

**Probe sensitivity**. When the current of 37 Hz and 0.88 μA (RMS value) is applied to the circuit according to Eqs. (5) and (6), the magnetic induction intensity between the two units is about 12 pT. This signal is the minimum magnetic induction intensity that can be detected, and the time and frequency domain of the signal are shown in Fig. 4. It is worth noting that the spike at 37 Hz is the detected signal, while the spike at 23 Hz is caused by environmental noise, which can be eliminated with a signal segmentation overlay, which we will discuss in part 3 of this section.

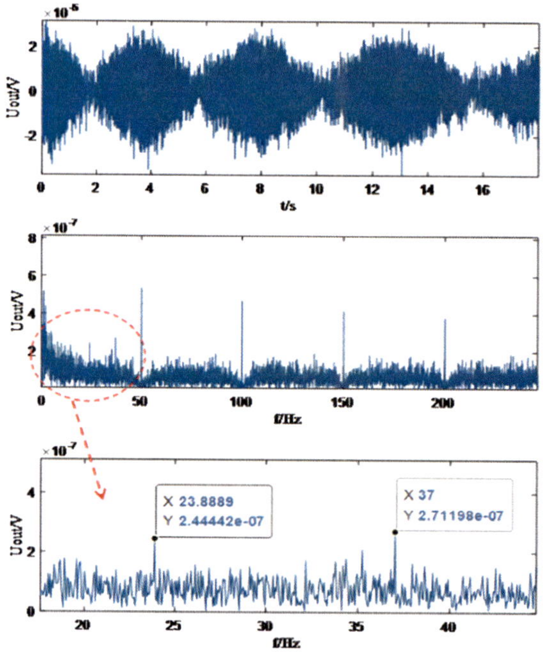


**Fig. 4.** The time and frequency domain of the probe output signal (B ≈ 12 pT, 37 Hz).

**Linearity**. Biomagnetic signal like (MEG and MCG) is low frequency and extremely weak. To test the linearity, we applied 37 Hz magnetic induction intensity (B) from 12 pT to 100 pT. And 100 pT peak to peak alternating magnetic field with the frequency from 9 to 200 Hz. Each signal was sampled for 20 s, and the linearity relationship diagram between output voltage and magnetic induction is shown in Fig. 5.

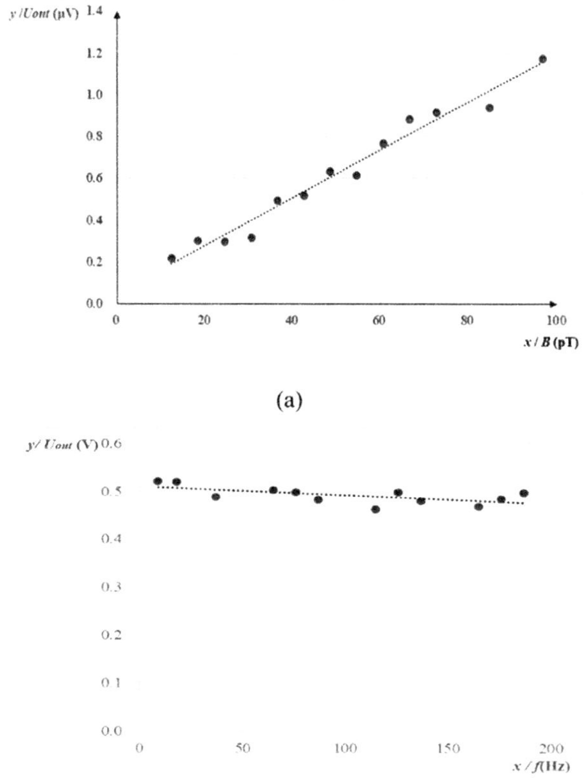


(a)

(b)

**Fig. 5.** **a** Linearity diagram of output voltage and magnetic amplitude. **b** Linearity diagram of output voltage and magnetic frequency.

**Signal Segmentation Superimposition.** Biological signals must be analyzed in both the time and frequency domain, for example, the magnetic field induced by a brainstem evoked potential, the waveform of which must be displayed. However, biomagnetic signals are extremely small and are easily drowned by noise, as shown in Fig. 4. Therefore, we applied a segmented superposition overlay to enhance the signal and reduce the noise.

First, the signal is segmented by a certain time interval, in the experiment we segmented by 1 s time interval. Then, the segmented signals are superimposed, and the stable signal becomes larger as the superimposition times increase, but the superimposed random noise does not change much or even becomes smaller after the process. As shown in Fig. 6, after 18 times of superposition, the 37 Hz signal can be seen in the time domain, at the same time, the interference at 23.889 Hz (shown in Fig. 4) is eliminated.

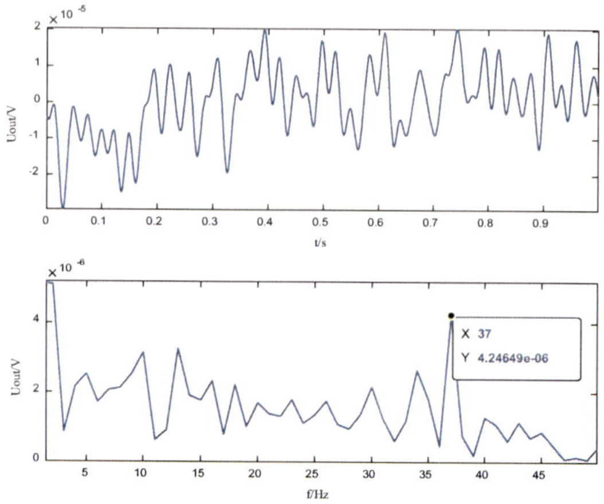


**Fig. 6.** The time and frequency domain of signal (B ≈ 12 pT, 37 Hz) after segmentation superimposition (times of superposition N = 18).

## 4 Conclusions and Discussions

The results show, the GMI gradient probe can detect a magnetic field signal as low as 12 pT in an unshielded environment. And the GMI gradient probe has good linearity in both amplitude and frequency in the biomagnetic field range. And the signal segmentation superimposition process can help to enhance the signal and reduce the background noises. The probe is a foundation for the development of biomagnetic sensors, the signal-to-noise ratio (SNR) must be further improved.

### 4.1 Noise

The sensitivity of the probe is determined by the noise the system made. A theoretical minimum magnetic noise spectral density of the amorphous wire is presented as follows [14]:

$$\beta = \sqrt{\frac{2\alpha k_B T}{\gamma M_s \pi D l}} \tag{7}$$

where $T$ is the temperature, $\alpha$ the magnetic damping constant, $k_B$ the Boltzmann constant, $\gamma$ the gyromagnetic ratio, and $M_s$ the saturation magnetization, $D$ and $\ell$ are the diameter and the length of the amorphous wire.

According to formula (7), at room temperature (20 °C), a Co-rich amorphous wire with length of 10 mm and diameter of 25 μm, the noise spectral density of which is about 10 fT. However in our tests, the background noises is much larger than the theoretical value, in the frequency band below 5 Hz, the noise can reach 30 pT. The possible causes of high background noise may be related to the interference generated by the signal generator connected to the industrial frequency power supply, or the working instrumentation in the laboratory. On the other side the noise is also produced by the probe, including the noise from deformation of the amorphous wire interface during welding, and the mismatch between the two units.

### 4.2 Sensitivity

The two parameters that affect the sensitivity are related to: $l/a$ and $\omega$. Theoretically, the value of length-to-radius ($l/a$) is the higher the better, but the length $l$ affects the size of the sensor, while the radius a is limited by the fabrication process of the amorphous filament material, and a small radius will lead to a higher noise spectral density ($\beta$), so the value of $l/a$ needs to be designed according to the application requirements. The frequency of the stimulation current ($\omega$) at the output is complex, to ensure a deep skin effect, a high frequency is needed, meanwhile, the frequency will affect $\mu$ and thus change the probe sensitivity. Therefore, it is necessary to test the probe to find the appropriate excitation frequency to achieve higher sensitivity.

**Acknowledgment.** Funding Information: The work was supported by National Natural Science Foundation of China (51977214).

## References

1. Lenz, J.: A review of magnetic sensors. Proc. IEEE **78**(6), 973–989 (1990)
2. Lenz, J., Edelstein, S.: Magnetic sensors and their applications. IEEE Sens. J. **6**(3), 631–649 (2006)
3. Speckmann, E.J.: Introduction of the neurophysiological basis of the EEG and DC potentials. In: Electroencephalography: Basic Principles, Clinical Applications, and Related Fields, pp. 15–26 (1993)
4. Kleiner, R., Koelle, D., Ludwig, F., Clarke, J.: Superconducting quantum interference devices. State Art Appl. **92**(10), 1534–1548 (2004)
5. Boto, E., Holmes, N., Leggett, J., et al.: Moving magnetoencephalography towards real-world applications with a wearable system. Nature **555**(7698), 657–661 (2018)
6. Chong, L., Jian, L., Zhen, Y., Tao, W., Yong, Z.: A low power micro fluxgate sensor with improved magnetic core. Microsyst. Technol. **19**, 591–598 (2013)
7. Huimin, S., Liang, H., Xin, F.: Integrated giant magnetoresistance technology for approachable weak biomagnetic signal detections. Sensors (Basel) **18**(1), 148 (2018)
8. Manh, H.P., Hua, X.P.: Giant Magnetoimpedance materials: fundamentals and applications. Prog. Mater. Sci. **53**(2), 323–420 (2008)
9. Uchiyama, T., Nakayama, S., Mohri, K., Bushida, K.: Biomagnetic field detection using very high sensitivity magnetoimpedance sensors for medical applications. Physica Status Solidi(A) **206**(4), 639–643 (2009)
10. Mohammed, A.K., Jian, S., Bodong, L., Aliexander, P., Jurgen, K.: Magnetic sensors—A review and recent technologies. Eng. Res. Express **3**, 022005 (2021)
11. Mohri, K., Uchiyama, T., Panina, L.V., Yamamoto, M., Bushida, K.: Recent advances of amorphous wire CMOS IC magneto-impedance sensors: innovative high-performance micromagnetic sensor chip. J. Sens. **2015**, 1–8 (2015)
12. Mohri, K., Honkura, Y., Panina, L.V., Uchiyama, T.: Super MI sensor: recent advances of amorphous wire and CMOS-IC magneto-impedance sensor. J. Nanosci. Nanotechnol. **12**(9), 7491–7495 (2012)

13. Xu, M., Han, C., Lu, H., Xiao, J., Tang, J., Zhou, Z.: The design of the biomagnetic field sensor without magnetic shielding. Int. J. Humanoid Rob. **16**(4), 87–10 (2019)
14. Panina, L.V., Mohri, K.: Magneto-impedance effect in amorphous wires. Appl. Phys. Lett. **65**(9), 1189–1191 (1994)

# A Single-Channel EEG Automatic Artifact Rejection Framework Based on Hybrid Approach

Xianbiao Zhong, Feilian Ren, Chengda Tong, Ying Wang, and Xingqun Zhao(✉)

School of Biological Science and Medical Engineering, Southeast University, Nanjing, China
ndt@seu.edu.cn

**Abstract.** Dealing with the physiological artifacts is a challenge in the period of recording electroencephalography (EEG), especially with a restricted number of channels. EEG contaminated with the Electromyogram (EMG) and electrooculogram (EOG) can affect the subsequent analysis. In order to more effectively reject the artifacts and not degrade the quality of the recorded EEG signals, a new framework with signal decomposed technology and blind source separation (BSS) is proposed. First, the framework detects and classifies EMG and EOG artifacts, and then uses CEEMDAN-CCA and SSA-SOBI methods to remove artifacts for EMG and EOG signals respectively. The method of removing the artifacts of EOG combines fuzzy entropy to distinguish the components of EOG. The methods are evaluated on semi-simulated dataset. Almost all the artifact fragments can be detected and type of the artifacts can be classified correctly. The two denoising algorithms achieve high correlation with the original signal under a low SNR condition. The results demonstrate the superior performance in single-channel EEG automatic artifact rejection.

**Keywords:** Automatic artifact rejection · Blind source separation · Single-channel EEG

## 1 Introduction

Electroencephalogram (EEG) is easily contaminated with physiological artifacts such as ElectroOlfactoGram (EOG) and Electromyogram (EMG) artifacts due to its weak amplitude, thus affecting the analysis of brain activity [1]. For single-channel artifact removal, a hybrid method combining with signal decomposition and blind source separation (BSS) has generally been used, such as WT-ICA [2], EEMD-CCA [3], etc. With the increase of wearable applications in recent years, the artifact suppression of single-channel or few channels of EEG has attracted many researchers' attention.

However, conventional hybrid methods can only solve single type of artifacts and lack of comparison with other algorithms for artifact removal. Besides, most algorithms need to manually identify artifacts. In this paper, a single-channel EEG automatic artifact rejection framework is proposed to detect and remove the EOG and EMG artifacts. In


G. Wang et al. (Eds.): APCMBE 2023, IFMBE Proceedings 103, pp. 79–86, 2024.
https://doi.org/10.1007/978-3-031-51455-5_10

the framework, an algorithm that can automatically identify artifacts and type classification is proposed and verified. To remove the EMG artifacts. The Complete Ensemble Empirical Mode Decomposed With Adaptive Noise [4] (CEEMDAN) combined with Canonical Correlation Analysis (CCA) is applied to remove the EMG artifacts. The Singular Spectrum Analysis (SSA) combined with Second Order Blind Identification (SOBI) and Fuzzy Entropy is applied to remove the EOG artifacts. The proposed algorithm is verified on the semi-simulated dataset, suggesting the capacity to identify and remove the artifacts.

## 2 Method

### 2.1 CEEMDAN-CCA

CEEMDAN is improved on the basis of EMD and solve the mixed model problem through adaptively adding the IMF component with auxiliary noise after EEMD decomposition into the signal to be decomposed. CEEMDAN can automatically decompose the signals into empirical mode components IMF according to the time scale characteristics of the signals, without setting any basis function in advance. CCA is a strong algorithm of BSS to remove EMG artifacts since the autocorrelation coefficient of EMG signal is very low compared with EEG signal.

In the paper, the CEEMDAN-CCA is implemented in 3 steps. First, the original signal is decomposed into a series of IMFs through CEEMDAN. Then input all the obtained IMFs into CCA. CCA takes the input IMFs and the unit delay version of IMFs as canonical correlation variables. It is further decomposed into a series of source component signals, sorted according to the autocorrelation coefficient. Step3 is to set the autocorrelation threshold coefficient, set the components whose autocorrelation coefficient is less than the threshold value to zero, and then multiply the inverse matrix of the decomposition matrix to obtain the reconstructed signal.

### 2.2 SSA-SOBI with Fuzzy Entropy

In the paper, SSA-SOBI is used to remove the EOG artifacts, which is also a decomposition component reconstruction algorithm. Singular spectrum analysis (SSA) is another powerful method for studying nonlinear time series data, which has emerged in recent years. It includes the following four steps: Embedding, SVD, Group and Reconstruct.

SOBI is a blind source separation algorithm based on independent component analysis. This algorithm rely on second-order statistics, and has faster operation speed and stability compared with the traditional ICA method.

The SSA-SOBI denoising process is similar to CEEMDAN-CCA, but the difference is that the IC component decomposed by SOBI needs to be distinguished. In order to realize automatic discrimination, Fuzzy entropy criterion is introduced here, which is a feature that can more reflect the complexity of the signal than the sample entropy.

### 2.3 The Detection and Denoise Framework

The Detection and Denoise Framework is shown as Fig. 1. The algorithm is divided into two parts: Detection Block and Denoise Block, including 4 steps:

- Step 1: Estimate the $STD_{all}$ of the original signals. The signal is uniformly calculated by taking N fragments and calculating the standard deviation $(std_i \ldots std_N)$, the fragments with excessive variance are excluded, and the remaining fragments are averaged as $STD_{all}$.
- Step 2: Traverse the sequence with 2s as the sliding window and 0.5s as the step size, and calculate the STD of each window.
- Step 3: Merge all adjacent fragments that meet condition $> N * STD_{all}$.
- Step 4: Determine the type of artifact by the Fuzzy Entropy and the canonical correlation coefficient.

In the Denoise Block, the CEEMDAN-CCA and SSA-SOBI combined with Fuzzy entropy is adopted to remove the EMG and EOG artifacts.

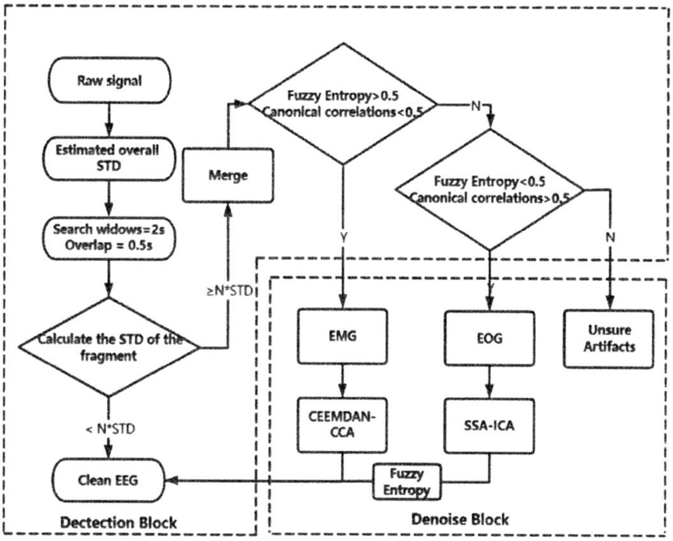


**Fig. 1.** The Detection and Denoise Framework

### 2.4 Data and Evaluation

The simulation and verification of the above algorithms are carried out on semi-simulated data sets. The EEGdenoiseNet dataset and the DEAP database are mainly used [5, 6]. The contaminated signals are generated by linearly mixing the pure EEG segments with EMG and EOG artifact segments, according to equation:

$$X_{mix} = X_{clean} + \lambda \cdot X_{artifact} \tag{1}$$

where $X_{mix}$ is the mixed EEG, $X_{clean}$ is the clean EEG, $X_{artifact}$ is the EMG or the EOG artifact, $\lambda$ is a parameter to control the signal-to-noise ratio (SNR) in the $X_{mix}$.

In this paper, SNR is defined as:

$$SNR = 10log_{10}\frac{RMS(X_{clean})}{RMS(\lambda \cdot X_{artifact})} \tag{2}$$

SNR levels range from −5 to 3 dB and for the convenience of presentation, the base number of SNR is taken as the abscissa (0.316, 0.398, 0.501, 0.631, 0.794, 1, 1.259, 1.58, 2).

In the Detection Block, the 40-segment EEG signal lasting for 63 s at 125 Hz from the DEAP database are selected as the long time series. For each experiment, two segments of EMG and two segments of EOG lasting for 2 s from the EEGdenoiseNet are randomly selected to add to $X_{clean}$. In the Denoise Block, 30 clean EEG signals from EEGdenoiseNet are randomly selected, and EMG or EOG artifact separately are added for each segment of signal.

In the Detection Block, the ADR is proposed to verify the ability of algorithm to recognize the location of artifacts. ADR is defined as:

$$ADR = \left(I_p \cap I_r\right)/I_r \tag{3}$$

where $I_p$ is the predicted interval of artifact, $I_r$ is the real artifact interval.

In the Denoise Block, the RRMSE and the correlation coefficient (CC) is use. RRMSE quantificationally measures the error between the denoised EEG and the real clean EEG. The smaller the RRMSE, the smaller the error between the de-noised EEG and the real EEG, and the better the effect of the noise reduction algorithm. CC is a measure of the ability to retain EEG information after noise reduction. The higher the CC, the more real EEG information contained in the de-noised EEG, and the stronger the noise reduction ability of the algorithm.

## 3 Results

### 3.1 Detection Block

The Fig. 2 shows one of the results of artifact detecting. EMG and EOG artifacts are added to the original signal with two segments respectively. The green rectangle represents the position of artifact fragments and the red rectangle represents the location of the artifact clip found. The SNR of the contaminated segment is equal to −3dB. The STD threshold N is set to 1.5, and the searching window is 2 s while slide window interval is 0.5 s. In the all 40 experiments, the average ADR is 1, suggesting all the artifact segment is detected.

Another part of the algorithm is to determine the corresponding artifact type. According to statistics, in all 160 artifact fragments, only 5 fragments are identified as other artifacts, the recognition accuracy up to 97%. Almost all the type of the artifacts are classified correctly.

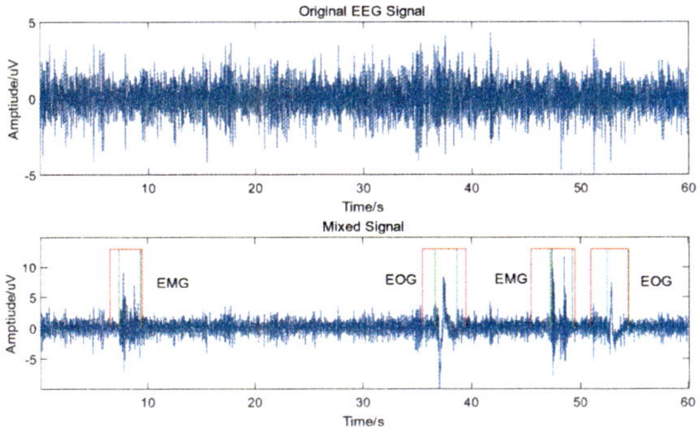


**Fig. 2.** A sample result of Detection Block

## 3.2 Denoise Block

For removing EMG artifacts, the CEEMDAN-CCA is applied to remove. The correlation coefficient threshold of CCA is set to 0.88, and the components that below the threshold is considered as EMG artifact and set to 0. In addition, to better demonstrate the performance of the CEEMDAN-CCA in removing EMG artifacts. Another recent algorithm SSA-CCA is implemented to compare with CEEMDAN-CCA. The correlation coefficient threshold of CCA is also set to 0.88.

The average results of 30 experiments using CEEMDAN-CCA and SSA-CCA to remove the EMG artifacts is shown in Fig. 3. The mean RRMSE of using CEEMDAN-CCA to denoise is slightly lower than that of SSA-CCA. The Fig. 3b shows that signal after noise reduction using CEEMDAN-CCA has the highest correlation with the original signal, which is significantly higher than SSA-CCA, especially in the case of low SNR. When SNR $= -5$dB, the CEEMDAN algorithm can reach a CC of 0.985 at most. The Fig. 3c, d show the best and worst denoising results in time domain respectively. It can be seen from Fig. 3c that the red curve representing the denoised signal has a high similarity with the pure signal. Figure 3d The inhibition of EMG in the second half of the signal is not obvious, resulting in a slightly lower overall correlation.

For each SNR of the mixed signal, SSA-CCA runs faster, shown in Table1. Therefore it may be more suitable for real-time application scenarios.

The evaluation of EOG artifact removal algorithm is similar to that of EMG artifact. For the SSA-SOBI, the window size of SSA is set to 55. A series of RC components are obtained after using the SSA for the mixed signals. Apply the SOBI to these RC components and calculate the Fuzzy entropy. In order to realize automatic operation, the Fuzzy entropy of each RC component is sorted, and the two components with the lowest Fuzzy entropy value are removed. The CEEMDAN-SOBI, WT-SOBI algorithms are realized as control. Three different hybrid algorithms are applied to denoise 30 randomly combined clean EEG and EOG artifacts. The parameter setting of the 3 algorithm and the running time is shown in the Table 1. The Operating environment is the same as that of the EMG artifact removal.

As is shown in Fig. 4a, b, SSA-SOBI algorithm has lower RRMSE and higher correlation coefficient at low SNR, and significantly higher than the signal not denoised. The WT-SOBI is similar to SSA-SOBI in the performance of denoising, even better

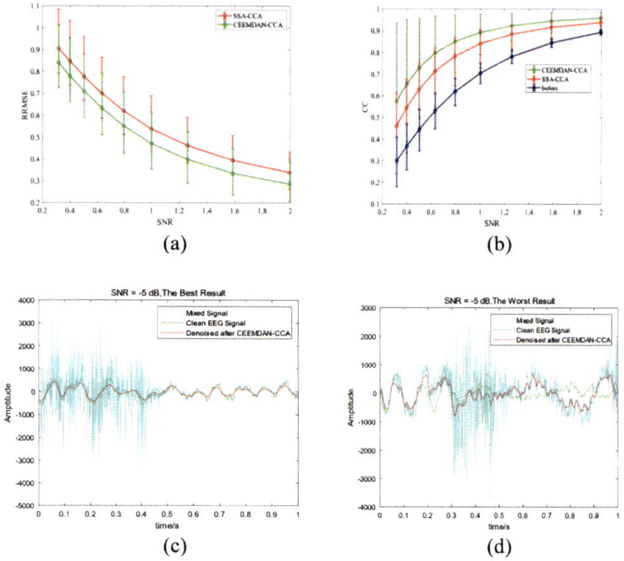

**Fig. 3.** The RRMSE-SNR curve (**a**), CC-SNR curve (**b**), the best (**c**) and worst result (**d**) in removing EMG artifacts

**Table 1.** The parameter of setting and the running time

| Algorithm | Parameter | Running time (s) |
|---|---|---|
| CEEMDAN-CCA | Nstd = 0.3<br>NR = 300<br>MaxIter = 1000<br>Correlation coefficient threthod = 0.88 | 3.95 |
| SSA-CCA | Window size = 125<br>Correlation coefficient threthod = 0.88 | 0.167 |
| SSA-SOBI | Window size = 55 | 2.47 |
| CEEMADN-SOBI | Nstd = 0.3<br>NR = 300<br>MaxIter = 1000 | 4.43 |
| WT-SOBI | Wavelet basis function = ‘db6’<br>Decomposition level = 8 | 0.41 |
| Fuzzy Entropy | Dim = 2, r = 0.2, n = 2 | – |

in high SNR. However, the algorithm based on wavelet decomposition requires prior knowledge, and need to adjust the wavelet basis function and decomposition level, which is not conducive to automatic processing. The Fig. 4a, b show the best result and worst results respectively using the SSA-SOBI when the SNR = −5 dB. In Fig. 4c, the red curve representing the denoised signal has a high similarity with the clean EEG.

In Fig. 4d, the performance of denoising if poor since there is still some EOG artifacts exist.

## 4 Conclusions

This paper evaluates the performance of the framework proposed in semi-simulated dataset. The experiment results show that, the EMG and EOG artifacts can effectively be detected and distinguished. Another advantage of artifact detection is that it can minimize the impact on clean EEG segments. In the Denoise Block, the CEEMDAN-CCA and SSA-SOBI are compared with other algorithms respectively. The results show that, the CEEMDAN-CCA can effectively remove the EMG artifacts and the SSA-SOBI also has high performance in removing EOG artifacts. In addition, the SSA-SOBI algorithm run fast since the SOBI is based on the SOS while the traditional ICA is based on the HOS, which allow the algorithm to be applied in the online system. In the next step, we will do further verification on real EEG data using our automatic detection algorithm in single-channel EEG recording.

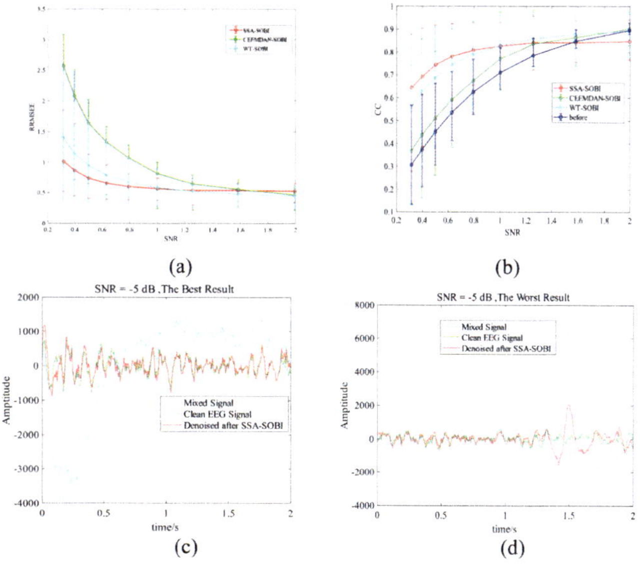


**Fig. 4.** The RRMSE-SNR curve (**a**), CC-SNR curve (**b**), the best (**c**) and worst result (**d**) in removing EMG artifacts

## References

1. Mumtaz, W., Rasheed, S., Irfan, A.: Review of challenges associated with the EEG artifact removal methods. Biomed. Signal Process. Contr. **68,** 102741 (2021)
2. Yasoda, K., Ponmagal, R.S., Bhuvaneshwari, K.S., Venkatachalam, K.: Automatic detection and classification of EEG artifacts using fuzzy kernel SVM and wavelet ICA (WICA). Soft Comput. **24**, 16011–16019 (2020). Smith J, Jones M Jr, Houghton L et al (1999) Future of health insurance. N Engl. J. Med. **965**, 325–329. https://doi.org/10.10007/s002149800025
3. Chen, X., Chen, Q., Zhang, Y., Wang, Z.J.: A novel EEMD-CCA approach to removing muscle artifacts for pervasive EEG. IEEE Sens. J. **19**(19), 8420–8431 (2018)
4. Bari, M.F., Fattah, S.A.: Epileptic seizure detection in EEG signals using normalized IMFs in CEEMDAN domain and quadratic discriminant classifier. Biomed. Signal Process. Contr. **58**, 101833 (2020)
5. Zhang, H., Zhao, M., Wei, C., Mantini, D., Li, Z., Liu, Q.: Eegdenoisenet: A benchmark dataset for deep learning solutions of eeg denoising. J. Neural Eng. **18**(5), 056057 (2021)
6. Koelstra, S., Muhl, C., Soleymani, M., Lee, J.S., Yazdani, A., Ebrahimi, T., ... Patras, I.: Deap: a database for emotion analysis; using physiological signals. IEEE Trans. Affect. Comput. **3**(1), 18-31 (2011)

# AGCN: Adaptive Graph Convolution Network with Hemibrain Differences of Resting-State EEG for Identifying Autism in Children

Wanyu Hu[1], Guoqian Jiang[1], Junxia Han[2](✉), and Xiaoli Li[3]

[1] School of Electrical Engineering, Yanshan University, Qinhuangdao 066004, China
m15978550205@163.com

[2] Beijing Key Laboratory of Learning and Cognition, School of Psychology, Capital Normal University, Beijing 100048, China

[3] State Key Laboratory of Cognitive Neuroscience and Learning, Beijing Normal University, Beijing 100875, China

**Abstract.** Early identification of autism in children has become a great concern due to the increasing prevalence of autism. Recently, EEG has become a promising tool to identify autistic children with some advanced signal processing and machine learning methods. However, it is still challenging to achieve accurate and reliable result due to the complexity of EEG signals. To this end, we propose a new adaptive graph neural network model by incorporating hemibrain differences (AGCN) of resting-state EEG to classify autistic children and typical developing (TD) children. First, a temporal feature learning module is designed to learn temporal dynamics of EEG signals. Then, to capture spatial correlations, we design an adaptive graph convolution network combined with spatial attention mechanism to learn the connectivity between nodes from the perspective of developmental abnormalities in the hemiencephalar and hemicerebral of autism. We collected a EEG dataset containing 45 ASD children and 45 typically developing (TD) children to evaluate our proposed method. Experimental results shown that our proposed method is superior to several baseline methods.

**Keywords:** Autism · Resting-state EEG · Hemibrain Differences · Adaptive Graph Convolution · Identification

## 1 Introduction

Autism spectrum disorder (ASD) is a developmental disorder appearing within the first three years of life. ASD is specifically manifested as language disorders, poor learning and imitation skills, narrow interests, intellectual abnormalities, and social communication disorders [1]. According to a report published in 2018 [2], the prevalence of autism is as high as 2.5%. At present, clinical diagnosis mainly relies on screening scales, which requires much expert experience and is time-consuming and labor intensive. Accordingly, there is an increasing need to perform automated identification of ASD in children to assist clinicians to make accurate and efficient diagnosis result.


G. Wang et al. (Eds.): APCMBE 2023, IFMBE Proceedings 103, pp. 87–94, 2024.
https://doi.org/10.1007/978-3-031-51455-5_11

In recent years, different objective diagnosis and evaluation techniques, such as functional magnetic resonance imaging (fMRI) [3], magnetoencephalogram (MEG) [4], electroencephalogram (EEG) and eye tracking [5] for ASD have been investigated. As a non-invasive measurement method with high temporal resolution and low cost, EEG has been widely studied to develop automated identification models with feature extractors and machine learning-based classifiers.For example, Heunis et al. [6] extracted improved multi-scale entropy for coherent analysis and recurrence quantification to classify resting EEG. Zhang et al. [7] fused EEG and eye tracking signals, first derived the synchronous measurement, information entropy and time-frequency characteristics of multi-channel EEG, and then classified them in combination with eye tracking records. Existing studies shown that deep learning methods achieved better performance than hand-crafted features.

Previous studies through the assessment of resting blood oxygen level dependence [8], functional magnetic resonance imaging research [9] have shown that autism has insufficient brain function connectivity, early overgrowth disrupts autism neural connections, and there are abnormal functional connections in and between cerebral hemispheres. Motivated by these studies, we attempt to incorporate the differences the left and right hemispheres of autism into deep learning model design, with the aim to automatically learn such differences the resting EEG data of autism and improve the identification performance.

The AGCN model proposed in this paper takes advantage of the differential characteristics of the left and right brains in autism. Firstly, the temporal features of the whole brain, left brain and right brain of autism are extracted by two-dimensional convolution, and then the adjacency matrix of the graph is obtained by adaptive learning based on the feature similarity, and then Chebyshev graph convolution learning spatial features is combined with spatial attention, and finally sent to the linear classifier for classification. Through specific experiments, the current mainstream and competitive resting EEG classification models are compared, and it is clearly shown that the performance of AGCN is better than other baseline models, with an accuracy rate of 91.11%. The combination of this model with left-right brain differences is visually illustrated.

## 2 Methodology

### 2.1 Data Collection and Preprocessing

In this study, a total of 90 children (45 ASD and 45 TD) aged 3–6 years volunteered to participate in the experiment. Children with ASD received diagnostic confirmation based on the Diagnostic and Statistical Manual of Mental Disorders, Fifth Edition (DSM-V). We collected resting-state EEGs of children using the 128-channel EGI HydroCel geodesic system (Eugen, Oregon, USA). During the collection process, each child was required to be seated in a comfortable chair with his or her eyes wide open while accompanied by a caregiver in a quiet room and that data collection lasts 5–10 min. The sampling frequency is 1000 Hz.

EEG data preprocessing was performed with EEGALB and MATLAB. The bad channel was first interpolated by selecting an artifact algorithm. According to the difference between the left and right brains, the channels in the central region were eliminated, and 46 channels were selected, mainly covering the left and right frontal lobes, the left and right temporal lobes, and the left and right occipital lobes.

### 2.2 Model Input

We selected EEG data for the first 30 s of each participant and divided the 90 participants into 2700 samples with a one-second segment. Each sample contains three branches: whole-brain, left-brain, and right-brain. We set the input $\boldsymbol{X} = [\boldsymbol{X}_a, \boldsymbol{X}_l, \boldsymbol{X}_r]$, $\boldsymbol{X}_a \in \mathbb{R}^{1 \times c \times t}$, $\boldsymbol{X}_l, \boldsymbol{X}_r \in \mathbb{R}^{1 \times \frac{c}{2} \times t}$, where $c$ is the number of whole brain channels, $\frac{c}{2}$ is the number of left and right hemisphere channels, $t$ is the sampling frequency. In this study $c = 46$, $\frac{c}{2} = 23$, and $t = 1000$.

### 2.3 Feature Extraction

(1) Temporal feature learning

Perform the following operations on the three sets of data entered. Whole-brain, left-brain, and right-brain data are defined $\mathbf{X}_a$, $\mathbf{X}_l$, and $\mathbf{X}_r$. We processed the samples into three-dimensional data and added a feature channel dimension specifically for convolutional layers. This allows only a single channel to learn temporal features, with no information crossing between channels. Let the scale of the convolution kernel $s = [1, 0.5t]$, the first is the channel dimension, the second dimension is the time dimension, set the time dimension to half of the sampling frequency, can capture frequency information of 2 Hz and above, suitable for EEG signals [10].

Convolutional layers are followed by an average pooling layer with a downsampling rate of 1/8 for the time dimension. Use the ReLU activation function for activation. Let the characteristics obtained by temporal feature learning be

$$\boldsymbol{X}'_{region} = \sigma_1\big(Avg\big(Conv2D\big(\boldsymbol{X}_{region}, s\big)\big)\big)$$

where, Avg(·) represents the average pooling layer, $\sigma_1(\cdot)$ represents the ReLU activation function, $\mathrm{X}_{\mathrm{region}}$ is the input data. $\mathrm{X}'_{\mathrm{region}} \in \mathbb{R}^{\mathrm{kernal} \times \mathrm{N} \times \mathrm{f}}$, region = {a, l, r}, where kernal is the number of convolution kernels used in the two–dimensional convolutional layer, $f$ is the number of features in the time dimension after learning and downsampling through the convolutional layer, $N$ is the number of nodes, $N \in \{c, \frac{c}{2}\}$.

(2) Adaptive graph learning

Unlike the study of fixed graphs, a non-fixed adjacency matrix is used in this paper to represent the graph. First, let the adjacency matrix is used in this paper to represent the graph. Let the adjacency matrix of the graph be $\boldsymbol{A}_{ij} = g\big(x_i, x_j\big)(i, j \in \{1, 2, \ldots, N\})$, used to represent node $\mathrm{x_i}$ and $\mathrm{x_j}$ connections. $\mathrm{g}\big(\mathrm{x_i}, \mathrm{x_j}\big)$ Can be learned by the learnable weight vector $\omega = (\omega_1, \omega_2, \ldots, \omega_f)^{\mathrm{T}}$. The convolution kernel feature layers obtained by all the previous convolutional layers are averaged. Get $\boldsymbol{X}^{mean}_{region} = (x_1^{region}, x_2^{region}, \ldots, x_N^{region}) \in \mathbb{R}^{N \times f}$. The adjacency matrix graph structure is thenlearned to be represented as

$$\boldsymbol{A_{ij}} = g\big(x_i, x_j\big) = \frac{\exp(ReLU(\boldsymbol{\omega}^T |x_j - x_i|))}{\sum_{i=1}^{N} \exp(ReLU(\boldsymbol{\omega}^T |x_j - x_i|))}$$

where the corrected linear unit ($ReLU$) is an activation function to guarantee that the $\boldsymbol{A}_{ij}$ is non-negative. Row weight vector $\omega$ is obtained by minimizing the loss function

$$\mathcal{L}_{graph} = \sum_{i,j=1}^{N} \|x_j - x_i\|_2^2 \boldsymbol{A}_{ij} + \lambda \|\boldsymbol{A}\|_F^2$$

where, $\|x_j - x_i\|_2^2$ is the distance between nodes, and it can be seen from the formula that the larger the distance between nodes, the smaller the $\boldsymbol{A}_{ij}$. Since the incomplete connection graph formed between the nodes, the second term in the formula is used to control the sparsity of figure $\boldsymbol{A}$, where $\lambda \geq 0$ is the regularization parameter.

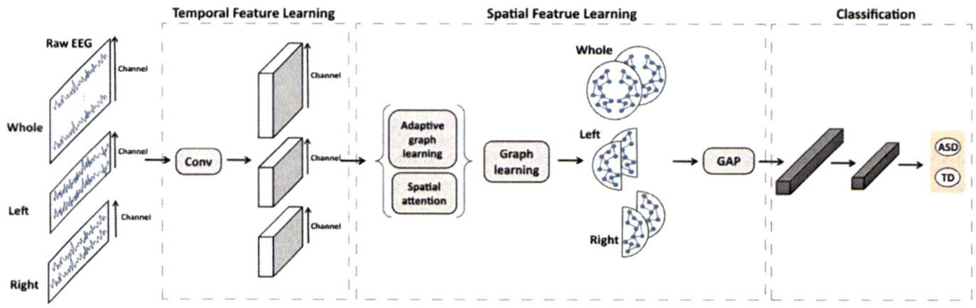


**Fig. 1.** The proposed autism auxiliary classification AGCN overall architecture. AGCN performed temporal and spatial feature extraction on resting EEG in autism, where spatial features were completed by adaptive graph convolution and graph learning with spatial attention

Adding a loss function to the adaptive graph stage can only calculate the loss inside that stage, so we define the loss function for the entire model as

$$\mathcal{L}_{loss} = \mathcal{L}_{CrossEntropy} + \mathcal{L}_{graph}$$

$$\mathcal{L}_{CrossEntropy} = -\frac{1}{B} \sum_{batch=1}^{B} \sum_{class=1}^{2} y_{batch,class} \log \hat{y}_{batch,class}$$

where $B$ represents the sample size and 2 indicates that this paper is a dichotomous model. $\boldsymbol{y}$ is the real label and $\hat{\boldsymbol{y}}$ is the label predicted by the model. In the final loss function, $\mathcal{L}_{graph}$ equivalent to a regularized term.

(3) Spatial attention

In graph convolutional learning, we also use the spatial attention mechanism [11] combined with Chebyshev polynomials for dynamic spatial feature learning. Spatial attention between nodes is defined as

$$\boldsymbol{Satt} = \boldsymbol{V} \cdot \sigma\left(\left(\boldsymbol{X}'_{region} \mathcal{Z}_1\right) \mathcal{Z}_2 \left(\mathcal{Z}_3 \boldsymbol{X}'_{region}\right)^T + \boldsymbol{b}\right)$$

$$\boldsymbol{Satt}'_{i,j} = Softmax(\boldsymbol{Satt}_{i,j})$$

where $\boldsymbol{V}, \boldsymbol{b} \in \mathbb{R}^{N \times N}$, $\mathcal{Z}_1, \mathcal{Z}_3 \in \mathbb{R}^{kernal}$, $\mathcal{Z}_2 \in \mathbb{R}^{f \times kernal}$, denote learnable parameters. Normalize $\boldsymbol{Satt}$ using *Softmax* to obtain $\boldsymbol{Satt}' \in \mathbb{R}^{N \times N}$.

(4) Spatial Graph Convolution

Spatial features use spectra-based graph convolution to learn the connections between whole-brain and hemi-brain nodes. Chebyshev graph convolution using polynomial of order K−1 [12] is defined as

$$\boldsymbol{F}_{region} = g_\theta *_G \boldsymbol{X}'_{region} = g_\theta(L)\boldsymbol{X}'_{region} = \sum_{k=0}^{K-1} \boldsymbol{Satt}'_{i,j}\boldsymbol{\theta}_k T_k(\tilde{L})\boldsymbol{X}'_{region}$$

where, $g_\theta$ represents the convolution kernel, $*_G$ represents the graph convolution operation, $\boldsymbol{\theta}_k \in \mathbb{R}^K$ represents the vector of Chebyshev's coefficients. $L = D - A$ is the Laplace matrix, $\boldsymbol{D} \in \mathbb{R}^{N \times N}$ is the degree matrix, $\tilde{L} = \frac{2}{\lambda_{max}}L - \boldsymbol{I}_N$, $\lambda_{max}$ is the maximum eigenvalue of the Laplace matrix, $T_k(\tilde{L})$ represents Chebyshev polynomial, and the corresponding features of the nodes are attention-weighted.

After learning the spatiotemporal features of $\boldsymbol{X}_a, \boldsymbol{X}_l, \boldsymbol{X}_r$, three feature map $F_a, F_l, F_r$ and then, stitching in the spatial dimension to obtain $\boldsymbol{feature}' = [\boldsymbol{F}_a, \boldsymbol{F}_l, \boldsymbol{F}_r] \in \mathbb{R}^{kernal \times 2c \times Filer}$), where Filter is the number of graph convolution kernels. Finally, after fusion through the global pooling layer and the final feature definition is

$$\boldsymbol{feature} = GAP(\boldsymbol{feature}')$$

where $GAP(\cdot)$ represents the global pooling layer, $\boldsymbol{feature} \in \mathbb{R}^{kernal}$.

(5) Classification

Next, the learned spatiotemporal features are sent to a linear classifier with two fully connected layers, which are output by the Softmax layer, and the probability of the sample being ASD or TD children is finally obtained.

The network structure of AGCN is shown in Fig. 1.

# 3 Result

## 3.1 Performance Evaluation

As described in Sect. 2, our proposed model consists of three inputs, namely whole brain, left brain and right brain. To investigate the effects of different inputs on identification performance, we design two model variants as follows

**AGCN-1**: One input using only whole brain data;
**AGCN-2**: Two inputs using only left and right brain data.

Table 1 summarizes the results of the comparison of the three different methods. Obviously, the accuracy of the extraction of left and right brain data features is much

**Table 1.** Ablation experiments

| | Accuracy (%) | STD (%) |
|---|---|---|
| AGCN | 91.11 | 6.33 |
| AGCN-1 | 82.88 | 6.16 |
| AGCN-2 | 89.41 | 6.28 |

higher than that of AGCN-1 using whole brain data alone, indicating that there is a significant difference in left and right brain features in autistic children. Comparing the accuracy of AGCN and AGCN-2, it was found that the accuracy of using left and right brain data and whole brain data was higher than that of using only left and right brain data, and the combination of global and local was better. Therefore, combining the left and right brain differences of autism can make AGCN achieve better results.

### 3.2 Compared With the State-of-the-Art Methods

In order to verify the performance of the proposed framework, we compare the results with this year's mainstream EEG classification networks. As shown in Table 2, AGCN is far superior in accuracy to the other three models. Moreover, from the results of comparative cross-verification, it is concluded that the accuracy of each fold of AGCN is higher than that of other models, so AGCN is the model with the best performance.

**Table 2.** Comparison with baseline approaches

| | AGCN | TSception [13] | EEGNet [10] | Shallow ConvNet [14] |
|---|---|---|---|---|
| Acc | 91.11% | 83.37% | 84.33% | 77.22% |
| std | 6.33% | 6.67% | 6.28% | 8.69% |

### 3.3 Visualization

We randomly selected thirty samples of one autistic child and one TD child to learn adjacency matrices, average them as adjacency matrices, and visualize them through heat maps. It is clear from Fig. 2 that the heat map is basically symmetrical, with different overall depths in the three brain regions. Moreover, comparing the upper and lower sets of pictures, it is not difficult to find that the depth of the left and right brain feature adjacency matrix obtained by autism convolution is more different.

### 3.4 Discussion

Under the same experimental conditions, our AGCN framework offers considerable advantages in accuracy and standard variance. Since autism has the problem of abnormal

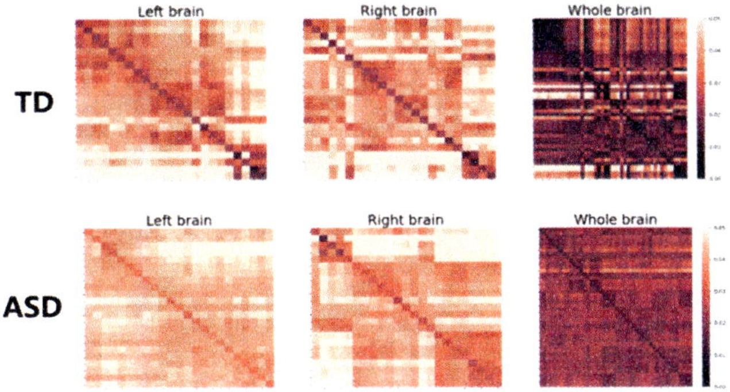


**Fig. 2.** Adjacency matrix heatmap of an adaptive graph

left and right brain connections and differences, the network performance is significantly improved after using this feature to design the network, and it is also very novel in the field of autism diagnosis. In exploring whether the performance improvement caused by the introduction of left and right brain division is related to the autism hemibrain, we use heat map to visualize the adaptive adjacency matrixs.

## 4 Conclusion

A new AGCN was proposed as an auxiliary diagnostic model based on resting-state EEG for automated ASD identification. Our proposed method incorporates the difference between the left brain and the right brain of ASD, which can better learn discriminative features from the characteristics of the whole brain and left and right hemispheres of EEG data. It is clear from the results that the proposed model is superior to other baseline networks. And it can also be seen that the left and right brain differential thoughts do have a significant improvement effect in the resting EEG data of autism. In summary, AGCN is suitable for deployment in medical systems to assist in efficient diagnostic and therapeutic services.

**Acknowledgement.** This work was supported in part by the National Natural Science Foundation of China under Grant 62003228 and Grant 61761166003, in part by the Science and Technology Development Project of Beijing Municipal Education Commission of China under Grant KM202010028019, and in part by the National Key Research and Development Program of China under Grant 2017YFC0820205.

## References

1. Kanner, L.: Autistic disturbances of affective contact. Nervous Child **2**(3), 217–250 (1943)
2. Christensen, D.L., Braun, K.V.N., Baio, J., Bilder, D., Charles, J., Constantino, J.N., ... Yeargin-Allsopp, M.: Prevalence and characteristics of autism spectrum disorder among children aged 8 years—autism and developmental disabilities monitoring network, 11 sites, United States, 2012. MMWR Surveillance Summaries **65**(13), 1 (2018)

3. Just, M.A., Keller, T.A., Malave, V.L., Kana, R.K., Varma, S.: Autism as a neural systems disorder: a theory of frontal-posterior underconnectivity. Neurosci. Biobehav. Rev. **36**(4), 1292–1313 (2012)
4. Precenzano, F., et al.: Electroencephalographic abnormalities in autism spectrum disorder: characteristics and therapeutic implications. Medicina (Kaunas) **56**(9), 419 (2020)
5. Han, J., et al.: A multimodal approach for identifying autism spectrum disorders in children. IEEE Trans. Neural Syst. Rehab. Eng. **30**, 2003–2011 (2022)
6. Heunis, T.M., Aldrich, C., de Vries, P.J.: Recent advances in resting-state electroencephalography biomarkers for autism spectrum disorder-a review of methodological and clinical challenges. Pediatr. Neurol. **61**, 28–37 (2016)
7. Zhang, S., Chen, D., Tang, Y., Zhang, L.: Children ASD evaluation through joint analysis of EEG and eye-tracking recordings with graph convolution network. Front. Hum. Neurosci. **15**, 651349 (2021)
8. Anderson, J.S., Druzgal, T.J., Froehlich, A., DuBray, M.B., Lange, N., Alexander, A. L., ... Lainhart, J. E.: Decreased interhemispheric functional connectivity in autism. Cerebral cortex **21**(5), 1134–1146 (2011)
9. Minshew, N.J., Williams, D.L.: The new neurobiology of autism: cortex, connectivity, and neuronal organization. Arch. Neurol. **64**(7), 945–950 (2007)
10. Lawhern, V.J., Solon, A.J., Waytowich, N.R., Gordon, S.M., Hung, C.P., Lance, B.J.: EEGNet: a compact convolutional neural network for EEG-based brain–computer interfaces. J. Neural Eng. **15**(5), 056013 (2018)
11. Guo, S., Lin, Y., Feng, N., Song, C., Wan, H.: Attention based spatial-temporal graph convolutional networks for traffic flow forecasting. In: Proceedings of the AAAI Conference on Artificial Intelligence, July, vol. 33, No. 01, pp. 922–929 (2019)
12. Defferrard, M., Bresson, X., Vandergheynst, P.: Convolutional neural networks on graphs with fast localized spectral filtering. Adv. Neural Inf. Process. Syst. **29** (2016)
13. Ding, Y., Robinson, N., Zeng, Q., Guan, C.: TSception: capturing temporal dynamics and spatial asymmetry from EEG for emotion recognition (2021)
14. Schirrmeister, R.T., et al.: Deep learning with convolutional neural networks for EEG decoding and visualization. Hum. Brain Mapp. **38**, 5391–5420 (2017)

# Recognition of VR Motion Sickness Level Based on EEG and Functional Brain Network

Chengcheng Hua[1(✉)], Lining Chai[1], Zhanfeng Zhou[1], and Rongrong Fu[2]

[1] School of Automation/C-IMER/CICAEET, Nanjing University of Information Science and Technology, Nanjing, China
huachengcheng@nuist.edu.cn

[2] Department of Electrical Engineering, Yanshan University, Qinhuangdao, China

**Abstract.** Virtual reality motion sickness (VRMS) is a common problem for VR players. To study the causes and cures of VRMS, the recognition of VRMS level is a precondition. So, we aim to study how VRMS modulates EEG in functional brain networks and extract EEG features to measure VRMS. In this study, 23 subjects are recruited and their EEG are collected when they are in VMRS induced by "VRQ test". We introduce a functional brain network approach based on empirical mode decompose and phase locking value to analysis the EEG, and recognize the VRMS level using graph-theoretic indexes and machine learning. The results suggest that the high frequency mode (about 30–40 Hz) of EEG has more significant features between low and high VRMS levels, and the classification accuracy in the task and the post-task rest states are up to 96.3% and 97.6% respectively. This work firstly reveals the effects of VRMS on the functional brain networks and provides a method to assess and guide the comfortable VR products design.

**Keywords:** Virtual reality motion sickness (VRMS) · EEG · Phase locking value (PLV) · Functional brain network (FBN)

## 1 Introduction

Virtual reality (VR) technology has developed rapidly in recent years and is widely used in entertainment, education, rehabilitation, training, etc. However, VR motion sickness (VRMS), a type of visually induced motion sickness, causes VR users to sweat, salivate, fatigued, dizzy and regurgitate. In more extreme cases, users may even experience vomiting, disorientation, poor posture-hand-eye coordination and prolonged reaction time [1]. Thus, VRMS presents serious safety and health risks to users and affects the VR industry.

Evaluation of VRMS level is a precondition in studies of VRMS mechanism and cures [2–4]. The self-assessment method had long been used to evaluate motion sickness in various simulators [5] like questionnaire. However, the questionnaire is susceptible to subjective judgments and cannot be conducted during a task. Physiological and behavioral methods such as: EGG, ECG, blood pressure, EOG, EDA, respiration, postural sway [1, 6–9] can be online collected, so many researches introduce them to evaluate


G. Wang et al. (Eds.): APCMBE 2023, IFMBE Proceedings 103, pp. 95–102, 2024.
https://doi.org/10.1007/978-3-031-51455-5_12

VRMS. However, they are not suitable for use alone [9], because they are susceptible to noise and may be related to other factors [6].

EEG has the advantages of non-invasive, non-interfering, and high temporal resolution. And the neural information contained in EEG signals can reflect human cognitive function and abnormal states such as fatigue, pain, pressure and motion sickness. Therefore, it has the potential to evaluate VRMS levels objectively. Jang et al. develop a VR scene with vections including pitch, yaw, roll, zoom in and zoom out. They compare SSQ and EEG rhythm absolute energy in three states: rest, VRMS exposure and recovery, and found significant contrasts in the $\alpha$ rhythm in the forehead, central area, top, occipital, and temporal regions after ANOVA analysis [10]. Lim et al. analyze the SSQ and EEG rhythm energy of subjects between baseline and VRMS states when they are in a simple flight VR task, and the study found a significant difference in $\theta$ energy in the frontal region. However, the relationship between SSQ and EEG is not analyzed [11]. Syed et al. investigate the temporal-frequency changes in the EEG energy associated with the visual-induced motion sickness level. The results show that the theta and beta rhythm energies differed between 2D and 3D [12].

To sum up, the current studies focused mainly on the power spectra, and the results are not uniform. Nevertheless, VRMS is caused by many and complex reasons [13, 14], so a simple EEG feature may not detect VRMS accurately, because it has multiple interpretations and is easily influenced. Functional brain network (FBN) is a frequent-used approach to investigate complex cognition states from the interactions among different brain regions [15] and has potential to measure VRMS severity. In this study, we focus on the EEG of subjects collected during and after a VRMS exposure task, then introduce empirical mode decomposition (EMD) and phase locking value (PLV) to compute FBNs [16]. Finally, we apply the Wilcoxon rank sum test to select VRMS-related FBN features and perform classification and T-distributed stochastic neighbor embedding (T-SNE) to verify those features.

## 2 Methods

### 2.1 VRMS Stimulation and Experimental Protocol

A VR scene named as "VRQ test" developed by Vectorush Studio is introduced to make four types of self-motion illusion (named as vection) for the subjects, e.g. moving forward, swing in the Roll axis, rotation in the Yaw axis and swing in the Pitch axis, as shown in Fig. 1. The experiment has 3 stages: Rest1, Task and Rest2. In Rest1 the subjects are recorded EEG for 2 min; Task is the VRMS exposure stage of 3 min; Rest2 is the after-task rest phase, in which the subjects are record 2 min of EEG. Rest1 is used as a baseline to eliminate the individual difference. For the safety and health of the subjects, the experiment is conducted in a sitting position and can be terminated any time the subject cannot tolerate the VRMS. Simulator Sickness Questionnaire (SSQ) [17] is conducted after the task to assess the subjective VRMS level of the subjects. According to the results, the median value, 25.96, is taken as a threshold to divide the subjects into two groups: low-SSQ (<25.96) and high-SSQ (>25.96), which are used as the labels of EEG data [17]. The experiment followed is in accordance with the ethical standards of the ethics committee of Qinhuangdao first hospital (2022A024) and with the Helsinki Declaration.

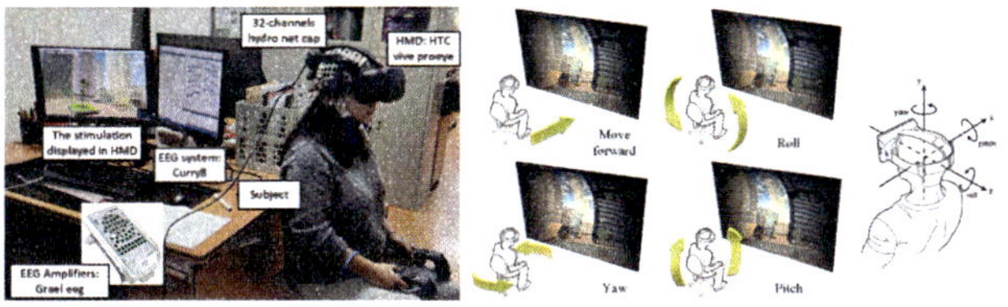


**Fig. 1.** Experimental scene with key devices and the VR scenes of vection

## 2.2 Subjects and EEG Data

A total of 23 subjects (20 male and 3 female, 22.8 ± 1.1 years old) are recruited for this study, and one male subject is discarded due to excessive noise in the EEG data. All subjects have normal hearing and the normal/corrected-to-normal vision, and no history of neurological disease and sign an informed notice before the experiment and have no report. Because the experiment may cause discomfort, the subjects have all the right to terminate the experiment at any time.

Neuroscan Grael EEG system is used to collect EEG signals in the experiment (Fig. 1), the EEG cap has 30 EEG electrodes. The sampling rate is 1024 Hz. The pre-processes of the raw EEG data include baseline-drifting correction, 50 Hz-notch filter to remove power frequency interference, manual removal of the parts with serious artifact interference and abnormal amplitude, ocular artifacts correction using ICA and EOG reference, and a band pass filter of 0.5–45 Hz.

## 2.3 Feature Extraction

PLV reflects the phase coupling among the electrodes [16, 18]. In FBNs, the electrodes are considered as the nodes, and the PLVs among the electrodes are considered as the edges. The EMD is used to decompose the EEG into different frequency components, and then the PLVs of the first four IMFs are computed separately. Then, the graph-theory indexes such as clustering coefficient (C), shortest path length (L), degree (D) and betweenness centrality (B) are used to quantify the FBNs [19]. We analyze the global and local FBN features, which stand for average FBN features of all nodes and FBN features of each node respectively. After calculating the FBN features above, the features of Rest1 are considered as the baseline to correct the FBN features in Rest2 and Task to decrease the influence caused by individual factors. The detail method is that we subtract the average features of Rest1 from the features of Rest2 and Task to obtain the new corrected features.

### 2.4 Feature Selection and Classification

There are 496 features consisting of four IMFs * four features * (30 nodes + one average node) in total, most of which contribute little to the recognition of VRMS, and the majority of features do not follow a normal distribution. Therefore, the Wilcoxon rank sum test is conducted to select features. Then useful FBN features are screened to distinguish the different VRMS levels: low and high-SSQ scores using EEG data in Task and Rest2 states. To verify the effect of the selected features, T-SNE [20] is introduced to visualize the separability and relevance to the VRMS level. After that, the classifications are performed using classification learner toolbox in MATLAB. We apply selected features as input and VRMS level (high- and low-SSQ) as the output to train those classifiers. The 10-fold cross-validations are conducted to assess the performance of the classifiers and the selected features.

## 3 Reulsts

### 3.1 Frequency Decomposition

The decomposition of the pre-processed EEG data by EMD gives 10 IMFs, of which the first four IMFs contain the most of the EEG components. Therefore, only the first four IMFs are used. The ranges of the instantaneous frequency of IMF1-4 are 30–40 Hz, 10–20 Hz, 4–8 Hz and 1–4 Hz respectively and correspond to $\gamma$, part $\alpha$ and part $\beta$, $\theta$ and $\delta$ rhythm respectively.

### 3.2 FBN Features

The brain maps of C and B of the different SSQ levels are given in Figs. 2 and 3. In Fig. 2, the bigger difference of Task between high and low-SSQ is in IMF1 and IMF2 than in other IMFs while that of Rest2 is in IMF1 and IMF3, which suggests that the features distinguishing high and low-SSQ may be in different frequency bands and the C in IMF1 are general-used in Rest2 and Task. The L and D behave similarly to C, because the L and C highly rely upon D. Summary the results of these three features, the high VRMS level weaken the connections among the nodes.

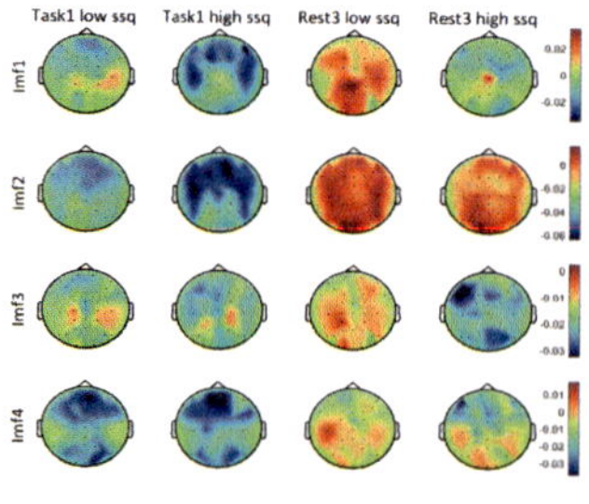


**Fig. 2.** Brain maps of C in different groups and different IMFs

In Fig. 3, the performance of the B is different from the other three local features. For Task, the B of high and low-SSQ in IMF1 show some lateralized features, and the B of high-SSQ focus in smaller number of nodes in IMF2 and IMF3. Different from Task, in Rest2, the B of high-SSQ are higher than those of low-SSQ in prefrontal and left frontal areas in IMF1, IMF2 and IMF3.

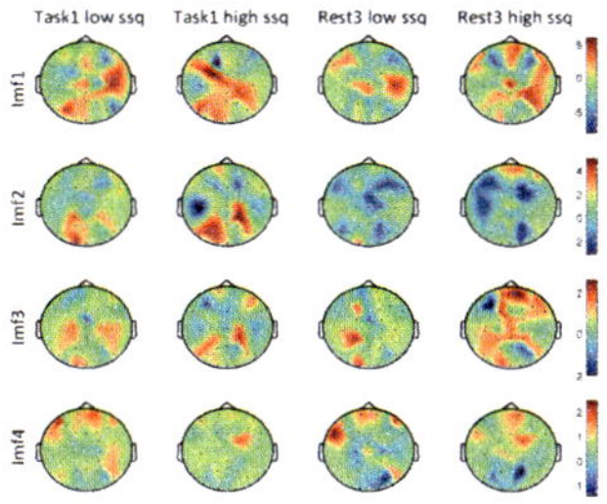


**Fig. 3.** Brain maps of B in different groups and different IMFs

### 3.3 Feature Selection and Classification

We hypothesize that the EEG features truly reflecting VRMS levels are consistent in the Rest2 and Task states, so the FBN features with p-values less than 0.0001 in both Rest2 and Task are selected as indicators of VRMS levels. The new feature set is shown in Table 1. The lower the frequency range an IMF contains, the less the significant features it has.

**Table 1.** Significant FBN features between low versus high-SSQ both in Rest2 and Task

| | B | C | D | L |
|---|---|---|---|---|
| IMF1 | FP1, F7, F3, F12, FC4, FT12, CZ, T8, P8, O1 | FP2, F11, F7, F3, FZ, F4, F8, F12, FC4, FT12, C3, CZ, T8, CP3, CPZ, CP4, P7, PZ, P4, P8, O1, OZ, O2, Global | F7, F3, FZ, F4, FC4, FT12, C3, CZ, T8, CP3, CPZ, CP4, P7, PZ, P4, OZ, O2, Global | FP1, FP2, F11, F7, F3, FZ, F4, FT11, FC4, FT12, C3, CZ, T8, CP3, CPZ, CP4, P7, PZ, P4, P8, O1, OZ, O2, Global |
| IMF2 | FP1, F3, T7, CZ, | F11, FT11, FC3, FC4, T7 | F11, FT11, FC3, FC4, T7, T8 | F11, F3, FT11, FC3, FC4, FT12, T7, T8, M2, O1, OZ, Global |
| IMF3 | FP1 | F3, FZ, FC3, T7, C3, T8 | F3, FZ, FC3, T7, C3, T8 | F3, FZ, FC3, T7, C3, T8 |
| IMF4 | FT11, C4, P7, P8 | None | None | None |

T-SNE is used to project the selected features mentioned above into a 3D space in Fig. 4. For Rest2 and Task, the results indicate that the low-SSQ samples are clearly distinguished from the high-SSQ samples, and the points are clustered into several groups.

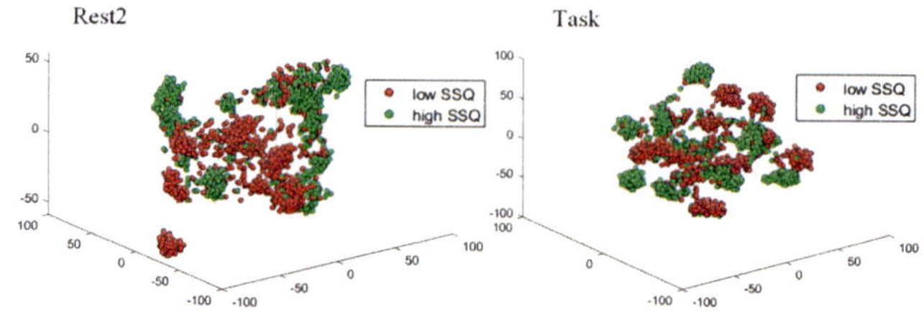


**Fig. 4.** T-SNE of selected features

Table 2 shows the classification results of the classifiers of the highest accuracy. The absolute and relative rhythm power and mRMR method are introduced as the reference. The best classifier for recognizing SSQ level using Rest2 data is boosted trees and the classification accuracy is 96.3%, while the best classifier using Task data is cubic SVM and the accuracy is 97.6%.

**Table 2.** The performance of the classifications

| | Approaches | Acc.(%) | Pre | Rec | F | AUC |
|---|---|---|---|---|---|---|
| Rest2 | Power + mRMR + Bagged Trees | 94.3 | 0.94 | 0.94 | 0.94 | 0.99 |
| | Our features + mRMR + Boosted Trees | 95.6 | 0.95 | 0.97 | 0.96 | 0.99 |
| | **Our selected features + Boosted Trees** | **96.3** | **0.95** | **0.98** | **0.96** | **1** |
| Task | Power + mRMR + Bagged Trees | 97.2 | 0.96 | 0.98 | 0.97 | 1.0 |
| | Our features + mRMR + Bagged Trees | 96.0 | 0.96 | 0.96 | 0.96 | 0.99 |
| | **Our selected features + Cubic SVM** | **97.6** | **0.98** | **0.97** | **0.98** | **1** |

## 4 Discussion

In this paper, we conduct an experiment to induce VRMS of subjects and collect their EEG and SSQ, introduce EMD and FBN methods to extract VRMS-related features, and verify those features through statistical methods and classifications. All the samples are divided into two levels of VRMS to find the EEG features related to the subjective VRMS severity shown in Table 1. This work has two major contributions: First, we analyze the VRMS-related FBNs build based on EEG using the EMDPL method, and the results prove that the EMDPL method is suitable to analyze VRMS-related EEG and the FBN features are potentially indicators to detect VRMS severity. Second, in order to optimize the feature set, there are three approaches performed: (1) the Wilcoxon rank sum test is used to analyze and select features; (2) the significant features in both Rest2 and Task are selected, and (3) the average FBN features of Rest1 are used to corrected the individual difference. The indicator of VRMS level based on EEG proposed in this work will provide guidance and recommendations for the developments of VR system to ensure more comfortable VR experience.

There are two drawbacks need to improve in the future: First, the subjects are gender imbalanced, so it is difficult to demonstrate in this study that VIMS-related brain functional network features are also presented in females. Then, there is only one SSQ result per subject, therefore, the results may be influenced by individual difference. Given that, we subtract the Rest1 features from Rest2 and Task to weaken the effect of the individual difference. However, the samples belong to same subject are still clustered together in Fig. 4b, c, which suggests that the individual difference is still influence the new features. To solve these problems, more gender-balanced subjects should be recruited and multiple VR scenarios should be introduced in the experiment for each subject.

## 5 Conclusions

In this paper, the EMD and PLV are used to analyze the comparison of FBN features before, during and after VRMS exposure experiments, as well as the comparison of EEG features between different SSQ levels (high and low-SSQ). The results show that the FBN features in high frequency are related to subjective VRMS level. Based on those, we select features to do the classification. The accuracy in Rest2 is up to 96.3%, the accuracy in Task is up to 97.65%, that suggest that the FBN features can be used to assess VRMS level.

**Acknowledgment.** We gratefully acknowledge the financial support from National Natural Science Foundation of China (62206130, 62073282), Natural Science Foundation of Jiangsu Province (BK20200821), and Startup Foundation for Introducing Talent of NUIST (2020r075). Thanks a lot for all the subjects and personnel of the experiments.

## References

1. Nalivaiko, E., Davis, S.L., Blackmore, K.L., Vakulin, A., Nesbitt, K.V.: Cybersickness provoked by head-mounted display affects cutaneous vascular tone, heart rate and reaction time. Physiol. Behav. **151**, 583–590 (2015)
2. Kim, J., Oh, H., Kim, W., Choi, S., Son, W., Lee, S.: A deep motion sickness predictor induced by visual stimuli in virtual reality. IEEE Trans. Neur. Netw. Learn. **33**, 554–566 (2022)
3. Kim, H.G., Lim, H.T., Lee, S., Ro, Y.M.: VRSA Net: VR sickness assessment considering exceptional motion for 360 degrees VR video. IEEE Trans. Image Process. **28**, 1646–1660 (2019)
4. Wang, Y., Chardonnet, J.R., Merienne, F.: VR sickness prediction for navigation in immersive virtual environments using a deep long short term memory model. In: 2019 IEEE Conference on Virtual Reality and 3D User Interfaces (VR) (2019)
5. Chang, E., Kim, H.T., Yoo, B.: Virtual reality sickness: a review of causes and measurements. Int. J. Hum-Comput. Interact. **36**, 1658–1682 (2020)
6. Gersak, G., Lu, H.M., Guna, J.: Effect of VR technology matureness on VR sickness. Multimed Tools Appl. **79**, 14491–14507 (2020)

7. Nam, Y., Hong, U., Chung, H., Noh, S.R.: Eye movement patterns reflecting cybersickness: evidence from different experience modes of a virtual reality game. Cyberpsychol. Behav. Soc. Netw. **25**, 135–139 (2022)
8. Kim, Y.Y., Kim, E.N., Park, M.J., Park, K.S., Ko, H.D., Kim, H.T.: The application of biosignal feedback for reducing cybersickness from exposure to a virtual environment. Presence-Teleoper. Virtual Environ. **17**, 1–16 (2008)
9. Keshavarz, B., Peck, K., Rezaei, S., Taati, B.: Detecting and predicting visually induced motion sickness with physiological measures in combination with machine learning techniques. Int. J. Psychophysiol. **176**, 14–26 (2022)
10. Jang, K.-M., Shin Woo, Y., Kyoon Lim, H.: Electrophysiological changes in the virtual reality sickness: EEG in the VR sickness. In: The 25th International Conference on 3D Web Technology, pp. 1–4 (2020)
11. Lim, H.K., et al.: Test-retest reliability of the virtual reality sickness evaluation using electroencephalography (EEG). Neurosci. Lett. **743**, 135589 (2021)
12. Naqvi, S.A.A., Badruddin, N., Jatoi, M.A., Malik, A.S., Hazabbah, W., Abdullah, B.: EEG based time and frequency dynamics analysis of visually induced motion sickness (VIMS). Aus. Phys. Eng. Sci. Med. **38**, 721–729 (2015)
13. Ng, A.K.T., Chan, L.K.Y., Lau, H.Y.K.: A study of cybersickness and sensory conflict theory using a motion-coupled virtual reality system. Displays **61**, 6 (2020)
14. Xu, W., Liang, H.-N., Zhang, Z., Baghaei, N.: Studying the effect of display type and viewing perspective on user experience in virtual reality exergames. Games Health J. (2020)
15. Bullmore, E., Sporns, O.: Complex brain networks: graph theoretical analysis of structural and functional systems. Nat. Rev. Neurosci. **10**, 186–198 (2009)
16. Aydore, S., Pantazis, D., Leahy, R.M.: A note on the phase locking value and its properties. Neuroimage **74**, 231–244 (2013)
17. Kennedy, R.S., Lane, N.E., Berbaum, K.S., Lilienthal, M.G.: Simulator sickness questionnaire: an enhanced method for quantifying simulator sickness. Int. J. Aviat. Psychol. **3**, 203–220 (1993)
18. Olejarczyk, E., Marzetti, L., Pizzella, V., Zappasodi, F.: Comparison of connectivity analyses for resting state EEG data. J. Neural Eng. **14**, 13 (2017)
19. Rubinov, M., Sporns, O.: Complex network measures of brain connectivity: Uses and interpretations. Neuroimage **52**, 1059–1069 (2010)
20. Van der Maaten, L., Hinton, G.: Visualizing data using t-SNE. J. Mach. Learn. Res. **9**, 2579–2605 (2008)

# Biomedical Imaging and Image Processing

# SRSA-Net: Separable ResUnit and Self-attention Optimized Network for Simultaneous Nuclei Segmentation and Classification in Histology Images

Ranran Wang[1], Yusong Qiu[3], Yong Zhang[3], and Hongming Xu[1,2](✉)

[1] School of Biomedical Engineering, Faculty of Medicine, Dalian University of Technology, Dalian, China
mxu@dlut.edu.cn
[2] Key Laboratory of Integrated Circuit and Biomedical Electronic System, Liaoning Province, Dalian, China
[3] Department of Pathology, Liaoning Cancer Hospital and Institute, Shenyang, China

**Abstract.** Automatic nuclei segmentation and classification plays an important role in histopathological image analysis. However, existing algorithms mainly targeting H&E images have not provided a satisfied performance in processing immunohistochemical (IHC) images. On this account, we propose a multi-task deep learning model termed as the SRSA-Net to simultaneously segment and classify cell nuclei in IHC images. The SRSA-Net adopts ResNet50 augmented depth-wise separable convolution within each ResUnit as the feature encoder. Three paralleled decoder branches consist of self-attention modules and a series of DenseUnit and upsampling operations to derive results of nuclei classification, distance map prediction and nuclei segmentation. The watershed algorithm is finally used as a post-processing step to split touching cell nuclei. Experiments have been performed on the IHC dataset with more than 9000 cell nuclei, which show that the proposed SRSA-Net outperforms state-of-the-art nuclei segmentation and classification models.

**Keywords:** Nuclei segmentation and classification · Self-attention · Depth-wise separable convolution · Immunohistochemical · Computational pathology

## 1 Introduction

Lung cancer has the highest incidence and mortality rate in the world, in which non-small cell lung cancer (NSCLC) accounts for 80%. The quantitative analysis of tumor immune microenvironment (TIME) of NSCLC patients can help pathologists to explore disease progression and tumor stage [1]. Immunohistochemical (IHC) image analysis plays a key role in quantifying the TIME. The basic principle of IHC staining technology replies on specific binding of antigen and antibody [2]. The discovery and application of abundant tumor-specific antibodies result in severe staining heterogeneity in IHC images, which


G. Wang et al. (Eds.): APCMBE 2023, IFMBE Proceedings 103, pp. 105–112, 2024.
https://doi.org/10.1007/978-3-031-51455-5_13

brings a great challenge for automatic IHC image analysis. Nowadays, pathologists examine digitized IHC images mainly based on subjective judgements and empirical knowledge, suffering from the strong subjectivity and large deviation [3]. Nuclei quantification is a fundamental procedure in IHC image analysis, which provides computed numerical values reflecting nuclear features to pathologists so as to recommend a more suitable therapeutic solution. Hence, the development of nuclei quantification algorithm in IHC images is of great significance to treatment recommendation for lung cancer patients.

The traditional nuclei segmentation or classification algorithms such as Otsu's thresholding [4] and random forest classifier [5] usually fail to provide robust results across multiplex IHC images. Moreover, these traditional algorithms cannot simultaneously perform nuclei segmentation and classification. Compared with traditional algorithms, deep learning model has a more flexible applicability in computational pathology, as the multi-task learning model can be applied to simultaneously segment and classify cell nuclei. Graham et al. [6] proposed a Hover-Net to achieve nuclei segmentation and classification, which utilizes markers obtained from horizontal and vertical distance maps to post-process nuclei detection and classification. Ghahremani et al. [7] employed the generative adversarial network to perform nuclei segmentation and classification. Yao et al. [8] proposed the PointNu-Net to segment and classify cell nuclei, which considers nuclear detection and classification as a key point heatmap regression task. Although these existing methods reported promising performances, they mainly focused on H&E stained images.

With the purpose of quantitative TIME analysis, we propose a multi-task deep learning model that can precisely delineate every nucleus and identity its type (i.e., negative or positive) in IHC images. The main contributions of this paper are as follows. (1) We propose a multi-task learning model termed as the SRSA-Net for simultaneous nuclei segmentation and classification in IHC images. (2) The SRSA-Net takes advantage of cascaded separable ResUnit in encoding features and exploits self-attention mechanism, upsampling and DenseUnit in decoding features. (3) Experiments conducted on the IHC dataset show that the SRSA-Net outperforms other state-of-the-art models in nuclei segmentation and classification.

## 2 Methods

The overview of our proposed SRSA-Net is shown in Fig. 1. The given image is input into an encoder for extracting feature maps. The feature maps are then sent to three decoder branches (i.e., NC, HV, and NP) to perform nuclei classification, distance map regression and nuclei segmentation, respectively. The distance maps are post-processed to get markers and then the marker-controlled watershed is used to process NP prediction to obtain the final nuclei segmentation. Based on NC prediction, the segmented nuclei are classified into either positive or negative type. Figure 2 shows detail architecture of the SRSA-Net that is presented in the following.

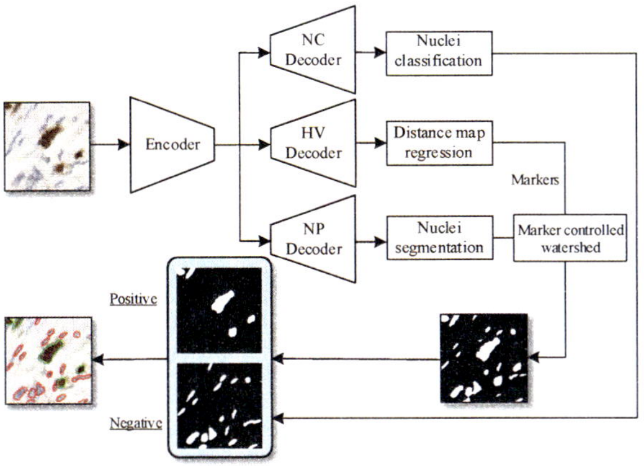


**Fig. 1.** Overview of our proposed SRSA-net.

### 2.1 Encoder

As shown in Fig. 2a, given an input image, it is first processed by the 7 × 7 convolution and then a series of Separable ResUnit blocks and a 1 × 1 convolution are applied for feature extraction, where *m* refers to the number of feature maps. As observed in Fig. 2d, our Separable ResUnit is designed by incorporating the ResUnit and Depth-wise Separable Convolution (DSC) [9]. The number of Separable ResUnit within each block is 3, 4, 6, 3, corresponding to 1, 2, 4 and 8 down-sampling levels, respectively.

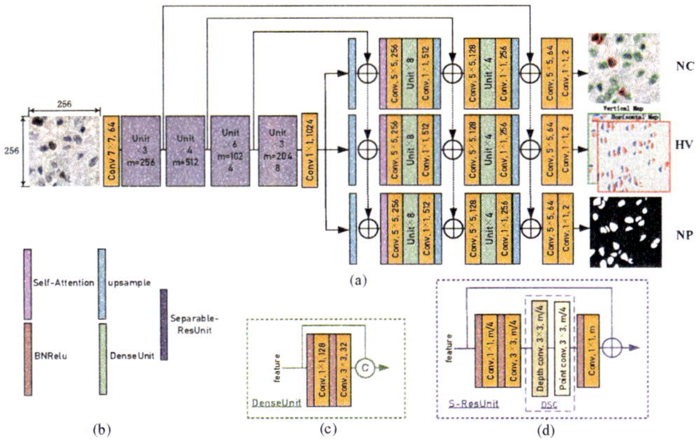


**Fig. 2.** Illustration of our SRSA-net. **a** SRSA-net architecture. **b** Illustration of different operations in (**a**). **c** DenseUnit. **d** Separable ResUnit.

### 2.2 Decoder

The feature maps from the same encoder are input to three paralleled decoder branches. In each decoder branch, feature maps from the third Separable ResUnit block and feature maps following the upsampling operation are firstly added and then processed by the Self-Attention block, a 5 × 5 convolution, a DenseUnit block and a 1 × 1 convolution. The stacked feature maps are upsampled and added with feature maps from the second Separable ResUnit block. Subsequently, a 5 × 5 convolution, a DenseUnit block and a 1 × 1 convolution are applied to perform feature decoding. Finally, the feature maps are upsampled and added with feature maps from the first Separable ResUnit block. The added feature maps are processed by a 5 × 5 convolution and a 1 × 1 convolution to generate the prediction (e.g., nuclei subtypes, nuclei detection and distance map regression).

The structure of the Self-Attention block [10] is shown in Fig. 3, where the calculation process can be divided into three steps:

(1) By using a 1 × 1 convolution operation, we obtain: Query ($Q$), Key ($K$) and Value ($V$), where the number of feature map channels for $Q$ and $K$ should be the same.
(2) The similarity is calculated by matrix multiplication of $Q$ and the transpose of $K$, which is then processed by the *softmax* function, i.e.,

$$A = softmax(QK^T) \tag{1}$$

(3) The attention map $A$ is multiplied with $V$ and then processed by a 1x1 convolution to get the final output feature maps F, i.e.,

$$F = conv(AV) \tag{2}$$

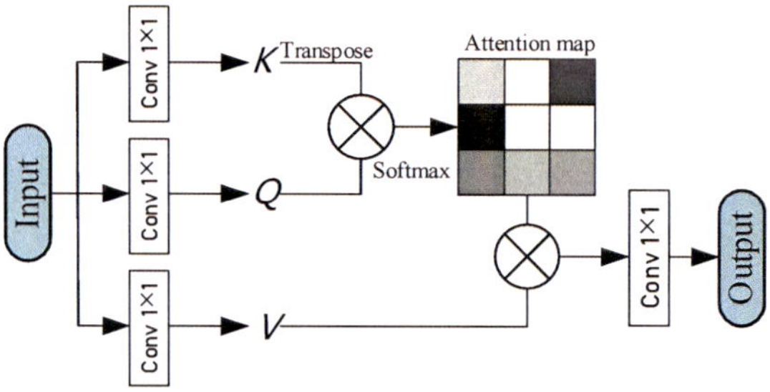


**Fig. 3.** Self-attention mechanism.

### 2.3 Loss Function

We take advantage of a general multi-task loss function [6] for optimization of our SRSA-Net. In addition to weighting parameters in three decoder branches, the weight parameters of encoder block also need to be updated. All weighting parameters are updated by using the following loss function that is defined as:

$$L = \lambda_a L_a + \lambda_b L_b + \lambda_c L_c + \lambda_d L_d + \lambda_e L_e + \lambda_f L_f \tag{3}$$

where $L_a$, $L_b$ are the mean squared errors computed by using predicted horizontal and vertical (HV) distances, gradient maps of HV distances and corresponding ground truths. $L_c$, $L_d$ separately denote cross-entropy loss and Dice loss in nuclei segmentation task with respect to the NP branch. $L_e$, $L_f$ separately denote cross-entropy loss and Dice loss in nuclei classification task with respect to the NC branch. $\lambda_{a...f}$ are hyperparameters, where $\lambda_b$ is set as 2 and the other weighting parameters are set as 1, by following the reference [6].

### 2.4 Post Processing

In HV distance maps, adjacent nuclear pixels belonging to different nuclear instances have a significant difference, which lays the fundamental to separate overlapping cell nuclei. Let us denote $p_x$, $p_y$ as the predicted HV distance maps, $H_x$, $H_y$ as the gradient maps computed from predicted HV distance maps by Sobel kernels. The maximum of HV gradient maps represents nuclear boundary, which is computed as:

$$S_m = max(H_x(p_x), H_y(p_y)) \tag{4}$$

According to the $S_m$, energy map $E$ and marker map $M$ are obtained and then applied to further separate overlapping cell nuclei, i.e.,

$$E = [1 - \tau(S_m, k)] \times \tau(q, h) \tag{5}$$

$$M = \sigma(\tau(q, h) - \tau(S_m, k)) \tag{6}$$

where $\tau(x, t)$ is a threshold function that set $x$ to 1 when the value is above $t$ or 0 otherwise. $q$ denotes nuclei pixel prediction and $\sigma$ is a rectifier that sets all negative values to 0. Note that $h$ and $k$ are empirically set as 0.5. The energy map $E$ and marker map $M$ obtained from this operation are applied to separate nuclei detection result output by the NP branch with the marker-controlled watershed algorithm.

## 3 Experiments

In this section, we first provide dataset and evaluation criteria used in our experiments, and then conduct ablation and comparison evaluations to illustrate the advantages of our SRSA-Net in nuclei segmentation and classification.

### 3.1 Dataset & Evaluation Criteria

*IHC dataset:* There are totally 256 IHC image patches selected from the tissue microarray (TMA) of NSCLC patients, of which 194, 36 and 35 images are used in training, validation and testing, respectively. Multiplex IHC stained images including CD3, CD20, CD38, CDK4, Cyclin-D1, Ki67, P53, CD34, CD68, D2-40, FAP, and SMA were collected from Liaoning Cancer Hospital and Institute in China. There are two categories of annotated cell nuclei: negative (blue color) and positive (brown color). There are in total 9,724 manually labeled cell nuclei in our IHC dataset.

*Evaluation criteria*: We use the ensemble Dice (Dice2) [11], Aggregated Jaccard Index (AJI) [12] and Panoptic Quality (PQ) [13] to evaluate nuclei segmentation performance, and the $F_c$ score of every nuclear type [6] to evaluate nuclei classification performance. In our experimentation, we denote the corresponding $F_c$ score as $F_c^n$ and $F_c^p$ for negative and positive cell nuclei, respectively.

### 3.2 Ablation Experiment

In order to evaluate the effect of different modules that are incorporated in our SRSA-Net, we conduct the following ablation experiments.

*SR-Net*: Using Separable ResUnit blocks to replace ResUnit blocks based on the Hover-Net [6];
*SRSA-Net*: Adding the Self-Attention mechanism before the first 5 × 5 convolution based on the SR-Net;
*SRSA-Net-II*: Adding the Self-Attention mechanism behind the first 5 × 5 convolution based on the SR-Net;
*SRSA-Net-III*: Adding Self-Attention layers before the first and the second 5 × 5 convolutions based on the SR-Net.

Table 1 lists ablation experiments on the IHC dataset. Among different configurations, the SRSA-Net achieves the overall best performance, with the highest values of Dice2 (0.758), AJI (0.627), PQ (0.625) and $F_c^p$ (0.735). This indicates the efficacy of the SRSA-Net that makes use of separable ResUnit blocks in encoder and self-attention blocks before the first 5 × 5 convolution in three decoders.

**Table 1.** Ablation experiments on the IHC dataset.

| | Segmentation | | | Classification | |
|---|---|---|---|---|---|
| | Dice2 | AJI | PQ | $F_c^n$ | $F_c^p$ |
| SR-Net | 0.754 | 0.626 | 0.622 | **0.794** | 0.730 |
| SRSA-Net | **0.758** | **0.627** | **0.625** | 0.792 | **0.735** |
| SRSA-Net-II | 0.736 | 0.600 | 0.592 | 0.776 | 0.653 |
| SRSA-Net-III | 0.713 | 0.550 | 0.529 | 0.718 | 0.663 |

### 3.3 Comparison Experiment

In order to further evaluate the efficacy of the SRSA-Net, we retrained and independently tested several generalized models including the U-Net [14], NucleiSegNet [15], Deeplabv3+ [16], and Hover-Net [6] on the IHC dataset. Comparative results are listed in Table 2, which show that the SRSA-Net provides significant improvements in nuclei segmentation and classification over comparative models. Note that U-Net, NucleiSeg-Net and Deeplabv3+ were only designed for nuclei segmentation, and hence they do not have classification evaluation results.

**Table 2.** Comparison experiments on the IHC dataset.

| | Segmentation | | | Classification | |
|---|---|---|---|---|---|
| | Dice2 | AJI | PQ | $F_c^n$ | $F_c^p$ |
| U-net [14] | 0.633 | 0.488 | 0.464 | 0.579 | 0.512 |
| NucleiSegNet [15] | 0.650 | 0.505 | 0.470 | 0.627 | 0.524 |
| Deeplabv3+ [16] | 0.719 | 0.575 | 0.546 | 0.656 | 0.563 |
| Hover-net [6] | 0.747 | 0.610 | 0.612 | 0.783 | 0.716 |
| SRSA-net | **0.758** | **0.627** | **0.625** | **0.792** | **0.735** |

Figure 4 Shows visual comparison results by using different deep learning models and ground truths on CDK4, CD20 and CD3 IHC images, respectively. We apply color-deconvolution to split channels and use dab-channel images to identify positive nuclei in U-Net, NucleiSegNet and Deeplabv3+ for visual comparison. As observed in Fig. 4. (e.g., regions with superimposed blue circles), the SRSA-Net has shown a superior capability in identifying small cell nuclei and splitting cell nuclei clusters in IHC images.

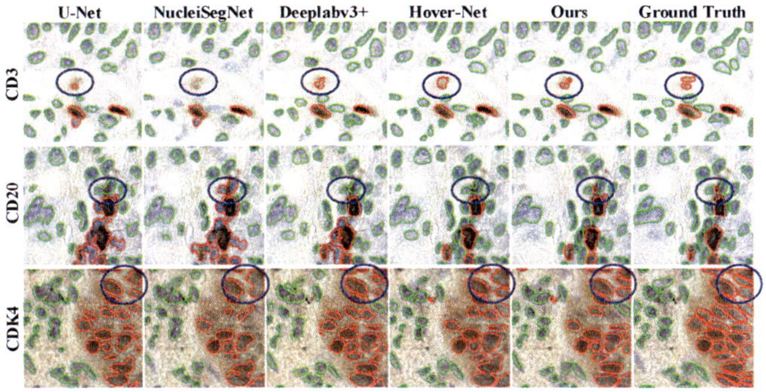


**Fig. 4.** Visual comparative results by using U-Net [14], NucleiSegNet [15], Deeplabv3+ [16], Hover-Net [6], SRSA-Net and ground truths on multiplex IHC images. Note that overlapped red, green contours highlight identified positive and negative cell nuclei in IHC images.

## 4 Conclusion

This paper presents a multi-task learning model termed as the SRSA-Net for simultaneous nuclei segmentation and classification in IHC images of NSCLC patients. The SRSA-Net is designed based on separable ResUnit and self-attention blocks, which help the model achieve state-of-the-art performance compared with other deep learning models. By using our proposed model, pathologists could effectively quantify the number and proportion of positive and negative cell nuclei in IHC images, which assists in quantifying the TIME of cancer patients for precise diagnosis and prognosis.

**Acknowledgment.** This study was supported by the National Key Research and Development Program of China (2022YFC3902100), the National Natural Science Foundation of China (82102135) and the Fundamental Research Funds for the Central Universities (DUT22YG114).

## References

1. Lu, C., et al.: Nuclear shape and orientation features from H&E images predict survival in early-stage estrogen receptor-positive breast cancers. Lab. Invest. **98**(11), 1438–1448 (2018)
2. Key, M.: Immunohistochemistry staining methods. In: Education Guide Immunohistochemical Staining Methods, 4th Edition, vol. 47 (2006)
3. Binnewies, M., et al.: Understanding the tumor immune microenvironment (TIME) for effective therapy. Nat. Med. **24**(5), 541–550 (2018)
4. Otsu, N.: A threshold selection method from gray-level histograms. IEEE Trans. Syst. Man Cybern. **9**(1), 62–66 (1979)
5. Breiman, L.: Random forests. Mach. Learn. **45**(1), 5–32 (2001)
6. Graham, S., et al.: Hover-net: Simultaneous segmentation and classification of nuclei in multi-tissue histology images. Med. Image Anal. **58**, 101563 (2019)
7. Ghahremani, P., et al.: Deep learning-inferred multiplex immunofluorescence for immunohistochemical image quantification. Nat. Mach. Intell. **4**(4), 401–412 (2022)
8. Yao K., et al.: PointNu-Net: simultaneous multi-tissue histology nuclei segmentation and classification in the clinical wild (2021). arXiv:2111.01557
9. Sifre, L., Stéphane, M.: Rigid-motion scattering for texture classification (2014). arXiv:1403.1687
10. Zhang, H., et al.: Self-attention generative adversarial networks. ICML. PMLR (2019)
11. Vu, Q.D., et al.: Methods for segmentation and classification of digital microscopy tissue images. Front Bioeng Biotech **53** (2019)
12. Kumar, N., et al.: A dataset and a technique for generalized nuclear segmentation for computational pathology. IEEE T Med Imaging **36**(7), 1550–1560 (2017)
13. Kirillov, A., et al.: Panoptic segmentation. In: Proceedings of the IEEE Conference on Computer Vision and Pattern Recognition, Germany (2019)
14. Ronneberger, O., Fischer, P., Brox, T.: U-net: convolutional networks for biomedical image segmentation. MICCAI. Springer, Cham (2015)
15. Lal, S., et al.: NucleiSegNet: robust deep learning architecture for the nuclei segmentation of liver cancer histopathology images. Comput Biol Med **128**, 104075 (2021)
16. Chen, L.-C., et al.: Encoder-decoder with atrous separable convolution for semantic image segmentation. In: Proceedings of the ECCV, USA, 2018 (2018)

# Developmental Pattern of Individual Morphometric Similarity Network in the Human Fetal Brain

R. Zhao[1], X. Xu[1], Z. Zhao[1], M. Li[1], R. Chen[1], Y. Shen[1], C. Sun[2], G. Wang[3], and D. Wu[1](✉)

[1] College of Biomedical Engineering & Instrument Science, Zhejiang University, Zheda Road, Hangzhou, China
danwu.bme@zju.edu.cn

[2] Department of Radiology, Institute of Geriatric Medicine, Beijing Hospital, National Center of Gerontology, Chinese Academy of Medical Sciences, Beijing, China

[3] Department of Radiology, Shandong Provincial Hospital, Shandong First Medical University, Jinan, China

**Abstract.** The development of cerebral cortex during the fetal period is complex yet well-coordinated. MRI-based morphological brain network provides a powerful tool for describing this process at a network level. Due to the challenges of in-utero MRI acquisition and image processing, the fetal brain morphological network has not been established. In this study, utilizing high-resolution in-utero MRI image, we constructed individual morphometric similarity network for each fetus based on multiple cortical features and characterized the spatiotemporal changes of morphological connections and the network topology. Edge analysis demonstrated a decline of morphological symmetry between hemispheres, especially for the parietal cortex. The limbic and parieto-occipital regions exhibited the most drastic changes of network connections. Graph theoretical analysis indicated that the small-world structure of the network appeared as early as 22 weeks and that the network topology exhibited an enhanced integration and reduced segregation during the prenatal period. In summary, this study provides an important evidence for understanding the normal development of fetal brain connectome during second-third trimester.

**Keywords:** Fetal brain · In-utero MRI · Morphometric similarity network · Small-world · Integration and segregation

## 1 Introduction

The development of cerebral cortex during fetal period is complex yet well-coordinated. A range of histogenetic processes occur successively, including neural proliferation and migration, axonal growth and dendritic differentiation [1]. These processes are coordinated between spatially distinct regions of cortex, resulting in the similar developmental trajectories of these regions.


G. Wang et al. (Eds.): APCMBE 2023, IFMBE Proceedings 103, pp. 113–120, 2024.
https://doi.org/10.1007/978-3-031-51455-5_14

The morphological brain network based on magnetic resonance imaging (MRI) provides a useful tool for describing these coordinated developments. In recent years, many studies on morphological brain network during the early development have emerged. These studies demonstrated a nonrandom modular organization and small-world topology of networks at birth [2, 3]. Further, an increasing segregation and decreasing integration in the structural covariance network (SCN) was observed during infancy and childhood (0–6 years) [4]. Although morphological network has been intensively investigated during infancy and childhood, configurations of fetal morphological network have not been established, probably due to the challenges in the data acquisition and processing. The only study using fetal specimens between 14 and 22 weeks indicated an immature and inefficient network organization with low integration and high segregation during the early second trimester [5].

SCN and morphometric similarity network (MSN) are two major types of morphological network. SCN that utilizes single cortical feature may exhibit inconsistent trends with different features [2–4]. Also, SCN usually performs at the group level and is unable to represent individual variability. The MSN approach using a combination of cortical features can avoid these problems, provide a comprehensive characterization of inter-regional morphological similarity and allow us to construct the individual network.

In this work, using 3T high resolution in-utero MRI, we constructed individual MSNs for fetuses from 22 to 39 weeks gestational age (GA). The developmental patterns of inter-regional connections during the second-to-third trimester were characterized. We also used the graph theoretical model to explore whether the small-world topology exist in the fetal brain and how network topology reorganize with prenatal development. For validation, this MSN pipeline was also applied to neonates from the developing human connectome project (dHCP) with postmenstrual age (PMA) at scan between 28 and 38 weeks.

## 2 Materials and Methods

### 2.1 Participants and Data Acquisition

We collected MRI data at Shandong Provincial Hospital from October 2019 to September 2021. Ethical approval and written informed parental consent from each subject were obtained.

T2-weighted images were acquired on 3.0 T Siemens MAGNEOM Skyra scanner (Siemens Healthcare, Erlangen, Germany) with an 18-channel body coil using HASTE sequence with the following parameters: repetition time = 800 ms, echo time = 113 ms, slice thickness = 2 mm, no slice gap, in-plane resolution = $1.1 \times 1.1$ mm$^2$, FOV = 280 $\times$ 280 mm$^2$. Each fetal brain was scanned several times in multiple orthogonal planes. Fetuses with radiological brain abnormalities (e.g., ventriculomegaly and asymmetrical ventricles) and visible motion artifacts on MR images were excluded. We finally included 91 fetuses within the GA range of 22.57–39 weeks (Fig. 1a).

### 2.2 Image Reconstruction and Preprocessing

The 3D volume was reconstructed from 2D stacks of multiple orientations. Briefly, we manually selected 2D multislice stacks with minimal inter-slice motion. Then, the fetal brain was extracted using brain location tool [6] and the N4 bias field correction was performed [7]. After that the 3D fetal brain volume was reconstructed from 2D stacks at 0.8mm isotropic resolution using NiftyMIC [6], with iterative slice-to-volume registration (SVR) and super-resolution reconstruction (SRR).

Image preprocessing was performed by a modified dHCP-structural-pipeline [8] (Fig. 1c). Briefly, the cortical gray matter (cGM) label was first segmented and manually refined. Then, the cortical surfaces were generated and a number of cortical morphological features were calculated, including mean curvature, gauss curvature, curvedness, sulcal depth, cortical thickness and surface area. Each fetal brain was parcellated utilizing the CRL atlas [9] which provided a set of 78 cortical regions. And the volume parcellation was then mapped to the surface space.

### 2.3 Morphometric Similarity Matrix (MSM)

Each cortical feature was averaged within each parcel and normalized (z-scored) across all parcels in each individual. Pearson's correlation between the vectors of cortical features from each pair of parcels was performed to obtain a 78 * 78 morphometric similarity matrix for each fetal brain (Fig. 1d).

### 2.4 Network Analysis

The edge strengths of contralateral homologous regions and the average edge strength of matrix were extracted. GA-dependent changes of all edges were evaluated using Pearson's correlation. At the node level, the numbers of edges with significantly GA-dependence (adjusted $p < 0.05$) were mapped to nodes, and we evaluated the correlations between GA and average nodal connection strengths (average of all edges connected to the node). All p-values were adjusted using the false discovery rate method.

Each matrix was binarized based on the 26–35% sparsity, where 26% was the minimum sparsity to ensure no isolated node in the network. The following properties were computed in GRETNA toolkit [10]: clustering coefficient (Cp); characteristic path length (Lp); small-worldness (sigma); global efficiency; local efficiency.

### 2.5 Validation Analysis

For validation, we included 42 preterm-born neonates from dHCP Release 3 with PMA at scan between 28 and 38 weeks (Fig. 1b) and compared the results with the fetal data.

## 3 Results

### 3.1 Development of Edges and Nodes in MSM

We observed a reduction of contralateral homologous connection strength in the whole brain, especially the parietal lobe (Fig. 2a) and a decline of the average edge strength of the matrix (Fig. 2b). Further, we evaluated the effects of GA on all edges of the matrix. The edges with the strongest positive correlation with GA were mainly between

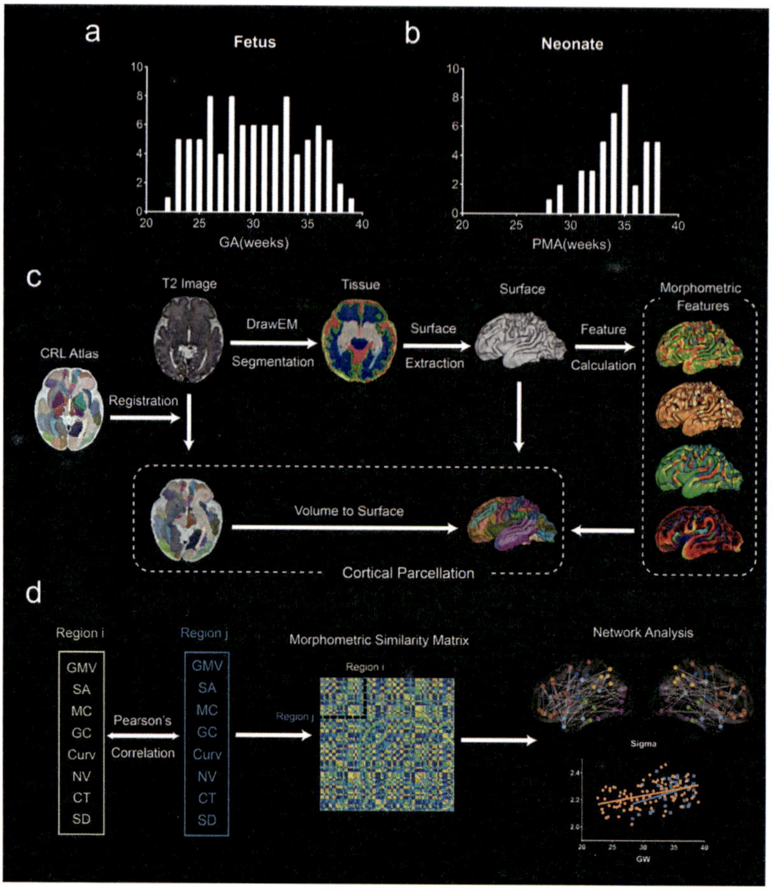


**Fig. 1.** The frequency distribution of GA for fetuses (**a**) and PMA at scan for dHCP neonates (**b**). (**c**) The processing pipeline of fetal brain MRI. (**d**) The construction and analysis of fetal brain MSN.

the temporal poles and the insula/the medial superior frontal gyri (Fig. 2c); while the edges with the strongest negative correlation were mainly between the cingulate gyri and the parahippocampal gyri/the temporal poles of the middle temporal gyri (Fig. 2d), illustrating the rapid development of the limbic regions.

At the node level, we found that more edges positively correlated with GA in the limbic regions (the parahippocampal gyri, the cingulate gyri, the olfactory cortices) (Fig. 2e) and more edges negatively correlated with GA in the parieto-occipital regions (the superior and inferior parietal gyri, the superior occipital gyri and the angular gyri) (Fig. 2f). The average nodal connection strength showed the similar spatial pattern (Fig. 2g). The nodes significantly positively correlated with GA mainly localized in the limbic cortex, while nodes negatively correlated with GA mainly localized in the parieto-occipital cortex.

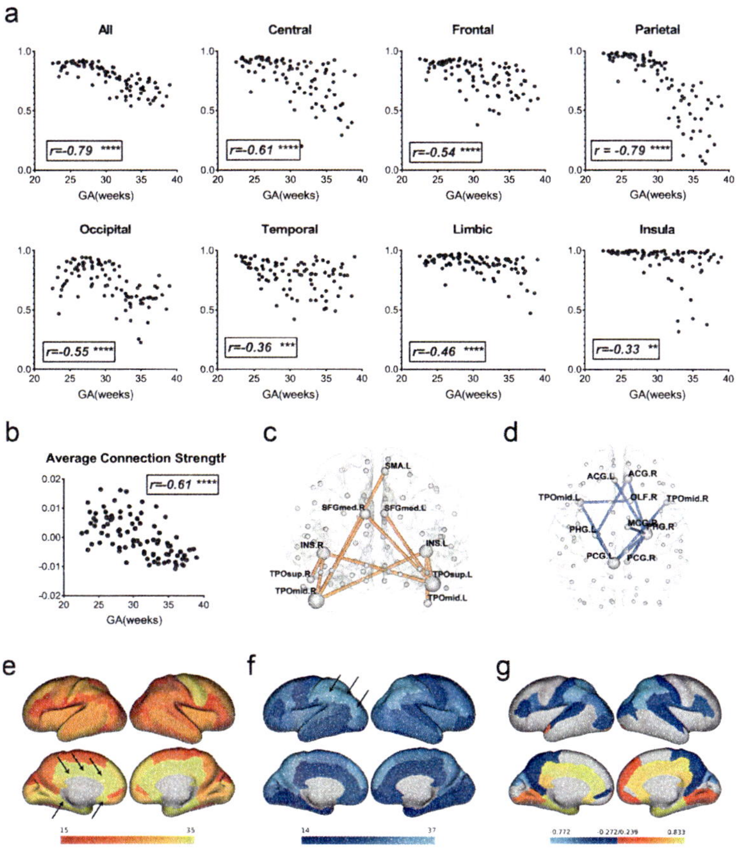


**Fig. 2.** **a** The GA-related changes of contralateral homologous connections between hemispheres in the whole brain and each cortical lobe. **b** The GA-related changes of whole-brain average connection strength. **c** Top ten edges with the strongest positive correlation with GA. **d** Top ten edges with strongest negative correlation with GA. **e** The number of edges that were significantly positively correlated with GA (adjusted $p < 0.05$) in each cortical parcel. **f** The number of edges that were significantly negatively correlated with GA (adjusted $p < 0.05$). **g** The correlation coefficients between GA and average connection strength of the nodes in each parcel. *P value < 0.05, **P value < 0.01, ***P value < 0.001, ****P value < 0.0001.

## 3.2 Development of Network Properties

The MSNs of all fetal brains showed sigma > 1, indicating the appearance of small-world topology before 22 weeks (the earliest GA in our study) (Fig. 3a). We found that Cp, Lp and local efficiency significantly decreased with GA and global efficiency significantly increased with GA, suggesting an enhanced integration and weakened segregation of the individual MSN during the prenatal period. The AUCs of network properties confirmed these findings (Fig. 3b). The results from fetal brain were also inline that from the neonatal brain.

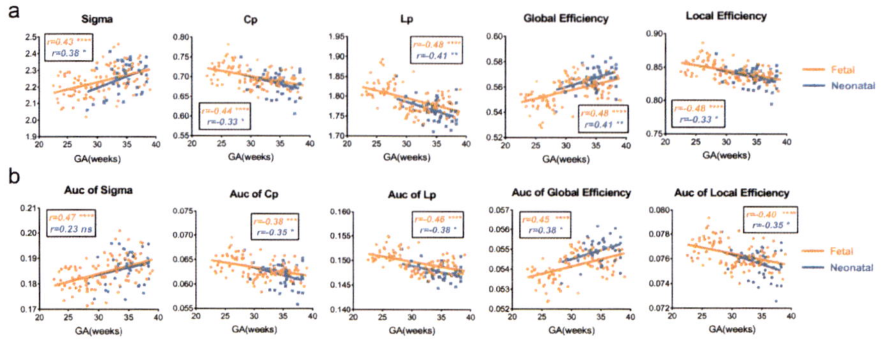


**Fig. 3.** **a** The development of network properties based on the 26% sparsity. **b** The development of the AUCs of network properties based on the 26–35% sparsities.

# 4 Discussion

## 4.1 Developmental Trajectories of Morphometric Similarity

Combining multiple cortical features, the MSN can integrate complementary developmental patterns to synthetically portray morphometric similarities between brain regions. We found the significant negative correlation between whole-brain average connection strength and GA, suggesting the further morphological differentiation and increasing structural complexity during the fetal period. By extracting the homologous morphological connections, we also proved that the structural asymmetry reported in the infant and adult study [11, 12] already existed during the second trimester.

The drastic changes of morphological connections were mainly associated with limbic and parieto-occipital regions. This finding may be linked with the asynchronous cortical folding and the different cortical growth rates between brain regions. The calcarine and parieto-occipital fissures and cingulate sulcus (outlining the developing limbic lobe) have appeared before the second trimester. In our previous study, the parietal lobe was proved to be the earliest develop [13]. Another study revealed that the parietal and occipital regions had greater volume increases during 20–28 weeks [14]. Further, more rapid development took place in the occipital cortex between 30 and 40 weeks PMA [15]. In a word, the timing and scale of cortical maturation during the fetal period can be reflected by GA-dependence of morphological profiles.

## 4.2 Small-World Structure of Fetal Brain

Another significant finding is that the small-world property of fetal morphological network is already present as early as 22 weeks, suggesting the coexistence of local specialization for segregation and global connection for integration in the fetal brain. In a previous study, structural covariance demonstrated the characteristic small-world topology in neonates [2]. This finding inspired us to explore when the small-world topology appears and how it develops in-utero. In functional networks and white matter networks, the earliest appearance of small-world architecture was found around 20 weeks [16, 17]. In terms of morphological connectome, Xu et al. established a SCN for fetal brain specimens between 14 to 22 weeks and found an immature and inefficient organizations during the early second trimester [5]. Notably, this conclusion was drawn from a qualitative comparison with term-born neonates. Overall, the configuration of prenatal morphological network has been not fully established. Our study filled this gap and verified the existence of small-world topology as early as 22 weeks (earliest GA in our study).

We further explored the dynamic reorganization of network during the prenatal period. We found an enhanced integration and reduced segregation of fetal brain network, which also were validated in the dHCP cohort. Xu et al. found that the fetal SCN had lower integration and higher segregation relative to the neonatal SCN [5], consistent with our findings. Possibly, long-range connections gradually emerge during the prenatal period, allowing for shortening the path length between distant nodes and accelerating global information transfer; while short-range connections within local communities are pruned, and some weak connections gradually disappear. Overall, this study provided complementary information of life-span development trajectories of brain network.

## 5 Conclusion

Using high-resolution in-utero MRI, we presented the first study of fetal morphological brain network and revealed the spatiotemporal developmental pattern of the morphometric similarity and the dynamic reorganization of the network topology. The drastic changes of network were mainly associated with the parieto-occipital and limbic regions. Graph theoretical analysis demonstrated the appearance of small-world organization as early as 22 weeks, and the network topology exhibited an enhanced integration and weakened segregation during the prenatal period. This study filled a gap in the prenatal brain network research and provided an important evidence for understanding fetal brain development in-utero.

## References

1. Kostović, I., Sedmak, G., Judaš, M.: Neural histology and neurogenesis of the human fetal and infant brain. Neuroimage **188**, 743–773 (2019)
2. Fan, Y., Shi, F., Smith, J.K., et al.: Brain anatomical networks in early human brain development. Neuroimage **54**, 1862–1871 (2011)
3. Nie, J., Li, G., Wang, L., et al.: Longitudinal development of cortical thickness, folding, and fiber density networks in the first 2 years of life. Hum. Brain Mapp. **35**, 3726–3737 (2014)
4. Woodburn, M., Bricken, C.L., Wu, Z., et al.: The maturation and cognitive relevance of structural brain network organization from early infancy to childhood. Neuroimage **238**, 118232 (2021)
5. Xu, F., Liu, M., Kim, S.Y., et al.: Morphological development trajectory and structural covariance network of the human fetal cortical plate during the early second trimester. Cereb. Cortex **31**, 4794–4807 (2021)
6. Ebner, M., Wang, G., Li, W., et al.: An automated framework for localization, segmentation and super-resolution reconstruction of fetal brain MRI. Neuroimage **206**, 116324 (2020)
7. Tustison, N.J., Avants, B.B., Cook, P.A., et al.: N4ITK: improved N3 Bias correction. IEEE Trans. Med. Imaging **29**, 1310–1320 (2010)

8. Makropoulos, A., Robinson, E.C., Schuh, A., et al.: The developing human connectome project: a minimal processing pipeline for neonatal cortical surface reconstruction. Neuroimage **173**, 88–112 (2018)
9. Gholipour, A., Rollins, C.K., Velasco-Annis, C., et al.: A normative spatiotemporal MRI atlas of the fetal brain for automatic segmentation and analysis of early brain growth. Sci. Rep. **7**, 476 (2017)
10. Wang, J., Wang, X., Xia, M., et al.: GRETNA: a graph theoretical network analysis toolbox for imaging connectomics. Front. Hum. Neurosci. **9** (2015)
11. Gilmore, J.H., Lin, W., Prastawa, M.W., et al.: Regional gray matter growth, sexual dimorphism, and cerebral asymmetry in the neonatal brain. J. Neurosci. **27**, 1255–1260 (2007)
12. Kong, X.-Z., Mathias, S.R., Guadalupe, T., et al.: Mapping cortical brain asymmetry in 17,141 healthy individuals worldwide via the ENIGMA Consortium. Proc. Natl. Acad. Sci. **115**, E5154–E5163 (2018)
13. Xu, X., Sun, C., Sun, J., et al.: Spatiotemporal atlas of the fetal brain depicts cortical developmental gradient. J. Neurosci. **42**, 9435–9449 (2022)
14. Rajagopalan, V., Scott, J., Habas, P.A., et al.: Local tissue growth patterns underlying normal fetal human brain gyrification quantified in utero. J. Neurosci. **31**, 2878–2887 (2011)
15. Moeskops, P., Benders, M.J., Kersbergen, K.J., et al.: Development of cortical morphology evaluated with longitudinal MR brain images of preterm infants. Plos One **10**, e0131552 (2015)
16. Song, L., Mishra, V., Ouyang, M., et al.: Human fetal brain connectome: structural network development from middle fetal stage to birth. Front. Neurosci. **11** (2017)
17. Turk, E., van den Heuvel, M.I., Benders, M.J., et al.: Functional connectome of the fetal brain. J. Neurosci. **39**, 9716–9724 (2019)

# Automatic Segmentation of Liver Tumor from Multi-phase Contrast-Enhanced CT Images Using Cross-Phase Fusion Transformer

Wencong Zhang[1], Yuxi Tao[2], Wei Liang[1], Junjie Li[1], Yingjia Chen[1], Tengfei Song[2], Xiangyuan Ma[1(✉)], and Yaqin Zhang[2]

[1] Department of Biomedical Engineering, College of Engineering, Shantou University, 243 Daxue Road, Shantou, Guangdong, China
zhyaqin@mail.sysu.edu.cn, maxiangyuan@stu.edu.cn

[2] Department of Radiology, The Fifth Affiliated Hospital of Sun Yat-Sen University, 52 East Meihua Road, New Xiangzhou, Zhuhai, China
{zhyaqin,zhyaqin}@mail.sysu.edu.cn

**Abstract.** Multi-phase contrast-enhanced CT images can provide abundant and complementary tumor information, and thus radiologists often use multi-phase images to assist in segmenting and diagnosing liver tumors. However, the current multi-stage liver tumor segmentation methods are based on convolutional neural networks (CNNs), which make them ineffective in extracting global information during the multi-phase information fusion process. In this study, we propose a novel multi-phase liver tumor segmentation approach using delayed phase images to aid in portal vein phase tumor segmentation. The proposed method employs a Transformer structure to extract both global information and local information of tumors, which contributes to the precise segmentation of tumor boundaries. More importantly, we design a cross-phase aggregator (CFA), which facilitates the bidirectional interaction of cross-phase features to take full advantage of the complementary information from multi-phase images. A dataset of 164 multi-phase abdominal CT scans was collected with Institutional Review Board approval to evaluate the performance of the proposed approach. The experimental results showed that the proposed approach can better utilize multi-phase information and is superior to several state-of-the-art methods. Ablation study is performed to further validate the effectiveness of each module in the proposed model. The proposed method has the potential to assist radiologists to locate more accurate liver tumors and improve their diagnosis efficiency.

**Keywords:** Multi-phase · Liver tumor segmentation · Deep learning · Transformer · Cross-phase aggregator

Xiangyuan Ma contributed equally to this work.


G. Wang et al. (Eds.): APCMBE 2023, IFMBE Proceedings 103, pp. 121–130, 2024.
https://doi.org/10.1007/978-3-031-51455-5_15

## 1 Introduction

Liver cancer is a severe and fatal form of cancer that affects millions of individuals across the globe [1]. As per the World Cancer Research Fund International's data from 2020, liver cancer ranks as the sixth most common cancer and third leading cause of cancer-related deaths globally [2]. Early detection of liver lesions is very crucial for effective liver cancer treatment. Traditionally, radiologists have detected and diagnosed tumors by manually segmenting liver tumors, which is time-consuming, difficult to produce, and susceptible to subjective personal experience. Therefore, it is essential to develop an automatic and accurate method for liver tumor segmentation.

Single-phase computed tomography (CT) images have been used to segment liver tumors in most existing liver tumor segmentation (LiTS) methods [3–8]. However, these methods often fail to achieve satisfactory results due to inherent problems such as low contrast of medical images and blurred tumor boundaries. Therefore, some multi-phase-based segmentation methods for liver tumors have been proposed [9–11]. Compared to single images, multi-phase images can provide rich and complementary information of tumors, in which tumor areas are different from other tissues in morphology or grayscale. The multi-phase contrast-enhanced CT images are acquired in four phases: the noncontract-enhanced (NC) phase, arterial (ART) phase, portal vein (PV) phase and delay (DL) phase. Among the four phases, the PV phase is the preferred stage for liver tumor segmentation because the maximum contrast between the tumor and the surrounding liver tissue occurs in the PV phase. However, not all types of tumors are evident in the PV stage, hence we also need to employ other phases to assist in the segmentation of liver tumors [10].

The current multi-phase liver tumor segmentation methods can be categorized in accordance with multi-phase fusion strategies: input-level fusion (ILF) methods [12], decision-level fusion (DLF) methods [12–14] and feature-level fusion (FLF) methods [8, 10, 11]. Under these three fusion strategies, the FLF methods can achieve the best performance because they exploited the features from multiple phases. Wu et al. [9] proposed an MW-UNet, which integrated different phases by weighting their features from hidden layers of U-Net [6]. Xu et al. [10] developed a PA-ResSeg model based on residual networks [15] that re-weights features from different phases using the channel-attention mechanism. Zhang et al. [11] modified the PA-ResSeg with a spatial aggregation module (SAM) and a uncertain region inpainting module (URIM) to further improve the performance of liver tumor segmentation. Although known FLF methods focus on inter-phase relationships, it is still difficult to fully utilize the key global cues between different phases due to the inherent limitations of CNNs in extracting features in local sliding windows.

In recent years, Transformer has shown excellent performance not only in natural language processing (NLP) tasks [16], but also in semantic segmentation [17–19]. Because the Transformer based methods are better at leveraging global information and modeling long-term dependencies than the CNN approach, some studies have begun to apply the Transformer approach to medical image analyzing tasks [18, 20]. These methods utilize the self-attention mechanism of transformers to selectively focus on important regions of the image, allowing for better global feature extraction and improved segmentation performance. Therefore, Transformer based architecture has the potential to better utilizes information from different phases.

In this study, we propose a framework for accurate liver tumors segmentation from multiphase contrast-enhanced CT images. Specifically, our method takes advantage of the complementary information from delayed phase (DL) images to assist in segmenting liver tumors in portal venous (PV) phase images. We introduce the Transformer architecture into the traditional encoder-decoder structure to facilitate the model to fully learn the explicit global information. More importantly, we design a cross-phase aggregator to better exploit the features from PV and DL phases for comprehensively multi-phase information fusion. Specifically, our contributions can be summarized as follows: (1) Based on the tokens-to-tokens vision Transformer (T2T-ViT) architecture, we build a symmetric Transformer Encoder-Decoder architecture with skip-connection. In the encoder, the local and global information is extracted by self-attention, and in the decoder, the local and global features are up-sampled to the input resolution for corresponding pixel-level liver tumor prediction. (2) The designed cross-phase aggregator that can efficiently utilize the complementary information from DL phase images to help the tumor segmentation in PV phase images.

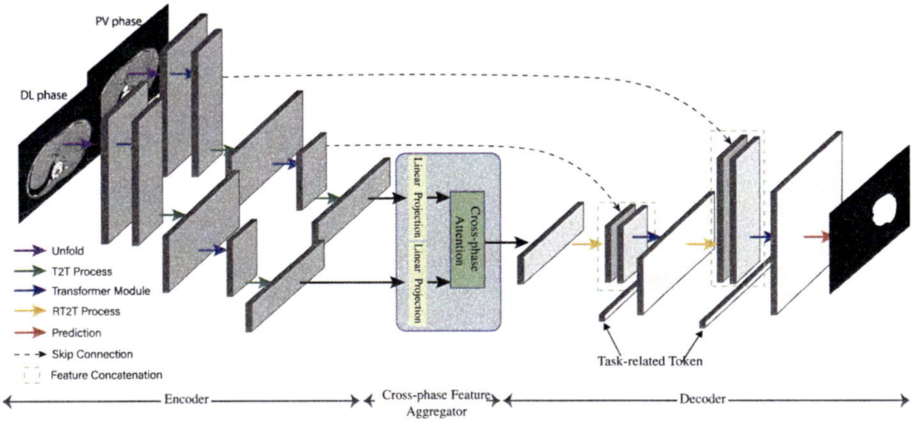


**Fig. 1.** Illustration of our proposed multi-phase liver tumor segmentation framework.

## 2 Method

In this paper, we propose a multi-phase liver tumor segmentation framework consisting of the encoder, cross-phase feature aggregator (CFA), decoder, and skip connection as Fig. 1. Tokens-to-tokens (T2T) strategy is used in the framework. Given input multi-phase (PV and DL phases) images and their multi-phase features are extracted utilizing the encoder. The multi-phase feature tokens generated in the encoder are interacted in the cross-phase feature aggregator, which also outputs feature tokens for the decoder. In the decoder, the Reverse T2T process gradually recovers the resolution of the features. In order to improve the capacity of global cue utilization and reduce tumor boundary ambiguity, we apply self-attention [16] in both the encoder and decoder. Furthermore, a task-related token and a skip connection mechanism assist in the recovery of finer segmentation results.

### 2.1 Encoder

Comparing the wide-applying convolution encoder module, we adopt the T2T-ViT model [17–19] as the backbone, and convolutional windowing similar to that in CNN is used to locally aggregate adjacent tokens, which helps model local features.

Giving the inputs of the PV phase and DL phase image, the encoder first unfolds these images into tokens by setting $k = 7, s = 3$ and $p = 3$. Then, we perform the T2T Transformer and T2T Process twice to obtain the two phases' feature tokens separately. The dimensions of the feature token in the three stages of the encoder can be expressed as $\mathrm{T}_i^{\mathrm{PV}} \in \mathbb{R}^{l_i \times c}$ and $\mathrm{T}_i^{\mathrm{DL}} \in \mathbb{R}^{l_i \times c}$, where PV and DL denote PV phase and DL phase, separately, $i = 1, 2, 3$, and $c = 64$.

**T2T Transformer**. For a particular input token from the preceding step, a linear projection is used to project the embedding dimension from c = 64 to d = 384. Then, it is processed by the self-attention block, as formulated:

$$\mathrm{T} = \mathrm{MLP}\left(\mathrm{MSA}\left(\mathrm{T}'\right)\right) \tag{1}$$

where MSA represents the multi-head-attention mechanism with layer normalization and MLP denotes multi-layer perceptron with layer normalization in the standard transformer.

**T2T Process**. As shown in Fig. 1, after obtaining the feature tokens from the T2T Transformer, we reshaped the feature tokens as an image $I$ in the spatial dimension. Then, $I$ is split into a $k \times k$ patch that uses the overlapping of $s$ and the zero padding of $p$ to fill the image boundary. finally, the patch is unfolded into tokens sequence and the length of the output token is defined as the below formula:

$$l_0 = \left[\frac{h + 2p - k}{k - s} + 1\right] \times \left[\frac{w + 2P - k}{k - s} + 1\right] \tag{2}$$

During the two times of the T2T Process, the patch size is set as $k = [3, 3]$, the overlapping is set as $s = [1, 1]$ and the padding size is set as $P = [1, 1]$.

### 2.2 Cross-Phase Feature Aggregator

The Cross-phase feature aggregator (CFA) is introduced to better fuse the feature tokens which are output by the encoder session from PV and DL. The CFA module contains three parts, first is the linear projection, the second is the cross-phase attention, and the third part is the concatenation of the cross-phase features. The encoder output initially passes via linear projection to project the dimension to d = 384. A modified cross-phase self-attention is used to help multi-phase feature interactions and the features obtained after the interactions are aggregated, formulated as:

$$F_{PV} = Attention(Q_{PV}, K_{DL}, V_{DL}) = softmax\left(\frac{Q_{PV}K_{DL}^{T}}{\sqrt{d}}\right)V_{DL} \tag{3}$$

$$F_{DL} = Attention(Q_{DL}, K_{PV}, V_{PV}) = softmax\left(\frac{Q_{DL}K_{PV}^{T}}{\sqrt{d}}\right)V_{PV} \tag{4}$$

$$T_M = MLP(Concat(F_{PV}, F_{DL})) \tag{5}$$

where Concat represents concatenation (superimposed on channel dimension) and MLP is the multi-layer Perceptron that is used to recover the dimensional size of the superimposed C-channel.

## 2.3 Decoder

The decoder in the proposed framework is designed to decode the patch token into a significant graph. Considering that directly adopting the low-resolution feature to perform segmentation prediction cannot achieve a satisfactory result, we introduce the decoder that consists of three main components, the first is RT2T Process that gradually up-sampled the main feature tokens, and the second is Task-related Transformer Module which is aimed to perform patch-task-attention between patch token and task-related token for better improve the segmentation performance. The last one is the Prediction that utilizes the high-resolution main feature tokens to perform liver tumor prediction.

**RT2T Process.** Given the input tokens, we adopt a linear projection to extend the embedding dimension from c to $ck^2$. Then, each token is treated as a k × k image patch with $s$ overlapping and the tokens are folded as an image with P zero-padding. finally, the generated image is reshaped back to the unsampled tokens.

**Task-Related Transformer Module.** Inspired by T2T-ViT [17–19], which introduces a class token to improve the classification accuracy, we also introduce a task-related token in our proposed model to help us improve the accuracy of liver tumor segmentation.

We first concatenate a low-level PV feature from the encoder with the multi-phase feature token from the cross-phase feature aggregator to generate the main feature tokens. Then, we introduce a task-related token $T_{ts}$, and concatenate it with the main feature tokens $T_i^M$. The concatenated tokens will be processed by Transformer module. The processed tokens are divided into task-related tokens and main-phase features.

For the overall processes of the decoder, we adopt the RT2T Process and Task-related Transformer Module twice to obtain the main feature tokens at the $\frac{1}{4}$ scale, and set $k = [1, 1]$, $s = [1, 1]$, and $p = [1, 1]$ in the two RT2T Processes. To recover the major feature tokens to full resolution, we project the embedding dimension of main feature tokens from $c$ to $ck^2$ ($k = 7$). Then we fold the tokens into an image, setting $k = 7$, $s = 3$, and $p = 3$. Finally, we use a linear projection to predict the final segmentation result.

# 3 Experiment and Discussion

## 3.1 Dataset

With Institutional Review Board approval (IRB) approval, a clinical multi-phase contrast-enhanced CT liver tumor dataset was collected in this study. The dataset includes 164 multi-phase abdominal CT scans. For the source hospital of the dataset, Sun Yat-Sen University's Third Affiliated Hospital contributes to 108 cases of multiphase abdominal CT scans, and Sun Yat-Sen University's Fifth Affiliated Hospital contributes to 56 cases of multiphase abdominal CT scans.

The typology of CT images we captured included the non-contrast phase, arterial phase, portal venous phase, and delay phase. Below Table 1 shows the details of the characteristic of CT scans.

**Table 1.** Characteristic of CT scans.

| Item | Data |
|---|---|
| Format | DICOM |
| Volume range | 34 ~ 679 |
| Dimension | 512 × 512 pixels |
| Voxel spatial resolution in thickness | 2.0 ~ 5.0 $mm^3$ |
| Pixel spacing range | 0.87 mm |

## 3.2 Preprocessing

The dataset is separated into 80 and 20% for training and evaluation.

For data pre-processing, first, all the input images are set as 224 × 224. Second, we set the limit of the intensity value between −80 and 220 HU. Third, normalization is performed on these scans to eliminate interference and solve abnormal data scale distribution.

## 3.3 Experiment Configuration

For the hyperparameters and training strategies for learning, the setting of the initial learning rate is 0.0001, using the Adam gradient descent with momentum for the optimizer in the model and the binary cross entropy loss is used. For the strategy in the learning rate, occurring a reduction in the learning rate up to 10 times when the loss of training stops falling and continues for 10 times.

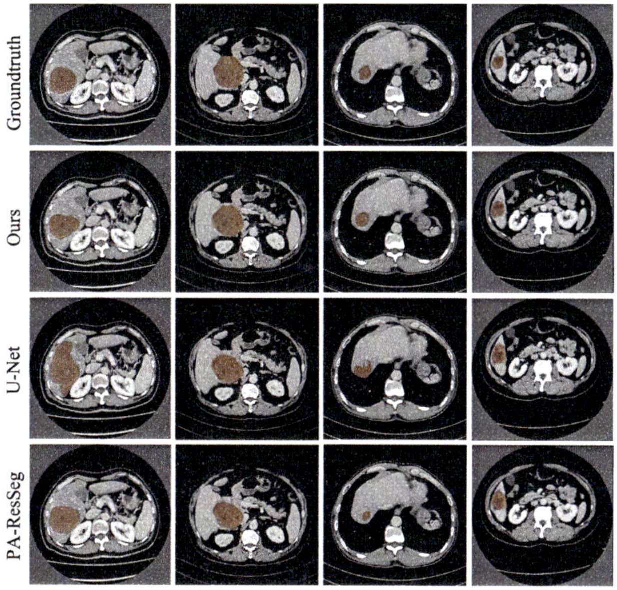


**Fig. 2.** Visual comparison between the state-of-the-art liver tumor segmentation methods and our proposed method.

### 3.4 Evaluation Metrics

We introduce three metrics for evaluation, which are Dice similarity coefficient (DSC), absolute relative volume difference (ARVD), and average symmetric surface distance (ASSD). First, the accuracy of segmentation is evaluated by the DSC and ARVD. Second, ASSD is capable to evaluate the segmentation distance error.

A great performance method is proven by high values of DCS and sensitivity with low values of ARVD and ASSD.

### 3.5 Comparison Study

We provide qualitative comparison results on the dataset, as shown in Fig. 2. We compare the ground truth with segmentation results of three methods—The original U-Net applies the PV phase images as input; PA-ResSeg which fuses the DL and PV phases as input; and our proposed method which fuses the DL and PV phases as input. In this example, our network achieves the best performance compared with the multi-phase segmentation method and the single-phase segmentation method, which demonstrates the validity of utilizing delay and portal vein images for segmentation.

U-Net and PA-ResSeg are both based on the traditional CNN architecture. The performance of PA-ResSeg is great but still exists some puzzle. The loss of high-frequency information in Up and Down-sampling operations, and low contrast between the tumor and surroundings result in blurred boundaries. In the proposed method, the structure of the Transformer has a wider perceptual area than the convolutional neural network, allowing for a more complete segmentation of the entire tumor region.

**Table 2.** Performance (MeanValue ± StandardDeviation) comparison of different methods on the multiphase contrast-enhanced liver tumor CT dataset.

| Methods | DSC (%) | ARVD (%) | ASSD (mm) |
|---|---|---|---|
| U-Net [6] | 86.63 ±1.64 | 7.41 ± 1.55 | 5.06 ± 1.90 |
| PA-ResSeg [11] | 89.78 ± 1.67 | 6.85 ± 1.54 | 4.05 ± 1.60 |
| Ours | 90.17 ± 1.77 | 6.71 ± 1.59 | 3.55 ±1.42 |

Table 2 shows the results of three evaluation metrics for different methods. Our proposed method achieved the best performance under the three metrics compared to the state-of-the-art CNN-based models, hence demonstrating the great effectiveness of our network. Both the U-Net and the PA-ResSeg prediction exist some blurred boundary issues. Instead, as the transformer has strong global properties and modal fusion capabilities, it allows the proposed method to better understand the information about the tumor, leading to the demonstration of better predictive capabilities.

### 3.6 Ablation Study

In the baseline testing phase, there occur two issues that should be improved. First, the baseline divides the image into multiple tokens and then uses multiple transformers to model the global picture, but this loses localization, and in fact, local information such as edges, lines, and textures are essential for the network to comprehend the visual information. Second, the attention backbone of the baseline contains redundancy and limited feature richness. Based on this, the RT2T module was added to iteratively reduce the length of Tokens, adding locality to simulate the local structural information of surrounding Tokens. CFA is added to help multi-phase feature interactions and multi-level token fusion is added to support low-level fine-grained information.

**Table 3.** Ablation study of proposed methods on the multi-phase contrast-enhanced liver tumor CT dataset. The baseline is the T2T-ViT model. "CFA" denotes the cross-phase feature aggregator. "RT2T" denotes the reverse token-to-token process. "F" denotes multi-level token fusion. (*MeanValue* ± StandardDeviation).

| Methods | DSC (%) | ARVD (%) | ASSD (mm) |
|---|---|---|---|
| Baseline | 82.13 ± 2.26 | 9.14 ± 1.91 | 8.85 ± 2.40 |
| +CFA | 83.01 ±1.98 | 7.21 ± 1.55 | 9.11 ± 2.37 |
| +CFA+RT2T | 87.55 ± 2.04 | 7.03 ± 1.64 | 5.05 ± 1.86 |
| +CFA+RT2T+F | 90.17 ± 1.77 | 6.71 ± 1.59 | 3.55 ±1.42 |

We conduct ablation studies to verify all our proposed model components. The experimental results of all the validation and results are shown in Table 3. The advantage of our method is shown in both DSC, ARVD, and ASSD. The step-by-step addition module shows that using boundary detection brings further performance gain in the perception of global information and edge characteristics.

### 3.7 Discussion

The results from the comparison study and ablation study demonstrate the proposed method achieved the best performance on all three-evaluation metrics for segmenting tumors of different sizes. The results indicate that our new method has good stability and thus possesses the ability for clinical application.

There are several reasons why our method outperformed other approaches. First, our backbone of T2T-ViT enables the network to extract local tumor details, which facilitates accurate segmentation of small regions. Second, our token module addresses the issue in ViT [21] that modeling local regions loses the line as well as edge information of the image and uses the CFA module to fuse multimodal tumor features and leads to more precise segmented tumor boundaries, particularly for small tumors.

Despite these strengths, our method still has some drawbacks. For instance, in the multiphase fusion stage, our multiphase data need to be strictly aligned, but the tumor location of different phases in the same location may be shifted due to the possible movement of the patient during the shooting. Future work will focus on finding algorithms that can achieve liver position alignment to obtain a finer tumor profile.

## 4 Conclusions

The transformer architecture is well-known for its robust self-attention mechanisms and has been widely adopted in various fields of deep learning in recent years. In our study, we design a symmetric Transformer Encoder-Decoder architecture with skip-connection to extract the multi-phase features and predict the liver tumor. More importantly, we introduce a cross-phase aggregator, which can assist the interaction of the PV phase feature and the DL phase feature. Extensive experiments on a clinical multi-phase contrast-enhanced CT liver tumor dataset have demonstrated that the proposed method outperforms state-of-the-art methods and highlights the promising potential of Transformers for liver tumor segmentation tasks.

**Acknowledgment.** This work is supported by Shantou University (STU Scientific Research Foundation for Talents: NTF21004) and Zhuhai Basic and Applied Basic Research Project Foundation, under Grant ZH22017003200001PWC.

## References

1. McGlynn, K.A., Petrick, J.L., El-Serag, H.B.: Epidemiology of hepatocellular carcinoma. Hepatology **73**, 4–13 (2021)
2. Sung, H., Ferlay, J., Siegel, R.L., et al.: Global cancer statistics 2020: GLOBOCAN estimates of incidence and mortality worldwide for 36 cancers in 185 countries. CA: a Cancer J. Clin. **71**, 209–249 (2021)

3. Han, X.: Automatic liver lesion segmentation using a deep convolutional neural network method (2017). arXiv:170407239
4. Bi, L., Kim, J., Kumar, A., et al.: Automatic liver lesion detection using cascaded deep residual networks (2017). arXiv:170402703
5. Bellver, M., Maninis, K.-K., Pont-Tuset, J., et al.: Detection-aided liver lesion segmentation using deep learning (2017). arXiv:171111069
6. Ronneberger, O., Fischer, P., Brox, T.: U-net: convolutional networks for biomedical image segmentation. Springer; pp 234–24 (2015)
7. Seo, H., Huang, C., Bassenne, M., et al.: Modified U-Net (mU-Net) with incorporation of object-dependent high level features for improved liver and liver-tumor segmentation in CT images. IEEE Trans. Med. Imaging **39**, 1316–1325 (2019)
8. Huang H, Lin L, Tong R et al (2020) Unet 3+: A full-scale connected unet for medical image segmentation, pp. 1055–1059. IEEE
9. Wu Y, Zhou Q, Hu H et al (2019) Hepatic lesion segmentation by combining plain and contrast-enhanced CT images with modality weighted U-Net, pp. 255–259. IEEE
10. Xu, Y., Cai, M., Lin, L., et al.: PA-ResSeg: a phase attention residual network for liver tumor segmentation from multiphase CT images. Med. Phys. **48**, 3752–3766 (2021). https://doi.org/10.1002/mp.14922
11. Zhang, Y., Peng, C., Peng, L., et al.: Multi-phase liver tumor segmentation with spatial aggregation and uncertain region inpainting, pp 68–77. Springer (2021)
12. Ouhmich, F., Agnus, V., Noblet, V., et al.: Liver tissue segmentation in multiphase CT scans using cascaded convolutional neural networks. Int. J. Comput. Assist. Radiol. Surg. **14**, 1275–1284 (2019)
13. Sun, C., Guo, S., Zhang, H., et al.: Automatic segmentation of liver tumors from multiphase contrast-enhanced CT images based on FCNs. Artif. Intell. Med. **83**, 58–66 (2017)
14. Raju, A., Cheng, C.-T., Huo, Y., et al.: Co-heterogeneous and adaptive segmentation from multi-source and multi-phase CT imaging data: a study on pathological liver and lesion segmentation, pp. 448–465. Springer (2020)
15. He, K., Zhang, X., Ren, S., et al.: Deep residual learning for image recognition, pp. 770–778 (2016)
16. Vaswani, A., Shazeer, N., Parmar, N., et al.: Attention is all you need. In: Advances in Neural Information Processing Systems, vol. 30 (2017)
17. Yuan, L., Chen, Y., Wang, T., et al.: Tokens-to-token vit: training vision transformers from scratch on imagenet, pp. 558–567 (2021)
18. Cao, H., Wang, Y., Chen, J., et al.: Swin-unet: unet-like pure transformer for medical image segmentation (2021). arXiv:210505537
19. Zheng, S., Lu, J., Zhao, H., et al.: Rethinking semantic segmentation from a sequence-to-sequence perspective with transformers, pp. 6881–6890 (2021)
20. Chen, J., Lu, Y., Yu, Q., et al.: Transunet: transformers make strong encoders for medical image segmentation (2021). arXiv:210204306
21. Dosovitskiy, A., Beyer, L., Kolesnikov, A., et al.: An image is worth $16 \times 16$ words: transformers for image recognition at scale (2020). arXiv:201011929

# Site Effects in Multisite Fetal Brain MRI: A Morphological Study of Early Brain Development

Xinyi Xu[1], Haoan Xu[1], Tianshu Zheng[1], Yutian Wang[1], Chi Zhou[1], Jiaxin Xiao[1,2], Ruike Chen[1], Mingyang Li[1], Cong Sun[3], Xianglei Kong[4], Qingqing Zhu[4], Hong Yu[5], Guohui Yan[6], Yu Zou[6], Jingshi Wang[5], Guangbin Wang[7], and Dan Wu[1(✉)]

[1] Department of Biomedical Engineering, College of Biomedical Engineering & Instrument Science, Zhejiang University, 38 Zheda Rd, Hangzhou, China
danwu.bme@zju.edu.cn

[2] School of Biomedical Engineering & Imaging Sciences, Faculty of Life Sciences and Medicine, King's College London, London, UK

[3] Department of Radiology, Institute of Geriatric Medicine, Beijing Hospital, National Center of Gerontology, Chinese Academy of Medical Sciences, Beijing, People's Republic of China

[4] Department of Radiology, Sir Run Run Shaw Hospital, Zhejiang University School of Medicine, Hangzhou, China

[5] Dalian Municipal Women and Children's Medical Center (Group), Dalian, China

[6] Department of Radiology, Women's Hospital, Zhejiang University School of Medicine, Hangzhou, China

[7] Department of Radiology, Shandong Provincial Hospital Affiliated to Shandong First Medical University, Jinan, Shandong, China

**Abstract.** Studies have shown that the non-biological site-related effects may induce bias in multisite neuroimaging studies among adults and adolescents. It is unknown how site effects would affect fetal brain MRI and which acquisition factors are critical in quantitative analysis. In this study, we identified site effects, including manufacture, field strength, in-plane resolution, and slice thickness on structural subcortical volume and cortical thickness measurements in normal fetuses. We also showed these site effects could be effectively removed with ComBat-GAM while preserving developmental patterns indicating that the harmonization procedure is necessary when combing multisite imaging data to study fetal brain morphological development.

**Keywords:** Multisite · Fetal brain · Morphological development · Harmonization · Cortical thickness


G. Wang et al. (Eds.): APCMBE 2023, IFMBE Proceedings 103, pp. 131–139, 2024.
https://doi.org/10.1007/978-3-031-51455-5_16

# 1 Introduction

*In-utero* fetal MRI plays an important role in the evaluation of normal or pathological brain development. Due to the challenges in fetal and maternal motions, the sample size in fetal brain MRI studies is typically small and the findings are not always consistent [1–4]. Combining data collected from multiple sites may improve the reliability of the results, but a major drawback in multisite studies is the non-biological site-related effects. Several studies have shown that field strength, manufacture, and software upgrade, as well as the acquisition protocol can introduce bias and variance in measurements of brain volume [5, 6] and cortical thickness [7–9] in adults and adolescents. However, how the site effects affect the analysis of fetal brain MRI remains unknown, given that fetal brain MRI requires complex volumetric reconstruction [10] before quantification. Thus the purpose of this study is to investigate the key acquisition factors on volume and cortical thickness measurements in normal fetal brains.

# 2 Materials and Methods

## 2.1 Data Acquisition

We acquired in-utero MRI from healthy fetal brains across four hospitals. The major site-specific acquisition factors were summarized in Table 1. Ethical approval was obtained from the Institutional Review Board at the local hospitals. All participants provided written informed consent. Note that 122 healthy fetuses included in Shandong Provincial Hospital (SPH) who underwent two MRI scans with different slice thicknesses were considered as two sites in the following analysis. All scans were obtained using T2-weighted fast spin-echo sequences (T2-HASTE imaging on Siemens scanners or ssFSE sequence on GE scanners), typically one scan in axial, coronal, and sagittal planes respectively except for SPH where 1–4 scans were acquired in each orientation. No maternal sedation was used.

## 2.2 Preprocessing

We used the same processing pipeline for all sites (Fig. 1). The 2D multi-slice stacks from multiple orthogonal orientations went through the preprocessing pipeline to obtain the high-resolution 1 mm isotropic 3D volumes using NiftyMIC that included stack selection, brain extraction, bias field correction, slice-to-volume registration (SVR) and super-resolution reconstruction (SRR) [10]. Regional segmentation of brain structures was performed using atlas-based segmentation using a three-stage registration (rigid, affine, and SyN) in ANTs [11]. Briefly, the fetal brain images were nonlinearly registered to the standard CRL atlas [12] at corresponding gestational ages (GA), and then the segmentations in the subject space were obtained by applying the inverse transformations to reference segmentations in CRL space. Here we focused on the volumes of hippocampus, amygdala, thalamus, caudate, putamen, cerebellum, internal capsule, corpus callosum, and midbrain. Vertex-wise cortical thickness measurements were computed using dHCP-structural-pipeline [13] which was modified to adapt to our fetal data (originally defined for neonates) based on cortical segmentation obtained using nnU-net [14], which was combined with the DrawEM-derived labels [15] to obtain regional thickness. All data were visually inspected for quality assurance before analyses.

**Table 1.** Key acquisition factors in the four fetal brain datasets.

| Site name | Location | Field strength (T) | Manufacture | Age | In-plane resolution ($mm^2$) | Slice thickness (mm) | No. participants |
|---|---|---|---|---|---|---|---|
| Shandong Provincial Hospital | Jinan | 3 | Siemens | 21.7–40 w | 1.09 × 1.09 | 2<br>4 | 122 |
| Dalian Municipal Women and Children's Medical Center | Dalian | 1.5 | GE | 23.8–34 w | 1.64 × 1.64 | 4 | 48 |
| Women's Hospital | Hangzhou | 1.5 | GE | 23–37 w | 0.74 or 0.7031 | 2–5 | 13 |
| Sir Run Run Shaw Hospital | Hangzhou | 1.5 | Siemens | 22–38 w | 1.0156 × 1.0156 | 4 | 36 |

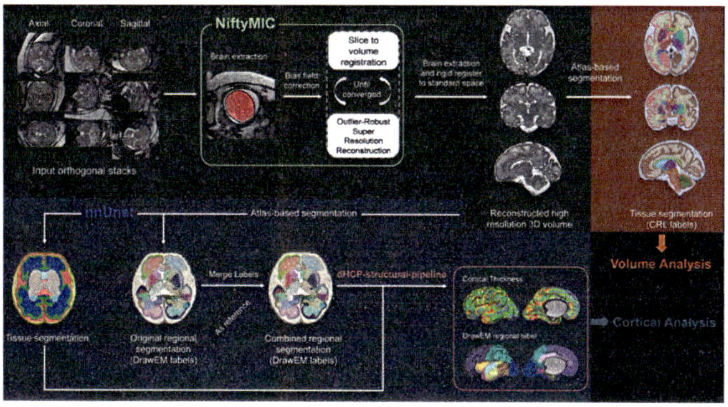


**Fig. 1.** Overview of data processing pipeline including fetal brain MRI reconstruction (green block) and quantification of regional brain volume (orange block) and cortical thickness (dark blue block).

## 2.3 Statistical Analysis

In order to study the effects of field strength, manufacture, in-plane resolution, and slice thickness on volume and cortical thickness measurements, we applied generalized additive models (GAMs) using restricted maximum likelihood with the GA as a potential nonlinear effect (REML, implemented in *mgcv* package [16]) in R (https://www.r-project.org/). After fitting GAM models to the morphological measurement in each ROI, we used the false discovery rate (FDR) approach [17] to correct for multiple comparisons across all ROIs.

For the removal of the site effects, we used ComBat-GAM harmonization procedure [18] to capture the age-related nonlinear change by fitting a GAM with a penalized smooth term, and GA was used as the biological variable as well as the only smooth term in the model (https://github.com/rpomponio/neuroHarmonize). The harmonized data underwent GAM again to evaluate the performance of ComBat-GAM.

## 3 Results

The influences of site effects on regional volumes are summarized in Table 2. GAM analysis revealed a significant slice thickness effect on the volume of internal capsule which was larger from the 4 mm slice thickness data than that from the 2 mm thickness (top row in Fig. 2a, b). Field strength had a significant impact on the volume of corpus callosum, with 1.5T scanners showing a larger volume than 3T scanners (bottom row in Fig. 2a, b). Regional volumes revealed no detectable influence from manufacture or in-plane resolution.

Table 2 shows that the effect of in-plane resolution on cortical thickness was significant in almost all cortical regions, except for the cingulate gyrus and left insular cortex. The cortical thickness of the whole brain and hemispheres was higher at lower in-plane resolution (Fig. 3a, b). The in-plane resolution had different effects on cortical thickness in various cortical regions, with the strongest effect on the left occipital lobe and the least impact on the right cingulate gyrus (Fig. 3d).

The site effects after ComBat-GAM harmonization are also presented in Table 2. Results demonstrated that all site effects that affected subcortical volumes and cortical thickness had been successfully eliminated (Figs. 2c and 3c).

## 4 Discussion

Multisite neuroimaging studies merge data from multiple MRI manufacturers, field strengths, and sequence parameters, and have to take into account the non-biological variances. We measured these impacts on measurements of volume and cortical thickness of normal fetuses using in-utero MRI.

We found that thicker slices or lower field strength led to higher subcortical volume measurements. These effects depended on specific regions which were also found in a previous study [6] that investigated scanner-related effects on subcortical volumes of adults.

In contrast, we found that in-plane resolution had a significant and widespread impact on cortical thickness, with lower resolution leading to an overestimation of cortical thickness. Fortin et al. found significant cortical thickness differences across different scanners and field strengths [7]. Auzias et al. stated that scanner-related variables would affect the outcome of cortical thickness abnormalities in ASD pathology [9]. The effect

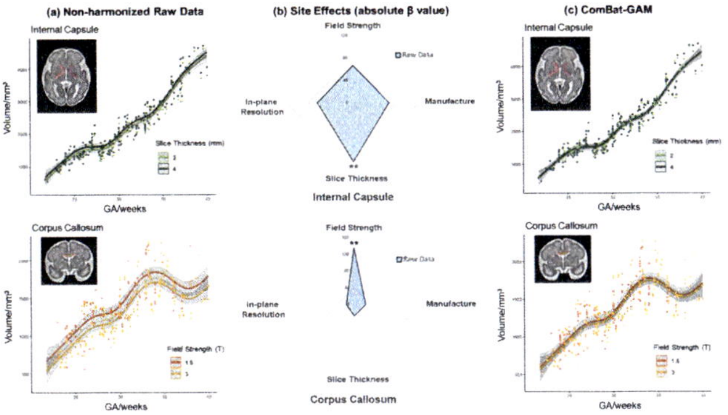


**Fig. 2.** Effects of manufacture, slice thickness, in-plane resolution, and field strength on volume measurements of representative ROIs. **a** Age-related changes in non-harmonized raw volume data using different slice thickness and field strength. **b** Radar charts showing site effects of manufacture, slice thickness, in-plane resolution, and field strength on the non-harmonized raw volume of the corresponding ROI. **c** Age-related changes of the harmonized volume data. * Adjusted p < 0.5, ** Adjusted p < 0.01.

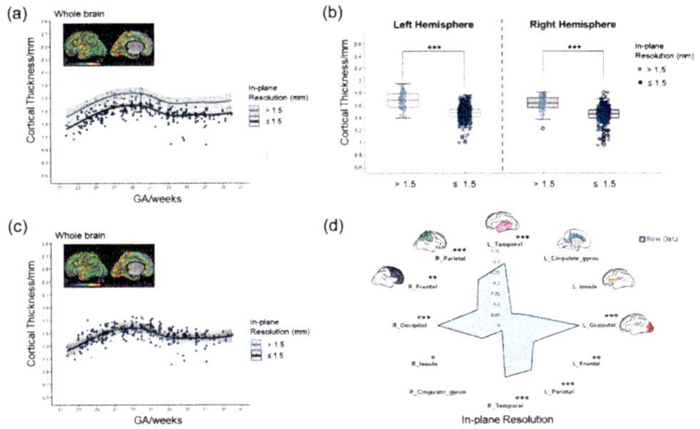


**Fig. 3.** Effects of in-plane resolution on cortical thickness. **a**, **c** Developmental trajectories of averaged cortical thickness of the whole brain over GA with non-harmonized raw data (**a**) and harmonized data (**c**). **b** Box plot showing in-plane resolution effects on averaged cortical thickness of left and right hemispheres. **d** Radar charts showing in-plane resolution effects on the raw cortical thickness of different cortical regions. * Adjusted P < 0.05, ** adjusted P < 0.01, *** adjusted P < 0.001.

of in-plane resolution was not separately pointed out in the two studies mentioned above, but it was included in the influence of scanner factors.

## 5 Conclusion

We investigated the effects of manufacture, field strength, in-plane resolution, and slice thickness on the regional volumes and cortical thickness of healthy fetuses across four centers. We found that the volume of subcortical brain structures depended on field

**Table 2.** Summary of site-related effects (β values) on regional volumes and cortical thickness before and after harmonization.

| | Non-harmonized raw data | | | | After ComBat-GAM harmonization | | | |
|---|---|---|---|---|---|---|---|---|
| | Field strength | Manufacture | Slice thickness | In-plane resolution | Field strength | Manufacture | Slice thickness | In-plane resolution |
| *Volume analysis* | | | | | | | | |
| Hippocampus | −45.124 | 5.534 | 4.344 | 48.375 | 4.853 | 49.991 | −9.61 | 41.42 |
| Amygdala | −2.175 | 3.631 | 2.887 | 3.792 | 4.697 | −7.46 | −1.234 | 3.555 |
| Thalamus | −132.49 | 134.62 | 67.08 | 81.33 | 17.073 | 91.586 | 9.188 | 155.676 |
| Caudate | −85.46 | 53.208 | 23.103 | −8.211 | 12.604 | −79.7 | −0.988 | 76.491 |
| Putamen | −75.22 | 292.33 | 117.82 | −138.59 | 15.162 | 9.573 | 30.176 | 16.472 |
| Cerebellum | −159.18 | 531.31 | 134.64 | −77.69 | 89.98 | 306.07 | −13.16 | 352.85 |
| IC | −66.45 | 65.51 | 105.87** | 64.2 | −4.299 | 57.452 | 35.747 | 94.864 |
| CC | 135.92** | 27.62 | −27.21 | 18.83 | −35.05 | −35.49 | −22.86 | 18.54 |
| Midbrain | −165.2 | 228.82 | 25.17 | −13.4 | −13.33 | 113.25 | −16.38 | 157.03 |
| *Cortical analysis* | | | | | | | | |
| Whole brain | −0.044 | 0.046 | −0.012 | 0.189*** | −0.003 | 0.006 | 0.001 | −0.005 |
| L_hemisphere | −0.022 | 0.031 | 0.000 | 0.207*** | 0.006 | 0.000 | 0.007 | −0.007 |
| R_hemisphere | −0.065 | 0.059 | −0.023 | 0.170*** | −0.012 | 0.012 | −0.005 | −0.001 |
| L_Temporal | −0.03 | 0.063 | −0.042 | 0.295*** | 0.001 | 0.008 | −0.014 | −0.026 |

(*continued*)

**Table 2.** *(continued)*

| | Non-harmonized raw data | | | | After ComBat-GAM harmonization | | | |
|---|---|---|---|---|---|---|---|---|
| | Field strength | Manufacture | Slice thickness | In-plane resolution | Field strength | Manufacture | Slice thickness | In-plane resolution |
| L_Cing_gyrus | −0.066* | −0.017 | 0.02 | −0.064 | −0.011 | −0.008 | 0.017 | 0.03 |
| L_Insula | −0.04 | −0.06 | −0.009 | −0.105 | 0.003 | −0.03 | 0.005 | 0.035 |
| L_Occipital | −0.06 | 0.095 | 0.011 | 0.349*** | −0.004 | 0.021 | 0.014 | −0.032 |
| L_Frontal | −0.037 | 0.008 | −0.033 | −0.153** | 0.003 | −0.009 | −0.007 | 0.017 |
| L_Parietal | 0.003 | 0.038 | 0.004 | 0.244*** | 0.024 | −0.002 | 0.013 | −0.007 |
| R_Temporal | −0.04 | 0.053 | −0.038 | 0.246*** | −0.003 | 0.006 | −0.011 | −0.009 |
| R_Cing_gyrus | −0.070* | −0.097 | 0.02 | 0.028 | −0.011 | −0.037 | 0.017 | 0.061 |
| R_Insula | −0.029 | −0.035 | −0.001 | −0.122* | 0.006 | −0.017 | 0.01 | 0.033 |
| R_Occipital | −0.075 | 0.122 | 0.003 | 0.314*** | −0.009 | 0.029 | 0.011 | −0.024 |
| R_Frontal | −0.026 | 0.008 | −0.033 | −0.150** | 0.008 | −0.008 | −0.007 | 0.014 |
| R_Parietal | −0.009 | 0.051 | −0.016 | 0.249*** | 0.017 | 0.001 | 0.003 | −0.008 |

* Adjusted $P < 0.05$, ** Adjusted $P < 0.01$, *** Adjusted $P < 0.001$. Abbreviation: IC = Internal Capsule, CC = Corpus Callosum, Cing = Cingulate

strength and slice thickness and was less sensitive to manufacture and in-plane resolution. In contrast, cortical thickness was highly influenced by in-plane resolution. These results demonstrate that it is important to take these factors into account when planning multisite or longitudinal studies. Meanwhile, ComBat-GAM can effectively remove nuisance variabilities associated with the acquisition while maintaining the age effects in volume and cortical thickness. Therefore, it is crucial to harmonize the data when analyzing multicenter fetal brains for morphological development.

## References

1. Clouchoux, C., Kudelski, D., Gholipour, A., et al.: Quantitative in vivo MRI measurement of cortical development in the fetus. Brain Struct. Funct. **217**, 127–139 (2012)
2. Habas, P.A., Scott, J.A., Roosta, A., et al.: Early folding patterns and asymmetries of the normal human brain detected from in Utero MRI. Cereb. Cortex **22**, 13–25 (2011)
3. Rajagopalan, V., Scott, J., Habas, P.A., et al.: Local tissue growth patterns underlying normal fetal human brain gyrification quantified in utero. J. Neurosci. **31**, 2878–2887 (2011)
4. Clouchoux, C., Du Plessis, A.J., Bouyssi-Kobar, M., et al.: Delayed cortical development in fetuses with complex congenital heart disease. Cereb. Cortex **23**, 2932–2943 (2013)
5. Takao, H., Hayashi, N., Ohtomo, K.: Effect of scanner in longitudinal studies of brain volume changes. J. Magn. Reson. Imaging **34**, 438–444 (2011)
6. Jovicich, J., Czanner, S., Han, X., et al.: MRI-derived measurements of human subcortical, ventricular and intracranial brain volumes: reliability effects of scan sessions, acquisition sequences, data analyses, scanner upgrade, scanner vendors and field strengths. Neuroimage **46**, 177–192 (2009)
7. Fortin, J.-P., Cullen, N., Sheline, Y.I., et al.: Harmonization of cortical thickness measurements across scanners and sites. Neuroimage **167**, 104–120 (2018)
8. Han, X., Jovicich, J., Salat, D., et al.: Reliability of MRI-derived measurements of human cerebral cortical thickness: the effects of field strength, scanner upgrade and manufacturer. Neuroimage **32**, 180–194 (2006)
9. Auzias, G., Takerkart, S., Deruelle, C.: On the influence of confounding factors in multisite brain morphometry studies of developmental pathologies: application to autism spectrum disorder. IEEE J. Biomed. Health Inform. **20**, 810–817 (2016)
10. Ebner, M., Wang, G., Li, W., et al.: An automated framework for localization, segmentation and super-resolution reconstruction of fetal brain MRI. Neuroimage **206**, 116324 (2020)
11. Avants, B.B., Epstein, C.L., Grossman, M., et al.: Symmetric diffeomorphic image registration with cross-correlation: evaluating automated labeling of elderly and neurodegenerative brain. Med. Image Anal. **12**, 26–41 (2008)
12. Gholipour, A., Rollins, C.K., Velasco-Annis, C., et al.: A normative spatiotemporal MRI atlas of the fetal brain for automatic segmentation and analysis of early brain growth. Sci. Rep. **7**, 476 (2017)
13. Makropoulos, A., Robinson, E.C., Schuh, A., et al.: The developing human connectome project: a minimal processing pipeline for neonatal cortical surface reconstruction. Neuroimage **173**, 88–112 (2018)
14. Isensee, F., Jaeger, P.F., Kohl, S.A.A., et al.: NnU-Net: a self-configuring method for deep learning-based biomedical image segmentation. Nat. Methods **18**, 203–211 (2021)
15. Makropoulos, A., Gousias, I.S., Ledig, C., et al.: Automatic whole brain MRI segmentation of the developing neonatal brain. IEEE Trans. Med. Imaging **33**, 1818–1831 (2014)
16. Wood, S.N.: Generalized additive models: an introduction with R. chapman and hall/CRC (2006)

17. Benjamini, Y., Hochberg, Y.: Controlling the false discovery rate: a practical and powerful approach to multiple testing 57, 289–300 (1995)
18. Pomponio, R., Erus, G., Habes, M., et al.: Harmonization of large MRI datasets for the analysis of brain imaging patterns throughout the lifespan. Neuroimage **208**, 116450 (2020)

# A Low-Power Variable Gain Amplifier Design with 70-DB Gain Range and 1.28-DB Gain Error for Ultrasound Imaging System

Jieyu Ma[1(✉)], Yuanyu Yu[1], Jiujiang Wang[2], Peng Un Mak[2], Hungchun Li[3], Liu Yu[4], Weibao Qiu[5], Sio Hang Pun[1], and Mang I. Vai[1]

[1] State Key Laboratory of Analog and Mixed-Signal VLSI, University of Macau, Avenida da Universidade, Macau, China
17843128286@163.com
[2] Department of Electrical and Computer Engineering, University of Macau, Macau, China
[3] Lingyange Semiconductor Inc. Zhuhai City, Guandong, China
[4] School of Microelectronics, University of Tianjin, Tianjin, China
[5] Paul C. Lauterbur Research Center for Biomedical Imaging Shenzhen Institute of Advanced Technology, Chinese Academy of Sciences, Shenzhen, China

**Abstract.** This work presents a Variable Gain Amplifier (VGA) design with low power consumption and dB-linear characteristic for the ultrasound (US) imaging system based on the cell-based topology. It compensates for the distance attenuation of the US echo signal by providing a variable gain that increases exponentially over time. By cascading several VGA building blocks, the gain range of the combined dB-linear VGA can be increased. Each VGA building block is designed by common source input MOS transistors working in the triode region to approximate an exponential function for high robustness and low power consumption. Designed in the 65 nm CMOS process, the presented VGA occupies 0.02 $mm^2$ and can regulate a linear gain variation range in decibels of 70 dB with $\pm 1.28$ dB maximum gain error. Meanwhile, more than 80 MHz of $-3$ dB bandwidth can be realized within the gain range. The total power consumption of the combined VGA is 0.384 mW with a 1.2 V supply voltage, and the input-referred voltage noise density is 20 nV/$\sqrt{}$Hz.

**Keywords:** CMOS variable gain amplifier · dB-linear · Ultrasound imaging · Cell-based topology · Low power amplifier

## 1 Introduction

The US imaging technique is a popular imaging modality in medical inspection commonly used in routine clinical applications due to its safety for humans. An ultrasound imaging system reconstructs the image of internal organs by transmitting an acoustic wave into the human body and analyzing the received echoes. A typical US imaging system, as shown in Fig. 1, consists of a high voltage (HV) pulser, a protection switch, a low noise amplifier (LNA)/transimpedance amplifier (TIA), a Time-Gain Compensation (TGC) module, a Low-Pass Filter (LPF), an Analog-to-Digital Converter (ADC) and an external back-end module.


G. Wang et al. (Eds.): APCMBE 2023, IFMBE Proceedings 103, pp. 140–148, 2024.
https://doi.org/10.1007/978-3-031-51455-5_17

Among the components of a typical US imaging system, a TGC module is generally needed to improve the obtained image's quality and relieve the stringent Dynamic Range (DR) requirement of the subsequent ADC. This dilemma originates as the US signal attenuates exponentially with distance when it travels within lossy human tissues. As a result, the US front-end amplifier receives strong echoes from nearby tissues and needs to amplify very weak echoes from deep inside tissues. Without proper correction, the US image will be either too bright in the near-surface region or too dark in the deep-inside region, as shown in Fig. 2a. On the contrary, a compensated image (Fig. 2b) can significantly improve the image quality for the deep-inside region.

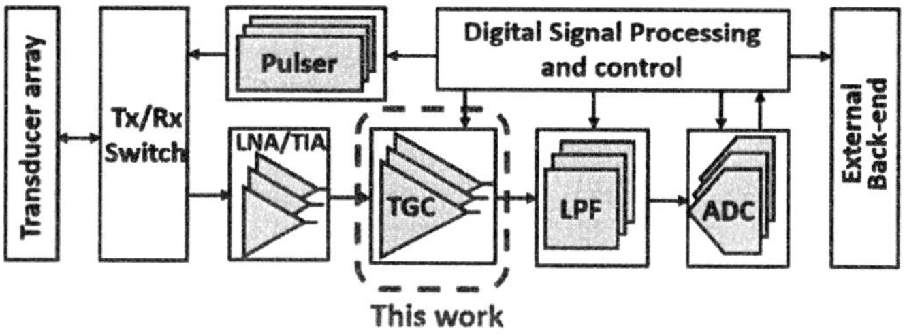


**Fig. 1.** System diagram of an ultrasound imaging system.

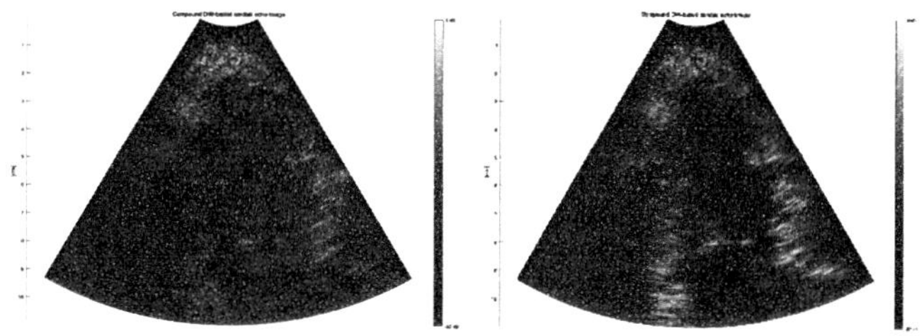

(a) (b)

**Fig. 2.** Simulated ultrasound image without TGC operation (**a**) and after TGC operation (**b**).

To realize a TGC, a Programmable Gain Amplifier (PGA) with digital control circuitry was mostly adopted [1, 2]. The implementation of a PGA is simple; however, a discrete gain step can lead to a transient response between steps, which will lead to artifacts in an ultrasonic image. Thus, a Variable Gain Amplifier (VGA) with continuous gain control is preferable in medical ultrasound applications. The critical issue of designing dB-linear VGA is to implement an exponential function. Although this can be easily achieved using the exponential characteristics of the bipolar technology [3, 4], it is better to implement it in a standard CMOS technology because of the lower integration cost.

Various approaches using MOS devices have been reported to achieve a dB-linear characteristic [5–10]. However, obtaining an accurate exponential function using MOS devices, which follow the square law, is difficult. When a small gain error was required, additional complex circuits were needed to implement the approximate exponential function, sacrificing area and power consumption. In addition, the dB-linear gain range has been significantly restricted to ensure the accuracy of the approximate exponential function.

In this paper, the cell-based structure has been used, as shown in Fig. 3a, in which the range of the combined VGA's dB-linear gain can be increased by cascading multiple VGA building blocks. Based on this structure, an efficient building block with low power consumption and small gain error is designed to optimize the overall performance of a VGA. This building block (Fig. 3b) adopts common source input MOS transistors working in the triode region to implement a good exponential approximation and active inductors in series with MOS resistors to extend its bandwidth [10]. This article is arranged as below. Section I discusses the design considerations and techniques for the efficient VGA building block, and Section III shows the simulation results. Finally, Section IV summarizes this paper.

## 2 Circuit Design and Methods

As illustrated in Fig. 3b, the VGA building block biases the input transistors $M_{1,2}$ in the triode region and is tuned by the gate voltage $V_{ctrl}$ that varies linearly with time to get the dB-linear gain. By providing a gate control voltage that varies linearly with time, the gain of VGA can vary exponentially with time(dB-linear gain). The active inductor is realized by transistors $M_{4,5}$, the gate of which is connected to the MOS resistors $M_N$ in series with the resistor $R_L$. By adjusting the DC bias voltage $V_{CN}$, the resistance of MOS resistor $M_N$ and the inductance of the active inductors can be changed accordingly. The transistor $M_3$ biased by the gate voltage $V_B$ provides a bias current for the circuit. The derived voltage gain of the presented VGA building block is

$$Av = g_{m1}R_{total} = \frac{\left(-x + \sqrt{x^2+1}\right)}{(c+x)} \approx \frac{\left(1 - x + \frac{x^2}{2}\right)}{(c+x)} \approx \frac{e^{-x}}{c+x} \tag{1}$$

$$x = \frac{(V_{G1} - V_{D1} - V_{TH1})}{\sqrt{\frac{2I_{D1}}{K_1}}} \tag{2}$$

*where* $c = \sqrt{K_5/K_1}$, $K = \mu C_{ox} W/L$, $\mu$ is the electron mobility for NMOS transistor, $C_{ox}$ is the equivalent capacitance of gate oxide, $W$ and $L$ represents the gate width and gate length of MOS transistor, respectively. $V_{TH1}$ is the threshold voltage.

Equation 1 indicates that a larger $c$ makes the denominator closer to a constant, and thus the approximate exponential gain will be more accurate. For the input differential pair, a small transistor requires a higher gate voltage range to attain larger $V_{ov}$(overdrive voltage) and $V_{ds}$(drain to source voltage) so that the triode region shrinks. As a result, the variation range of gain is compressed, and the error is decreased as c increases. On the contrary, a large input transistor can increase the gain range of the circuit.

In this design, the tail current affects the power consumption and gain characteristics. A high gate voltage of input transistors is required for a small tail current to ensure $M_{1,2}$ operate in the triode region. Therefore, the control voltage range is shortened, which

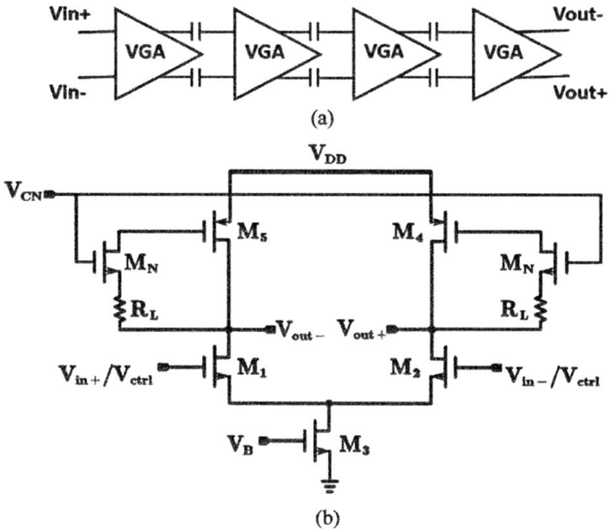


**Fig. 3.** The proposed cell-based VGA for the US imaging system. The design comprises four identical VGA building blocks. (b) The architecture of the VGA building block. $V_{ctrl}$ is the DC bias voltage for $M_{1,2}$, $V_{CN}$ is the DC bias voltage for $M_N$

leads to a restricted gain range. For a large tail current, the gain range becomes larger due to the extension of the triode region. To reduce power consumption while keeping the gain error small and the gain range large, a tail current of 80 μA is selected for the VGA building block. The VGA building block is designed, and its parameters are listed in Table 1.

**Table 1.** Key parameters of the VGA building block.

| Parameters | $W_1$ | $W_5$ | $I_d$ | $W_N$ | $R_L$ |
|---|---|---|---|---|---|
| VGA building block | 3 μm | 0.45 μm | 80 μA | 2 μm | 2 kΩ |

## 3 Results

The circuit design and simulation were implemented in the TSMC 65 nm CMOS process. From the simulation result, a building block consumes only 0.096 mW, and the combined dB-linear VGA consumes only 0.384 mW by cascading four VGA building blocks. The frequency response of the building block and dB-linear VGA under gate bias voltage $V_{ctrl}$ from 1.05 to 1.19 V has been simulated. The −3 dB bandwidth of the combined dB-linear VGA is over 80 MHz under the highest gain control with a load capacitance of 1 pF.

The simulated gain characteristics of the VGA building block and the combined VGA are presented in Fig. 4. Figure 4a shows that the gain of the building block is dB-linear over the variation range from −16.6 to 0.8 dB with a maximum dB-linear error of 0.32 dB (Fig. 4b). The gain of combined VGA achieves a range from −66.5 to 3.5 dB (Fig. 4c) with a maximum gain error of 1.28 dB (Fig. 4d). Although the gain is almost negative, this work is intended to implement a VGA with a wide gain variation range with minimum gain error to compensate for the distance attenuation of US echoes. The preamplifier of the US imaging system can boost the overall gain to the positive range.

The simulated gain characteristics of the VGA building block and the dB-linear VGA with five typical temperatures, −40, −20, 27, 80, and 125 °C, are shown in Fig. 5. From Fig. 5a, c, temperature variation slightly affects the gain range of both the VGA building block and the combined dB-linear VGA. Temperature variations have little effect on the gain error, as shown in Fig. 5b, d.

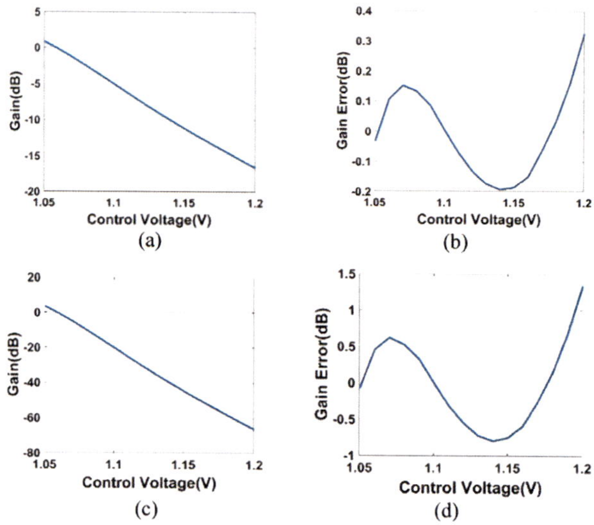


**Fig. 4.** The gain characteristic of the VGA building block and the combined VGA. **a** The dB-linear gain of the VGA building block with respect to the control voltage; **b** the dB-linear gain error of the building block; **c** the gain of the combined VGA with respect to the control voltage; **d** the gain error of the combined VGA

To verify the effect of process deviation on the dB-linear function. Figure 6 presents Monte-Carlo simulation results for 100 runs. The figure shows that gain variations are small for the VGA building block, but gain variations are significant for the combined dB-linear VGA. The mean maximum gain error of the VGA building block is 0.51 dB, and the standard deviation is 0.29 dB for 100 Monte Carlo runs. The VGA's mean maximum gain error is 2.05 dB, and the standard deviation is 1.18 dB.

Table 2 presents a summary and comparison between this design with previous state-of-the-art literary designs. Compared to other VGAs, the power consumption of this design is further saved. A smaller gain error is achieved while the gain range is

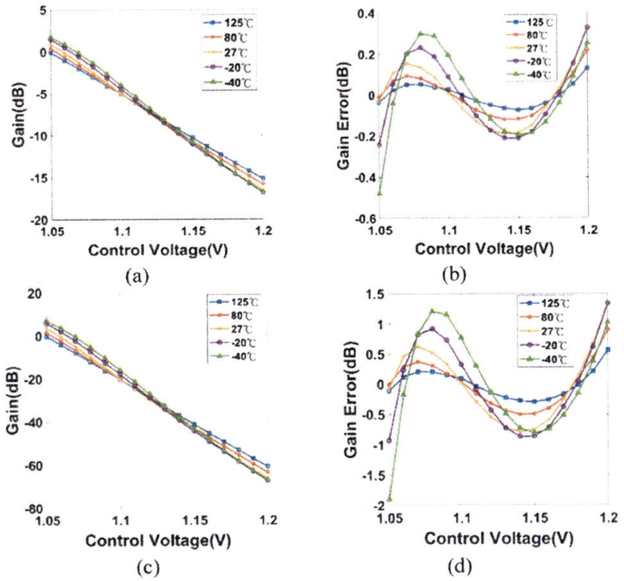


**Fig. 5.** The performances of the VGA building block and the combined dB-linear VGA over temperature. **a** The variation of the gain of the VGA building block over temperature variation; **b** the gain errors of a VGA building block subject to temperature variation; **c** the variation of the gain of the combined VGA over temperature variation; **d** the gain errors of the combined VGA subject to temperature variation

maintained. Although the noise of this VGA design is large, the noise of the front end of the US imaging system is determined by the first stage—the readout preamplifier, which is usually an LNA. Last but not least, the bandwidth is maintained, which results from the active inductors. In conclusion, the presented VGA design outperforms the previous literary works.

## 4 Discussion

To obtain a high-quality ultrasound image, VGA with a large gain range and small gain error is required to compensate well for the US echo attenuation. This VGA design achieved a 70 dB gain range benefiting from cascading several VGA building blocks. But the disadvantage of cascading is the accumulation of the gain error and power consumption. So this work is intended to implement an excellent VGA building block with minimum gain error and power consumption. The difficulty of designing such a VGA building block in a standard CMOS technology is to implement an accurate exponential approximation because the intrinsic nature of MOS transistor is not an exponential characteristic. This paper carefully analyzed each MOS transistor of the entire circuit, and the source of gain error has been found. By carefully selecting the circuit parameters, the gain error of each building block has been reduced to only 0.32 dB, resulting in 1.28 dB gain error of the whole VGA. Moreover, the bandwidth of the VGA

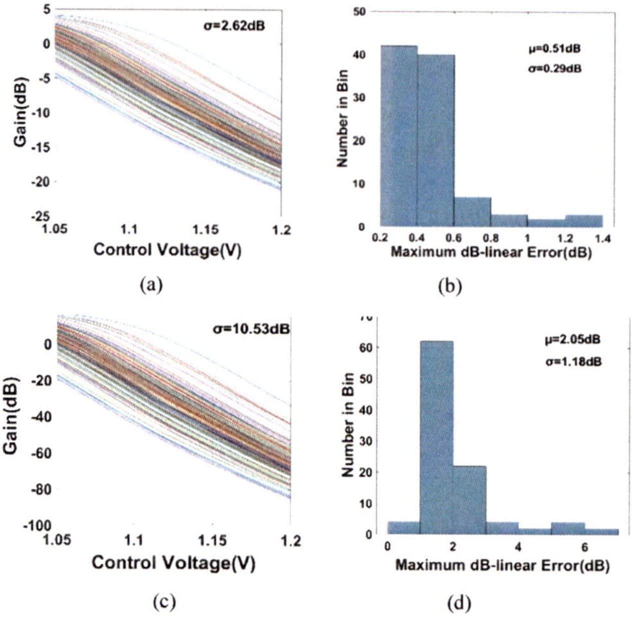


**Fig. 6.** Monte Carlo simulation results for 100 runs of the VGA building block and the combined dB-linear VGA. **a** Simulated gain of the VGA building block with respect to the control voltage; **b** histogram of maximum gain error of the VGA building block for 100 Monte Carlo runs; **c** simulated gain of the combined VGA with respect to the control voltage; **d** histogram of maximum gain error of the combined VGA for 100 Monte Carlo runs.

is larger than 80 MHz, which is suitable to be applied to high-frequency US applications, such as ophthalmic imaging, dermatology imaging, and intravascular imaging.

With a gain range of 70 dB, gain error of 1.28 dB, and bandwidth of 80 MHz, the VGA can perfectly compensate for the ultrasound echo attenuation of most ultrasound imaging application scenarios. For example, in intravascular imaging, the attenuation coefficient of ultrasound propagation in the blood is 0.15 dB/cm/MHz. For 50 MHz high-frequency ultrasound, this VGA can compensate the ultrasonic attenuation of more than 9 cm propagation distance, which means that tissue located at a depth of 4.5 cm can be clearly visualized.

The power consumption of the whole VGA is only 0.384 mW, reducing the power consumption burden of the entire ultrasound imaging system and facilitating the implementation of handheld US devices. Although this paper only presents the simulation results, we can see the excellent robustness of this VGA design from the temperature simulation and Monte Carlo simulation results. Further measurement is required to verify the final performance.

**Table 2.** Performance comparison with previous state-of-the-art designs

| | [7] 2013 | [9] 2016 | [10] 2020 | [5] 2022 | This work |
|---|---|---|---|---|---|
| dB-lin. Gain (dB) | 50 | 22 | 40 | 37 | 70 |
| Gain error (dB) | 0.5 | 0.3 | 1 | 1.4 | 1.28 |
| BW (MHz) | 14.8 | 2200 | 4000 | 3.1 | 80 |
| IRN (nV/$\sqrt{}$Hz) | 3.5@4 MHz | – | – | 8.6@2 MHz | 20@50 MHz |
| Supply (V) | 1.2 | 1.2 | 1.2 | 1.8 | 1.2 |
| Power (mW) | 2.16 | 3.48 | 3.5 | 0.96 | 0.384 |
| Technology (nm) | 65 | 65 | 65 | 180 | 65 |

## 5 Conclusions

In this paper, we presented a design of the dB-linear VGA cascading four VGA building blocks for the US imaging system. This work, departing from the theoretical analysis of the architecture, successfully reached an efficient design as the basic building block for VGA. As a consequence, the overall power consumption of the dB-linear VGA is 0.384 mW, while the achieved linear gain variation range in decibels is 70 dB with a maximum gain error of 1.28 dB. Moreover, the proposed design is robust to temperature variations, process mismatch, and variations, as shown from the temperature simulation results and 100 Monte Carlo runs. It is believed that the presented design can be adequately applied to high-frequency US imaging applications.

**Acknowledgment.** This work was funded by the National Key R&D Program of China (No. 2020YFB1313502) and funded by the Shenzhen-Hong Kong-Macau S&T Program (Category C) of SZSTI (SGDX20201103094002009) and funded by the University of Macau (File no. MYRG2020-00098-FST, MYRG2022-00111-IME) and funded by The Science and Technology Development Fund, Macau SAR (File no. 0144/2019/A3, 0022/2020/AFJ, SKL-AMSV (FDCT-funded), SKL-AMSV-ADDITIONAL FUND, SKL-AMSV(UM)-2020-2022) and funded by the Lingyange Semiconductor Incorporated, Zhuhai.

## References

1. Cho, S.-E., et al.: A single-stage 37 dB-linear digitally-controlled variable gain amplifier for ultrasound medical imaging. IEIE J. Semi-Cond. Technol. Sci. **14**, 579–587 (2014)
2. Attarzadeh, H., et al.: A low-power high-dynamic-range receiver system for in-probe 3-D ultrasonic imaging. IEEE Trans. Biomed. Circuits Syst. **11**, 1053–1064 (2017). https://doi.org/10.1109/TBCAS.2017.2716836
3. Lee, H.D., et al.: A wideband CMOS variable gain amplifier with an exponential gain control. IEEE Trans. Microw. Theory Tech. **55**, 1363–1373 (2007). https://doi.org/10.1109/TMTT.2007.896787
4. Alegre, J.P.: SiGe analog circuit for an 802.11a WLAN direct conversion receiver. IEEE Trans. Circuits Syst. II Exp. Briefs **56**, 93–96 (2009). https://doi.org/10.1109/TCSII.2008.2010173

5. Um, J.-Y.: A compact variable gain amplifier with continuous time-gain compensation using systematic predistorted gain control. IEEE Trans. Circuits Syst. II Exp. Briefs **69**, 274–278 (2022). https://doi.org/10.1109/TCSII.2021.3090424
6. Duong, Q.-H., et al.: A 95-dB linear low-power variable gain amplifier. IEEE Trans. Circuits Syst. I Regul. Pap. **53**, 1648–1657 (2006). https://doi.org/10.1109/TCSI.2006.879058
7. Choi, I., et al.: Accurate dB-linear variable gain amplifier with gain error compensation. IEEE J. Solid-State Circuits **48**, 456–464 (2013). https://doi.org/10.1109/JSSC.2012.2227606
8. Liu, H., et al.: Cell-based variable-gain amplifiers with accurate dB-linear characteristic in 0.18 μm CMOS technology. IEEE J. Solid-State Circuits **50**, 586–596 (2015). https://doi.org/10.1109/JSSC.2014.2368132
9. Liu, H., et al.: A wideband analog-controlled variable-gain amplifier with dB-linear characteristic for high-frequency applications. IEEE Trans. Microw. Theory Tech. **64**, 533–540 (2016). https://doi.org/10.1109/TMTT.2015.2513403
10. Kong, L., et al.: Design of a wideband variable-gain amplifier with self-compensated transistor for accurate dB-linear characteristic in 65 nm CMOS technology. IEEE Trans. Circuits Syst. I Regul. Pap. **67**, 4187–4198 (2020). https://doi.org/10.1109/TCSI.2020.2995725

# Group Information Guided Smooth Independent Component Analysis Method for Brain Functional Network Analysis

Yuhui Du[1(✉)], Chen Huang[1], Yating Guo[1], Xingyu He[1], and Vince D. Calhoun[2]

[1] School of Computer and Information Technology, Shanxi University, Wucheng Road No. 92, Taiyuan City, Shanxi Province, China
duyuhui@sxu.edu.cn

[2] Tri-Institutional Center for Translational Research in Neuroimaging and Data Science (TReNDS), Institute of Technology, Georgia State University, Emory University, Atlanta, GA, USA

**Abstract.** Independent component analysis (ICA) is widely used for extracting brain functional network (FN) from fMRI data, but the low signal-to-noise ratio in fMRI data makes FNs contain a lot of noise. Previous methods that remove the noise-related components obtained from ICA to reconstruct fMRI largely depend on the trained models and fail to directly optimize FN. Here, based on our previously proposed group information guided ICA (GIG-ICA), we incorporate a smoothness term to construct a multi-objective function so as to effectively remove the noises in FNs in addition to guaranteeing the independence and correspondence of FNs. Importantly, different kinds of noises can be handled independently or jointly, adaptively or knowledge-based. We validate our method using both the simulated and real fMRI data. Using the simulated data added with different noises, the spatial accuracy of FNs obtained by our method (named GIG-sICA) is higher than that obtained by the original GIG-ICA. Using fMRI data of 134 healthy controls and 123 schizophrenia patients, our method yields greater group differences in most FNs compared with GIG-ICA. In summary, our method is effective in extracting smooth and accurate brain FNs with less noise, and helpful to identify stable biomarkers and predict mental illnesses.

**Keywords:** fMRI · Independent component analysis · Multi-objective optimization · Smoothness and denoising

## 1 Introduction

Independent component analysis (ICA) is a widely used data-driven method for brain functional network (FN) analysis using functional Magnetic Resonance Imaging (fMRI) data [1]. However, the non-neuronal signals such as head movements, physiological noise, and scanner artifacts can make the obtained FNs contain a lot of noise, which interferes with brain disease-related studies in identifying network-level biomarkers and leads to some false conclusions [2].


G. Wang et al. (Eds.): APCMBE 2023, IFMBE Proceedings 103, pp. 149–156, 2024.
https://doi.org/10.1007/978-3-031-51455-5_18

In order to denoise the fMRI data and resulting FNs, previous studies often first decompose fMRI data by ICA, then the noise-related independent components (ICs) are identified and removed from the fMRI data. And last, the cleaned fMRI data are used to extract meaningful ICs reflecting FNs. In the ICA-based denoising methods, the identification of noise ICs can be performed manually, which is time-consuming and depends on the experience [3], or by using machine learning based classification [4], which largely depends on the classifier type, features for training model, and the training data. For example, Salimi et proposed the FIX, which uses distinct features to train a multi-level classifier to detect noise ICs, but the model training needs the hand-classification of a sufficient number of training datasets [5]. Pruim et developed the ICA-AROMA, which is mainly used to reduce motion effects due to the used features [6]. Van et optimized the combination of the ICA-AROMA and aCompCor which can identify the motion and physiological noise well, but their combination methods are diverse, and different combinations produce very different results [7]. In addition to the limited generalization ability of the built models in denoising other data, these methods did not optimize FNs themselves to directly denoise the FNs.

In this paper, we propose a group information guided smooth ICA (GIG-sICA) based on our previously proposed GIG-ICA [8] to explicitly optimize the smoothness of FNs in addition to optimizing the independence and correspondence of FNs. By adding a graph regularization term to form a multi-objective function, GIG-sICA clusters voxels with similar characteristics into the same FN so as to learn accurate and realistic FNs. GIG-sICA can remove most of the noises in the gray matter (GM), white matter (WM), cerebrospinal fluid (CSF), and brain edge (BE) independently or jointly, adaptively or knowledge-based by incorporating and combining 13 voxel features. Compared to the original GIG-ICA, GIG-sICA extracts more smooth and accurate FNs on the simulated data and yields greater group differences between 134 healthy controls (HC) and 123 schizophrenia patients (SZ) in the noise-free FNs. Both of the results validate that GIG-sICA is a promising method for brain FN analysis.

## 2 Materials and Methods

We first briefly introduce the GIG-ICA method and then describe our proposed GIG-sICA in detail. After that, we state how we evaluate our method and compare it with GIG-ICA using both the simulated data and real fMRI data.

### 2.1 GIG-ICA Method

GIG-ICA can simultaneously guarantee the independence of individual-subject FNs and the correspondence of FNs across subjects. The method primarily includes the following two steps, i.e., the IC computation at group and subject levels.

First, the group ICs (GICs) are extracted. For the fMRI data of all subjects, the two-level principal component analysis (PCA) are used to reduce dimension along the time points. Then, the group-level ICA is performed to decompose the reduced data, resulting in the GICs.

Second, the GICs are used as guidance in the subject-level ICA to compute individual ICs using a multi-objective function, as formulated in (1).

$$\max\begin{cases} J(Y_i) = \{E[G(Y_i)] - E[G(v)]\}^2 \\ U(Y_i) = E(Y_i * R_i) \end{cases} \tag{1}$$

The terms $J(Y_i)$ and $U(Y_i)$ are the independence measure (i.e., negative entropy) of the component $Y_i$ and the correspondence measure between $Y_i$ and $R_i$. Here, $Y_i = W_i^T \cdot \tilde{X}$ is the estimated $i$th IC, $\tilde{X} = \left(\tilde{X}_1, \tilde{X}_2, \cdots, \tilde{X}_M\right)^T$ is whitened vectors of fMRI data. $R_i$ is the $i$th GIC with zero mean and unit variance. $M$ is the number of time points. $v$ is a Gaussian variable with zero mean and unit variance. $G(\cdot)$ represents any non-quadratic function, $E(\cdot)$ denotes the mathematical expectation. In GIG-ICA, the unmixing matrix $W_i$ is iteratively optimized by the gradient ascent method to obtain each IC for each subject. Among the resulting ICs, some meaningful ICs representing the FNs can be used for further study.

## 2.2 GIG-sICA Method

Inspired by GIG-ICA, GIG-sICA incorporates a graph regularization term based on the carefully designed voxel features to construct a multi-objective function, which can extract smooth and noise-free FNs in addition to the original advantages of GIG-ICA. Figure 1 shows the framework of GIG-sICA, which includes two steps stated in Sects. 1 and 2 and the design of voxel features is included in Sect. 3.

*Section 1: Calculation of GICs*

Our method estimates the GICs first based on the fMRI data of all subjects. The calculation of GICs is as same as that in GIG-ICA. In this paper, the Infomax ICA [9] is used for the group-level ICA. To obtain reliable GICs, ICASSO is used to cluster the results of multiple ICA runs (20 times).

*Section 2: Construction and optimization of the multi-objective function*

In the second step, the individual ICs are computed using a multi-objective optimization based on the GICs.

Specifically, our multi-objective function as formulated in (2) is constructed to simultaneously optimize the independence, correspondence, and smoothness of the FNs.

$$\max\begin{cases} K(Y_i) = \frac{2}{\pi} \cdot \arctan\left(d \cdot \{E[G(Y_i)] - E[G(v)]\}^2\right) \\ F(Y_i) = E(Y_i \cdot R_i) \\ T(Y_i) = e^{\frac{-Tr(Y_i \cdot L \cdot Y_i')}{t}} \end{cases} \tag{2}$$

The $K(Y_i)$ and $F(Y_i)$ are the normalized independence and correspondence measures, which are consistent to that in GIG-ICA. The $T(Y_i)$ is a graph regularization term that we add to optimize the smoothness of ICs. $Tr(\cdot)$ denotes the trace of matrix, $L = D - Q$ is a Laplace matrix. The basic idea of our method is to design a series of voxel features that are used to compute the adjacency matrix $Q$ and the degree matrix $D$, reflecting the

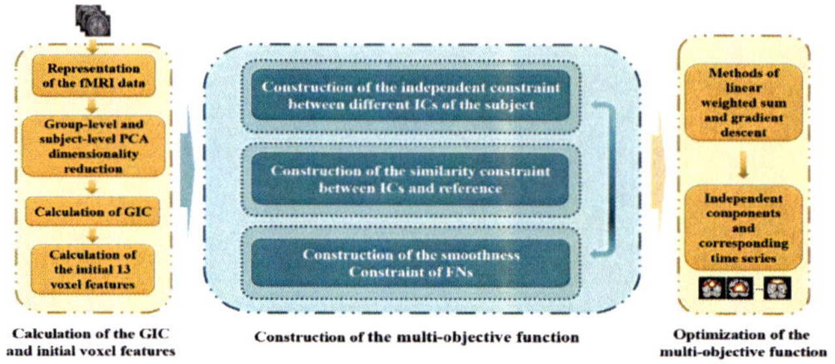


**Fig. 1.** The block diagram of GIG-sICA.

between-voxel relations. By adding the $T(Y_i)$, the smoothness between voxels can be achieved. In addition, $d$ and $t$ are the hyperparameters that are automatically determined in our method.

After constructing the multi-objective function, we use the linear weighted sum method to express the total objective function as Formula (3) to realize the optimization problem.

$$A_i^* = argmax[a \cdot K(Y_i) + b \cdot F(Y_i) + \mathrm{c} \cdot T(Y_i)] \\ s.t. a + b + \mathrm{c} = 1 \tag{3}$$

where $a$, $b$, $c$ are the weight parameters. Their different values reflect the preference for the independence, correspondence, and smoothness of ICs. We performed the experiments with the weight parameters of $a = b = 0.3$ and $c = 0.4$.

Here, we derive Eq. (3) to obtain an iterative expression, which is shown in (4). Then, the gradient ascent method is used to optimize the IC iteratively.

$$g = \mathrm{a} \cdot \nabla k(Y_i) + \mathrm{b} \cdot \nabla F(Y_i) + \mathrm{c} \cdot \nabla T(Y_i) \tag{4}$$

$$d = \frac{g}{||g||} \tag{5}$$

where $||\cdot||$ is the norm of the vector $g$. According to Formula (5), we can get the iteration direction $d$. And we use the backtracking method to determine the iteration step. We set an initial step and determine whether the sufficient ascent condition is currently met, stop if so, otherwise halve the step size and judge again until the sufficient ascent is met. Besides, we set a threshold parameter $\partial = e^{-2}$, if the difference between the total objective function value obtained by iteration and the initial value is greater than $\partial$, the feature values are updated according to the IC obtained by this iteration. If not, the feature values are kept and the iteration continues.

*Section 3: The design of voxel features*

In our method, we design a total of 13 voxel features that can cover the mostly common noises in fMRI data to remove different noises in FNs. We categorize those features into four groups. Three groups of features both include the activation states, the mean value and the mean similarity of activation states, which differ noise from meaningful voxels by the spatial localization of CSF, WM and BE separately so as to remove the noise in

CSF, WM and BE. The fourth group of features includes the connected region of voxels, the voxel degree, the mean value, and mean similarity of voxel degrees, which distinguish noise and meaningful voxels by their differences such as the size, space distance, and the z-scores to remove the noise in GM. Regarding each group of features, an adjacency matrix is computed to reflect the between-voxel similarity from a certain angle, yielding $Q_1$, $Q_2$, $Q_3$, and $Q_4$. As mentioned above, these features can be independently or jointly applied in our method. When the four groups of features are used jointly, the adjacency matrix can be $Q = Q_1 + Q_2 + Q_3 + Q_4$. Then, L can be computed to construct the smoothness term so as to achieve denoising.

### 2.3 Validation and Evaluation Experiments

*Section 1: Evaluation based on simulated datasets*

We first generated a group of initial simulated data using the SimTB toolbox [10] and then added four types of noises to generate four groups of data for examination. In the initial data, every subject included 150 time points, 148 × 148 voxels, and 8 ICs. We generated WM and CSF masks based on the IC templates in the SimTB and added noise at the corresponding positions for each IC to obtain two groups of data. Moreover, we generated a BE mask and added a BE-related noise for each IC. For the fourth group of data, we randomly added two block noises in each IC that did not coincide with the above three positions to simulate the noises in GM.

Experiments on the four groups of simulated data were conducted using GIG-ICA and GIG-sICA. The number of ICs was set to 8, and we respectively used four groups of voxel features to compute L and construct the smoothness term, which corresponds to removing noise in the four groups of simulated data. After obtaining the FNs, we visualized the FNs with their corresponding ground truth and calculated the spatial accuracy to verify the denoising ability of our methods. Particularly, the spatial accuracy of an individual FN was measured by the Pearson correlation coefficient between the estimated FN and its corresponding ground truth [8].

*Section 2: Evaluation based on real fMRI datasets*

Our method was conducted on the fMRI data of 134 HC and 123 SZ to verify the denoising capability in FNs. It was expected that resulting smooth FNs could help reveal more interesting and important biomarkers of SZ. The data preprocessing process was consistent with that in [8].

The number of ICs was set to 20 for both GIG-ICA and GIG-sICA. For evaluation, we visualized the estimated ICs with their common GICs to verify the denoising capability of our method. For each method, we performed two-sample t-test on the estimated ICs to assess the group differences between HC and SZ. In detail, one-sample t-tests were done on all brain voxels to identify the important regions and then a two-sample t-test was applied to these regions between HC and SZ. Then, to compare the group differences obtained by GIG-ICA and GIG-sICA, we performed additional two-sample t-tests on the positive and absolute value of negative T values separately obtained by the former two-sample t-tests to verify whether the group differences from GIG-sICA are more evident than that from GIG-ICA.

# 3 Results

## 3.1 Results of the Simulated Data

As displayed in Fig. 2, our method removes the noise in WM, CSF, and BE completely as well as most of the noise in GM. In general, our method yields smoother FNs than GIG-ICA regardless of data with any kind of noise. Figure 3 shows the spatial accuracy of FNs obtained by GIG-ICA and GIG-sICA. It is seen that most of the spatial accuracy of FNs obtained by GIG-sICA is higher than that obtained by GIG-ICA.

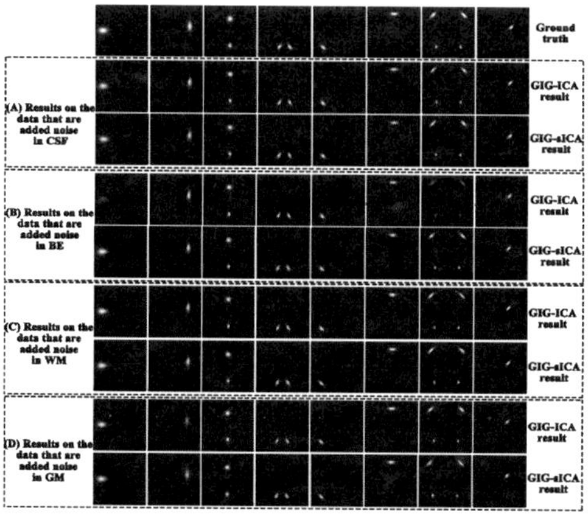


**Fig. 2.** **(A)–(D)** The FNs of one subject estimated from the four groups of simulated data by GIG-ICA and GIG-sICA. In each group, the FNs extracted by GIG-ICA and GIG-ICA are shown on above and below respectively. Ground truth: the 8 FNs of the subject simulated by simTB.

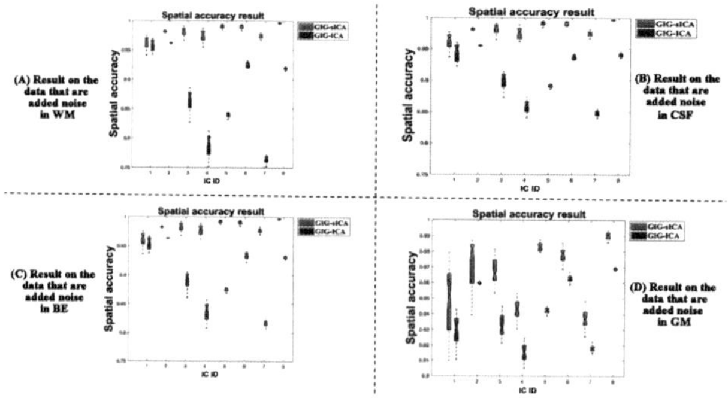


**Fig. 3.** **(A)–(D)** Spatial accuracy of FNs extracted from four groups of simulated data. The red and blue boxplots reflect the spatial accuracy of FNs from GIG-sICA and GIG-ICA, respectively.

### 3.2 Results of the Real Data

We randomly select a subject out of 134 HC to show the FNs obtained by GIG-ICA and GIG-sICA. Figure 4 shows three randomly selected FNs, suggesting that our method successfully removes most of the noises in GM, WM, CSF, and BE, and extracts smooth and realistic FNs.

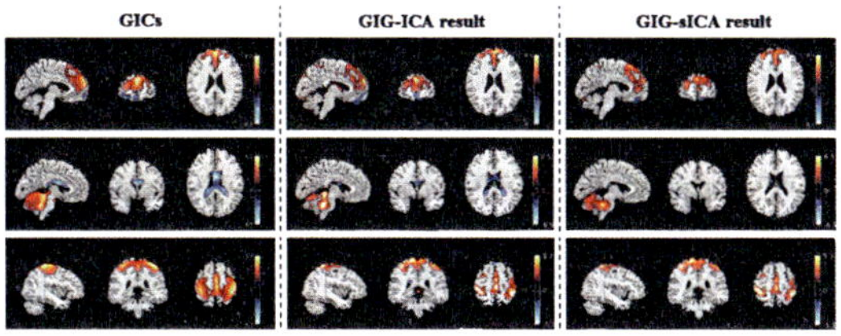


**Fig. 4.** Three of the twenty GICs and corresponding three FNs estimated by the GIG-ICA and GIG-sICA of one subject.

Figure 5 shows the T-values and absolute T-values obtained by the two-sample t-test. In general, our method yields greater group differences in two-thirds of the FNs compared with GIG-ICA. And on the default mode network, salience network and sensorimotor system, the group differences obtained by our method are significantly greater than GIG-ICA.

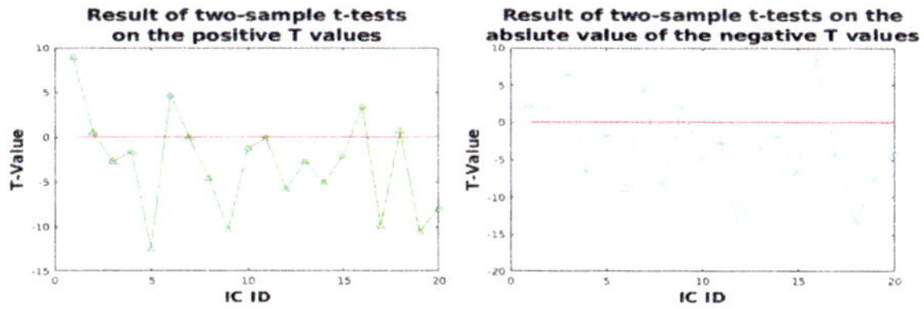


**Fig. 5.** Results of the two-sample t-test on the positive and absolute value of negative T values. The red line represents 0, the points above the red line indicate that the FNs estimated by the GIG-ICA have greater group differences, conversely, the FNs estimated by the GIG-sICA have greater group differences.

## 4 Discussion

ICA has been an important tool in analysis of brain networks using fMRI data, but the non-neuronal signals in fMRI can make the obtained FNs contain a lot of noise. Exiting ICA-based methods achieve denoising by reconstructing fMRI data, which do not optimize FNs directly and are constrained by the trained models. In contrast, our method adds a smoothness term to construct the multi-objective function, where the voxel features are used to enable the method to estimate accurate FNs and denoise. The spatial accuracy and visualized FNs of simulated data show that most of the spatial accuracy of FNs obtained by our method is higher than that obtained by GIG-ICA, and our method succeeds in removing most of the noise in WM, CSF, GM and BE. Generally, our method yields greater group differences between HC and SZ, which may result in more accurate and reliable biomarkers.

Compared with the existing ICA-based denoising methods, our method directly optimizes FNs and avoids the model dependency problem. Compared with GIG-ICA, our method can estimate smoother and more accurate FNs. In the future, the voxel features for the construction of the smoothness term can be extended according to the actual situations in the data.

## 5 Conclusions

In conclusion, we have proposed a new ICA method named GIG-sICA for studies of fMRI data. Experiments based on both simulated and real fMRI data have demonstrated that great performance can be achieved by GIG-sICA with respect to functional network smoothness and denoising, the spatial accuracy of the network, as well as group difference detection. GIG-sICA is effective and promising to extract noise-free FNs and is helpful to identify reliable biomarkers and study brain diseases.

**Acknowledgement.** This work was supported by National Natural Science Foundation of China (Grant No. 62076157 and 61703253 to Yuhui Du), Fund Program for the Scientific Activities of Selected Returned Overseas Professionals in Shanxi Province (to Yuhui Du), the 1331 Engineering Project of Shanxi Province of China.

## References

1. Yang, W., Pilozzi, A., Huang, X.: An overview of ICA/BSS-based application to Alzheimer's brain signal processing. Biomedicines **9**(4), 386 (2021)
2. De Blasi, B., Caciagli, L., et al.: Noise removal in resting-state and task fMRI: functional connectivity and activation maps. J. Neural Eng. **17**(4), 046040 (2020)
3. Griffanti, L., Douaud, G., et al.: Hand classification of fMRI ICA noise components. Neuroimage **154**, 188–205 (2017)
4. Kam, T.E., Zhang, H., et al.: A deep learning framework for noise component detection from resting-state functional MRI. In: Proceedings of the international conference on medical image computing and computer assisted intervention, vol. 11766, pp. 754–762 (2019)
5. Salimi-Khorshidi, G., et al.: Automatic denoising of functional MRI data: combining independent component analysis and hierarchical fusion of classifiers. Neuroimage **90**, 449–468 (2014)
6. Pruim, R.H.R., et al.: ICA-AROMA: a robust ICA-based strategy for removing motion artifacts from fMRI data. Neuroimage **112**, 267–277 (2015)
7. Van Schuerbeek, P., De Wandel, et al.: (2022) The optimized combination of aCompCor and ICA-AROMA to reduce motion and physiologic noise in task fMRI data. Biomed. Phys. Eng. Express **8**(5) (2022)
8. Du, Y., Fu, Z., Xing, Y., et al.: Evidence of shared and distinct functional and structural brain signatures in schizophrenia and autism spectrum disorder. Commun. Biol. **4**(1), 1073 (2021)
9. Wei, P., Bao, R., et al.: Comparing the reliability of different ICA algorithms for fMRI analysis. Plos One **17**(6), e0270556 (2022)
10. Erhardt, E.B., Allen, E.A., Wei, Y., et al.: SimTB, a simulation toolbox for fMRI data under a model of spatiotemporal separability. Neuroimage **59**(4), 4160–4167 (2012)

# An Attention Guided Multi-scale Network with Channel-Enhanced Transformer for Coronary Arteries Segmentation

Jinzhong Yang[1,2], Peng Hong[2], Bu Xu[1], Yaojun Chen[1], Lisheng Xu[1,2,3](✉), Chengbao Peng[2], Yu Sun[4], and Benqiang Yang[4]

[1] College of Medicine and Biological Information Engineering, Northeastern University, Shenyang 110169, China
xuls@bmie.neu.edu.cn

[2] Neusoft Research of Intelligent Healthcare Technology, Co. Ltd., Shenyang 110169, China

[3] Key Laboratory of Medical Image Computing, Ministry of Education, Shenyang 110169, China

[4] Department of Radiology, General Hospital of North Theater Command, Shenyang 110169, China

**Abstract.** Coronary artery disease is a major cause of mortality and morbidity. Automatic segmentation of the coronary artery is a key step in the diagnosis of coronary artery disease. This study aims to propose an attention guided multi-scale fusion network with channel-enhanced Transformer for automatic segmentation of coronary arteries on coronary computed tomography angiography (CCTA). To improve the segmentation performance, an attention guided multi-scale fusion (AGMF) module and channel-enhanced transformer (C-Trans) module are proposed. The AGMF can effectively extract and fuse multi-layer features to locate and segment multiple small coronary arteries accurately. Specifically, the AGMF module not only can extract representative coronary artery features in the encoding process but also can accurately locate and segment coronary arteries in the decoding process. To select the effective channel features, the C-Trans is introduced to obtain the channel features with token. This module can effectively screen out the channel features in each layer of U-net to improve the accuracy of segmentation. Experimental results show that our proposed method obtains the IoU of 0.6996 and the Dice of 0.8224, which are more than 1% higher than the existing model. From the results, it is found that our proposed network outperforms the state-of-the-art 2D coronary artery segmentation method.

**Keywords:** Coronary arteries segmentation · Attention guided · Multi-scale fusion · Channel-transformer

## 1 Introduction

Coronary artery disease (CAD) remains the leading cause of mortality in the upper-middle and high-income countries [1, 2]. Coronary computed tomography angiography (CCTA) has been embraced as a non-invasive and accurate imaging modality for detection and exclusion of CAD [3]. Segmenting coronary arteries fastly and accurately is a


G. Wang et al. (Eds.): APCMBE 2023, IFMBE Proceedings 103, pp. 157–167, 2024.
https://doi.org/10.1007/978-3-031-51455-5_19

prerequisite for CCTA to evaluate coronary artery lesions. There are some challenges for the automatic segmtation of coronary arteries in CCTA images. For example, there is weak boundary between coronary arteries and surrounding tissues in the CCTA [4, 5]. The coronary arteries present the characteristics of strip and fuzzy boundary in the CCTA cross-sectional view with aortic root. The coronary arteries around the pericardium are scattered and have various shapes.

The deep learning has been widely used in medical image segmentation and achieved excellent performance, such as three-dimensional (3D) U-net [6, 7], 3D U-net with global feature [4], improved 3D Dense U-net [8, 9], and V-net [10]. To improve the accuracy of coronary artery segmentation, a two-stage 3D U-net method is implemented to segment the heart region first, and then segment the coronary artery [11]. However, this two-stage segmentation method has high computational complexity. To reduce the computational complexity, a two-stage strategy in which 2D and 3D networks are fused for coronary arteries segmentation [12]. However, these methods ignore the local positioning information of the small coronary artery. To obtain accurate coronary artery location information, Fu et al. used the Mask R-CNN to segment the coronary arteries after locating them [13]. Mirunalini et al. realized coronary artery segmentation by first identifying the location of the coronary artery and then using U-net network with a residual module (Resnet) [14]. These studies are to determine the position of the coronary artery first and then segment the coronary artery, instead of using a deep learning network for end-to-end processing of the entire segmentation task. To locate the coronary artery features in the deep learning network model, Cheung et al. used a U-net with deconvolution in the decoder (Decnet) [15]. In addition, Zhu et al. utilized a feature fusion net (FFnet) of temporal and spatial features to achieve accurate coronary artery segmentation [16]. However, the above methods do not screen feature segmentation which is prone to mis-segmentation.

To reduce mis-segmentation results, a multi-scale fusion block of layered convolution with residual is built to link local vessel segments together within a single convolution block [17]. However, the receptive field can be enlarged in the process of multi-layer convolution, ignoring the positioning and segmentation of small objects. To focus on small objects when segmenting multiple coronary arteries, an attention guided multi-scale fusion module was proposed in this study. From the perspective of the channel characteristics of skip connection, the U-net is relatively simple and does not screen the characteristics in the channel. The coronary artery discontinuity occurs when the coronary arteries are segmented. Transformers are strong enough to capture long-range dependencies within the input [18]. Therefore, the channel transformer (C-Trans) was used to skip the connection [19].

The main contributions of the article can be summarized as:

1. A novel coronary artery segmentation network, attention guided multi-scale transformer (AGMT), is proposed. The semantic information of different receptive fields in each convolution layer is extracted by taking full advantage of multi-scale convolution, which reduces the loss of information, improving the problem that small vessels are difficult to locate and recognize.
2. A channel transformer (C-Trans) structure is introduced to exchange the simple skip connection in the U-net structure, to screen out the useful features in the channel. In

addition, this module is used to eliminate the problem of inconsistent decoding features between the Transformer and U-net to achieve accurate automatic segmentation.

# 2 Method

In this section, the preprocessing used to reduce the influence of lungs on coronary artery segmentation is described first. Then the AGMT segmentation network structure is described. Finally, the attention-gated multi-scale module and the C-Trans module proposed in the segmentation network are introduced.

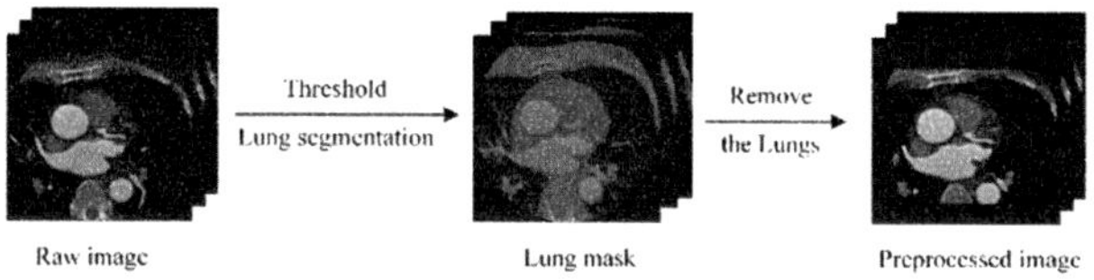


**Fig. 1.** The general framework for preprocessing, where the red part is the lung mask established after threshold segmentation.

*A. Data Preprocessing*

The data preprocessing is shown in Fig. 1. In the CCTA, the CT value of the lung area is low, showing a large black area. To suppress the influence of the lung area around the coronary, we preliminarily extract the mask of the lung area in the CT image. However, this method can only segment the black lung area in the CT image and cannot include the pulmonary artery that is close to the coronary artery CT value. Therefore, some small pulmonary arteries were removed by morphological closure operation (expansion before corrosion). The method of the 8-connected domain is used to refine the lung mask.The largest connected domain is retained. And then, the lung mask was removed from the raw image to obtain preprocessed image.

*B. Network Architecture*

To segment coronary arteries from CCTA, an attention guided multi-scale transformer (AGMT) with U-net architecture as the backbone is designed to locate different coronary arteries, as shown in Fig. 2. The whole encoder part is composed of 4 convolution modules and 3 attention guided multi-scale fusion (AGMF) modules. The convolution module is composed of a 3 × 3 convolutional layer, batch normalization two dimension (BatchNorm2d) layer, and nonlinear rectified linear unit (ReLU) activation layer. The AGMF module is a multi-layer convolution framework to enlarge the receptive field while adding attention-gated multi-scale fusion between the corresponding convolution layers. The channel-enhanced transformer is used to screen the useful features of each layer in the encoder to the decoder. The decoder includes 4 upsampling layers, 3 AGMF modules, and a sigmoid activation function.

The AGMF block is shown in Fig. 3. After a 1 × 1 convolutional layer, the features are evenly divided into 4 feature groups named $x_i$, $i = 1, 2, 3, 4$. The feature size of each

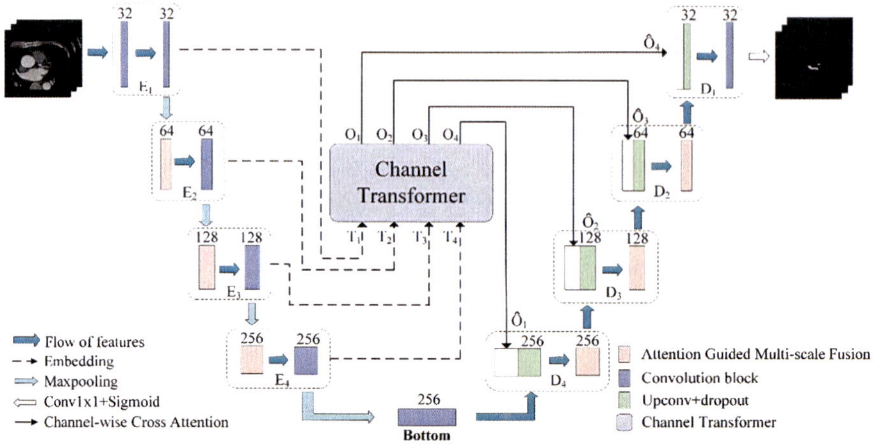


**Fig. 2.** Overall architecture of the proposed attention guided multi-scale Transformer. This transformer model is an end-to-end coronary arteries segmentation network. The designed attention guided multi-scale fusion effectively locate the different shape of the coronary arteries. Every convolution kernel is 3 × 3.

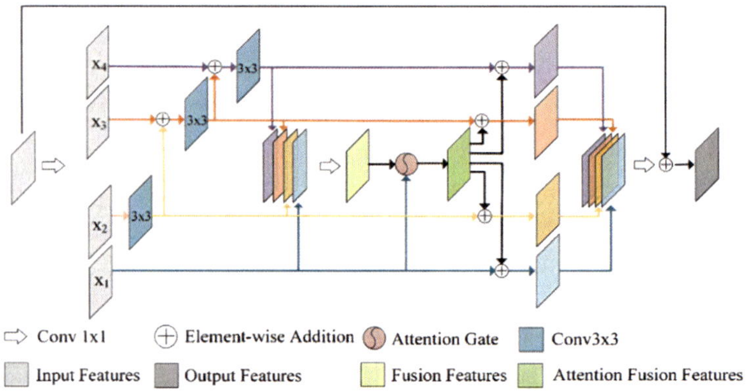


**Fig. 3.** Illustration of attention guided multi-scale fusion (AGMF) architecture. The designed AGMF adopts several 3 × 3 convolution to increase the number of scales. The features of different scales are fed to the attention gate after the fusion of 1 × 1 convolution. Fusing attention-enhanced all features, the output features are refined by residual learning.

group of $x_i$ is the same as the input feature. Except for $x_1$, the sum of each $x_i$ and $x_{i-1}$ are fed to the 3 × 3 convolution, followed by BatchNorm2d and ReLU. This process can be formulated as:

$$f(x_i) = \begin{cases} x_i,\ i = 1 \\ Conv_3(x_i),\ i = 2 \\ Conv_3(x_i + f(x_{i-1})),\ i = 3, 4 \end{cases} \tag{1}$$

where $Conv_3$ denotes convolution with 3 × 3 kernel size.

To prevent the loss of small target areas from being ignored during segmentation, the attention gate is adopted to refine the segmentation of small target areas after these features are fused through the $1 \times 1$ convolution. In the attention module, the input image called $x_1$ contains more shallow edge information, while the fused feature map contains deeper semantic contextual information. Therefore, the convolution operations of different convolution kernels are used to distribute the weights of different features to accurately locate and segment small coronary artery. After obtaining $F$ and $I$ with different weights, the attention feature map $C$ is obtained by feature addition and fusion. After $C$ is convoluted by $k_l$ with $1 \times 1$ convolution kernel, the $C$ is fed to the ReLU activation function and the $k_*$ with $7 \times 7$ convolution kernel to obtain the attention factor $\alpha_*$, which enhances the global features of vessels and retains the contextual features of small blood vessels. After $\alpha_*$ performs sigmoid, the final attention factor can be obtained. The output $O$ is obtained by multiplying the final attention factor and the input image.

After screening out the features of attention, these features are sent into each multi-scale convolution block for fusion. The formula is as follows:

$$f^{'}(x_i) = f(x_i) + O, i = 1, 2, 3, 4 \tag{2}$$

$$y = x + Conv_1\Big(Concat\Big(f^{'}(x_i)\Big)\Big), \; i = 1, 2, 3, 4 \tag{3}$$

where $x$ represents the input feature of AGMF. The y represents the output feature of AGMF. $Conv_1$ denotes convolution with $1 \times 1$ kernel size. Concat represents feature fusion in the manner of concatenate in AGMF.

Channel Transformer (C-Trans) consists of a channel-wise cross fusion transformer (CCT) and a channel-wise cross attention (CCA). The structures of the two-channel-wise cross modules are shown in Fig. 4. CCT fuses multi-level encoding features, including multi-scale feature embedding, multi-channel cross-attention, and multi-layer perceptron. Multi-scale feature embedding is to change specific 4-layer encoding features into 2D patch sequences to mark the positions of features of each scale as $T_1$, $T_2$, $T_3$, and $T_4$. The patch size is set to 16. The marking feature sizes of each layer are 1, 1/2, 1/4, and 1/8 of the patch. Then, the features at the marked location are transferred to a multi-head channel cross-attention module. Since key ($K$) and value ($V$) need to be calculated in the multiple-head attention, the features of $T_1$, $T_2$, $T_3$, and $T_4$ are concatenated as $K$ and $V$. The output feature $O$ is calculated by Formula (4). Finally, the output results are screened out more useful channel output characteristics through a multi-layer perceptron (MLP) with residual structure (a multi-layer perceptron with 2, 4, 8, and 12 layers of Layer Normalization and a combination of MLP), which transmitted into CCA.

$$O = \sigma\left[\psi\left(\frac{Q_i^T \times K}{\sqrt{T_\Sigma}}\right)\right] \times V^T \tag{4}$$

where $T_\Sigma = T_1 + T_2 + T_3 + T_4$, $\sigma$ represents the Sigmoid function, $\psi$ represents the Instance Normalization

CCA can fuse the semantic features between C-Trans and U-net decoders. The output features $O$ marked by CCT are upsampled and convolved to a feature block with the

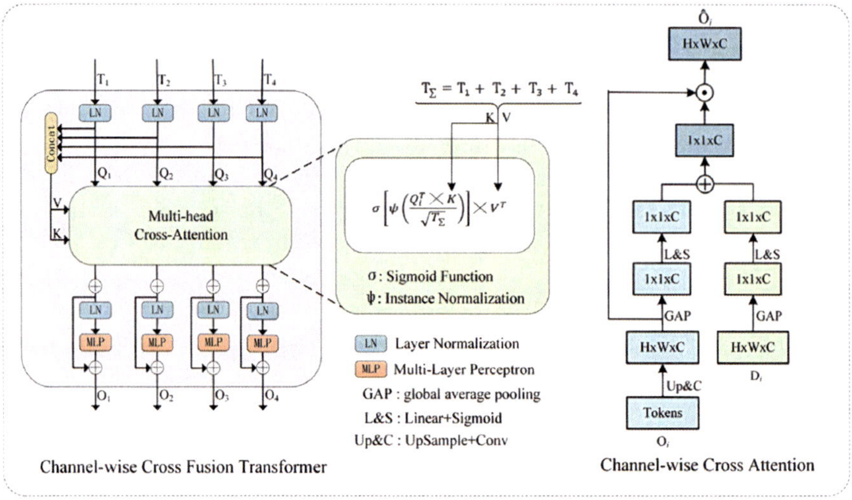


**Fig. 4.** The mentioned Channel Transformer module in AGMT, which includes channel-wise cross fusion transformer and channel-wise cross attention.

same size as the decoded feature. This feature block and decoding feature block $D$ are spatially compressed through global average pooling (GAP) so that global features can be embedded. Channel output features and decoding features embedded in global features generate feature blocks with the same scale through linear layer weight and Sigmoid function. And the two feature blocks are combined to obtain channel feature blocks with encoding information. The channel feature $\widehat{O}$ is obtained by multiplying the feature block with the encoding information and the original channel feature.

## 3 Experiments and Results

All the experiments are implemented with Python 3.8 and Pytorch 1.10.1 on four Tesla V100 with 32G memory. The learning rate is initially set to $1\text{x}10^{-4}$. The epoch is set to 50. The batch size is set to 16. The optimizer selects Adam. The loss function selects the mixed loss function of Dice loss and binary cross entropy (BCE) loss. The segmentation input image size is 512 * 512.

*A. Dataset and evaluation metrics*

The CCTA Data is composed of 81 subjects collected from the General Hospital of the North Theater Command in Shenyang, China. Data annotation is finished by three experienced radiologists. Among a total of 81 subjects, 65 cases were used for training. The accuracy of the algorithm was verified through 8-fold cross-validation. 16 cases were used for testing.

IoU, Dice, Recall, and Precision are used as indicators to evaluate segmentation performance. The defined expressions are as follows:

$$IoU = \frac{TP}{FP + TP + FN} \tag{5}$$

$$Dice = \frac{2TP}{FP + 2TP + FN} \tag{6}$$

$$Recall = \frac{TP}{TP + FN} \tag{7}$$

$$Precision = \frac{TP}{TP + FP} \tag{8}$$

where true positive (TP) represents the true positive segmentation result. False positive (FP) represents the false positive segmentation results. False negative (FN) represents the false negative of segmentation results.

*B. Comparative experiment*

**Table 1.** The segmentation results of various models on CCTA Data

| Model | IoU | Dice | Recall | Precision |
|---|---|---|---|---|
| U-net [6] | 0.6799 | 0.8085 | 0.7683 | 0.7964 |
| FFnet [16] | 0.6819 | 0.8100 | 0.7501 | 0.8013 |
| Decnet [15] | 0.6861 | 0.8130 | 0.7659 | 0.8061 |
| MAUnet [20] | 0.6284 | 0.7707 | 0.7615 | 0.7353 |
| LVSnet [17] | 0.6848 | 0.8121 | 0.7671 | 0.8003 |
| Resnet [14] | 0.6850 | 0.8121 | 0.7563 | **0.8255** |
| AGMT | **0.6996** | **0.8224** | **0.7733** | 0.8225 |

In the comparison experiment, the AGMT was compared with U-net [6], Multi-stage attention U-net (MAUnet) [20], FFnet [16], Decnet [15], Resnet [14], and liver vessel segmentation net (LVSnet) [17]. In the Table 1, the AGMT achieved the best results in all evaluation indicators. IoU of AGMT was 0.6996, which was 0.0197 higher than U-net's IoU. Dice of AGMT was 0.8224, which was 0.0139 higher than U-net's Dice. Recall of AGMT was 0.7733, which was 0.005 higher than U-net's Recall. Precision of AGMT was 0.8225, which was 0.0261 higher than U-net's Precision.

As shown in Fig. 5, Three 2D visualization results are selected from the aortic root to the apex. With aortic influence, the segmentation result of the AGMT has fewer false positive points than FFnet, Decnet, and Resnet. At the bifurcation of the anterior descending branch and the circumflex branch of the coronary artery, AGMT segmentation results are more accurate than FFnet segmentation results, and fewer false positives than Decnet and Resnet segmentation results.The AGMT can be used accurately locate this small coronary artery, but AGMT's sgmentation is not as much as Resnet segmentation. Compared with FFnet, Decnet, and Resnet, the AGMT can segment multiple small coronary shapes with coronary artery ostium more accurately. The AGMT's results at the posterior branch of the right coronary artery have fewer false positives than FFnet's results.

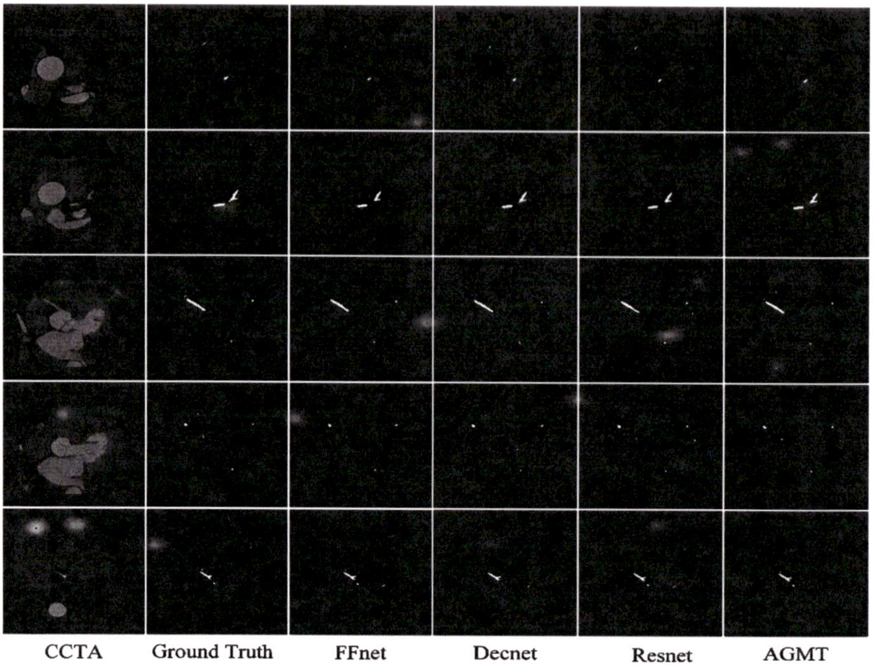


**Fig. 5.** 2D cross-sectional view results of the coronary artery on CCTA Data.

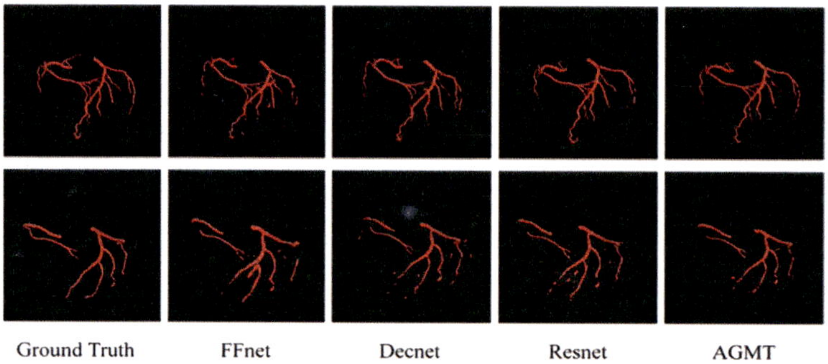


**Fig. 6.** 3D visualization results of comparative experiments on CCTA Data

In the 3D visualization results, two kinds of coronary arteries are selected based on the number of coronary artery branches. The first case is the coronary artery with more branches, and the second one is the coronary artery with fewer branches. It can be found from Fig. 6 that in the first segmentation case, the 3D result of AGMT is more accurate than that of the FFnet segmentation. The coronary arteries segmented by AGMT have fewer false positive points than that segmented by Decnet. The coronary arteries segmented by AGMT have more branches than those segmented by Resnet. In the second case of less-branch coronary artery segmentation, the coronary arteries segmented by AGMT are more accurate than those segmented by FFnet. Compared with the Decnet segmentation results, the segmentation results of the AGMT have fewer false positive points, especially the segmentation results of the AGMT at the end of the coronary artery are more accurate. Compared with Resnet segmentation results, the segmentation results of the AGMT have better continuity at the end.

## 4 Discussion

Automatic segmentation of coronary arteries from CCTA images is of great significance in the diagnosis of coronary artery diseases. In the study of coronary artery segmentation, many algorithms can make mistakes. A Transformer based on AGMF is proposed to improve the segmentation accuracy. Compared with the 2D U-net, AGMT uses the advantage of the Transformer to capture long-distance global features. Compared with the FFnet, AGMT can segment more coronary artery branches. Compared with the Dec-net, AGMT reduced the false positive rate of coronary artery. Compared with the Resnet, AGMT can segment more coronary artery branches. AGMT has achieved satisfactory results in most cases. However, there are still some limitations. As shown in the 3D visualization results, there are still some discontinuities in the coronary artery segmentation. In future work, we will consider how to make the coronary artery segmentation more continuous and complete by combining the coronary artery geometry information with the deep learning network.

## 5 Conclusion

In this paper, a AGMT with the AGMF and the C-Trans is proposed for the coronary artery segmentation. The C-Trans uses a cross multi-head attention to select useful context features, making up for the lack of small vessel location features in the U-net decoding part. The AGMF effectively extracts multi-scale vascular features, reducing the occurrence of false predictions. From the results, it is found that the AGMT outperforms the existing 2D coronary artery segmentation networks.

**Acknowledgments.** This work was supported by the Liaoning Provincial 'Selecting the Best Candidates by Opening Competition Mechanism' Science and Technology Program (No.2022JH/10400004). This study was also supported by the National Natural Science Foundation of China (No. 62273082 and No. 61773110), the Natural Science Foundation of Liaoning Province (No. 20170540312 and No. 2021-YGJC-14), the Basic Scientific Research Project (Key Project) of Liaoning Provincial Department of Education (LJKZ00042021), the Fundamental Research Funds for the Central Universities (No. N2119008), and the Shenyang Science and Technology Plan Fund (No. 21–104-1–24, No. 20–201-4–10, and No. 201375). We gratefully acknowledge the kind assistance of Yanan Wu and Chengbao Peng in article structure and writing logic.

## References

1. Roth, G.A., et al.: Global burden of cardiovascular diseases and risk factors, 1990–2019: update from the GBD 2019 study. J. Am. Coll. Cardiol. **76**(25), 2982–3021 (2020)
2. Knuuti, J., Revenco, V.: 2019 ESC Guidelines for the diagnosis and management of chronic coronary syndromes. Eur. Heart J. **41**(5), 407–477 (2020)
3. Schoepf, U.J., Becker, C.R., Ohnesorge, B.M., Yucel, E.K.: CT of coronary artery disease. Radiology **232**(1), 18–37 (2004)
4. Gu, J., Fang, Z., Gao, Y., Tian, F.: Segmentation of coronary arteries images using global feature embedded network with active contour loss. Comput. Med. Imaging Graph. **86**, 101799 (2020)
5. Y. Lei et al., "Automated coronary artery segmentation in coronary computed tomography angiography (CCTA) using deep learning neural networks," in Medical Imaging 2020: Imaging Informatics for Healthcare, Research, and Applications, 2020, vol. 11318: SPIE, pp. 279–284
6. Ronneberger, O., Fischer, P., Brox, T.: U-net: Convolutional networks for biomedical image segmentation. In: International Conference on Medical image computing and computer-assisted intervention, pp. 234–241. Springer (2015)
7. W. Huang et al., "Coronary artery segmentation by deep learning neural networks on computed tomographic coronary angiographic images," in 2018 40th Annual international conference of the IEEE engineering in medicine and biology society (EMBC), 2018: IEEE, pp. 608–611
8. Pan, L.S., Li, C.W., Su, S.F., Tay, S.Y., Tran, Q.V., Chan, W.P.: Coronary artery segmentation under class imbalance using a U-Net based architecture on computed tomography angiography images. Sci. Rep. **11**(1), 1–7 (2021)
9. Song, A., et al.: Automatic coronary artery segmentation of CCTA images with an efficient feature-fusion-and-rectification 3D-UNet. IEEE J. Biomed. Health Inform. **26**(8), 4044–4055 (2022)
10. Tian, F., Gao, Y., Fang, Z., Gu, J.: Automatic coronary artery segmentation algorithm based on deep learning and digital image processing. Appl. Intell. **51**(12), 8881–8895 (2021)
11. C. Dong, S. Xu, and Z. Li, "A novel multistage deep learning solution for automatic coronary arteries segmentation from CCTA," Journal of the American College of Cardiology, vol. 77, no. 18_Supplement_1, p. 3224, 2021
12. Gu, L., Cai, X.C.: Fusing 2D and 3D convolutional neural networks for the segmentation of aorta and coronary arteries from CT images. Artif. Intell. Med. **121**, 102189 (2021)
13. Y. Fu et al., "Mask R-CNN based coronary artery segmentation in coronary computed tomography angiography," in Medical Imaging 2020: Computer-Aided Diagnosis, 2020, vol. 11314: SPIE, pp. 1047–1052
14. P. Mirunalini, C. Aravindan, A. T. Nambi, S. Poorvaja, and V. P. Priya, "Segmentation of Coronary Arteries from CTA axial slices using Deep Learning techniques," in TENCON 2019–2019 IEEE Region 10 Conference (TENCON), 2019: IEEE, pp. 2074–2080
15. Cheung, W.K., et al.: A computationally efficient approach to segmentation of the aorta and coronary arteries using deep learning. IEEE Access **9**, 108873–108888 (2021)
16. Zhu, H., Song, S., Xu, L., Song, A., Yang, B.: Segmentation of coronary arteries images using spatio-temporal feature fusion network with combo loss. Cardiovasc. Eng. Technol. **13**(3), 407–418 (2022)
17. Yan, Q., et al.: Attention-guided deep neural network with multi-scale feature fusion for liver vessel segmentation. IEEE J. Biomed. Health Inform. **25**(7), 2629–2642 (2020)
18. K. Han et al., "A survey on vision transformer," IEEE transactions on pattern analysis and machine intelligence, 2022

19. Wang, H., Cao, P., Wang, J., Zaiane, O.R.: Uctransnet: rethinking the skip connections in u-net from a channel-wise perspective with transformer. Proceedings of the AAAI Conference on Artificial Intelligence **36**(3), 2441–2449 (2022)
20. S. Li, J. Zhang, C. Ruan, and Y. Zhang, "Multi-stage attention-unet for wireless capsule endoscopy image bleeding area segmentation," in 2019 IEEE International Conference on Bioinformatics and Biomedicine (BIBM), 2019: IEEE, pp. 818–825

# A Specularity Suppression Algorithm for Endoscope Image Conforming to Weber-Fechner Law

Changlin Liu[1] and Gang He[1,2](✉)

[1] School of Computer Science and Technology, Southwest University of Science and Technology, Mianyang, China
ganghe@swust.edu.cn

[2] NHC Key Laboratory of Nuclear Technology Medical Transformation (Mianyang Central Hospital), Mianyang, China

**Abstract.** During the process of endoscopic examination, there may be specularity in the image caused by insufficient illumination, and the internal surface of the workpiece has a specular reflection or other reasons. It creates difficulties for further image analysis. The existing algorithms have poor generalization for endoscopic images, and some algorithms' design problems may cause the image's original features to be treated as specularity and processed. Therefore, we propose a specularity suppression algorithm for endoscope images conforming to Weber-Fechner Law using a single image to obtain a better visual image and reduce the impact of the specularity on further image analysis. Make the gray value the operand to suppress the specularity and the region impacted by it. The algorithm can protect the suppressed area when suppressing the specularity. Experimental results show that the proposed algorithm has a better adaptability to suppress the specularity of the endoscopic images, which can retain more pixels unaffected by the specularity.

**Keywords:** Endoscope · Specularity Suppress · Weber-Fechner Law · Single-image Processing

## 1 Introduction

At present, endoscopes have been used in many fields, such as medical and industrial fields. It is used for various internal body inspection that is difficult to be observed directly by the human eyes, the implementation of surgery, and the internal inspection of industrial workpieces, etc. [1–6]. Due to the use of the light sources when using the endoscope collects images, the specular reflection of these light sources, which is used for lighting up the dark environment, occurs on the smooth surface or the surface has a high reflection rate, which will produce the specularity that impacts further image analysis. Therefore, a specularity suppression algorithm is proposed in this paper to weaken and suppress the influence of these specularities in the images.


G. Wang et al. (Eds.): APCMBE 2023, IFMBE Proceedings 103, pp. 168–179, 2024.
https://doi.org/10.1007/978-3-031-51455-5_20

The existence of the specular reflection is inevitable. In the actual situation, the object's surface will appear as a diffuse reflection, and at the same time, there will also be a specular reflection. The appearance of specular reflection will cover up the original details and features of the object surface, and some additional features will appear which are not inherent features of the object [7]. On the other hand, many algorithms in computer graphics, computer vision, and image processing assume that the image to be processed has a perfectly diffuse surface and take the values of the location impacted by specular reflection as outliers [8]. Such an assumption limits the algorithm's use of images under certain conditions to some extent.

At present, existing research can be divided into two main categories: the first is multi-image processing, and the other is single-image processing. The first type is mainly based on multiple images of the same object. Taking the facts as the basic information from these images, an image without specular reflection can be obtained by using these different positions' real information of the same object contained in multiple pictures. The second category of methods has been used to isolate or remove specular reflections using only one image under certain assumptions. However, due to the problem of using assumptions mentioned earlier in this paper, this kind of method does not perform well in the test of the endoscopic image that has specularity. In general, the results of using multiple images will be better than the results of using only one image. For the single-image processing method, no additional data can supplement the information on the position impacted by the specularity. Therefore, it is challenging to use single-image processing to solve this problem [9]. For multiple-image processing, that is the best way to remove the specularity completely. So most of the method to remove the specularity is this type. Zhu et al. proposed a polarization-based method to do this. It uses a polarizing filter To capture images at different polarization angles [10]. This method not only needs a polarizer but also has high requirements for the angle adjustment of the polarizer and the control of the exposure time during the test. Feng et al.'s algorithm is also a multiple-image processing method. It uses the Dichroic Reflection Model(DRM), which is also one of the most popular reflection models, and the total variation optimization with a light field camera [11]. Although this approach has promising experimental results, it requires a light field camera. This greatly reduces the applicable scenarios of the algorithm. At present, most of the research on single-image processing is carried out according to the DRM [9, 12–18]. The DRM assumes that reflection is composed of surface reflection components and interface reflection components. Because there are many assumptions, it has a low generalization ability [19]. Especially for the endoscopic images with specularity under the actual working conditions used in the test in this paper, there are no obvious advantages to these methods.

This paper focuses on using a single image to suppress the specularity of the endoscopic image. In this paper, we take the gray value of each pixel as the operation object to propose a specularity suppression algorithm for endoscopic images conforming to Weber-Fechner Law. Based on retaining more correct and effective information as required by the industry. Suppress specularity and affected areas as much as possible. Improve the discernability of the available information in a single image and prevent the appearance of false contours. The remaining parts of this paper are organized as follows: the second part will introduce the specularity suppression algorithm for endoscopic images conforming to Weber-Fechner Law. The third part is compared with other typical single image processing algorithms (SSIM and PSNR are the comparison indicators), as well as the comparison of visual perception. Finally will make a summary of the algorithm.

## 2 Proposed Algorithm

Weber-Fechner Law describes that the amount of difference in the same stimulus must reach a certain proportion to cause the difference in human perception. Weber's law can be expressed as:

$$\frac{\Delta I}{I} = K \tag{1}$$

where I is the brightness of the background around the object, delta I is the minimum sensory difference, and K is the Weber ratio.

On this basis, Fechner took the continuous difference threshold as a unit of measurement for the change of sensory quantity and deduced:

$$S = Klg(I) + C \tag{2}$$

where S is a sensory quantity, K is a constant. I is a physical quantity, and C is an integral constant. This formula relates sensory quantities to physical quantities; that is, the increase of sensory quantities lags behind the increase of physical quantities, the increase of physical quantities in a geometric series, and mental quantities in an arithmetic series.

According to the Weber-Fechner law, the relationship between physical and psychological quantities, and our analysis of the gray value of the endoscopic images which have the specularity on it, to ensure the effectiveness of specularity suppression without impacting the normal gray value region, we propose to use tanh function and Softplus function, two activation functions commonly used in deep learning, as the basis to construct the mapping function so that the changing trend of the physical quantity is consistent with the changing trend of the psychological quantity to suppress the specularity.

The activation function is a continuous and differentiable nonlinear function. It has the advantages of simple function expression, high computational efficiency, and the range of its derivative function in a suitable interval. These properties make the deformation of the activation function highly controllable, and it is easy to make the mapping function achieve the desired effect with only a few parameters. Because single image processing has certain limitations on the actual information at the specularity, and to meet the requirements of the workpiece detection on the authenticity of the image, the method proposed in this paper is mainly for the gray value processing, the specularity and the impacted area of the appropriate gray transformation, to compress the gray value of the specularity and the impacted pixels around it, to achieve the purpose of specularity suppression. The main reason for using these two activation functions simultaneously is that the tanh function has the linear region of the low input value and the compression region of the high input value in line with our expectations. Combined with the Softplus function, the input data can be well distinguished into excited and non-excited so that the mapping function can start from the threshold and the above part can be well compressed. The part below the threshold keeps the original value unchanged. The curves of the two functions used simultaneously are smooth curves, which can reduce the generation of false contours to a certain extent.

The hyperbolic tangent function (tanh) is a common Sigmoid-type activation function. The closer the input value is to 0, the more linear the graph will be. The Sigmoid type function also has the property of saturation at both ends, which means that the derivative of the Sigmoid type function tends to 0 as the input value tends to plus or minus infinity. This helps to restrict the input and output to a fixed interval.

$$tanh(x) = \frac{e^x - e^{-x}}{e^x + e^{-x}} \tag{3}$$

For the image with specularity, the gray value of the specularity should be at the rightmost end of the gray value histogram of the whole image, and the gray value of the area seriously affected by the specularity should be greater than a certain threshold. Therefore, in image processing, according to the characteristics of Eq. (3), it can be applied as follows: when the input is less than a certain threshold, the mapping result can keep the original value as much as possible; when the input is more significant than a certain threshold, the input value can be compressed.

To introduce the limiting effect of the threshold on the algorithm so that the linear and compressed regions of tanh can produce different adaptive changes to the gray values of different pixel points of different images, we choose to introduce the Softplus function into the tanh function using the properties of the Softplus function.

$$Softplus(x) = log\left(1 + e^x\right) \tag{4}$$

The Softplus function can be seen as a smooth Rectifie (ReLU) function, the most frequently used activation function. According to its function curve, it is clear that the Softplus function has the property of suppressing smaller inputs. In particular, when the input is less than 0, it makes the output value 0, which is in line with our expectation that a threshold will differentiate the input grayscale values. At the same time, the function curve is different from the ReLU function with obvious turning points. The function image of the Softplus function is excessively smooth, which also facilitates us in preventing the generation of false contours.

After the combination of formulas (3) and (4) is deformed, the mapping function obtained by applying them to the gray value is as follows:

$$y = x \times (1 - tanh(\alpha \times Softplus(x - \lambda)) \times \beta) \tag{5}$$

where x is the gray value of a pixel of the input image, $\alpha$ is the value of the controller of the tanh curve, that is, the amount of controller tanh curve for lateral stretching. After many experiments, its optimal value should be 0.003 ~ 0.005. $\lambda$ is the threshold value, so that the input value less than the threshold value after Softplus function processing can make the input value in the part of the tanh function curve below the threshold $\lambda$ falls in the part of the curve close to linear, more significant than the threshold $\lambda$ falls in the compressed part of the tanh function curve, $\lambda$ is determined by the overall gray value of the input image mean value and the standard deviation of the gray value of the input image. $\beta$ is then the parameter that controls the amount of compression of the algorithm. The flow of algorithm is shown in Fig. 1.

Figure 2 shows the effect of the three parameters $\alpha$, $\lambda$, and $\beta$ on the function with grayscale values 0 to 255 as inputs. Where the larger $\alpha$ is, the more obvious the mapping function is for compression, and the same is true for $\beta$. As for the threshold value $\lambda$, it is obvious from the figure that for different $\lambda$, the input value below the threshold value can maintain good linearity in the output, and the compression starts above the threshold value, and the more significant difference between the input value and the threshold value, the more obvious the compression on the output value.

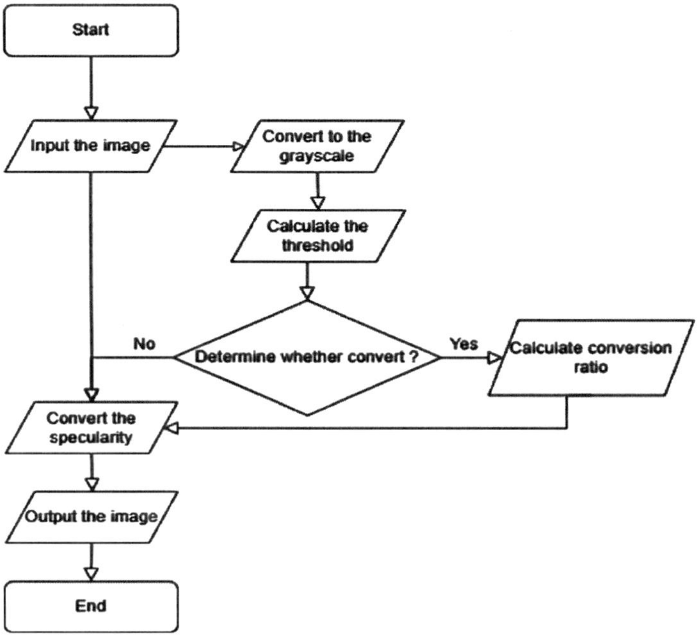


**Fig. 1.** Algorithm flow

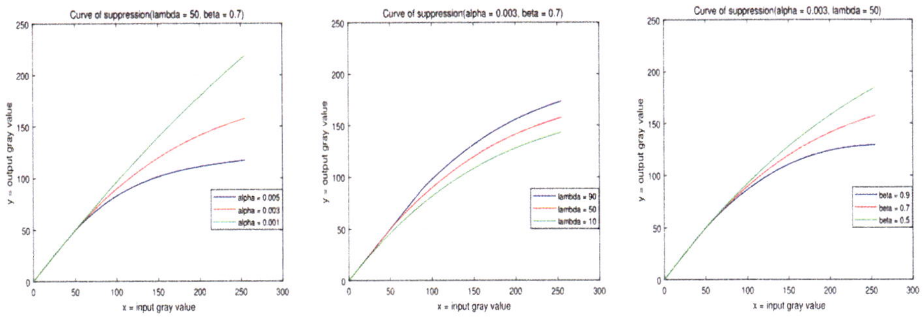


**Fig. 2.** Comparison of different parameters

```
Algorithm: A Specularity Suppression Algorithm for Endoscope Image Conforming to Weber-Fechner Law
Input: A data matrix X for a specularity image.
Output: Processed image
G = grayscale(X); // Convert the RGB to the grayscale;
O = G
Compute the λ for grayscale;
for i in Row(G)
 for j in Colum(G)
  if G[ i, j ] ≥ λ
    Compute the converting ratio a
    G[ i, j ] = G[ i, j ] * a //Compute the result each pixel
  end
 end
end
X[ , ,1] = X[ , , 1] .* (G ./ O) // Compute the R Channel each pixel
X[ , ,2] = X[ , , 2] .* (G ./ O) // Compute the G Channel each pixel
X[ , ,3] = X[ , , 3] .* (G ./ O) // Compute the B Channel each pixel
Output the X
```

## 3 Experiment

To verify the effectiveness of the proposed algorithm for specularity suppression, a specularity suppression algorithm for endoscope images conforming to Weber-Fechner Law proposed in this paper was compared with four existing single-image specularity processing algorithms [9, 14, 15, 17] from two indicator evaluation and visual perception. The environment used in the experiment is MATLAB R2022a for image analysis and calculation, using 12th Gen Intel(R) Core(TM) i9-12900H 2.50 GHz CPU, 32.0 GB RAM, NVIDIA GeForce RTX 3080Ti Laptop GPU with 64-bit Windows 11. In human visual perception, it is not sensitive enough to large-area color changes, but it is relatively more sensitive to differential changes of edges. Therefore, it isn't easy to objectively evaluate the algorithm's performance by only using a visual comparison [9]. The Peak Signal-to-Noise Ratio (PSNR) is used to circumvent this problem. PSNR mainly judges the difference between images in terms of pixels, considering all an image's pixels. At the same time, Structural Similarity (SSIM) was used to evaluate the objective indicators of the image jointly. The qualitative and quantitative evaluation of image evaluation are complementary, so comparing visual sensory aspects is also carried out at the end of this part.

The four algorithms [9, 14, 15, 17] in the references are mainly implemented by using a Matlab algorithm toolkit organized by Ramos on GitHub [20]. In these four algorithms, two parameters need to be set for the method of Akashi et al. [17] involved: the sparse regularization factor is set to $\lambda$ as 3, and the convergence criterion is set to exp(−15). And the function parameters in the method proposed in this paper are set to $\alpha$ as 0.003, $\lambda$ using the average of the grayscale values of the images (to improve the algorithm's ability to adapt to different images), and $\beta$ as 0.7.

## 3.1 PSNR and SSIM

The data sets used for the indicator evaluation were mainly derived from three frames of video images (Figs. 3, 4 and 5) of the endoscope under actual working conditions from Youtube (www.youtube.com/watch?v=Zo9jAuwtdLw), and the obtained three frames were synthesized by adding distinct specularity for the following indicators compared.

Table 1 compares the proposed algorithm's effect and the other four algorithms in specularity suppression. From the results of the evaluation of the indicators, it can be seen that the peak signal-to-noise ratio (PSNR) and structural similarity (SSIM) are worse on all three images in Yang's using bilateral filtering algorithm [15]. The proposed algorithm in this paper has an average improvement of 29.20% in PSNR and 7.37% in SSIM compared to the other four algorithms. The results show that the proposed algorithm performs better than the other three algorithms on the three endoscopic specularity synthesis images of the actual working conditions.

**Table 1.** Indicators comparison results

| | | Akashi | Shen | Yamamoto | Yang | **Proposed** |
|---|---|---|---|---|---|---|
| Figure 3 | PSNR | 25.19 | 22.74 | 22.74 | 20.13 | **26.73** |
| | SSIM | 0.9343 | 0.9426 | 0.9430 | 0.9035 | **0.9850** |
| Figure 4 | PSNR | 26.64 | 21.05 | 21.05 | 20.34 | **30.17** |
| | SSIM | 0.9311 | 0.9210 | 0.9212 | 0.8994 | **0.9905** |
| Figure 5 | PSNR | 26.76 | 21.98 | 21.97 | 19.72 | **29.49** |
| | SSIM | 0.9269 | 0.9250 | 0.9254 | 0.8811 | **0.9906** |

## 3.2 Visual Comparison Experiment

To compare visual processing effects, we add two images (One from www.youtube.com/watch?v=I8S27Gd30g8 and another image using the endoscope) to the evaluation of the indicators.

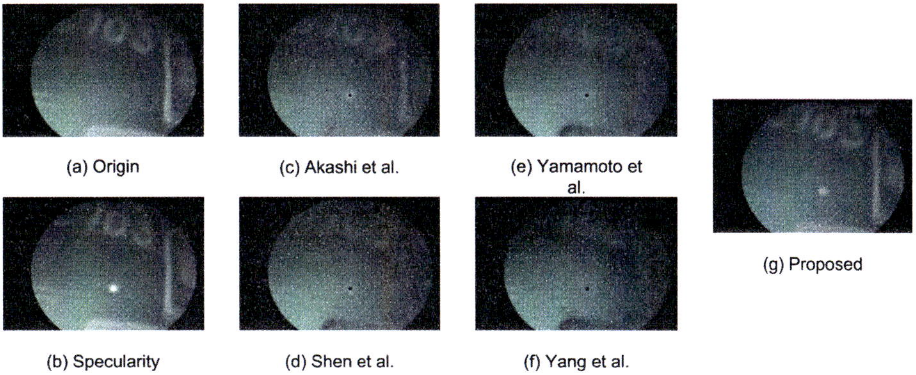


**Fig. 3.** **a** is the original image, **b** is the image after adding specularity, **c–f** are the results of four existing algorithms, and **g** is the proposed algorithm in this paper.

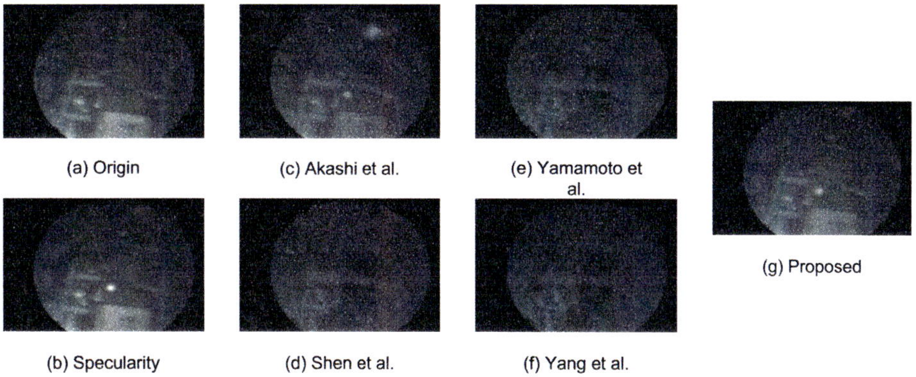


**Fig. 4.** **a** is the original image, **b** is the image after adding specularity, **c–f** are the results of four existing algorithms, and **g** is the proposed algorithm in this paper.

According to Fig. 3, 4, 5, 6 and 7, it is obvious that the algorithm proposed in this paper has obvious advantages for the image processing ability under the actual working condition, which not only suppresses the influence of specularity on the image but also avoids the generation of false contour and the distortion of the image. In contrast, Shen et al.'s algorithm [14], using intensity ratio, and Yamamoto et al.'s algorithm [9], using a high-emphasis filter and similarity function to separate the specularity, showed severe distortion of the images on the results of the processing of the five test images, losing most of the detailed information of the images. At the same time, obvious false contours were produced, as seen in Figs. 3, 4 and 5. Akashi et al.'s algorithm [17], which uses sparse non-negative matrix factorization, does not cause severe image distortion. Still, there is significant noise in the images processed by their algorithm. In contrast, in Fig. 7, Akashi et al.'s algorithm cause a change in the color of the image details while also showing an excess of suppressed specularity in Fig. 3. Compared to the algorithm proposed in this paper, the images processed by the algorithm of Akashi et al. have a certain degree of degradation in sharpness compared to the original images. As for the

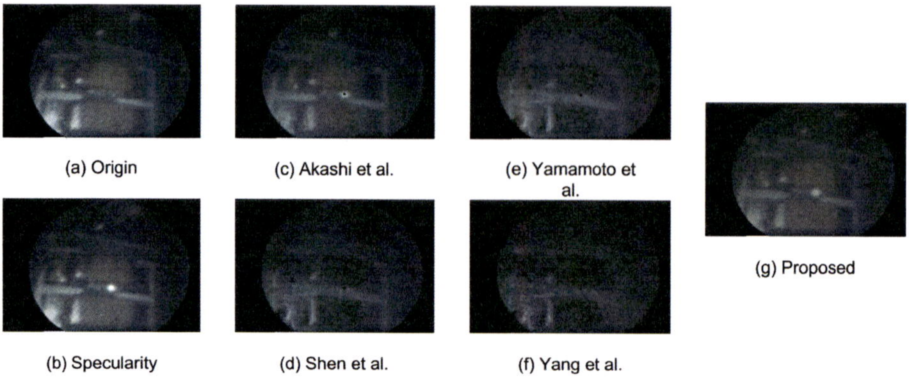


**Fig. 5.** **a** is the original image, **b** is the image after adding specularity, **c–f** are the results of four existing algorithms, and **g** is the proposed algorithm in this paper.

images processed by Yang et al.'s algorithm using bilateral filters [15], only Fig. 6 did not produce more serious distortion. Still, its suppression of specularity was insignificant, and serious distortion was observed in the remaining four images.

The proposed endoscopic image specularity suppression algorithm conforming to the Weber-Fechner law can show more obvious performance advantages for endoscopic image processing. While suppressing the specularity, it does not change the information of the remaining normal pixels, prevents the generation of false contours, retains more image details, and does not introduce the interference of new noise, which does not affect the image sharpness.

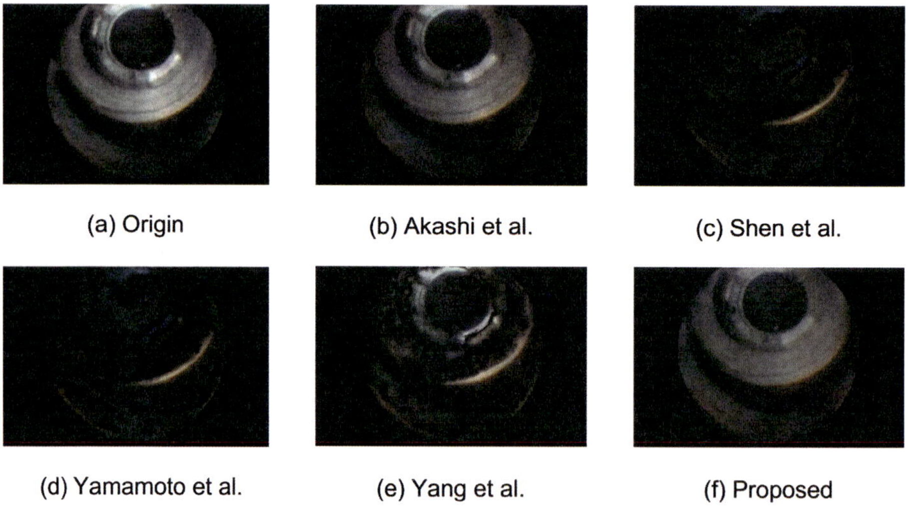


**Fig. 6.** Visual comparison experiment image **a** is the original image **b**, **c** are the results of four existing algorithms, and **f** is the proposed algorithm in this paper.

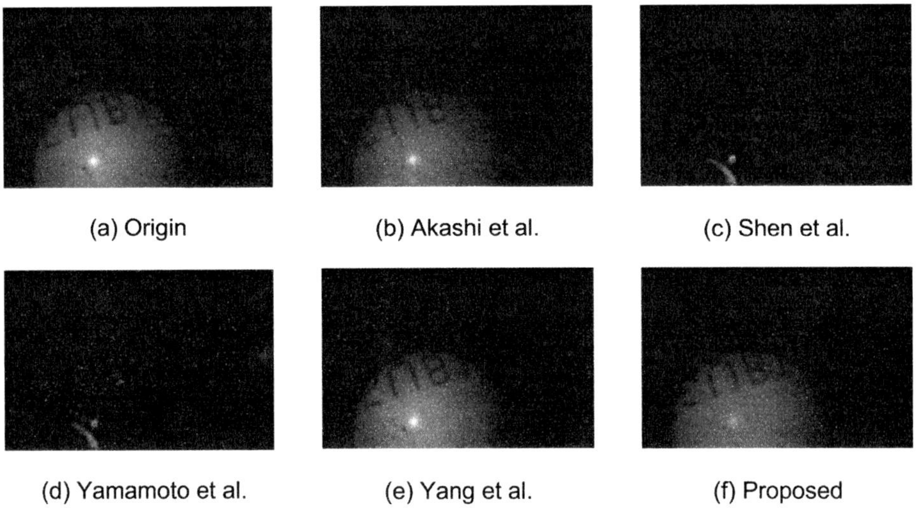


**Fig. 7.** Visual comparison experiment image **a** is the original image **b**, **c** are the results of four existing algorithms, and **f** is the proposed algorithm in this paper.

# 4 Conclusion

This paper has proposed a new specularity suppression algorithm for endoscope images conforming to Weber-Fechner Law. To suppress the specularity in endoscopic images by the time it protects the normal region's pixels, we use the tanh and the Softplus functions, which can make it possible to meet our expectations. Each function we used in the proposed algorithm has a smooth curve. This characteristic makes it avoid generating false contours. According to the experimental results, it's obvious that the proposed algorithm in this paper has a better effect in terms of specularity suppression. The indicators have increased more than the other four algorithms. While for the visual comparison experiment results, the proposed algorithm's affection is the best of the five algorithms we used in the comparison experiment. It will not generate false contours in the endoscopic images or destroy them. The evaluation of the indicators significantly evidences the algorithm's adaptability to endoscopic images. It can improve the peak signal-to-noise ratio (PSNR) and the structural similarity (SSIM) by using the threshold to limit the processing range of the pixels for distinguishing between the normal pixels and the specular pixels.

However, according to the mapping function of our algorithm, it is obvious that the use of a threshold to limit the processing range of the algorithm makes it possible to show strong suppression on images where there is a significant difference between the gray value of the spot and the affected area and the normal pixel area. Still, if this difference is small, the processing capability is reduced. How to improve the effect of spot suppression and increase the robustness and generalization is the next direction that needs to be studied by the algorithms for specularity removal or specularity suppression.

**Acknowledgments.** This work was financially supported by Sichuan Science and Technology Program(NO.2020YFS0454, NO.2020YFS0318), NHC Key Laboratory of Nuclear Technology Medical Transformation (MIANYANG CENTRAL HOSPITAL)(Grant No.2021HYX031).

## References

1. Xu, T., Chen, Z., Jiang, Z., Huang, J., Gui, W.: A Real-Time 3D Measurement System for the Blast Furnace Burden Surface Using High-Temperature Industrial Endoscope. Sensors **20**(3), 869 (2020). https://doi.org/10.3390/s20030869
2. Wurster, L.M., Ginner, L.: Endoscopic optical coherence tomography with a flexible fiber bundle. J. Biomed. Opt. **23**(06), 1 (2018). https://doi.org/10.1117/1.JBO.23.6.066001
3. Vercauteren, T.: Image registration and mosaicing for dynamic In vivo fibered confocal microscopy, p. 173
4. Orth, A., Ploschner, M., Wilson, E.R., Maksymov, I.S., Gibson, B.S.: Optical fiber bundles: Ultra-slim light field imaging probes. Sci. Adv., vol. 5, no. 4, p. eaav1555. https://doi.org/10.1126/sciadv.aav1555
5. Han, J.-H., Lee, J., Kang, J.U.: Pixelation effect removal from fiber bundle probe based optical coherence tomography imaging. Opt. Express **18**(7), 7427 (2010). https://doi.org/10.1364/OE.18.007427
6. Ding, P., Ma, Q.S., Li, C.Y., Yao, H.Y.: Spatially adaptive context-based wavelet shrinkage for borescope image denoising," presented at the Sixth International Symposium on Instrumentation and Control Technology: Signal Analysis, Measurement Theory, Photo-Electronic technology, and Artificial Intelligence, Beijing, China, Nov. 2006, p. 63570J. https://doi.org/10.1117/12.716903
7. Ping Tan, Long Quan, and S. Lin, "Separation of Highlight Reflections on Textured Surfaces," in 2006 IEEE Computer Society Conference on Computer Vision and Pattern Recognition - Volume 2 (CVPR'06), New York, NY, USA, 2006, vol. 2, pp. 1855–1860. doi: https://doi.org/10.1109/CVPR.2006.273
8. Artusi, A., Banterle, F., Chetverikov, D.: A Survey of Specularity Removal Methods. Computer Graphics Forum **30**(8), 2208–2230 (2011). https://doi.org/10.1111/j.1467-8659.2011.01971.x
9. Yamamoto, T., Nakazawa,A.: General Improvement Method of Specular Component Separation Using High-Emphasis Filter and Similarity Function, vol. 7, no. 2, p. 11 (2019)
10. Zhu, Z., Xiang, P., Zhang, F.: Polarization-based method of highlight removal of high-reflectivity surface. Optik **221**, 165345 (2020). https://doi.org/10.1016/j.ijleo.2020.165345
11. Feng, W., Li, X., Cheng, X., Wang, H., Xiong, Z., Zhai, Z.: Specular highlight removal of light field based on dichromatic reflection and total variation optimizations. Opt. Lasers Eng. **151**, 106939 (2022). https://doi.org/10.1016/j.optlaseng.2021.106939
12. Shen, H.-L., Zhang, H.-G., Shao, S.-J., Xin, J.H.: Chromaticity-based separation of reflection components in a single image. Pattern Recogn. **41**(8), 2461–2469 (2008). https://doi.org/10.1016/j.patcog.2008.01.026
13. Yoon, K., Choi, Y., Kweon, I.S.: Fast Separation of Reflection Components using a Specularity-Invariant Image Representation. In: 2006 International Conference on Image Processing, Atlanta, GA, 2006, pp. 973–976. https://doi.org/10.1109/ICIP.2006.312650
14. Shen, H.-L., Zheng, Z.-H.: Real-time highlight removal using intensity ratio. Appl. Opt. **52**(19), 4483 (2013). https://doi.org/10.1364/AO.52.004483
15. Yang, Q.: Real-Time Specular Highlight Removal Using Bilateral Filtering. In: Computer Vision – ECCV,: Vol. 6314. Berlin, Heidelberg: Springer, Berlin Heidelberg **2010**, 87–100 (2010). https://doi.org/10.1007/978-3-642-15561-1_7

16. Tan, R.T., Ikeuchi, K.: Separating reflection components of textured surfaces using a single image. IEEE Trans. Pattern Anal. Machine Intell. **27**(2), 178–193 (2005). https://doi.org/10.1109/TPAMI.2005.36
17. Akashi, Y., Okatani, T.: Separation of reflection components by sparse non-negative matrix factorization. Comput. Vis. Image Underst. **146**, 77–85 (2016). https://doi.org/10.1016/j.cviu.2015.09.001
18. Shen, H.-L., Cai, Q.-Y.: Simple and efficient method for specularity removal in an image. Appl. Opt. **48**(14), 2711 (2009). https://doi.org/10.1364/AO.48.002711
19. van de Weijer J, Beigpour S The dichromatic Reflection model: future research directions and applications, p. 5
20. Ramos, V.: SIHR: a MATLAB/GNU Octave toolbox for single image highlight removal. JOSS **5**(45), 1822 (2020). https://doi.org/10.21105/joss.01822

# Semantic Segmentation of Medical Images Based on Knowledge Distillation Algorithm

Hanqing Liu[1,2], Fang Li[1,3], Jingyi Yang[1], Xiaotian Wang[1], Junling Han[1], Jin Wei[4], and Xiaodong Kang[1](✉)

[1] School of Medical Technology, Tianjin Medical University, Tianjin, China
kxd2004@163.com
[2] Department of Radiology, Chongqing University Cancer Hospital, Chongqing, China
[3] The Beijing Prevention and Treatment Hospital of Occupational Disease for Chemical Industry, Beijing, China
[4] Tianjin Third Central Hospital, Tianjin, China

**Abstract.** (1) Background: Since the advent of convolutional neural networks, they have been employed in various fields. Nevertheless, the calculation cost must be considered for the automatic deep learning analysis. A novel strategy was proposed to improve the segmentation performance without adding additional parameters by transferring pre-trained prior knowledge information in medical scenes. (2) Methods: we accessed knowledge distillation to train a teacher and student network simultaneously, then introduced the best weight of the teacher to distill the student network, contributing to the distillation loss function. The effectiveness was verified with two segmentation convolutional neural network structures. (3) Result: the mean Acc, mIoU, Dice, and Kappa of the distilled network in three medical datasets were increased by 0.18 percent, 1.25 percent, 1.62 percent, and 0.79 percent, respectively. (4) Conclusions: the dark knowledge was transformed from a deeper network to a lightweight one that can enhance the segmentation significantly without additional elements.

**Keywords:** Semantic Segmentation · Knowledge Distillation · Ultrasonic image · Deep learning

## 1 Introduction

Computer vision is the discipline of how machines can learn to see, and it simulates the human brain's visual system to comprehend or describe an image into various semantic scenes. In the early development of computer vision, image analysis rested on traditional machine learning [1–4], a subset of artificial intelligence that over-rely on predefined features. Designing and extracting handcrafted features is extremely labor-intensive and somewhat subjective, making individual errors easy. Furthermore, traditional methods show poor performance in terms of robustness and generalization in that they lack semantic information in capturing image features.


G. Wang et al. (Eds.): APCMBE 2023, IFMBE Proceedings 103, pp. 180–196, 2024.
https://doi.org/10.1007/978-3-031-51455-5_21

With Internet technology's emergence and rapid development, the requirements for efficiently analyzing massive data are continuously increasing. Moreover, computer processing is increasingly powerful because of hardware improvement. In this circumstance, the feature extraction strategies of convolutional neural network-based rise to the occasion.

They have enabled tremendous advancements and presented a breakthrough possibility for medical development. Semantic segmentation, as one of the computer vision tasks, seeks to assign each pixel in an image to one of several predefined classes, essentially pixel-level image classification. Therefore, lesions can be outlined from normal areas in medical datasets. Zhang et al. [5] embed a one-stage neural network in ultrasound equipment based on knowledge distillation and a structured lightweight neural network to detect breast lesions with a sensitivity of 89.25%, specificity of 96.33%, and mAP of 0.85. Aleksandar et al. [6] incorporated an attention block into a U-Net to increase the likelihood of capturing radiologists' visual attention. The experiment revealed a Dice similarity coefficient of 90.5% and potential for robustness in other organs. Davood et al. [7] used a CNN training and ensemble strategy to segment easy and complicated transrectal ultrasound images. The method produced a Dice score of $93.9 \pm 3.5\%$, which significantly alleviated the likelihood of segmentation mistakes. Some deep learning approaches were involved in cardiac segmentation, which can quantify cardiac function as a basis for clinical diagnosis, and good progress has been made [8, 9]. Shen et al. [10] proposed segmentation of the femur and tibia bones based on pure dilated residual U-Net. The novel method has a greater performance with fewer parameters, higher accuracy, and converges more rapidly. Faster and more accurate scene-paring algorithms can accelerate the development of both domains; high resolution and quick response are imperative. Clinical participants must deal with massive amounts of images largely dependent on their diagnostic experience, and computer-aided diagnosis systems show great promise. Therefore, knowledge distillation provides a lightweight and sensitive clinical application model that can speed up diagnosis without adding extra calculations or be transplanted to portable devices for bedside clinical rounds.

Some algorithms pursue accuracy improvement while neglecting to account for computational cost and complexity. Model compression was presented to solve the above concerns, provided that a lightweight model can achieve the same performance as a larger model. It includes parameter pruning and sharing [11–13], low-rank factorization [14, 15], transferred compact convolutional filters [16], and knowledge distillation [17]. A stronger model is trained to maintain accuracy when speeding up operations, then transferring the prior information into a lightweight model.

This paper proposed a semantic segmentation method in medical datasets based on knowledge distillation, Resnet-50 and Resnet-18 were regarded as the teacher and student networks for feature extraction. Firstly, we accessed knowledge distillation to train teacher and student networks; secondly, we introduced the best weight of teacher to distill student, which introduced the distillation loss function; finally, the effectiveness was verified with two segmentation convolutional neural network structures.

## 2 Related Work

### 2.1 Deeplabv3+

DeepLab architectural variants have been proposed to counter Google, whereas Deeplabv3 + is a semantic segmentation network [18] based on deeplabv3 (shown in Fig. 1). A simple and effective decoder is added to refine the segmentation outcomes, especially along the objects' border, implemented by combining the spatial pyramid pool module or Encoder-Decoder structure.

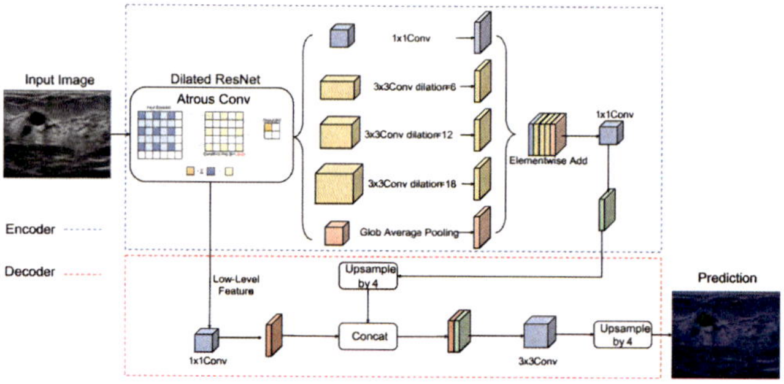


**Fig. 1.** The schematic illustration of Deeplabv3+

(1) Encoder: backbone and Atrous Spatial Pyramid Pooling (ASPP) [19] constitute the encoder module, which is a feature extraction block that captures essential information. Dilated Resnet plays the role of backbone for feature extraction in this paper. Dilated convolution (shown in Fig. 2) replaces the standard kernel to extend the reception field in Resnet. Dilated convolution, unlike standard kernel, is discontinuous and does not calculate all pixels. Equation (1) is the definition of a dilated convolution:

$$H_{out} = \frac{H_{in} + 2P - [D * (K - 1) + 1]}{S} + 1 \quad (1)$$

where $H_{in}$ and $H_{out}$ be the input and output size, $P$ the be padding size, $D$ the be dilated rate, $K$ the be kernel size, and $S$ the be stride.

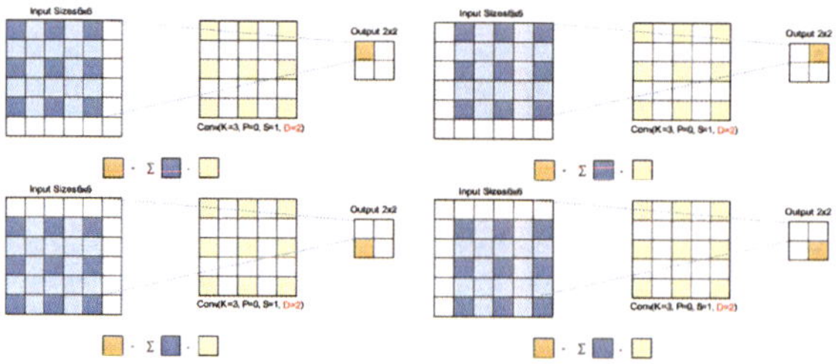

**Fig. 2.** Structure of dilated convolutional kernel

The extracted feature map is then fed into ASPP (shown in Fig. 3) to acquire advanced features. ASPP carries out a resampling method with different dilated rates for capturing spatial detail at multi-scale. It comprises five parallel layers: a 1 × 1 convolution, a glob average pooling layer, and three 3 × 3 convolutional layers with dilated rates of 6, 12, and 18.

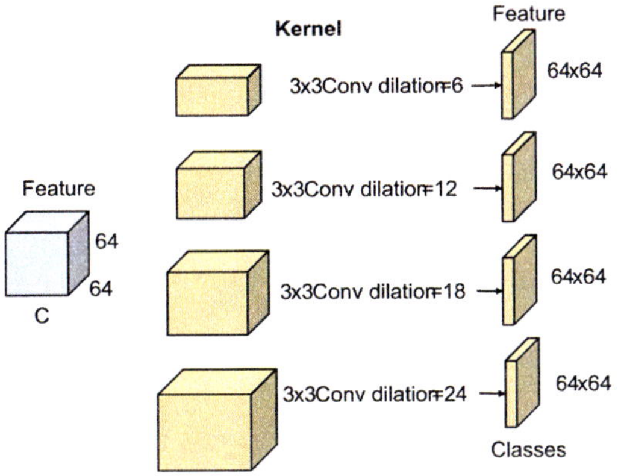


**Fig. 3.** Structure of Atrous Spatial Pyramid Pooling

Different receptive fields can be obtained through different padding and dilated rates, and multi-scale information can be extracted. The essence of ASPP pooling is adaptive average pooling, it only needs to specify the final output size, kernel size, and stride can be neglected. Each feature map is compressed 1 × 1, and the global features are obtained. Features obtained in the previous step are then delivered to a 1 × 1 convolution for further extraction and dimension reduction.

(2) Decoder: it progressively down-samples the input images and reduces feature map resolution to capture high-level detail of the scene. The decoder reconstructs the segmentation map of size equal to the original images from the small encoder feature map and gradually recovers boundary information. The decoder unit includes three steps below: firstly, low-level features with detailed information are adjusted by 1 × 1 convolution, changing the output dimension; secondly, advanced features with fused semantic information from ASPP after four times upsampling (bilinear interpolation) restored resolution; finally, the two features are concatenated, then fed into 3 × 3 convolution and four times to restore image resolution to receive output prediction.

## 2.2 SFNet

High-resolution and rich semantic features can be generated through atrous convolution and feature pyramid, requiring redundant calculation. The performance improvement of semantic segmentation networks is to gather multi-scale high-level semantic information and maximize the restoration of previously extracted image features. SFNet [20] (shown in Fig. 4) gets inspiration from the semantic flow and feature alignment across feature maps of adjacent levels. Between the decoder and the convolution, a Flow Alignment

Module (FAM) (shown in Fig. 5) is established to broadcast rough features and refined features with high resolution, which improves coding accuracy while also retaining high efficiency by optimizing the operation of transmitting semantic information from deep to shallow layers.

The overall network structure is shown in Fig. 4. The encoder and decoder follow a path with a growing number of feature map channels and a step-by-step reduction in image size. In the encoding path, Resnet serves as the backbone network for the down-sampling operation. Then Pyramid Pooling Module (PPM) makes a liaison between the encoder and the decoder, preserving the global contextual information. After receiving the information, the decoder merges the high and low-level features to generate a prediction map with constant resolution.

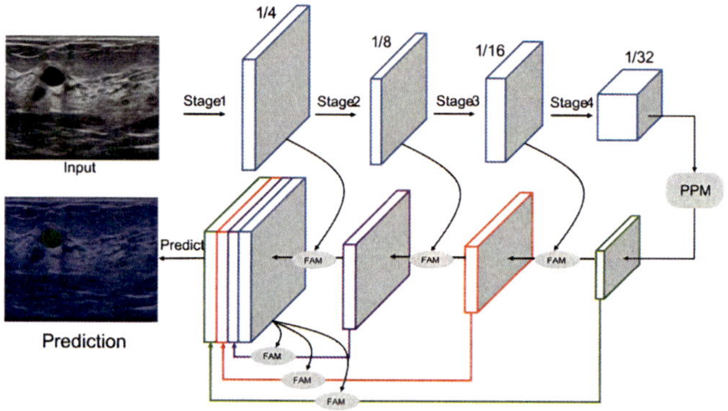


**Fig. 4.** The schematic illustration of SFNet.

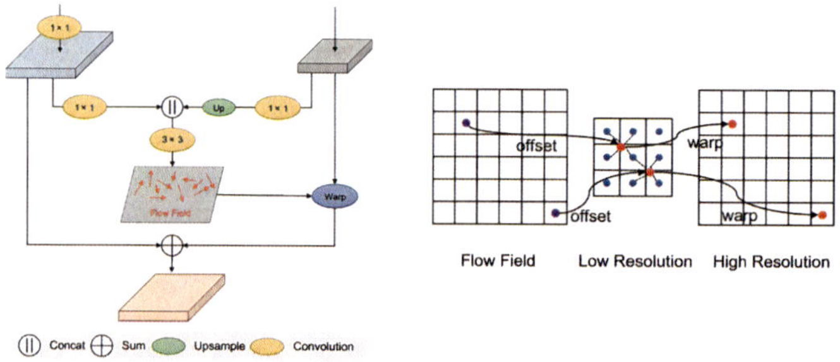


**Fig. 5.** Structure of Flow Alignment Module

The FAM is introduced to align the feature map information between each resolution layer and superimpose the high and low-level feature maps after the semantic flow alignment. The final prediction map's information is derived from the upsampling information of each stage. Similarly, the FAM module is embedded in each stage's feature map upsampling procedure to ensure semantic information alignment. FAM is designed to achieve the directional flow of semantic information from low-resolution high-semantic information feature maps to high-resolution low-semantic information feature maps between the multi-level feature extraction layers of the feature pyramid.

FAM replaces the traditional bilinear interpolation module for the feature map across adjacent levels of its feature pyramid. As illustrated in Eq. (2), the feature maps concatenate to be $F_l$ and $F_{l-1}$. Two feature maps with equal resolution are constructed following bilinear upsampling, and the semantic flow field is predicted after features concatenation.

$$\Delta_{l-1} = conv_l(cat(F_l, F_{l-1})) \tag{2}$$

As indicated in Eq. (3), any position $p_{l-1}$ of the spatial grid of the upper-level feature map is mapped to the corresponding position pl of the next level by an additive operation.

$$p_l = \frac{p_{l-1} + \Delta_{l-1}(p_{l-1})}{2} \tag{3}$$

Finally, based on differentiable bilinear interpolation, the $p_l$ neighborhood is approximated as $F_l$ $(p_{l-1})$ following interpolation, as shown in Eq. (4).

$$\tilde{F}_l(p_{l-1}) = F_l(p_l) = \sum_{p \in N(p_l)} \omega_p F_l(p) \tag{4}$$

The FAM is a lightweight and trainable module containing only one convolutional layer. The embedded upsampling path manifests the feature offset between the layers of traditional feature pyramid networks. The issue of feature misalignment at different resolution layers has been fixed, showing advanced performance in the semantic segmentation network.

### 2.3 Knowledge Distillation

In recent, knowledge distillation extension has concentrated on compressing deep neural networks. It proposes an approach for retaining accuracy by transferring knowledge from the deep network to a shallow one when compressing the deep model [21]. Furthermore, knowledge distillation can be extended to different tasks by transferring knowledge from one model to another. Especially the distillation method was described as a teacher-student strategy in which a high-accuracy deep network trained for a certain task instructs shallower student networks on the same task.

An extensive teacher network generally supervises a small student network: the student network simulates the teacher, transfers dark knowledge from the teacher, and enhances the generalization capabilities of the student. This approach usually improves performance and obtains a competitive or superior student performance without a distillation strategy. It ensures that the small model improves performance significantly with the same quantity of parameters and even achieves an accuracy index similar to the large model. The core concept is how to transfer the dark knowledge learned from the teacher network to the student, allowing the SoftMax of student and teacher to be close to each other.

The traditional strategy to train a neural network is to find a loss function that strives to be as close to the ground truth as possible. The loss function is being used to reduce neural network costs. Hinton et al. [17] applied the teacher network prediction as a soft "label", merged it with the ground truth as a "hard label", and replaced the L2 loss with the proposed temperature cross-entropy loss. The logits of an extensive deep model are used as the teacher's knowledge in a generic knowledge distillation.

In conventional model training, the loss is calculated from the model forward and real label computation output, and then the gradient backpropagation is performed. The teacher model has only forward computation in standard model distillation training. In contrast, the student model has forward computation and backpropagation. There are multiple losses to guide the student model for training: the output of the student model forward computation and the real label are computed to get the regular loss; the output of the student model forward computation and the output of the teacher model forward computation are calculated to get the distillation loss.

We combined the teacher and student into a new network (shown in Fig. 6), which outputs the prediction distributions of the student and teacher. Meanwhile, the gradient of the entire network of the teacher was fixed, whereas the student could perform normal backpropagation. Finally, we converted the logits of the two models into soft labels after the SoftMax activation function, then used JS scatter of both soft labels as loss functions for distillation model training. When selecting teacher and student, we choose Resnet-50 and Resnet-18. The distillation output will not be very beneficial if there is a significant structural difference between the teacher and student models throughout the distillation process. The teacher model with higher accuracy also dramatically impacts the results with the same structure. Weighting the distill loss (corresponding to Soft-target) and the student loss yields the loss function for the distillation process, as indicated in Eq. (5).

$$L = \alpha L_{soft} + \beta L_{hard} \tag{5}$$

where $\alpha$ is the weight of $L_{soft}$, and $\beta$ is the weight of $L_{hard}$.

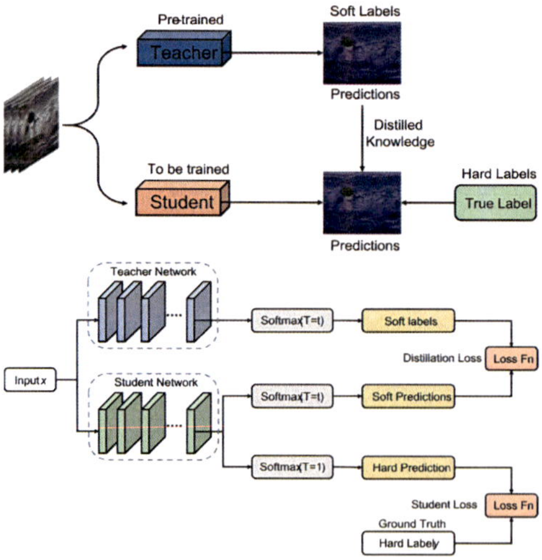


**Fig. 6.** The schematic illustration of knowledge distillation.

(1) The SoftMax distribution generated by the teacher model at high temperatures is utilized as the soft target. The teacher and student models are both simultaneously input to the transfer set. The first part of the loss function $L_{soft}$ is the SoftMax output of the student model at the same temperature and the cross-entropy of the Soft-target, which is shown in Eq. (6):

$$L_{soft} = -\sum_{j}^{N} p_j^T \log(q_j^T) \tag{6}$$

where $p$T i refers to the value of the teacher model's SoftMax output over class $i$ at a temperature equal to $T$. $q$T i refers to the value of the student's SoftMax output over class $i$ at a temperature equal to $T$. The formula is as follows.

$$p_i^T = \frac{\exp(v_i/T)}{\sum_k^N \exp(v_k/T)}$$
$$q_i^T = \frac{\exp(z_i/T)}{\sum_k^N \exp(z_k/T)}$$

where $v_i$ is the teacher's logits, $z_i$ is the student model's logits, and $N$ is the total number of labels.

(2) The SoftMax output of the student model with $T = 1$ and the cross-entropy of the ground truth is the loss function $L_{hard}$.

$$L_{hard} = -\sum_{j}^{N} c_j \log(q_j^T) \tag{8}$$

where $T$ stands for temperature, and it has the following attributes: this formula is SoftMax, which outputs the probability of each category according to logit if $T$ is set to be 1; If $T$ is near 0, the largest value will be closer to 1, and the other values will be close to 0, simulating to one-hot coding; the distribution of the output results will be smoother if $T$ is larger, which is equal to a role of smoothing.

## 3 Result

### 3.1 Evaluation Metrics

The following indicators represented evaluation metrics in this paper: Accuracy (Acc), mean Intersection over Union(mIoU), Dice coefficient, and Kappa.

Equations (9) and (10) indicate Acc and mIoU. Acc refers to the ratio of the proportion of pixels accurately predicted by the category to the total sum of pixels in the image. Higher Acc implies better model quality.

$$Acc = \frac{TP + TN}{TP + TN + FP + FN} \tag{9}$$

mIoU is the ratio of intersection and union of the prediction and ground truth. It then takes their mean value when the inference computation is performed independently for each dataset category.

$$mIoU = \frac{1}{k+1}\sum_{i=0}^{k}\frac{p_{ii}}{\sum_{j=0}^{k}p_{ij}+\sum_{j=0}^{k}p_{ji}-p_{ii}} = \frac{1}{k+1}\sum_{i=0}^{k}\frac{TP}{FN+FP+TP} \tag{10}$$

where $i$ be ground truth, $j$ be predicted segmentation, $p_{ij}$ be the prediction $i$ as $j$. Figure 7 depicts the confusion matrix for the four values listed above.

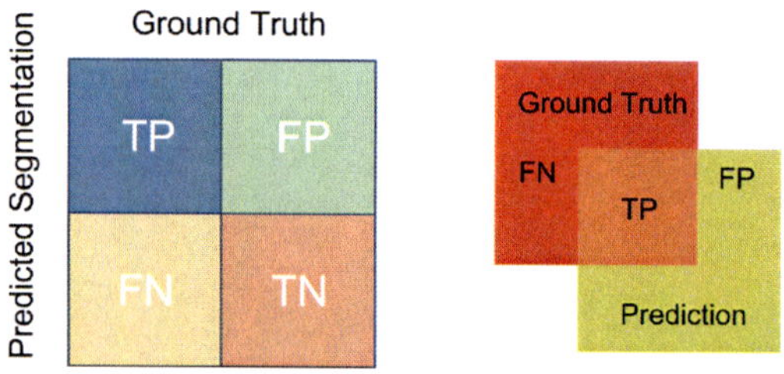


**Fig. 7.** Confusion matrix

Kappa is used to quantify the influence of classification and test consistency. Its calculation depends on the confusion matrix, with values ranging from –1 and 1 and generally greater than 0. Kappa is positively correlated with the quality of the model. Equation (11) shows Kappa, where $P_0$ and $P_e$ are the classifier's and random classifier's accuracy, respectively.

$$Kappa = \frac{p_o - p_e}{1 - p_e} \tag{11}$$

The dice coefficient is a segmentation metric that is an ensemble similarity measure function. It is commonly used to calculate the similarity of two samples and has a value range of [0,1]. Dice is also positively correlated with the model quality as well.

$$Dice = \frac{2|X \cap Y|}{|X| + |Y|} \tag{12}$$

where $X$ is the true value, i.e., the region in the image that needs to be segmented, and $Y$ be the predicted value, i.e., the region in which the deep learning network predicts the will be segmented.

### 3.2 Establishing Dataset

Three medical published datasets were used in this paper: ultrasonic mammary nodules from Kaggle, ultrasonic thyroid nodules and optic disc from Baidu Aistudio. Each image has its corresponding label.

The mammary nodules dataset was compiled in 2018 and included 780 images from 600 female patients aged 25 to 75. The image size was 500 × 500 pixels and saved as a PNG file. There were three categories: benign, malignant, and normal. Normal images were removed from the final dataset, leaving 645 images; the thyroid nodule dataset was uploaded in 2020 in BMP format, with 250 images chosen for the study; the optic disc dataset contained 381 BMP format. The above datasets are divided into the training, validation, and test sets with 7:2:1.

Deeplabv3 + and SFNet were the two segmentation networks used in this experiment on the three datasets mentioned above. Renset-50 and Renset-18 represent the teacher and student networks, respectively.

### 3.3 Analysis

We utilized Deeplabv3+ and SFNet to segment three datasets in the literature, and the distilled strategies were carried out on the student network. The promotion between distilled and student networks needs to be a concern indeed There is a result table, folding line charts, and visualization for each segment network. The tables demonstrates four metrics with Acc, mIoU, Kappa, and Dice for Deeplabv3+ (shown in Table 1) and SFNet (shown in Table 2) in each dataset, respectively. The relationship between acc, mIoU, and loss with epochs was divided into three portions in folding line charts. We randomly chose three distinct images for each visualization to compare segmentation performance.

**Table1.** Evaluation Indicators Comparison of Deeplabv3 + (%)

| Dataset | Type | Acc | mIoU | Kappa | Dice |
|---|---|---|---|---|---|
| Mammary | Teacher | 97.14 | 82.28 | 79.27 | 89.63 |
| | Student | 96.72 | 80.59 | 77.57 | 88.78 |
| | Distilled | **96.83(↑0.11)** | **81.53(↑0.94)** | **77.57** | **88.78** |
| Thyroid | Teacher | 98.74 | 95.92 | 95.80 | 97.90 |
| | Student | 97.24 | 91.47 | 90.94 | 95.47 |
| | Distilled | **97.55(↑0.31)** | **92.37(↑0.9)** | **91.94(↑1.0)** | **95.97(↑0.5)** |
| Optic Disc | Teacher | 99.61 | 93.33 | 92.90 | 96.45 |
| | Student | 99.57 | 88.68 | 87.29 | 93.65 |
| | Distilled | **99.67(↑0.10)** | **91.50(↑2.82)** | **90.74(↑3.45)** | **95.37(↑1.72)** |

The distilled model's Acc and mIoU improved by 0.11 percent and 0.94 percent over the student model based on the deeplabv3 + model in the mammary dataset. The distilled model outperformed the student model by 0.31 percent, 0.9 percent, 1.0 percent, and 0.50 percent for the four assessment measures Acc, mIoU, Kappa, and Dice, respectively, in the thyroid dataset. The distilled model outperformed the student model on every assessment metric in the optic disc dataset, improving by 0.10 percent, 2.82 percent, 3.45 percent, and 1.72 percent on Acc, mIoU, Kappa, and Dice.

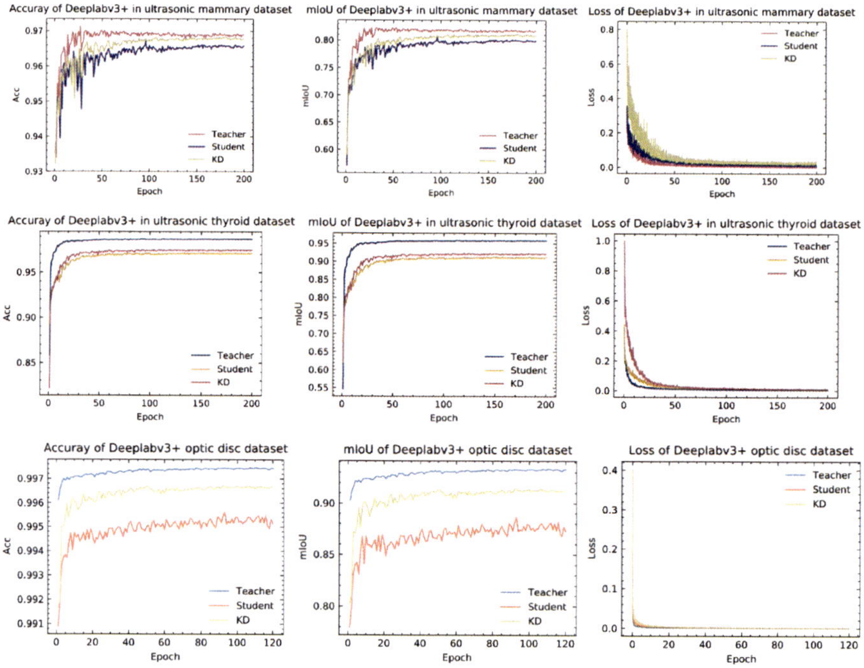


**Fig. 8.** The line chart of Acc, mIoU and loss with epoch on Deeplabv3 +

Figure 8 depicts Acc, mIoU, and loss in turns from left to right. Between the teacher and student model in Acc and mIoU, the distilled model is higher than the student in medical datasets. The distilled student model does not reveal a substantial difference. The loss function's fall indicates if the model has reached convergence. All models can match the data well in loss figures.

Figure 9, 10 and 11 shows the visualization of deeplabv3 + in the mammary, thyroid, and optic disc, including row image, masks, teacher network, student network, and distilled network in each visualization from left to right. The teacher and student network had serrated edges in the third mammary visualization, while the distilled network was relatively smoothly at the edges. The first thyroid depiction exhibited a concave notch, with the edge of the teacher and student roughly complete. The distilled network fitted the object's outlines better than the student in total segmentation performance.

In the mammary dataset, the distilled model's Acc, mIoU, Kappa, and Dice improved by 0.22 percent, 0.94 percent, 1.34 percent, and 0.66 percent over the student using the

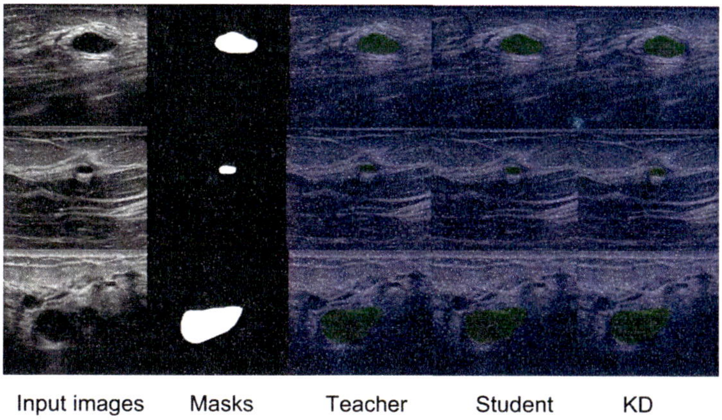


**Fig. 9.** Visualization of deeplabv3 + tested in the ultrasonic mammary dataset

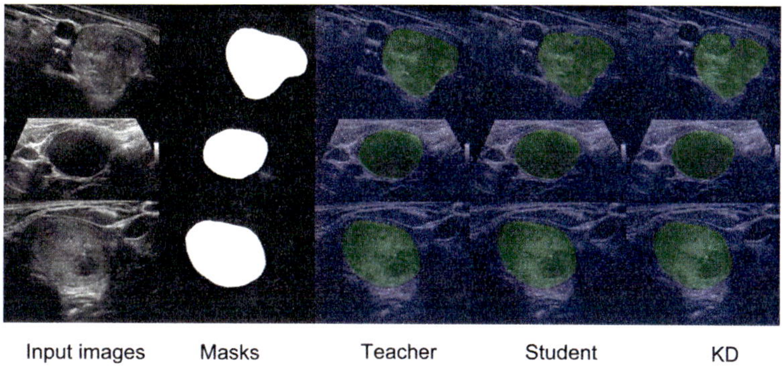


**Fig. 10.** Visualization of deeplabv3 + tested in ultrasonic thyroid dataset

SFNet model. The distilled model outperformed the student model by 0.3 percent, 0.88 percent, 0.97 percent, and 0.48 percent for the four assessment measure Acc, mIoU, Kappa, and Dice in the thyroid dataset. The distilled model outperformed the student model on every assessment metric in the optic dataset, improving by 0.04 percent, 1.01 percent, 2.95 percent, and 1.39 percent on Acc, mIoU, Kappa, and Dice.

From left to right, Fig. 12 illustrates Acc, mIoU, and loss of SFNet. The curves are similar to Deeplabv3 +, with the distilled model in acc, mIoU, and loss curves between teacher and student, with some improvement on the student.

Figures 13, 14 and 15 shows the visualization of SFNet in mammary, thyroid, and optic disc datasets, including raw images, masks, teacher, student, and distilled network from left to right. Overall, all three networks are segmented fairly well, with minimal variation between student and distilled network visualization.

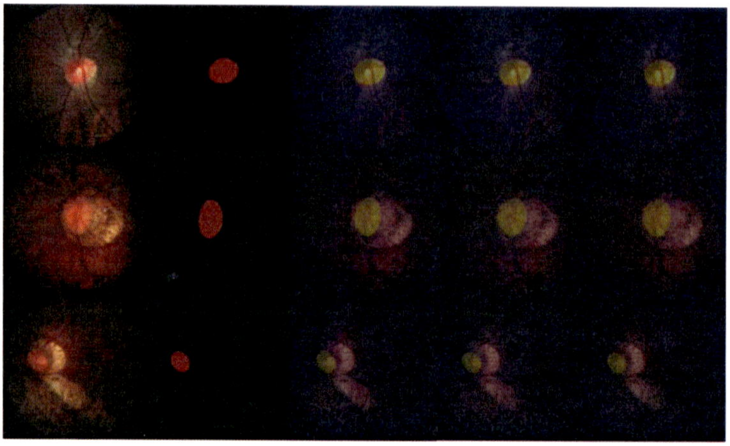


**Fig. 11.** Visualization of deeplabv3 + tested in optic disc dataset

**Table 2.** Evaluation Indicators Comparison of SFNet (%)

| Dataset | Type | Acc | mIoU | Kappa | Dice |
|---|---|---|---|---|---|
| Mammary | Teacher | 96.98 | 81.94 | 79.00 | 89.90 |
| | Student | 96.63 | 80.28 | 76.33 | 88.17 |
| | Distilled | **96.85(↑0.22)** | 81.22(↑**0.94**) | 77.67(↑**1.34**) | 88.83(↑**0.66**) |
| Thyroid | Teacher | 98.77 | 96.23 | 95.92 | 97.96 |
| | Student | 97.90 | 93.40 | 93.08 | 96.54 |
| | Distilled | **98.20(↑0.3)** | **94.28(↑0.88)** | **94.05(↑0.97)** | **97.02(↑0.48)** |
| Optic Disc | Teacher | 99.74 | 93.61 | 93.19 | 96.59 |
| | Student | 99.63 | 90.48 | 87.78 | 93.97 |
| | Distilled | **99.67(↑0.04)** | **91.49(↑1.01)** | **90.73(↑2.95)** | **95.36(↑1.39)** |

## 4 Discussion

We validated three datasets with two deep learning networks based on knowledge distillation. The results show that the distilled model improves the mean Acc, mIoU, Dice, and Kappa by 0.18 percent, 1.25 percent, 1.62 percent, and 0.79 percent based on the student network improvement in visualization. Overall, the distilled model outperformed the student and matched the teacher. However, the distilled method fluctuated from time to time during the training process, which could be related to the datasets' quality and the model's parameters.

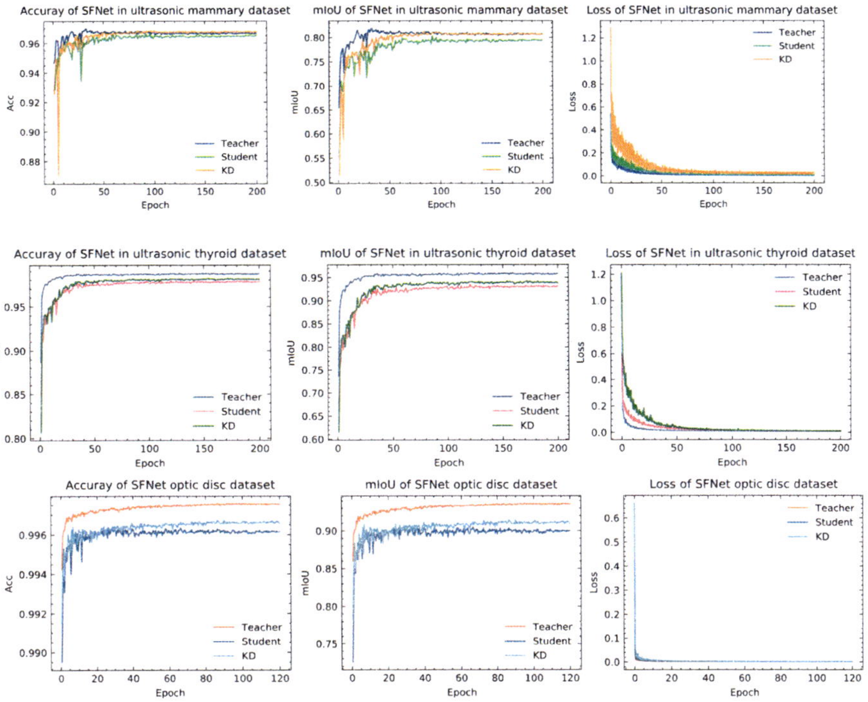


**Fig. 12.** The line chart of Acc, mIoU and loss with epoch on SFNet

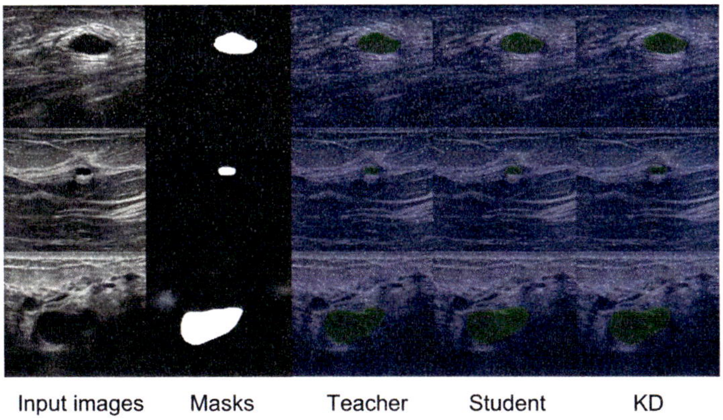


**Fig. 13.** Visualization of SFNet tested in the ultrasonic mammary dataset

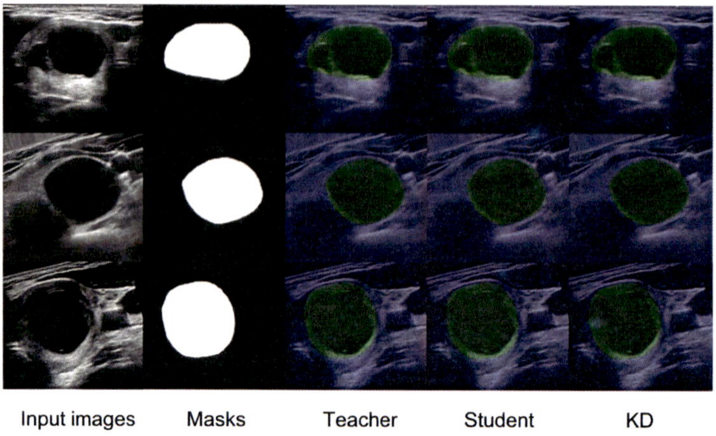


**Fig. 14.** Visualization of SFNet tested in ultrasonic thyroid dataset

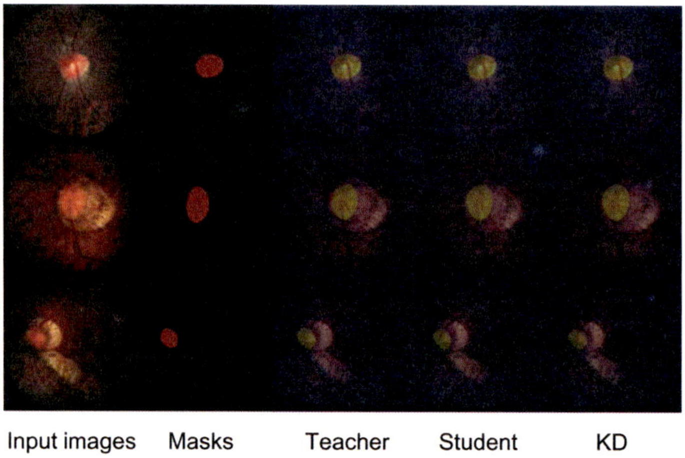


**Fig. 15.** Visualization of SFNet tested in optic disc dataset

## 5 Conclusion

A knowledge distillation-based image segmentation method was proposed, which transfers dark information from a trained teacher to a student network in feature extraction. The segmentation performance is significantly improved to a certain extent without revising any structure and parameter quantity of the student network. Computer-aided diagnosis systems involve diseases classification and detection, knowledge distillation is also suitable for those science. Some lightweight networks can be inferred into portable devices for bedside clinical rounds and speed up clinical diagnosis. However, in curve graphs, curves fluctuate in some datasets, indicating that there may be some issues, such as a lack of images or data imbalance. Therefore, we should focus on improving the quality of datasets and applying knowledge distillation in additional networks in the future.

**Acknowledgements.** This work was supported by the Beijing-Tianjin-Hebei Collaborative Innovation Project (17YEXTZC00020).

**Data Availability** Data is openly available in a public repository. The data that support the findings of this study are openly available in the ultrasonic mammary nodules dataset at [https://www.kaggle.com/datasets/aryashah2k/breast-ultrasound-images-dataset]; ultrasonic thyroid nodules dataset at [https://aistudio.baidu.com/aistudio/datasetdetail/64663] and optic disc dataset at [https://aistudio.baidu.com/aistudio/datasetdetail/19469].

## References

1. Waddle, S.L., Juttukonda, M.R., Lants, S.K., et al.: Classifying intracranial stenosis disease severity from functional MRI data using machine learning. J. Cereb. Blood Flow Metab. **40**, 705–719 (2020)
2. HSU, K.-C., Lin, C.-H., Johnson, K. R., et al.: Autodetect extracranial and intracranial artery stenosis by machine learning using ultrasound. Comput. Biol. Med. 116: 103569 (2020)
3. Araki, T., Jain, P.K., Suri, H.S., et al.: Stroke risk stratification and its validation using ultrasonic echolucent carotid wall plaque morphology: a machine learning paradigm. Comput. Biol. Med. **80**, 77–96 (2017)
4. Saba, L., Jain, P.K., Suri, H.S., et al.: Plaque tissue morphology-based stroke risk stratification using carotid ultrasound: a polling-based PCA learning paradigm. J. Med. Syst. **41**(6), 1–31 (2017)
5. Zhang, X., Lin, X., Zhang, Z., et al.: Artificial intelligence medical ultrasound equipment: application of breast lesions detection. Ultrason. Imaging **42**(4–5), 191–202 (2020)
6. Vakanski, A., Xian, M., Freer, P.E.: Attention-enriched deep learning model for breast tumor segmentation in ultrasound images. Ultrasound Med. Biol. **46**(10), 2819–2833 (2020)
7. Karimi, D., Zeng, Q., Mathur, P., et al.: Accurate and robust deep learning-based segmentation of the prostate clinical target volume in ultrasound images. Med. Image Anal. **57**, 186–196 (2019)
8. Wang, W., Wang, Y., Yuwei, W.T.L., et al.: Quantification of full left ventricular metrics via deep regression learning with contour-guidance. IEEE Access, 7: 47918–47928 (2019)
9. Hongyang, Z., Wenxue, Z., Weihao, S., et al.: Automatic segmentation of the cardiac MR images based on nested fully convolutional dense network with dilated convolution. Biomed. Signal Process. Control **68**, 102684 (2021)
10. Shen, W., Xu, W., Zhang, H., et al.: Automatic segmentation of the femur and tibia bones from X-ray images based on pure dilated residual U-Net. Inverse Problems & Imaging **15**(6), 1333–1346 (2021)
11. Wu, J., Leng, C., Wang, Y., et al.: Quantized convolutional neural networks for mobile devices. In: Proceedings of the 2016 IEEE Conference on Computer Vision and Pattern Recognition. Las Vegas, NV, USA, 4820–4828 (2018)
12. Han, S., Pool, J., Tran, J., et al.: Learning both weights and connections for efficient neural networks. In: Proceedings of the 2015 Proceedings of the 28th International Conference on Neural Information Processing Systems. Montreal, Canada: MIT Press, 2015: 1135–1143
13. Wang, Y., Xu, C., Xu, C., et al.: Packing convolutional neural networks in the frequency domain. IEEE Trans. Pattern Anal. Mach. Intell. **41**(10), 2495–2510 (2018)
14. Denton, E., Zaremba W, Bruna J, et al. Exploiting linear structure within convolutional networks for efficient evaluation. In: Proceedings of the 2014 Proceedings of the 27th International Conference on Neural Information Processing Systems. Montreal, Canada: MIT Press, 2014: 1269–1277

15. Yu, X., Liu, T., Wang, X., et al.: On compressing deep models by low rank and sparse decomposition. In: Proceedings of the 2017 IEEE Conference on Computer Vision and Pattern Recognition. Honolulu, HI, USA, 7370–7379 (2017)
16. Zhai, S., Cheng, Y., Lu, W., et al.: Doubly convolutional neural networks [C]// Proceedings of the 2016 Proceedings of the 30th International Conference on Neural Information Processing Systems. Barcelona, Spain: Curran Associates Inc., 1090–1098 (2016)
17. Hinton, G., Vinyals, O., Dean, J.: Distilling the knowledge in a neural network. 1503.02531 (2015)
18. Chen, L.-C., Papandreou, G., et al.: Encoder-decoder with atrous separable convolution for semantic image segmentation. Proceedings of the 2018 European conference on computer vision (ECCV). Munich, Germany: Springer, 2018: 801–818
19. Chen, L.-C., Papandreou, G., Kokkinos, I., et al.: Deeplab: Semantic image segmentation with deep convolutional nets, atrous convolution, and fully connected crfs. IEEE Transactions on Pattern Analysis and Machine Intelligence, 2017, 40(4): 834–848
20. Li, X., You, A., Zhu Z, et al.: Semantic flow for fast and accurate scene parsing. In: Proceedings of the 2020 European Conference on Computer Vision. Glasgow, UK: Springer, Cham, 2020: 775–793
21. Gou, J., Yu, B., Maybank, S.J., et al.: Knowledge distillation: A survey. Int. J. Comput. Vision **129**, 1789–1819 (2021)

# Combined Evaluation of T1 and Diffusion MRI Improves the Noninvasive Prediction of H3K27M Mutation in Brainstem Gliomas

Ne Yang[1], Xiong Xiao[2], Guocan Gu[2], Xianyu Wang[1], Liwei Zhang[2], and Hongen Liao[1(✉)]

[1] Department of Biomedical Engineering, School of Medicine, Tsinghua University, Beijing, China
liao@tsinghua.edu.cn

[2] Department of Neurosurgery, Beijing Tiantan Hospital, Capital Medical University, Beijing, China

**Abstract.** Objective: To establish an individualized predictive model to identify patients with brainstem gliomas (BSGs) at high risk of H3K27M mutation with the inclusion of diffusion MRI (dMRI). Methods: A cohort of 126 patients with BSGs were respectively included. Local tumor radiomics features were extracted from T1 images, and global brain connectomics features were extracted from dMRI data. A machine learning-based individualized H3K27M mutation prediction model was generated with a nested cross validation strategy. Additionally, two predictive signatures were established using the elastic net method, and simplified logistic models were built using multivariable logistic regression analysis. Results: 21 radiomics features and 52 topological properties of brain structural connectivity network were selected to construct a machine learning-based H3K27M mutation prediction model, which achieved an accuracy of 92.11% (AUC = 0.9246) in the validation cohort. T1- and dMRI-based signatures were generated and the combined multivariate logistic model was built, which achieved an AUC of 0.8783 in the validation cohort. Conclusion: dMRI is valuable in prediction of H3K27M mutation in BSGs. Combining multiple MRI sequences and clinical features, the established models have good performance.

**Keywords:** Brainstem gliomas · H3K27M · Diffusion magnetic resonance imaging · Machine learning

## 1 Introduction

Brainstem gliomas (BSGs) are defined as gliomas originated from midbrain, pons or medulla and they are a group of heterogeneous tumors [1]. The 2016 WHO began to integrate the status of H3K27M mutation to assist in classification, diagnosis and prognostic prediction of BSGs [2]. BSGs with this mutation show significant poorer responses to treatments and prognosis. Because of the critical neurofunctions of brainstem, surgical managements are very challenging and may induce fatal complications. Noninvasive methods will be valuable if they can reliably detect H3K27M mutations.


G. Wang et al. (Eds.): APCMBE 2023, IFMBE Proceedings 103, pp. 197–204, 2024.
https://doi.org/10.1007/978-3-031-51455-5_22

Radiomics has recently gathered attention, which extracts more information from medical images and is able to noninvasively capture tumor heterogeneity [3–5]. It is worth noting that almost all the existing radiomics researches are based on local tumor morphometric features, ignoring that the brain connections could also be associated with molecular indicators [6, 7]. Previous reports indicated that the dMRI-derived whole brain structural connectivity measurements can sensitively reflect the differences between different molecular types in brain diseases. However, its potential in predicting H3K27M mutation in BSGs was seldomly reported.

Thus, we aimed to develop and validate a machine learning-based model for preoperative prediction of H3K27M mutation in BSGs, using both the radiomics features and connectomics features. Moreover, we developed two easy-to-use signatures for H3K27M mutation prediction, based on multi-parametric MRI-derived features, respectively. To the best of our knowledge, this is the first study to do H3K27M mutation prediction from the perspective of brain connectivity.

# 2 Materials and Methods

## 2.1 Patient Enrollment

This study was approved by the Institutional Review Board of Beijing Tiantan Hospital. A retrospective analysis (Fig. 1) was performed on patients with histological diagnosis of BSG, who were surgically treated in Beijing Tiantan Hospital from December 2016 to June 2021. Finally, a total of 126 patients were identified, including 75 with H3K27M-mutant tumors and 51 with H3K27-wildtype tumors. The included patients were randomly assigned to either the primary cohort (n = 88) or the validation cohort (n = 38).

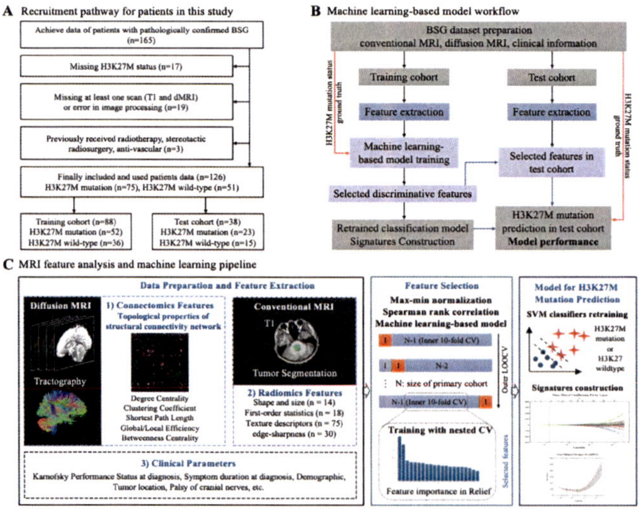


**Fig. 1.** Workflow of necessary steps in current study

All MRI data were obtained with a 3.0 T scanner, including sagittal three-dimensional T1-weighted (3D-T1: TR = 6.6 ms, TE = 3 ms, slice thickness = 1 mm, in-plane resolution = 1 × 1 mm), and axial diffusion-weighted imaging (DWI: TR = 4000 ms, TE = 87.8 ms, with b values of 0/1000/2000 s/mm$^2$ along 1/48/48 gradient directions, slice thickness = 2.5 mm, in-plane resolution = 2.27 × 2.27 mm).

### 2.2 Radiomics Feature Extraction

Firstly, T1 images preprocessing was conducted similarly as Pan's report [4]. Then, the tumor contour of BSG was delineated manually by two neurosurgeons in each source 3D-T1 image, using 3D Slicer. After that, the largest sagittal tumor slice was used to extract the ROI of BSG. In total, 137 local tumor radiomics features were extracted. These consisted of 107 features extracted automatically by using PyRadiomics [8] on the basis of shape and size, first-order intensity, and second-order texture descriptors, and 30 edge-sharpness features as Pan's report [4].

### 2.3 Connectomics Feature Extraction

The FSL [9] and MRtrix3 [10] were used to analyze DWI data, including (1) *bet* command: brain tissue extraction, (2) *eddy* command: eddy-current correction, (3) *dwi2fod* command: fiber orientation distributions estimation, and (4) *tckgen* command: probabilistic streamlines tractography.

To quantify alterations in the brain's white matter connections, connectomics features were extracted on the basis of structural connectivity (SC) among cortical parcellation, termed topological properties of SC. First, to construct brain SC networks, a merged brain cortical parcellation atlas from the MNI space was mapped to each individual tractography in respective native diffusion space. Specifically, the merged brain atlas parcellated the brain into 132 regions based on AAL atlas and Harvard-Oxford atlas. Then, the count of streamlines between each pair of brain regions was used to construct SC networks. Finally, six network topology properties [11] were extracted for each brain region, including degree centrality, shortest path length, clustering coefficient, global/local efficiency, and betweenness centrality.

### 2.4 Machine Learning-Based H3K27M Mutation Prediction

In the training process, feature selection was carried out to identify a small number of informative features in the primary cohort, from the extracted radiomics and connectomics features separately. First, all feature values were normalized. Then, Spearman correlation analysis between each feature and H3K27M genotype was performed. Next, combination of Relief algorithm [12] and SVM model with parameter tuning conducted by cross-validation (CV), was then applied to select H3K27M mutation status-related features.

Specifically, since the limited number of samples, a nested CV strategy was performed for parameter optimization and feature selection. In the primary cohort, during each outer LOOCV loop, the inner 10-fold CV was performed to train the optimal classification model with selection of the best parameters through grid search. The model parameters include weight threshold for feature selection with Relief, hyperparameter of SVM classifier. The features retained in at least 75 of the 88 outer loops were selected as the most robust imaging biomarkers. The most discriminative features thus selected and some preoperative clinical features were used to retrain a final model in the complete primary cohort. The selected features from both T1-based radiomics features and dMRI-based connectomics features were used to train two SVM models, respectively. Finally, the respective SVM classifier scores were weighted averaged to produce the final H3K27M mutation prediction results jointly. The validation cohort was used to evaluate the model performance using the ROC curve, AUC value, accuracy, sensitivity and specificity.

### 2.5 Radiomics and Connectomics Signatures Construction

To facilitate clinical practice, the elastic net method [13] was used to perform signature construction, based on removing redundant predictors from the above selected features. Firstly, H3K27M mutation status-related features with nonzero coefficients were selected from the primary cohort. Then, a linear combination of selected features weighted by their respective coefficients was used to generate a radiomics signature and a connectomics signature. Further, several simplified logistic models of the probability of H3K27M mutation were built based on the constructed signatures and several clinical variables, using multivariable logistic regression analysis. The discrimination performances were evaluated in the validation cohort and quantified by the AUC value.

## 3 Results

### 3.1 Feature Extraction and Feature Selection

Totally, 137 T1-based radiomics features, 792 dMRI-based connectomics features, and 20 clinical features were extracted for each subject. Of the 949 analyzed features, 366 had a $P < 0.05$ oof Spearman correlation, among which 21 radiomics and 52 connectomics features with high discriminative ability for H3K27M mutation prediction were selected through machine learning-based model training. The statistical comparison results between two groups based on a two-tailed Mann Whitney U test are provided.

For T1-derived radiomics features, 21 most stable features were selected from the primary cohort, all of which showed significant differences between H3K27M-mutant and H3K27-wildtype cases (Fig. 2). These key radiomics features included 6 shape, 3 edge-sharpness, 11 texture, and 1 intensity features. For dMRI-derived connectomics features, a set of brain regions were found with different network topology properties between H3K27M-mutant and H3K27-wildtype groups (Fig. 3). In total, 52 topological properties of brain SC network were selected. Of note, almost all involved regions exhibit significantly lower nodal properties in H3K27M-mutant groups, while the shortest path length was significantly higher in H3K27M-mutant groups.

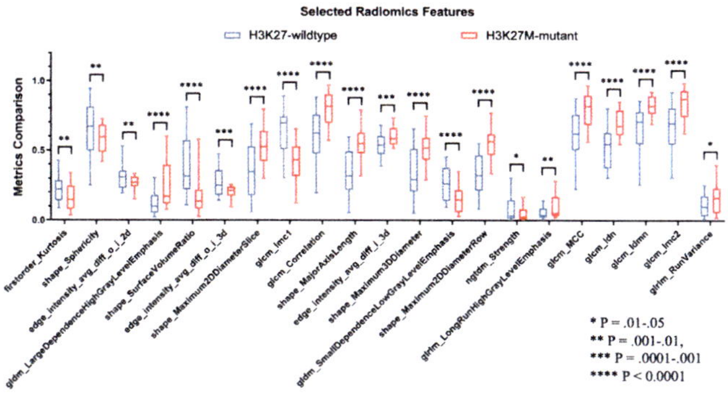


**Fig. 2.** The distribution of selected radiomics features

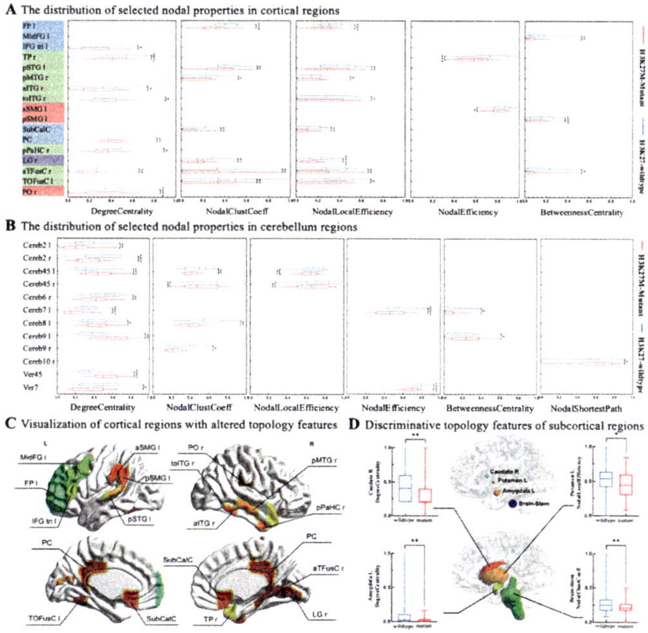


**Fig. 3.** Discriminative brain regions and structural connectivity network-based topology properties with predictive ability

## 3.2 Machine Learning-Based Model Prediction Performance

First, we evaluated H3K27M mutation prediction performance using features from single modality. As shown in Table 1, Image characteristics showed significantly improved H3K27M mutation prediction, as compared with clinical parameters. Also, connectomics-based methods achieved both higher accuracy and higher AUC than radiomics-based methods. Second, we performed experiments based on multi-modal

**Table 1.** H3K27M mutation prediction performance in the validation cohort

| Method | ACC | AUC | SEN | SPE |
|---|---|---|---|---|
| Clinical-only | 68.42% (26/38) | 0.7971 (0.6569, 0.9373) | 56.52% (13/23) | **86.67%** (13/15) |
| T1-RAD | 81.58% (31/38) | 0.8319 (0.7039, 0.9599) | 86.96% (20/23) | 73.33% (11/15) |
| dMRI-CON | 84.21% (32/38) | 0.8812 (0.7737, 0.9886) | 86.96% (20/23) | 80.00% (12/15) |
| T1 + Clinical | 84.21% (32/38) | 0.8638 (0.7486, 0.9790) | 82.61% (19/23) | **86.67%** (13/15) |
| dMRI + Clinical | 89.47% (34/38) | 0.8928 (0.7909, 0.9946) | **95.65%** (22/23) | 80.00% (12/15) |
| **Ours** | **92.11%** (35/38) | **0.9246** (0.8398, 1) | **95.65%** (22/23) | **86.67%** (13/15) |

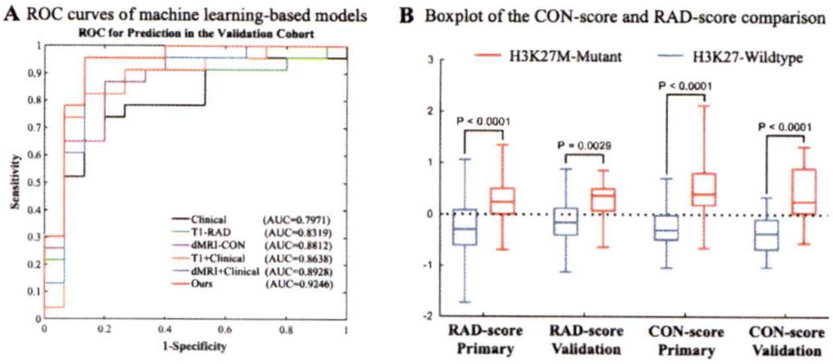


**Fig. 4.** The diagnostic performance in predicting H3K27M genotype

information. As can be seen, the multi-modal information can help improve the prediction performance, indicating the benefits of integrating local radiomics, global connectomics and traditional clinical features. Our final model achieved the best performance in the validation cohort (ACC = 92.11%, AUC = 0.9246) for preoperative H3K27M mutation prediction. The ROC curves for H3K27M mutation status prediction in the validation cohort are shown in Fig. 4a.

### 3.3 Diagnostic Validation of Simplified Models

11 H3K27M mutation status-related connectomics features, and 6 radiomics features with nonzero coefficients in the elastic net model, were selected from the primary cohort. The generated signatures were significantly associated with H3K27M genotype (Fig. 4b). Three preoperative clinical parameters were selected based on the univariate logistic regression analysis, namely preoperative KPS, muscle strength and palsy of cranial nerves. Then, several multivariable logistic models of the probability of H3K27M

mutation were built. The connectomics model yielded an AUC of 0.8551 in the validation cohort, which was higher than that of the radiomics model (AUC = 0.8348), and that of the clinical model (AUC = 0.7594). Moreover, the combined model showed the highest discrimination (AUC = 0.8783) between H3K27M-mutant and H3K27-wildtype subgroups in BSGs.

## 4 Discussion and Conclusion

The present study maybe the first to perform H3K27M mutation prediction in BSGs using both T1-based radiomics features and dMRI-derived brain connectomics features.

Recently, a few radiomics studies have been carried out to predict BSG-associated molecular pathological statuses. Our findings were in line with previous radiomic studies showing that the shape and textural features of structural MRI are potentially useful for H3K27M mutation prediction [3–5]. A major limitation of the traditional radiomics is ignoring the impact of BSGs on the other brain areas. Some findings indicated that the mutation of H3K27M can increase the invasion of adjacent structures along the white matter [1]. In this study, global connectomics features were extracted from dMRI data to characterize the BSGs' influence on the changes in brain connection, and our results suggest that the topological properties of the brain SC network in H3K27M-mutant group are more severely damaged than H3K27-wildtype patients.

Considering that both the tumor appearance and brain connections could be associated with H3K27M mutation, we reasonably infer that local radiomics and global connectomics features may provide different perspectives for the prediction. In this work, our joint machine learning-based model demonstrated adequate discriminative ability in the validation cohort (accuracy = 92.11%, AUC = 0.9246).

In conclusion, dMRI is valuable in prediction of H3K27M mutation of BSGs and connectomics analysis is a promising approach. Upon which, the proposed noninvasive machine learning-based prediction model, incorporating radiomics features, connectomics features and clinical parameters, showed satisfying efficacy and may facilitate preoperative evaluation of H3K27M mutation in BSGs. In addition, the simplified models can help clinicians to identify high-risk patients with H3K27M mutation early before surgery. These evaluation results may help improve clinical decision making.

**Acknowledgment.** The authors acknowledge supports from Beijing Municipal Natural Science Foundation (7212202), National Natural Science Foundation of China (82027807, U22A2051), National Key Research and Development Program of China (2022YFC2405200), Institute for Intelligent Healthcare, Tsinghua University (2022ZLB001), and Tsinghua-Foshan Innovation Special Fund (2021THFS0104).

## References


1. Chen, L.H., Pan, C., Diplas, B.H., et al.: The integrated genomic and epigenomic landscape of brainstem glioma. Nat. Commun. **11**(1), 3077 (2020). https://doi.org/10.1038/s41467-020-16682-y
2. Wesseling, P., Capper, D.: WHO 2016 Classification of gliomas. Neuropathol. Appl. Neurobiol. **44**(2), 139–150 (2018). https://doi.org/10.1111/nan.12432
3. Hua, T., Zhuo, Z., Duan, Y., et al.: Prediction of H3 K27M-mutant in midline gliomas by magnetic resonance imaging: a systematic review and meta-analysis. Neuroradiology **64**(7), 1311–1319 (2022). https://doi.org/10.1007/s00234-022-02947-4
4. Pan, C.C., Liu, J., Tang, J., et al.: A machine learning-based prediction model of H3K27M mutations in brainstem gliomas using conventional MRI and clinical features. Radiother. Oncol. **130**, 172–179 (2019). https://doi.org/10.1016/j.radonc.2018.07.011
5. Wu, C., Zheng, H., Li, J., et al.: MRI-based radiomics signature and clinical factor for predicting H3K27M mutation in pediatric high-grade gliomas located in the midline of the brain. Eur. Radiol. **32**(3), 1813–1822 (2022). https://doi.org/10.1007/s00330-021-08234-9
6. Li, Y., Liu, B., Hou, B., et al.: Less efficient information transfer in Cys-allele carriers of DISC1: a brain network study based on diffusion MRI. Cereb. Cortex **23**(7), 1715–1723 (2013). https://doi.org/10.1093/cercor/bhs167
7. Chen, L., Zhang, H., Lu, J., et al.: Multi-Label Nonlinear Matrix Completion with Transductive Multi-Task Feature Selection for Joint MGMT and IDH1 Status Prediction of Patient with High-Grade Gliomas. IEEE Trans. Med. Imaging **37**(8), 1775–1787 (2018). https://doi.org/10.1109/TMI.2018.2807590
8. van Griethuysen, J.J.M., Fedorov, A., Parmar, C., et al.: Computational Radiomics System to Decode the Radiographic Phenotype. Cancer Res. **77**(21), e104–e107 (2017). https://doi.org/10.1158/0008-5472.CAN-17-0339
9. Jenkinson, M., Beckmann, C.F., Behrens, T.E., et al.: Fsl. Neuroimage **62**(2), 782–790 (2012). https://doi.org/10.1016/j.neuroimage.2011.09.015
10. Tournier, J.D., Smith, R., Raffelt, D., et al.: MRtrix3: A fast, flexible and open software framework for medical image processing and visualisation. Neuroimage **202**, 116137 (2019). https://doi.org/10.1016/j.neuroimage.2019.116137
11. Wang, J., Wang, X., Xia, M., et al.: GRETNA: a graph theoretical network analysis toolbox for imaging connectomics. Front. Hum. Neurosci. **9**, 386 (2015). https://doi.org/10.3389/fnhum.2015.00386
12. Robnik-Šikonja, M., Kononenko, I.: Theoretical and empirical analysis of ReliefF and RReliefF. Mach. Learn. **53**(1), 23–69 (2003)
13. Tibshirani, R.: Regression shrinkage and selection via the lasso: a retrospective. Journal of the Royal Statistical Society: Series B (Statistical Methodology) **73**(3), 273–282 (2011)

# Liver Segmentation with MT-UNet++

Sijing Yang[1], Peng Sun[2], Yongbo Liang[1], Xin Song[2], and Zhencheng Chen[1](✉)

[1] School of Life and Environmental Science, Guilin University of Electronic Technology, Guilin, China
chenzhcheng@163.com

[2] School of Electronic Engineering and Automation, Guilin University of Electronic Technology, Guilin, China

**Abstract.** Liver cancer is the third leading cause of death in the world, and its mortality rate ranks second in China. Accurate liver segmentation is considered to be the key to help doctors diagnose and treat liver tumors. However, at present, the difference of patients, liver morphology and noise interference in the image are the three major challenges of liver image segmentation, which leads to unsatisfactory segmentation accuracy. To this end, considering the cost of medical data labeling and the large number of CT images that need to be processed, we propose a new semi-supervised architecture, called MT UNet ++. This architecture is based on the average teacher-assisted learning mechanism, and introduces two improved versions of the same UNet++, acting as teachers and students, to learn and self-correct a certain proportion of the labeled data in the input model. In addition, combined with data enhancement and confidence learning denoising, the liver tumor segmentation is realized. When the proportion of marked data is 30%, the method is tested on the LITS2017 dataset. The dice similarity coefficient is 95.80%, the intersection and combination ratio is 90.57%, and the hausdorff distance is 4.26 mm. The test results show that this method is effective for liver CT image segmentation. At the same time, the research of semi-supervised learning methods has increasingly become a trend.

**Keywords:** Liver segmentation · Diagnosis and treatment · MT-UNet++ · Data augmentation · Confidence denoising

## 1 Introduction

The liver is the largest organ in the human body, located on the right side of the abdomen and under the chest, and is the key center of many physiological processes, such as decomposing toxic substances, regulating blood volume and providing support for the immune system [1]. According to the data given by the World Health Organization in 2020, liver cancer ranks the third in the global mortality rate, and its mortality rate ranks the second in China [2]. Early detection and early treatment are important measures to improve the survival rate of patients. Liver imaging plays a key role in the diagnosis and treatment of liver cancer. Among them, computer tomography (CT) has strong resolution, fast imaging and wide range. It has high sensitivity and specificity for the


G. Wang et al. (Eds.): APCMBE 2023, IFMBE Proceedings 103, pp. 205–216, 2024.
https://doi.org/10.1007/978-3-031-51455-5_23

detection of liver tumors, and the diagnostic accuracy of liver cancer can reach more than 90%. Liver CT image segmentation refers to distinguishing the normal liver tissue and tumor lesion areas in the CT image. Clinically, accurate segmentation of CT images by doctors to get the liver and lesion area is the basis of lesion detection, accurate location, differential diagnosis, treatment planning and prognosis judgment. However, there are many problems, such as the huge number of medical images, the difference of patients, and the existence of noise on CT images obtained by different devices, which lead to manual labeling time-consuming, not universal, and difficult to distinguish by human eyes.

Although scholars have carried out a series of work in the field of liver CT image segmentation [3, 4, 15–20]. In 2022, Li et al. [21] proposed a model of simultaneous expansion and convolution using ResNetXt50 as the backbone, achieving liver segmentation with a dice coefficient of 93.38% for the LITS 2017 public dataset. In addition, Shukla et al. [22] proposed a 2.5D VNet-WGAN with a liver segmentation coefficient of 94.02% on the 3DIRCADb dataset. However, there are many challenges in the segmentation of liver. First, the morphology of liver and liver tumors is diverse, and the clinical manifestation of tumors on CT images is a number of tissue regions with different sizes and irregular shape and structure on and around the liver organs. The boundary distribution of these regions is relatively fuzzy, and the internal density of small tumors is similar, Most of them are lower than the surrounding normal liver parenchyma, and when the tumor is large, its density may be uneven due to internal necrosis or calcification; Second, the difference of CT value between most liver tumors and normal liver tissue is very small; Third, different performance equipment, different operators and other factors will have noise impact on imaging. Three major challenges lead to poor performance of tumor segmentation accuracy; Secondly, most of the existing methods are fully supervised, which means that a large amount of labeled data is required, otherwise over-fitting problems will easily occur; Third, due to the cost of labeling, semi-supervised and even unsupervised methods have become a research hotspot. The above three factors increase the difficulty of segmentation of liver and liver tumor on CT images. Therefore, it is of great significance to establish an effective computer-aided model to learn human visual perception mechanism and automatically and efficiently analyze and process liver CT images to reduce doctors' workload, improve diagnosis and treatment efficiency and save patients' costs.

## 2 Method

### 2.1 Dataset

This paper uses the LITS 2017 public data set [23] (LITS17), with a total of 201 cases (131 training sets and 70 test sets). It is the largest and most authoritative public data set in the field of liver and tumor segmentation of CT images presently. It comes from 7 medical centers and uses CT machines of different models and protocols to sample abdominal CT volume data. The details are shown in Table 1.

**Table 1.** The introduction of LITS2017 Dataset

| Parameter | Value |
|---|---|
| Data format | .nii |
| Axial resolution of CT section/mm | 0.56–1.00 |
| Layer thickness/mm | 0.69–5.00 |
| Spatial size of CT axial section | 512 × 512 |
| Slice quantity/piece | 91–1024 |
| Number of different CT tumors | 1–75 |
| Tumor volume range/$mm^3$ | 38– 349 |

### 2.2 Data Augmentation

Our data enhancement operations include three-dimensional rotation, mirroring and adding random noise. Rotating the data in three-dimensional space is beneficial for the model to fully learn the features of different spatial directions in the training set and is very beneficial for liver identification, which is a complex target with no fixed direction and different shapes, to improve the generalization. In addition, noisy data is added to improve the robustness of the model. It is worth noting that we cut the data to [128, 128, 128] and normalized it before input. The format is converted from two NII files of a patient to one h5 file. After conversion, the file memory ratio is significantly reduced, as shown in Table 2.

**Table 2.** The size comparison before and after data conversion

| File properties | Before | Later | |
|---|---|---|---|
| Format | nii (volume) | nii (segmentation) | h5 (both) |
| Size/MB | 37.5–493 | 30.7–243 | 8.8–50 |

### 2.3 Architecture

In order to improve the accuracy of liver CT image segmentation and reduce the cost of data annotation, we designed a semi-supervised learning method named MT-UNet++ (Mean Teacher UNet++). The architecture is shown in Fig. 1. The framework takes the average teacher-assisted learning mechanism as the starting point, and introduces confidence learning [24] to denoise the CT image of liver tumor segmentation. The innovation of MT-UNet++ lies in: first, the improved version of UNet++ plays the role of teacher and student respectively. The improved version of UNet++is shown in Fig. 2. The moving index average (EMA) updates the learning weight and completes the self-correction process of segmentation; Second, compared with the original UNet++, we added an adder and removed the jump dense connection layer of the first layer. The adder is used to collect the output feature map of each layer through upsampling and convolution operation to the first layer, making full use of the image feature information. Thirdly, the up-sampling plus convolution method replaces the most original deconvolution operation of UNet++, which can eliminate the artifacts caused by the stack of deconvolution layers, and finally achieve the goal of improving the segmentation accuracy.

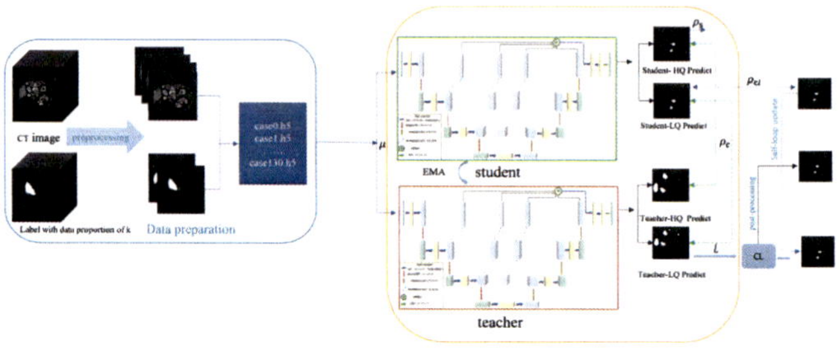


**Fig. 1.** Liver segmentation process of the proposed method

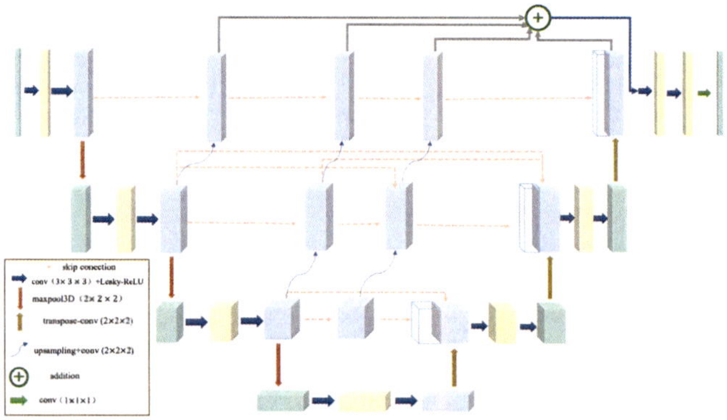


**Fig. 2.** An improved version of UNet++

## 2.4 Loss Function

Loss refers to the sum of the errors of all samples. The weight of the neural network is optimized by the gradient of the loss function during training. The total loss of this structure is the weighted sum of the labeled data $\rho_s$, disturbance consistency loss between labeled and unlabeled $\rho_c$ and learning loss of denoising module $\rho_{cl}$ as in formula (1), $k_1$ and $k_2$ is the weight coefficient. $\rho_s$, $\rho_c$, $\rho_{cl}$ is respectively defined as shown in Formula (2), (3) and (4).

$$loss = \rho_s + k_1\rho_c + k_2\rho_{cl} \tag{1}$$

$$\rho_s = 0.5CL + 0.5DL + 1FL + 0.5BL \tag{2}$$

$$\rho_c = \frac{1}{mnq}\sum_{i-0}^{m-1}\sum_{j-0}^{n-1}\sum_{k-0}^{q-1}[I(i,j,k) - K(i,j,k)]^2 \tag{3}$$

$$\rho_{cl} = 0.5FL + 0.5CL \tag{4}$$

$$k_1 = \begin{cases} e^{-5\times(1-\frac{t}{L})^2}, L = 400(t \le L) \\ 1, (t > L) \end{cases} \tag{5}$$

$$k_2 = \begin{cases} 0(epoch < 4000) \\ 0.5(epoch \ge 4000) \end{cases} \tag{6}$$

In the above formula, cross entropy loss function [25] (CL) measures the difference between two different probability distributions in the same random variable. Dice loss [26] (DL) focuses on mining the foreground area. Focal loss [27] (FL) can be used to reduce the weight of samples that are easy to classify, so that the model focuses more on samples that are difficult to classify during training. The boundary loss [28] (BL) adopts the form of distance measurement in the contour space rather than the region space, and integrates on the boundary between regions, which can alleviate the related problems of region loss in the highly unbalanced segmentation problem. $t$ is the number of training steps, $L$ is the length of ramp, and *epoch* is the number of iterations.

## 3 Result

In terms of evaluating the accuracy of the model method, we choose the dice similarity coefficient [29] (DSC), intersection over union ratio [30] (IOU) and hausdorff distance [31] (HD). IOU is defined as the ratio of intersection and union, and HD is the maximum distance from one set in space to the nearest point in another set. The calculation of the three indicators is shown in formula (7), (8) and (9) respectively.

$$DSC = \frac{2|\text{prediction} \cap \text{groundtruth}|}{|\text{prediction}| + |\text{groundtruth}|} \tag{7}$$

$$IOU = \frac{|\text{prediction} \cap \text{groundtruth}|}{|\text{prediction} \cup \text{groundtruth}|} \tag{8}$$

$$HD(A, B) = max\{h(A, B) - h(B, A) \tag{9}$$

$$h(A, B) = max_{a\in A}max_{b\in B}||a - b|| \tag{10}$$

The method relies on the deep learning framework and runs on four 12GB TITAN XP. The important training parameters are shown in Table 3. The training set and the number of iterations can be reduced by a certain percentage if the hardware is constrained, but these processes may have some impact on the segmentation accuracy.

In the experiment, when the LITS17 is divided, training and test sets are selected randomly and 20 of them are used as the test set. Then, the three indicators of liver segmentation using the MT-UNet++model and the visualization results of each patient's liver

**Table 3.** Important training parameter

| Parameter | Value |
|---|---|
| Optimizer | Adam |
| Learning Rate | 0.001, decrease progressively |
| Batch Size | 8 |
| Epoch | 10000 |

segmentation can be obtained through testing. To visually display, we use ITK-SNAP software [32] to display original CT images and manually labeled data of corresponding CT layers. Figure 3 shows the axial, sagittal, and coronal images of a certain layer in four patients. As illustrated in Fig. 4, it contains only preprocessed CT images, annotated data, and final prediction results. Figure 5 displays the segmentation result of this method for consecutive 12 layers (from layer 25 to 36) in three directions of the patient numbered 125. Meanwhile, we also compared our method with existing classical liver segmentation methods [5–18], and the results obtained are shown in Table 4.

Here is a brief introduction to those networks. First, UNet++superimposes and integrates features at different levels to obtain receptive fields of different sizes, preventing information loss of large objects' edge and small objects themselves due to sampling in the deep network. Second, The U-shaped structure and jump connection in UNet enable it to utilize both high-level and low-level features in image segmentation, making it the most widely used method in the field of medical image segmentation at present. Third, CeNet is proposed to solve the problem of spatial information loss caused by continuous aggregation and step convolution operations. Fourth, in order to extract spatial information between pixels in CT images, a spatial channel convolution and iterative extension learning strategy are proposed in the Channel UNet network, where spatial channel convolution appears in the sampling module. Fifth, Attention UNet adds an attention mechanism. Its encoder and decoder are connected by dense jumps. Attention gates are used in nested convolutional blocks to selectively merge different layer features during decoding. Sixth, the characteristic of ResNet34 UNet is that the encoder uses a pre trained ResNet34 encoding, and the decoder uses a decoding similar to UNet, which was first applied to automatic extraction of satellite image paths. Besides, Fcn8s, KiUNet, SegNet, and R2UNet have also been tested experimentally on the dataset.

It can be seen from Fig. 3 that some liver edges in the original CT image data have low contrast. Therefore, during the experimental design, in addition to the basic operations of image processing, we also conducted noise addition operations to better fit the model.

Compared to Fig. 3, the CT image in Fig. 4 undergoes a series of operations such as cropping, rotating, and horizontally flipping. This has two benefits: first, it lessens the influence of unrelated regions on segmentation prediction results, enabling the model to concentrate on learning features from the "liver" organ; and second, it relieves the strain on hardware brought on by high iterations. Moreover, the comparison results in Fig. 4 also show that though the method described in this paper has some processing issues with specific image details, the segmentation of the liver is remarkably consistent with the "gold standard".

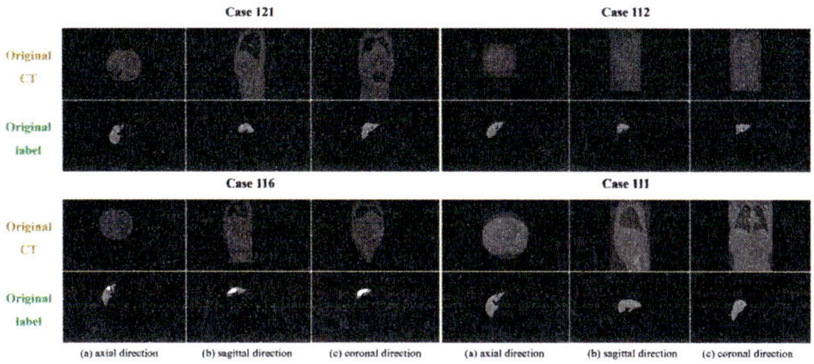


**Fig. 3.** The presentation of raw data from 4 patients

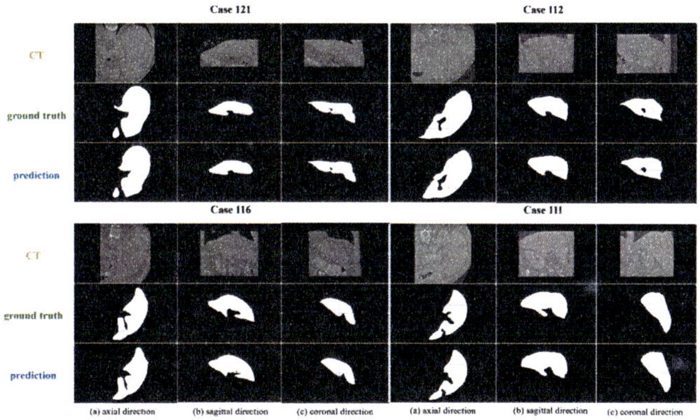


**Fig. 4.** The comparison between partial prediction and groundtruth

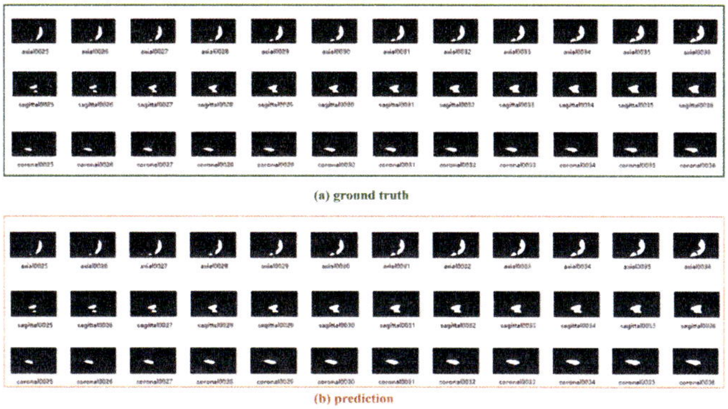


**Fig. 5.** The comparison of liver segmentation results of a patient's CT image with 12 consecutive layers

According to the Fig. 5, the predicted results of the model are in good agreement with the liver region labeled by the doctor. This continuous and correct segmentation result also indicates that the interlayer information of the CT image has been fully utilized.

**Table 4.** The results of liver segmentation

| Method | Annotated proportion (%) | Metric | | |
|---|---|---|---|---|
| | | DSC(%) | IOU(%) | HD (mm) |
| MT-UNet++ | 30 | 95.80 | 90.57 | 4.26 |
| UNet++ [5] | 100 | 93.83 | 88.49 | 6.43 |
| UNet [6] | 100 | 93.36 | 87.66 | 6.99 |
| CeNet [7] | 100 | 93.13 | 87.18 | 6.79 |
| Channel UNet [8] | 100 | 92.91 | 86.82 | 7.05 |
| Attention UNet [9] | 100 | 92.33 | 85.82 | 7.41 |
| Resnet34 UNet [10] | 100 | 91.07 | 83.63 | 6.74 |
| Fcn8s [11] | 100 | 90.46 | 82.60 | 7.36 |
| KiUNet [12] | 100 | 85.49 | 64.38 | 9.35 |
| SegNet [13] | 100 | 78.21 | 61.07 | 10.86 |
| R2UNet [14] | 100 | 68.58 | 52.78 | 11.37 |
| EAR-U-Net [15] | 100 | 95.20 | – | – |
| 3D RP-UNet [16] | 100 | 92.20 | – | – |
| TCSM [17] | 10 | 93.30 | – | – |
| semi-supervised UNet [18] | 20 | 86.83 | – | – |

*Note*: '–' means that the author of the original text has not given data

From the above statistical data in Table 4, we are told that UNet and some classical variant networks derived from it perform well in segmentation, among which the original UNet++ led with 93.83% of DSC. However, compared with it, our model increased the DSC score by 1.97% to 95.80%. It is worth noting that at this time, the proportion of this method in labelled samples is only 30%. With fewer marked samples, the segmentation accuracy is almost the same as that of the full-supervised method and even better than most full-supervised methods and some semi-supervised methods. This shows the effectiveness of our semi-supervised method in improving segmentation accuracy. Of course, data enhancement, confidence learning and model fusion are indispensable.

## 4 Discussion

The discrepancies between the prediction results marked in Fig. 6 and the gold standard are mainly shown in a few of small edge parts. The blue dotted line indicates the correct segmentation edge, and the red dotted line indicates the differential segmentation result. This is probably due to the discontinuity within the liver region having a bad impact on the boundary segmentation of the region, in another word, sometimes the discontinuous inflection point location in the target region is judged as the region. For this problem, there are two main solutions: one is to use an edge detector and add the discontinuous supervisory signal to the target function [33]; the other is to use the information of the orientation field to enhance the pixel association and refine the segmentation [34].

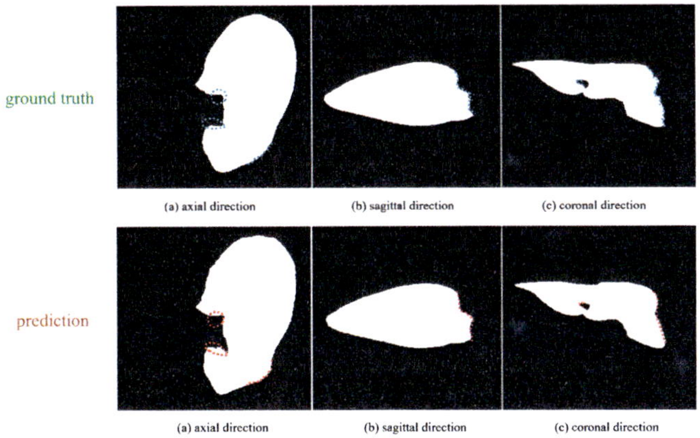


**Fig. 6.** The difference display of model segmentation

## 5 Conclusions

In this paper, we explore the advantages of our method compared with the recent fully supervised and semi-supervised methods. MT-UNet++is based on the average teacher-assisted learning mechanism, uses two improved UNet++models as teachers and students, rotates, mirrors and adds noise to the input data, and combines confidence learning to remove noise. Compared with the full supervision method, the model we designed achieves the same or even higher segmentation accuracy with less label data, which has foreseeable value in solving the cost of data labeling and improving the efficiency of doctors' diagnosis and treatment; Compared with semi-supervised method, this method improves the segmentation accuracy by 2.5%.

In the future work, we will focus on dealing with smaller segmentation targets and seek to integrate conditional random fields, attention mechanisms or other in-depth learning methods to further improve segmentation accuracy. Please look forward to it.

**Acknowledgment.** This work was supported in part by the Guangxi Innovation Driven Development Project (2019AA12005), National Major Instrument Development Project (61627807) and National Natural Science Foundation of China (81873913).

## References


1. Bray, F., Fer lay J, Soerjomataram I, et al.: A global cancer statistics 2018: GLOBOCAN estimates of incidence and mortality worldwide for 36 cancers in 185 countries. Ca-Cancer J Clin **68**(6), 394–424 (2018). https://doi.org/10.3322/caac.21492[InlineImageRemoved]
2. IARC (2021) Latest global cancer data: Cancer burden rises to 19.3 million new cases and 10.0 million cancer deaths in 2020. https://gco.iarc.fr/today/home
3. Shukla, P.K., Zakariah, M., Hatamleh, W.A., et al.: AI-DRIVEN novel approach for liver cancer screening and prediction using cascaded fully convolutional neural network. J Healthc Eng (2022). https://doi.org/10.1155/2022/4277436
4. Chen, Y., Zheng, C., Hu, F., et al.: Efficient two-step liver and tumour segmentation on abdominal CT via deep learning and a conditional random field. Comput. Biol. Med. **150**, 106076 (2022). https://doi.org/10.1016/j.compbiomed.2022.106076
5. Zhou, Z., Rahman Siddiquee, M.M., Tajbakhsh, N., et al.: Unet++: A nested u-net architecture for medical image segmentation, DLMIA and ML-CDS 2018 Proc. vol. 11045. Springer International Publishing, Granada, Spain **2018**, 3–11 (2018). https://doi.org/10.1007/978-3-030-00889-5_1
6. Ronneberger, O., Fischer, P., Brox, T.: U-net: Convolutional networks for biomedical image segmentation, MICCAI 2015 Proc.vol.9351. Springer International Publishing, Munich, Germany **2015**, 234–241 (2015). https://doi.org/10.1007/978-3-319-24574-4_28
7. Gu, Z., Cheng, J., Fu, H., et al.: Ce-net: Context encoder network for 2d medical image segmentation. IEEE Trans. Med. Imaging **38**(10), 2281–2292 (2019). https://doi.org/10.1109/TMI.2019.2903562
8. Chen Y, Wang K, Liao X, et al (2019) Channel-Unet: a spatial channel-wise convolutional neural network for liver and tumors segmentation
9. Front Genet 10:1110 DOI https://doi.org/10.3389/fgene. 2019.01110
10. Li, C., Tan, Y., Chen, W., et al.: ANU-Net: Attention-based Nested U-Net to exploit full resolution features for medical image segmentation. Comput Graph-UK **90**, 11–20 (2020). https://doi.org/10.1016/j.cag.2020.05.003
11. Buslaev, A., Seferbekov, S., Iglovikov, V., et al.: Fully convolutional network for automatic road extraction from satellite imagery, CVPRW 2018 Proc. IEEE, Salt Lake City, UT, USA **2018**, 207–210 (2018). https://doi.org/10.1109/CVPRW.2018.00035
12. Darshik, A.S., Dev, A., Bharath, M., et al.: Semantic segmentation of spectral images: A comparative study using FCN8s and U-NET on RIT-18 dataset, ICCCNT Proc. IEEE, Kharagpur, India **2020**, 1–6 (2020). https://doi.org/10.1109/ICCCNT49239.2020.9225461
13. Valanarasu, J.M.J., Sindagi, V.A., Hacihaliloglu, I., et al.: Kiu-net: Towards accurate segmentation of biomedical images using over-complete representations, MICCAI 2020 Proc. vol 12264. Springer International Publishing, Lima, Peru **2020**, 363–373 (2020). https://doi.org/10.1007/978-3-030-59719-1_36
14. Badrinarayanan, V., Kendall, A., Cipolla, R.: Segnet: A deep convolutional encoder-decoder architecture for image segmentation. IEEE Trans. Pattern Anal. Mach. Intell. **39**(12), 2481–2495 (2017). https://doi.org/10.1109/TPAMI.2016.2644615
15. Alom, M.Z., Yakopcic, C., Hasan, M., et al.: Recurrent residual U-Net for medical image segmentation. J Med Imaging **6**(1), 014006 (2019). https://doi.org/10.1117/1.JMI.6.1.014006
16. Wang, J., Zhang, X., Lv, P., et al.: Automatic liver segmentation using EfficientNet and Attention-based residual U-Net in CT. J Digital Imaging **1–15**,(2022). https://doi.org/10.1007/s10278-022-00668-x
17. Czipczer, V., Manno-Kovacs, A.: Adaptable volumetric liver segmentation model for CT images using region-based features and convolutional neural network. Neurocomputing **505**, 388–401 (2022). https://doi.org/10.1016/j.neucome.2022.07.024

18. Li, X., Yu, L., Chen, H., et al.: Transformation-consistent self-ensembling model for semisupervised medical image seg-mentation. IEEE Trans Neural Netw Learn Syst **32**(2), 523–534 (2020). https://doi.org/10.1109/TNNLS.2020.2995319
19. Han, K., Liu, L., Song, Y., et al.: An Effective Semi-supervised Approach for Liver CT Image Segmentation. IEEE J. Biomed. Health Inform. **26**(8), 3999–4007 (2022). https://doi.org/10.1109/JBHI.2022.3167384
20. Zhang, D., Chen, B., Chong, J., et al.: Weakly-supervised teacher-student network for liver tumor segmentation from non-enhanced images. Med. Image Anal. **70**, 102005 (2021). https://doi.org/10.1016/j.media.2021.102005
21. Meng, L., Tian, Y., Bu, S.: Liver tumor segmentation based on 3D convolutional neural network with dual scale. J. Appl. Clin. Med. Phys. **21**(1), 144–157 (2020). https://doi.org/10.1002/acm2.12784
22. Li, L., Ma, H.: RDCTrans U-Net: A Hybrid Variable Archi-tecture for Liver CT Image Segmentation. IEEE Sens. J. **22**(7), 2452 (2022). https://doi.org/10.3390/s22072452
23. Shukla, P.K., Zakariah, M., Hatamleh, W.A., et al.: AI-DRIVEN novel approach for liver cancer screening and prediction using cascaded fully convolutional neural network. J Healthc Eng **2022**,(2022). https://doi.org/10.1155/2022/4277436
24. Rezaei, M., Yang, H., Meinel, C.: Recurrent generative adversarial network for learning imbalanced medical image semantic segmentation. Multimed Tools Appl **79**(21–22), 15329–15348 (2020). https://doi.org/10.1007/s11042-019-7305-1
25. Xu, Z., Lu, D., Wang, Y., et al.: Noisy labels are treasure: mean-teacher-assisted confident learning for hepatic vessel segmentation, MICCAI 2021 Proc. vol. 12901. Springer International Publishing, Strasbourg, France **2021**, 3–13 (2021). https://doi.org/10.1007/978-3-030-87193-21
26. Ho, Y., Wookey, S.: The real-world-weight cross-entropy loss function: Modeling the costs of mislabeling. IEEE Access **8**, 4806–4813 (2019). https://doi.org/10.1109/ACCESS.2019.2962617
27. Sudre C H, Li W, Vercauteren T, et al (2017) Generalised dice overlap as a deep learning loss function for highly unbalanced segmentations, DLMIA and ML-CDS 2017, Proc. vol. 10553, Springer International Publishing, Québec, Canada, pp 240–248 DOI https://doi.org/10.1007/978-3-319-67558-9_28
28. Lin, T.Y., Goyal, P., Girshick, R., et al.: Focal loss for dense object detection. IEEE Trans. Pattern Anal. Mach. Intell. **42**(2), 318–327 (2020). https://doi.org/10.1109/TPAMI.2018.2858826
29. Kervadec, H., Bouchtiba, J., Desrosiers, C., et al.: Boundary loss for highly unbalanced segmentation. Med. Image Anal. **67**, 101851 (2021). https://doi.org/10.1016/j.media.2020.101851
30. Lee, R.: Dice Measures of the Amount of Ecologic Association Between Species. Ecology **26**(3), 297–302 (1945). https://doi.org/10.2307/1932409
31. Rezatofighi, H., Tsoi, N., Gwak, J.Y., et al.: Generalized intersection over union: A metric and a loss for bounding box regression, CVPR2019 Proc. IEEE COMPUTER SOC, Long Beach, CA, USA **2019**, 658–666 (2019). https://doi.org/10.1109/CVPR.2019.00075
32. Taha, A.A., Hanbury, A.: An efficient algorithm for calculating the exact Hausdorff distance. IEEE TPAMI **37**(11), 2153–2163 (2015). https://doi.org/10.1109/TPAMI.2015.2408351
33. Paul, A., Yushkevich, J.P., et al.: User-guided 3D active contour segmentation of anatomical structures: Significantly improved efficiency and reliability. Neuroimage **31**(3), 1116–1128 (2006). https://doi.org/10.1016/j.neuroimage.2006.01.015

34. Chu, J., Chen, Y., Zhou, W., et al.: Pay more attention to discontinuity for medical image segmentation, MICCAI 2020 Proc.vol.12264. Springer International Publishing, Lima, Peru **2020**, 166–175 (2020). https://doi.org/10.1007/978-3-030-59719-1_17
35. Cheng, F., Chen, C., Wang, Y., et al.: Learning directional feature maps for cardiac mri segmentation, MICCAI 2020 Proc. vol 12264. Springer International Publishing, Lima, Peru **2020**, 108–117 (2020). https://doi.org/10.1007/978-3-030-59719-1_11

# Background Interference Removal Algorithm for PIV Preprocessing Based on Improved Local Otsu Thresholding

Mengbi Xu[1], Gang He[1,2(✉)], and Jun Wen[1]

[1] School of Computer Science and Technology, Southwest University of Science and Technology, Mianyang, China
ganghe@swust.edu.cn

[2] NHC Key Laboratory of Nuclear Technology Medical Transformation (MIANYANG CENTRAL HOSPITAL), Mianyang, China

**Abstract.** In the Particle Image Velocimetry, due to background light fluctuation, noise interference, voltage fluctuation and other factors, there will be noise interference of different intensities in the background of the collected image. However, the existing image preprocessing methods cannot handle this situation well.In this paper, a PIV image background interference removal algorithm based on improved neighborhood Otsu processing is proposed. The algorithm proposed in this paper separates the particle image from the background interference through the adaptive neighborhood improved Otsu threshold segmentation method, and uses the common PIV analysis tools PIVLab and paraPIV to analyze the flow field after the interference is removed. The experimental results demonstrated that the proposed algorithm can obviously improve the quality of PIV results in terms of both PSNR and SSIM in the case of the background light interference, and the increasement of average performance is nearly 50 percent when comparing with traditional preprocessing algorithms, which solves the problem of large flow field analysis error caused by poor background light removal effect in the case of irregular grating and other background light interference only using traditional preprocessing.

**Keywords:** PIV · PIV image preprocessing · Otsu threshold method · Moving average threshold

## 1 Introduction

Particle Image Velocimetry is an optical measurement technique where the velocity field of an entire region within the flow is measured simultaneously. It is used to obtain the instantaneous velocity and related characteristics in the fluid and it is also a non-contact measurement. It can measure the flow field in the plane or volume instantaneously without disturbing the flow or fluid characteristics. The measurement accuracy is high [1], and the measurement range is large. Therefore, many articles involve the realization and


G. Wang et al. (Eds.): APCMBE 2023, IFMBE Proceedings 103, pp. 217–231, 2024.
https://doi.org/10.1007/978-3-031-51455-5_24

technical optimization of PIV in all aspects [2–5]. At the same time, because of these advantages of PIV, it has a very wide range of applications. In medicine, models can be made to study various fluids in blood vessels, such as studying the in vitro feasibility of shunt effect in aneurysm model [6] and measuring the flow velocity in blood vessel model [7], wind tunnel velocity test aerodynamic experiment [8], and water velocity measurement [9–11] (such as general fluid mechanics research, hull design, rotating machinery, channel flow), etc. In a PIV experiment, by releasing tracer particles small enough and assumed to faithfully follow the flow dynamics in the fluid, we illuminate the fluid with these particles and take high-speed video, and can calculate the speed and direction of the fluid under study by observing the displacement of tracer particles between different images. The PIV equipment is composed of fluid control equipment, CCD camera, laser, synchronizer, water storage tank, and tracer particle seeding equipment. The fluid control equipment is composed of circulating pipeline, piston cylinder, hydraulic resistance, hydraulic capacity, liquid storage tank, pulsating motor and peristaltic pump. The peristaltic pump transports the fluid, and the piston cylinder, hydraulic resistance, hydraulic capacity and pulsating motor reduce the noise of the fluid and change the fluid amplitude and waveform. The emitted laser forms sector light through the equipment composed of mirror and cylindrical mirror, so as to illuminate a thin layer of liquid. You can make the camera capture the position of the seeded particles in the cross section. The CCD camera captures the trajectory of the tracer particles at a frame rate of thousands frames per second, which is convenient to realize image correlation with algorithm. The synchronizer is used to control the camera, laser and the fluid being studied, and generate the fluid with specific speed and waveform required for the experiment. The schematic diagram of PIV Experimental equipment is shown in Fig. 1.

In particle image velocimetry, the images taken by our high-speed camera need to go th rough three steps to get the final flow field: image preprocessing, image correlation [12, 13], and image post-processing [14–16]. The effect of image preprocessing determines the accuracy of correlation between each particle in the process of image correlation. Generally, our image preprocessing uses high-pass [ 17], Intensity Capping [18]and Contrast Limited Adaptive Histogram Equalization (CLAHE) [ 19] to denoise, remove the over bright spots that affect the results and enhance the bright spots. In most cases, these three pretreatmen t methods can get better and accurate results, such as the application in the experimental study of Wake Vortex [20]. How ever, when facing some special and specific problems, it is necessary to find a special image preprocessing method for this situation to get more a ccurate results, such as PIV measurement of flow around an arbitrary moving free surface [21] and accurate partic le image velocity measurement near the moving wall [22].

Traditional preprocessing methods can achieve good results in several backgrounds, such as halo background, solid color background and gradient background. However, the existing traditional preprocessing methods cannot achieve the ideal results when the light emitted by the laser is uneven or there is power frequency interference and grating. In each query window, the particles affected by the grating will mislead the cross-correlation calculation due to the light dark difference, and may therefore get a large number of wrong velocity vectors. For our flow field analysis, the only useful information in the image is particles in the image. Therefore, from the perspective of

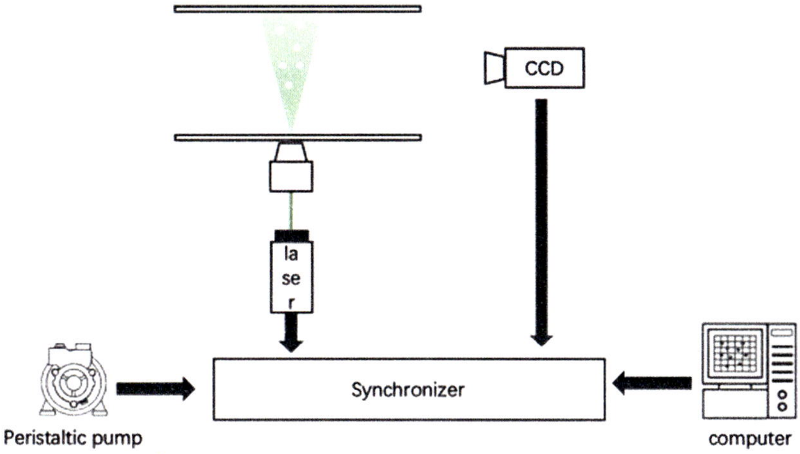


**Fig. 1.** Schematic diagram of PIV Experimental Equipment

image preprocessing of PIV image by removing the background, we propose a new algorithm for preprocessing PIV image to solve the background interference in this case.

# 2 Methodology

## 2.1 Preprocessing in PIV

### 2.1.1 Contrast Limited Adaptive Histogram Equalization

CLAHE is a variant of adaptive histogram equalization in which the contrast amplification is limited, so as to reduce this problem of noise amplification. It operates on small areas of the image and in each block, the most frequent intensity of the image histogram is distributed to the whole range of the data. Therefore, the low exposure region and the high exposure region are optimized independently. By limiting the height of local histogram to limit the enhancement amplitude of local contrast, so as to limit the amplification of noise and the over enhancement of local contrast, CLAHE can significantly improve the probability of detecting effective vectors in experimental images, which is applied in various fields of image processing [21–24].

### 2.1.2 High-Pass

In the frequency domain, the image with low frequency shows that it is relatively smooth, because the gray value change in the smooth place is small, while the image with high frequency is usually edge or noise, because these places are often abrupt changes in gray value. While in the PIV image uneven illumination will lead to low-frequency background information, which can be removed by applying high-pass filter, which mainly retains the high-frequency information of particle illumination. The filter emphasizes the particle information in the image and suppresses any low-frequency information in the image. It is also widely used in image processing [25, 26].

### 2.1.3 Intensity Capping

A common error source in particle image velocimetry is the bright spot in the image. The feature of these bright spots is that the intensity of gray is much greater than the average intensity of the image, which is usually produced by the strong scattering of seed particles. The displacement of the bright spot can dominate the cross-correlation calculation in the query window, and therefore the obtained velocity vector can be biased. This algorithm uses an efficient and easy way to implement image enhancement process to improve the particle image velocimetry results when bright spots appear, so that the deviation caused by bright spots is reduced. This process is called "intensity capping", which imposes an upper limit specified by the user on the gray intensity of the image. Intensity capping can significantly increase the number of effective vectors in experimental image pairs and reduce the displacement error in simulated image analysis. Compared with other particle image velocimetry image enhancement techniques, intensity capping provides competitive performance, low computational cost, easy implementation, and minimal image modification.

## 2.2 Cross Correlation Operation

The most sensitive part of a DPIV analysis is the cross-correlation algorithm: small sub images of an image pair are cross correlated to derive the most probable particle displacement in the interrogation areas. In essence, the cross-correlation is a statistical pattern matching technique that tries to find the particle pattern from interrogation area A back in interrogation area B. This statistical technique is implemented with the discrete cross correlation function:

$$R(k,l) = \sum^{\infty}\sum^{\infty} x(m,n)y(m+k,n+l) \tag{1}$$

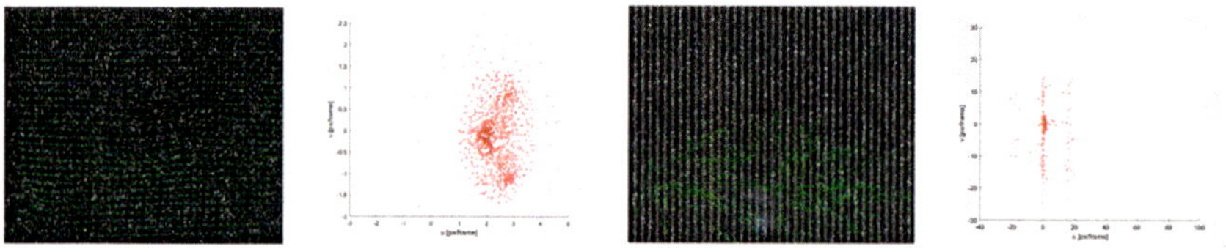

(a) (b) (c) (d)

**Fig. 2.** Diagram of the influence of background interference. **a** and **c** are the flow fields obtained without and with grating; **b** and **d** are the distributions of all vector u and v values without and with grating).

X is a fixed point of the original graph and Y is the point of the next graph. Find the Y vector that maximizes R through the independent variables K and l, then y (m + k, n + l) is considered as the target point. When there is uneven distribution of light spot and brightness on the image, it may occur: the pixel point x is in the bright (dark) position on the image, and the pixel point y to which X moves on the next image is in the dark (bright) position. In this case, the R obtained by using formula (1) is likely to be a false peak, so as to obtain the error vector field that is significantly different from the original image as shown in Fig. 2. 100% of the vectors have a great error in the vector speed, and 12% of the vectors have a deviation of more than 45° in the vector direction. The three traditional PIV image preprocessing methods we usually use cannot solve this problem. Therefore, this paper proposes a method to solve this kind of problem by removing the background.

### 2.3 Algorithm

The basic idea of Otsu [27] threshold method is to use a threshold to divide the data in the image into two categories. In one category, the grayscale of the image pixels is less than this threshold, and in the other category, the grayscale of the image pixels is greater than or equal to this threshold. If the variance of the gray level of pixels in these two classes is the largest, it indicates that the obtained threshold is the best threshold. The greater the interclass variance between background and foreground, the greater the difference between the two parts of the image. When part of the foreground is misclassified into background or part of the background is misclassified into foreground, the difference between the two parts will become smaller. Therefore, the segmentation that maximizes the variance between classes means the minimum misclassification probability.

However, in the face of the image obscured by the speckle gray mode, or the image with grating, the effect of removing the background with the ordinary threshold method will become very poor. Moving average method is a kind of variable threshold processing, which is relative to global threshold processing. Global threshold processing refers to calculating a fixed threshold according to the whole picture. If each pixel in the picture is greater than this value, it is considered as the foreground, otherwise it is the background. The variable threshold refers to that there are different thresholds in each pixel point or pixel block in the picture. If the pixel point is bigger than its corresponding threshold, it is considered as the foreground. Moving average method is a linear Z-shaped scanning of the entire image, and a threshold will be generated at each point. The image will be segmented by comparing the gray value at this point with the threshold calculated at this point. The algorithm is shown as follows:

$$m(k+1) = \frac{1}{n} \sum_{i=k+2-n}^{k+1} z_i \tag{2}$$

where z k + 1 represents the gray value of the point encountered in step k + 1 in the scanning sequence, m (k) is the pixel value of the k-th point of the input image, and n is the customized parameter representing the number of points used to calculate the average. The algorithm flow chart is shown in Fig. 3.

When sinusoidal grating of different thicknesses is added to the picture, as shown in Fig. 4 (using the experimental results obtained by PIVLab [28]), when coarse grating is added (Fig. 4a), good results can still be obtained by using the traditional preprocessing method. However, when the grating we use is brighter and dense enough (Fig. 4b), the traditional image preprocessing method will lead to too large vector deviation. This is

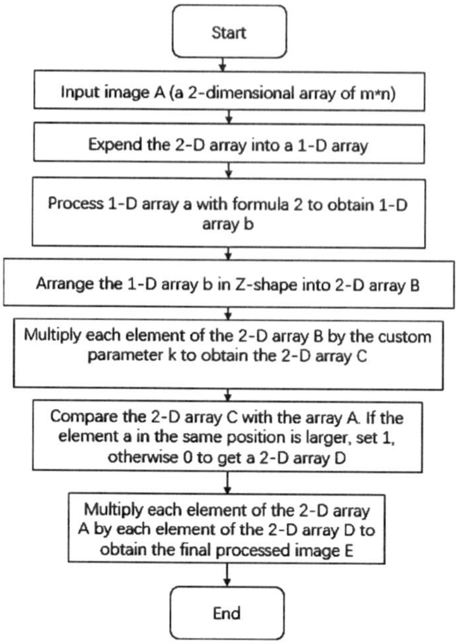


**Fig. 3.** Flow chart of movingthresh algorithm

because the thinner the grating, the higher the probability that a pixel of the previous image and the target point of the next image will be bright and dark. Therefore, we can try to use the moving average threshold for preprocessing. When the grating is horizontal (Fig. 4c), the impact on the image is small, because the vector itself is mostly horizontal, so the probability of light and shade changes before and after the pixel moves will be very small.

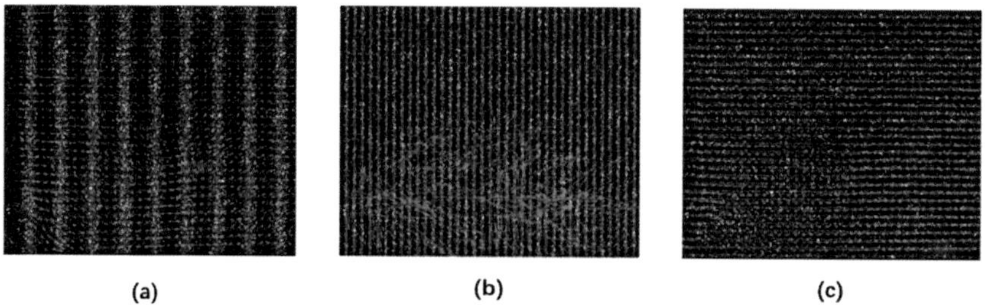


**Fig. 4.** Three typical background interference. **a** is horizontal sinusoidal interference with larger spacing. **b** is horizontal sinusoidal interference with smaller spacing and higher intensity. **c** is vertical sinusoidal interference with smaller spacing and higher intensity).

Therefore, it is proposed to apply the moving average threshold to PIV image preprocessing, so as to remove the grating on the basis of retaining the original image information, so that the position of each pixel before and after changing is not affected by the difference of light and shade.

### 2.3.1 The Selection of Function Parameters of Moving-Thresh Method in Preprocessing PIV Images

The range of concern for calculating the average threshold: n takes 2–3 times the pixel size of particles, which will not lose the foreground because it is too small, nor will it be affected by the light spot if it is too large.

### 2.3.2 Evaluation Standard

SSIM: Structural similarity is a standard to measure the similarity of two images. Given the sum of two images, the structural similarity of the two images can be calculated according to formula (3):

$$SSIM(x, y) = \frac{(2\mu_x\mu_y + c_1)(2\sigma_{xy} + c_2)}{(\mu_x^2 + \mu_y^2 + c_1)(\sigma_x^2 + \sigma_y^2 + c_2)} \quad (3)$$

$\mu_x$ is the mean value of x, $\mu_y$ is the mean value of y, $ó_x$ is the variance of x, $ó_y$ is the variance of y, $ó_{xy}$ is the covariance of x and y.c1 = (k1L)2, c2 = (k2L)2 are constants used to maintain stability. L is the dynamic range of pixel values. k1 = 0.01, k2 = 0.03. SSIM ranges from -1 to 1. When two images are identical, the value of SSIM is equal to 1.

PSNR: Peak Signal-to-Noise Ratio. For two images K and I with the size of m*n, the mean square error (MSE) is defined as:

$$MSE = \frac{1}{mn}\sum_{i=0}^{m-1}\sum_{j=0}^{n-1}[I(i,j) - K(i,j)]^2 \quad (4)$$

PSNR is defined as:

$$PSNR = 10 \cdot \log_{10}\left(\frac{MAX_I^2}{MSE}\right) \quad (5)$$

where MSE is obtained by formula (4), and MAXI is the maximum possible pixel value of the picture. When two pictures are identical, the value of PSNR is infinite.

## 2.4 Results and Discussion

This algorithm uses PIVLab and paraPIV [29] which are two common PIV images processing tools to verify the effect of this algorithm, and uses SSIM [30]and PSNR to compare the processing results of this algorithm and the traditional three preprocessing methods under horizontal and dense grating with different densities. The software used in the experiment is matlab2018, and the data set used in the experiment come from http://www.PIVchallenge.org/, which is a competition website about PIV. There are 6 types of interference: horizontal, vertical and inclined grating (high-density and low-density). The parameters of three traditional image preprocessing algorithms high-pass, intensity capping and contract limited adaptive histogram equalization (CLAHE) take the default value, and the parameter n of movingthresh (f, n, b) of this algorithm takes 4 and b takes 0.8.

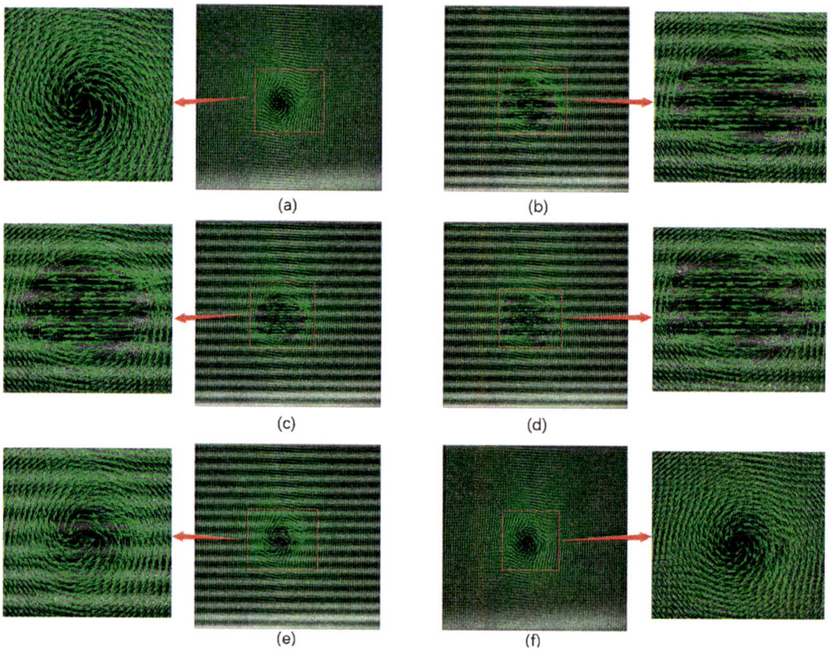


**Fig. 5.** Vector field obtained by PIVLab in 6 cases. **a** Initial image. **b** Adding grating without preprocessing. **c** CLAHE preprocessing. **d** Intensity capacity preprocessing. **e** High-pass preprocessing. **f** Processing by this algorithm).

### 2.4.1 Aircraft Wake Vortex

The image data is the aircraft in the landing configuration (DLR Avast half model) (u = 60 m/s, and the mainstream direction is perpendicular to the light plate plane) for the experimental study of the formation of wake vortices after transportation. This measurement position is 1.64 m behind the wingtip and 170 mm in view × 140 mm. Image is selected as strong gradient, image density loss and particle image size change are common problems in many PIV applications in large wind tunnels.

### 2.4.2 High Density Grating

The experimental results obtained by various high-density grating are similar. Here are the experimental results obtained by transverse low-density grating. The vector field obtained from PIVLab is shown in Fig. 5. Figure 5a shows the vector field obtained from the initial image, Fig. 5b shows the vector field obtained without preprocessing after adding a grating, Fig. 5c shows the vector field obtained by CLAHE after adding a grating, Fig. 5d shows the vector field obtained by intensity capacity after adding a grating, Fig. 5e shows the vector field obtained by high-pass after adding a grating, and Fig. 5f shows the vector field obtained by processing with this algorithm after adding a grating, The red box is used to select the areas with large vector deviation in many processing results for the method.

Using SSIM and PSNR evaluation standard, the vector field obtained from the original image is compared with the vector field obtained by adding grating without preprocessing, the vector field obtained by CLAHE after adding grating, the vector field obtained by intensity capping after adding grating, the vector field obtained by high-pass filtering after adding grating, and the vector field processed by this algorithm after adding grating. The picture uses Fig. 5 and the results of paraPIV experiment. Table 1 is the evaluation results of the images obtained by PIVLab and Table 2 is the evaluation results of the images obtained by paraPIV.

**Table 1.** Evaluation results of image processed by transverse high density grating obtained by PIVLab

| Preprocessing algorithm | SSIM | PSNR |
|---|---|---|
| Original image | 1 | Inf |
| Add grating | 0.1328 | 12.6775 |
| CLAHE | 0.1356 | 12.7114 |
| Intensity Capping | 0.1314 | 12.6594 |
| High-pass | 0.7526 | 17.4079 |
| Our algorithm | 0.8525 | 21.0431 |

According to Tables 1 and 2, after adding transverse dense grating, the image similarity is greatly reduced, and only high-pass is effective in improving this algorithm for the three traditional image preprocessing methods, while the other two image preprocessing algorithms have little effect in improving this situation, and our algorithm has greatly improved this situation. Figure 6 is the original image and the overall distribution of u, v, velocity and u, v of the respective vectors of the image using our algorithm to remove the transverse low-density grating, where u is the transverse velocity of the vector and v is the longitudinal velocity of the vector. It can be seen that the range of each value is very close to the distribution law except for a few deviations. The average v value in the original image is 3.2525, the average v value of the processed image is 3.2466, the deviation is 0.1817%, the average u value is 2.7963, and the average u value of the processed image is 2.8009, the deviation is only 0.1642%.

**Table 2.** Evaluation results of image processed by transverse high density grating obtained by paraPIV

| Preprocessing algorithm | SSIM | PSNR |
|---|---|---|
| Original image | 1 | Inf |
| Add grating | 0.4456 | 14.8573 |
| CLAHE | 0.4495 | 14.9568 |
| Intensity Capping | 0.4334 | 14.5803 |
| High-pass | 0.8152 | 20.1103 |
| Our algorithm | 0.9179 | 26.7623 |

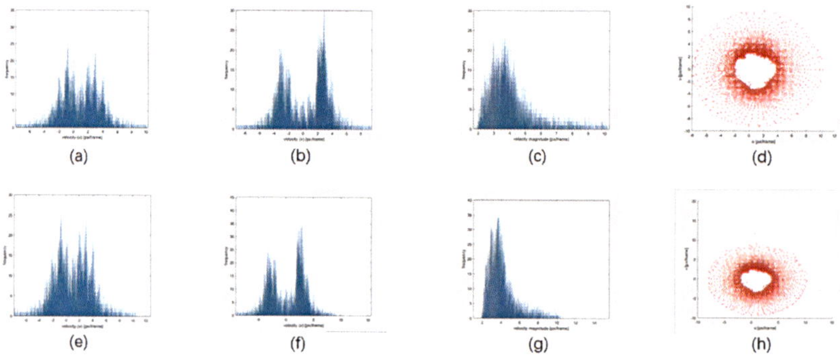

**Fig. 6.** Diagram of u, v and velocity overall distribution. **a, e** original diagram and the numerical frequency distribution diagram of all vectors after grating processing in the longitudinal direction, **b, f** are the numerical frequency distribution diagram of the original diagram and all vectors after grating processing in the transverse direction, **c, g** are the numerical frequency distribution diagram of all vectors in the vector velocity after the original diagram and grating processing, and **d, h** are the distribution diagram of u and v values of all vectors after the original diagram and grating processing, respectively)

### 2.4.3 Low Density Grating

The experimental results obtained by various high-density grating are similar. Here are the experimental results obtained by longitudinal high-density grating.

The vector field obtained from PIVLab is shown in Fig. 7. Figure 7a shows the vector field obtained from the initial image, Fig. 7b shows the vector field obtained without preprocessing after adding a grating, Fig. 7c shows the vector field obtained by CLAHE after adding a grating, Fig. 7d shows the vector field obtained by intensity capacity after adding a grating, Fig. 7e shows the vector field obtained by high-pass after adding a grating, and Fig. 7f shows the vector field obtained by processing with this algorithm after adding a grating.

Table 3 is the evaluation results of low-density grating images obtained by PIVLab. Figure 8 is the original image and the overall distribution of u, v, velocity and u, v of the respective vectors of the image using this algorithm to remove the transverse low-density

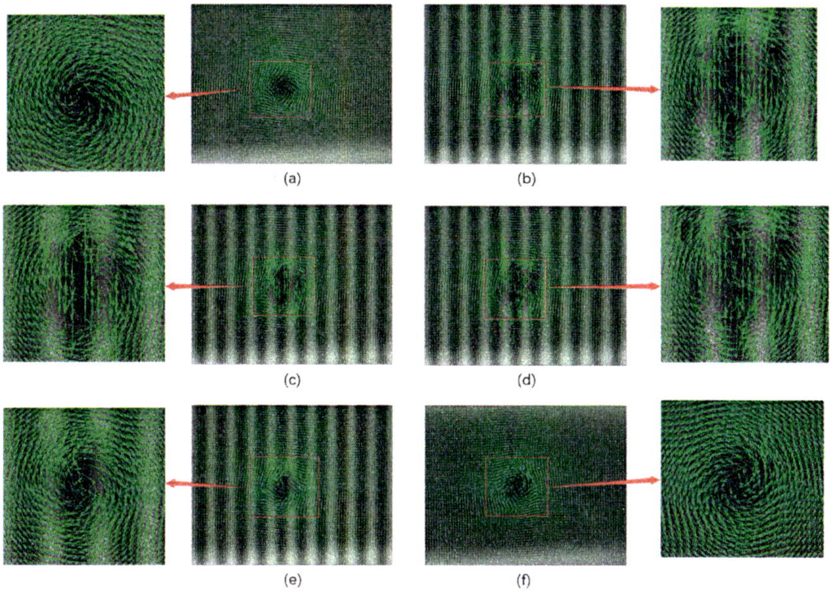


**Fig. 7.** Vector field obtained by PIVLab in 6 cases. **a** Initial image. **b** Adding grating without preprocessing. **c** CLAHE preprocessing. **d** Intensity capacity preprocessing. **e** High-pass preprocessing. **f** Processing by this algorithm

grating, where u is the transverse velocity of the vector and v is the longitudinal velocity of the vector. It can be seen that the range of each value is very close to the distribution law except for a few obvious deviations. The average v value in the original image is 3.2525, the average v value of the processed image is 3.2552, the deviation is 0.083%, the average u value is 2.7963, and the average u value of the processed image is 2.8095, the deviation is 0.472%.

Observing the data of several groups of experimental results, it can be seen that for the common flow field of aircraft wake vortex, after adding various types of grating, the vector field calculation of the area in the center of the flow field will produce a large deviation, while the traditional preprocessing method only has a certain effect of image preprocessing of high-pass, and the processing effect of CLAHE and intensity capacity is almost not. Our algorithm obviously achieves better preprocessing effect under various grating, and is very close to the original vector field.

### 2.4.4 Shear Field

The flow field is a computer-generated shear field, which is also one of the common flow fields. We also generated horizontal and vertical grating for preprocessing experiments. The flow field generated by the experiment is obtained by PIVLab. The experimental results are shown in Fig. 9, in which Fig. 9a is the vector field obtained from the initial image, Fig. 9b is the vector field obtained by adding grating without preprocessing, Fig. 9c is the vector field obtained by CLAHE after adding grating, and Fig. 9d is the vector field obtained by intensity capping after adding grating Fig. 9e shows the vector

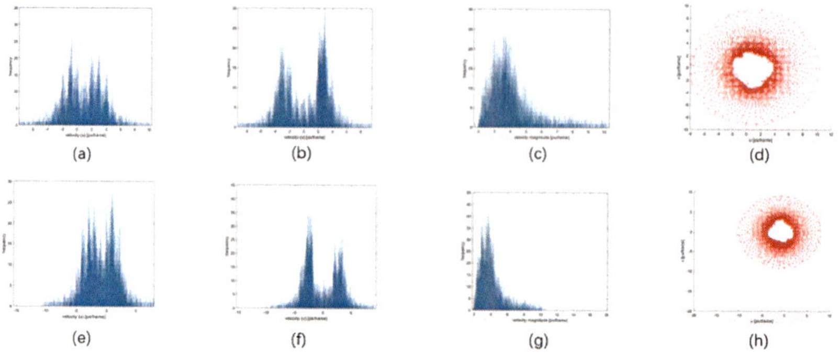

**Fig. 8.** Diagram of u, v and velocity overall distribution. **a** and **e** original diagram and the numerical frequency distribution diagram of all vectors after grating processing in the longitudinal direction, **b**, **f** are the numerical frequency distribution diagram of the original diagram and all vectors after grating processing in the transverse direction, **c**, **g** are the numerical frequency distribution diagram of all vectors in the vector velocity after the original diagram and grating processing, and **d**, **h** are the distribution diagram of u and v values of all vectors after the original diagram and grating processing, respectively

**Table 3.** Evaluation results of image processed by transverse low density grating obtained by PIVLab

| Preprocessing algorithm | SSIM | PSNR |
|---|---|---|
| Original image | 1 | Inf |
| Add grating | 0.7274 | 16.9910 |
| CLAHE | 0.7561 | 17.3542 |
| Intensity Capping | 0.7152 | 16.7736 |
| High-pass | 0.7823 | 18.2368 |
| Our algorithm | 0.8571 | 21.1210 |

field obtained by high-pass after adding grating, Fig. 9f shows the vector field obtained by processing with this algorithm after adding grating, and Fig. 9g, h mainly show that the transverse grating has no large image on the image.

It can be seen from the Fig. 9 that for the shear field where the vectors are almost parallel, the horizontal grating is parallel to the direction of the vector, so the addition of the grating has no effect on the calculation of the shear field vector, and the longitudinal grating will affect the direction of very few vectors and the size of all vectors.

Table 4 shows the evaluation results using the image obtained from the experimental results in Figs. 9, and 10 shows the u, v value distribution of the vector field of the original image and the processed image. It can be seen that our algorithm still gets good results. The average v value in the original image is 0.2828, the average v value of the processed image is 0.2753, the deviation is 3.536%, the average u value is 1.4792, and the average u value of the processed image is 1.4838, the deviation is 0.311%.

**Table 4.** Evaluation results of image processed by PIVLab

| Preprocessing algorithm | SSIM | PSNR |
|---|---|---|
| Original image | 1 | Inf |
| Add grating | 0.6594 | 23.2453 |
| CLAHE | 0.6552 | 23.1201 |
| Intensity Capping | 0.6567 | 23.1603 |
| High-pass | 0.6638 | 23.3924 |
| Our algorithm | 0.8151 | 24.8383 |

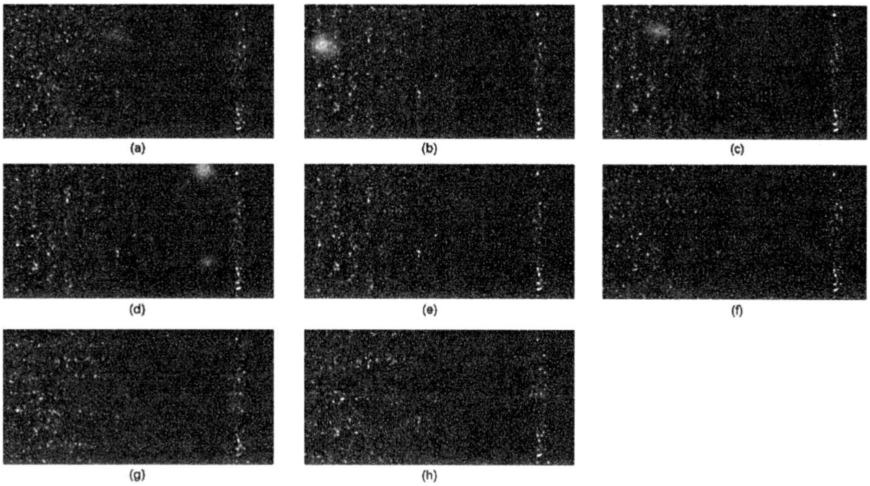


**Fig. 9.** Vector field obtained by PIVLab in 8 cases. **a** Initial image **b** Adding grating without preprocessing. **c** CLAHE preprocessing. **d** Intensity capacity preprocessing. **e** High-pass preprocessing. **f** Processing by this algorithm. **g** Transverse dense grating without processing. **h** Transverse sparse grating without processing

# 3 Conclusions

Due to light fluctuation, noise interference, voltage change and other reasons, the background of PIV image will have different intensity of noise interference. In this paper, a PIV image background interference removal algorithm based on improved neighborhood Otsu processing is proposed, which solves the problem of large flow field analysis error caused by poor background light removal effect when there is irregular grating and other background light interference with traditional preprocessing only. By testing the images in PIV challenge data set, processing with traditional PIV preprocessing algorithms such as CLAHE, intensity capacity, high-pass, etc., and analyzing the flow field in PIV analysis software such as PIVLab, paraPIV, etc. The results of the flow field are evaluated by SSIM, PSNR. The algorithm proposed in this paper is used in the experimental flow

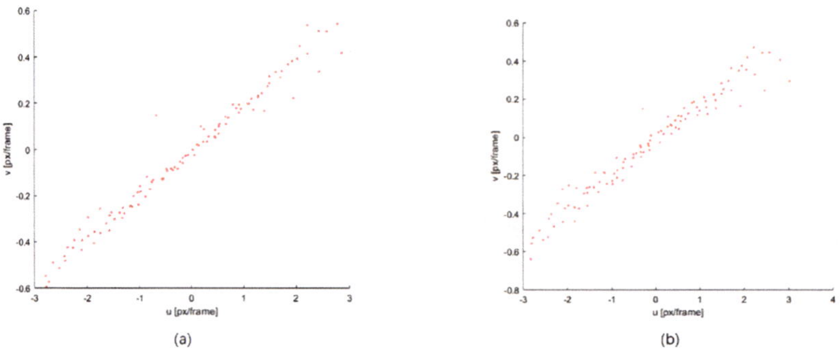


**Fig. 10.** Diagram of u and v value distribution. **a** u, v value distribution of the original vector field. **b** u, v value distribution of the original vector field after this algorithm

field (aircraft wake vortex) and the synthetic flow field (shear field). Both SSIM and PSNR show obvious advantages (an average increase of more than 50%), indicating the effectiveness of this algorithm in dealing with the background grating type interference of PIV images.

**Acknowledgment.** This work was financially supported by Sichuan Science and Technology Program(NO.2020YFS0454, NO.2020YFS0318), NHC Key Laboratory of Nuclear Technology Medical Transformation (MIANYANG CENTRAL HOSPITAL)(Grant No.2021HYX031).

## References

1. Adrian, R.J.: Dynamic ranges of velocity and spatial resolution of particle image velocimetry. Measurement Sci. Technol. 8(12):1393–1398(6) (2015)
2. Fleury, V., Bailly, C., Jondeau, E., et al.: Space Time Correlations in Two Subsonic Jets Using Dual Particle Image Velocimetry Measurements. AIAA J. **46**(10), 2498–2509 (2015)
3. Markus, R., Jurgen, K., Wereley, S.T., et al.: Particle image velocimetry : a practical guide. Experimental Fluid Mechanics **255**(3), 160–162 (2017)
4. Tauro, F., Pagano, C., Phamduy, P., et al.: Large-Scale Particle Image Velocimetry From an Unmanned Aerial Vehicle. IEEE
5. B M B A , A R D , C N G D B , et al. Borescopic particle image velocimetry in bubbling gas–solid fluidized beds. Particuology, 43:66–75 (2019)
6. Clauser, J., Knieps, et al.: A Novel Plasma-Based Fluid for Particle Image Velocimetry (PIV): In-Vitro Feasibility Study of Flow Diverter Effects in Aneurysm Model. Annals of Biomedical Engineering the Journal of the Biomedical Engineering Society (2018)
7. Bando, Y., Oishi, M., Oshima, M.: PIV Measurement of Deformation of the Wall and Internal Flow Structure of the Elastic Vascular Model[J]. Journal of the Visualization Society of Japan **1**(2), 1061 (2008)
8. Gil-Prieto D , Zachos P , Macmanus D G , et al. Convoluted Intake Distortion Measurements Using Stereo Particle Image Velocimetry. Aiaa Applied Aerodynamics Conference (2017)
9. Legleiter, C.J., Kinzel, P.J., Nelson, J.M.: Remote measurement of river discharge using thermal particle image velocimetry (PIV) and various sources of bathymetric information[J]. J. Hydrol. **554**, 490–506 (2017)

10. Raben, J.S., Hariharan, P., Robinson, R., et al.: Time-Resolved Particle Image Velocimetry Measurements with Wall Shear Stress and Uncertainty Quantification for the FDA Nozzle Model[J]. Cardiovasc. Eng. Technol. **7**(1), 7–22 (2016)
11. Morton, C., Yarusevych, S., Scarano, F.: A tomographic particle image velocimetry investigation of the flow development over dual step cylinders[J]. Phys. Fluids **28**(2), 2011–2022 (2016)
12. Huang, H., Dabiri, D., Gharib, M.: On errors of digital particle image velocimetry. Measurement Science and Technology, 8(12):1427–1440(14) (1997)
13. Stamhuis, E.J.: Basics and principles of particle image velocimetry (PIV) for mapping biogenic and biologically relevant flows[J]. Aquat. Ecol. **40**(4), 463–479 (2006)
14. Raffel, M., Willert, C.E., Scarano, F., et al.: Post-processing of PIV Data. Springer, Berlin Heidelberg (2018)
15. Shi, B., Wei, J., Zhang, Y.: Phase discrimination and a high accuracy algorithm for PIV image processing of particle-fluid two-phase flow inside high-speed rotating centrifugal slurry pump[J]. Flow Meas. Instrum. **45**, 93–104 (2015)
16. Dong, S., Hui, M.: Chebyshev spectral method and Chebyshev noise processing procedure for vorticity calculation in PIV post-processing. Experimental Thermal and Fluid Science, 2001, 24(1)
17. Gonzalez, R.C., Woods, R.E.: Digital image processing[J]. IEEE Trans. Acoust. Speech Signal Process. **28**(4), 484–486 (1980)
18. Shavit, U., Lowe, R.J., Steinbuck, J.V.: Intensity Capping: a simple method to improve cross-correlation PIV results[J]. Exp. Fluids **42**(2), 225–240 (2007)
19. Zuiderveld K . Contrast Limited Adaptive Histogram Equalization[J]. Graphics Gems, 1994:474–485
20. Fu, X.X., Liu, J.S., Wang, J.W., et al.: Application of Image Preprocessing on PIV Experimental Study of Wake Vortex Interactive Instability[J]. Appl. Mech. Mater. **696**, 85–91 (2015)
21. Park, J., Im, S., Sung, H.J., et al.: PIV measurements of flow around an arbitrarily moving free surface[J]. Exp. Fluids **56**(3), 56 (2015)
22. Lv, J., Wang, F., Xu, L., et al.: A segmentation method of bagged green apple image[J]. Sci. Hortic. **246**, 411–417 (2019)
23. Wang J , Li X , Zhang Z , et al. Application of image technology to simulate optimal frequency of automatic collection of volumetric soil water content data[J]. Agricultural Water Management, 2022, 269
24. Jucheng, Zhang, Yonghua, et al. HF-SENSE: an improved partially parallel imaging using a high-pass filter.[J]. Bmc Medical Imaging, 2019
25. Liaw J J , Lu C P , Huang Y F , et al. Improving Census Transform by High-Pass with Haar Wavelet Transform and Edge Detection[J]. Sensors, 2020, 20(9):2537.sensors journal, 2018
26. Zhu Y , Jia L , Bai Y , et al. Image preprocessing method for particle image velocimetry (PIV) image interrogation near a fluid-solid surface[C]// Aps Meeting. APS Meeting Abstracts, 2014
27. Ostu N , Nobuyuki O , Otsu N . A thresholding selection method from gray level histogram. 1979
28. Thielicke W , Stamhuis E J . PIVlab – Towards User-friendly, Affordable and Accurate Digital Particle Image Velocimetry in MATLAB[J]. Journal of Open Research Software, 2014, 2(1)
29. Wang C , Wang C . ParaPIVlab: PIVlab in Parallel. 2017
30. Wang Z , Bovik A C , Sheikh H R , et al. Image quality assessment: from error visibility to structural similarity[J]. IEEE Trans Image Process, 2004, 13(4)

# Development of the Fetal Brain Structural Connectivity Based on In-Utero Diffusion MRI

Ruike Chen[1], Xinyi Xu[1], Ruoke Zhao[1], Mingyang Li[1], Cong Sun[2], Guangbin Wang[3], and Dan Wu[1](✉)

[1] Department of Biomedical Engineering, College of Biomedical Engineering and Instrument Science, Zhejiang University, Hangzhou, China
danwu.bme@zju.edu.cn

[2] Department of Radiology, Beijing Hospital, National Center of Gerontology, Institute of Geriatric Medicine, Chinese Academy of Medical Sciences, Beijing, China

[3] Department of Radiology, Shandong Provincial Hospital Affiliated to Shandong First Medical University, Jinan, China

**Abstract.** Extensive cortico-cortical connections emerge in the fetal brain during the second-to-third trimester with the rapid development of white matter fiber pathways. However, the early establishment and prenatal development of the brain's structural network are not yet understood. In this work, we used in-utero diffusion MRI data of fetuses from 26 to 38 gestational weeks to build the fetal brain structural connectivity networks (SCN). Graph theory was adopted to investigate the developmental patterns of the fetal brain SCN. Network analyses revealed increasing global and local efficiency, modularity, and small worldness of the fetal brain during development. We observed the strengthening of short-range cortico-cortical connections and the weakening of long-range connections, reflecting the distinct developmental events of short and long-range fiber pathways during the studied period. The fetal brain SCN underwent complicated changes during the late-second-to-third trimester. The findings of this study provided valuable information on the early developmental patterns of brain cortico-cortical structural connectivity.

**Keywords:** Fetal brain · Diffusion MRI · Structural connectivity network · Normal development

## 1 Introduction

Neuronal pathways of the fetal brain develop rapidly during the second-to-third trimester, forming early cortico-cortical structural connections [1]. A few studies of structural connectivity networks (SCN) reported growing network strength and increasing efficiency during early brain development based on post-mortem fetuses or preterm-born neonates [2–4]. Some studies also observed adult-like properties such as small-worldness and rich-club organizations in the developing brains [3, 5]. However, none of the previous studies reported the development of cortico-cortical connectivity networks in-utero due


G. Wang et al. (Eds.): APCMBE 2023, IFMBE Proceedings 103, pp. 232–237, 2024.
https://doi.org/10.1007/978-3-031-51455-5_25

to the lack of data and the technical challenges of fetal motion. In this work, we aim to collect in-utero diffusion MRI (dMRI) data to build the SCN of the fetal brain from the second-to-third trimester and to decipher its developmental patterns.

## 2 Material and Methods

We enrolled a total of 161 pregnant women at Shandong Provincial Hospital under the approval of the Institutional Review Board. The fetuses were scanned in-utero at gestational age (GA) from 26 to 38 weeks (W) on a 3T Siemens scanner using a dMRI sequence with $b = 600$ s/mm$^2$, 30 gradient directions, 8 non-diffusion-weighted images, and two averages. The in-plane resolution was $1.73 \times 1.73$ mm$^2$ and the slice thickness was 4 mm. 139 scans were included for further processes after excluding those with large motion, noise, or other abnormalities. Reconstructed images with poor quality were excluded and 114 remained for SCN analysis (see Fig. 1).

Raw dMRI data was preprocessed in MRtrix3, allowing denoising, eddy-current distortion correction, between-volume motion correction, and bias removal [6]. Images were slice-to-volume-registered and reconstructed to 1.2 mm isotropic resolution using SVRTK [7]. We estimated each subject's fiber orientation distribution (FOD) function for probabilistic tractography [8, 9]. SIFT2 was performed to reweight streamlines according to the underlying FOD [10]. Seventy-eight cortical regions of interest (ROIs) were obtained as the nodes of SCN, by merging the CRL fetal brain parcellations [11] with the cortical tissue label from our previously published fetal brain atlas [12] that was transformed into subject space. The edges were calculated by the sum of streamline weights between every two nodes, normalized by nodal volumes.

Global efficiency (*Eglob*), mean local efficiency (*Eloc*), shortest path length (*Lp*), and network modularity were calculated using the GRETNA 2.0 toolbox implemented in MATLAB (https://www.nitrc.org/projects/gretna/). The clustering coefficient (*CC*) was calculated by an algorithm suitable for weighted connectomes [13]. Small-worldness was measured by

$$SW = \frac{CC_{norm}}{Lp_{norm}} \tag{1}$$

where $CC_{norm}$ and $Lp_{norm}$ are the *CC* and *Lp* normalized by the mean *CC* and *Lp* of the network's 100 degree-matched random networks. We then performed Pearson's correlation analysis between each network property and GA, as well as between each edge's strength and GA. All statistical analyses with p-values $<0.05$ after FDR correction were considered significant.

## 3 Results

We observed rapid changes in network properties in the fetal brain SCN. Both *Elogb* and *Eloc* of the network increased significantly over GA. The modularity also showed significant growth, reflecting an increase in intra-module connections compared to between-module ones. *SW* was found above 1 throughout the late-second-to-third gestational

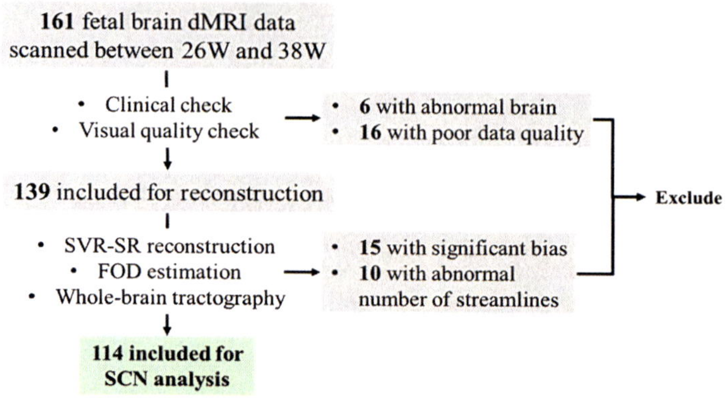


**Fig. 1.** Data inclusion flowchart. Diffusion MRI data of 161 fetuses were scanned. 139 scans were included for image reconstruction and 114 remained for SCN analysis after the quality check.

trimester and increased with GA since $CC_{norm}$ increased while $Lp_{norm}$ remained stable (see Fig. 2), which means that small-world property existed over the studied period and strengthened.

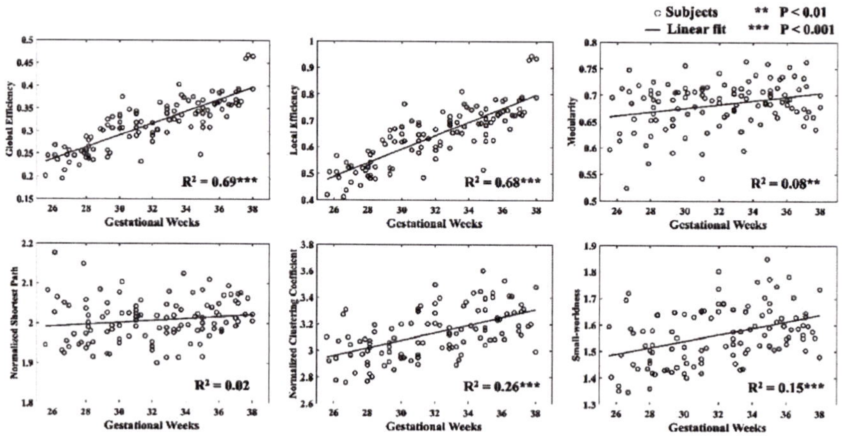


**Fig. 2.** Network properties of fetal brain structural connectivity network during 26–38 weeks of gestation. Global and local efficiency, modularity, normalized clustering coefficient, and small-world index increased significantly with gestation, while the normalized shortest path length remained unchanged.

The edge strength changed heterogeneously across regions. Short-range connectivity in the frontal and occipital cortices and those connecting the limbic nodes with their neighboring regions increased most significantly. Some of the long-range edges mainly connected to the anterior brain decreased significantly. The decrease in edge strength along the cingulum pathways was the most prominent (see Fig. 3).

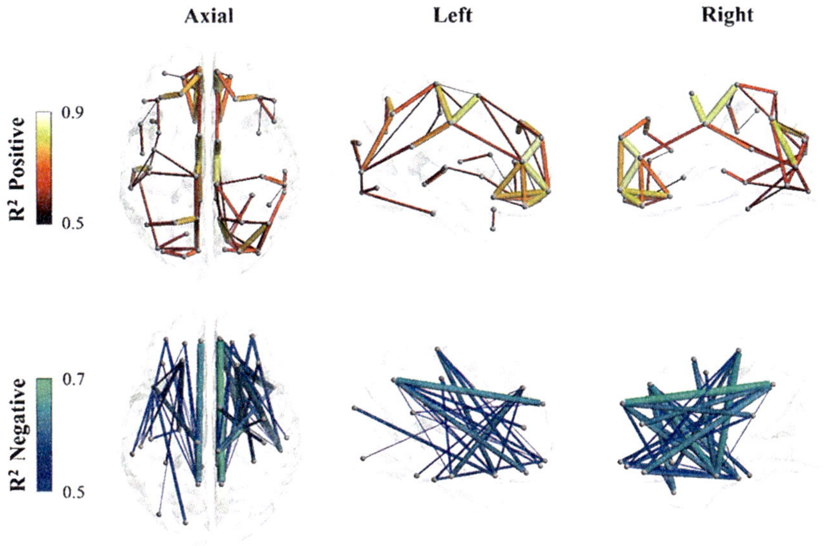


**Fig. 3.** Edges with significantly changed strength during 26–38 weeks of gestation. Pearson's correlation between edge strength and GA showed strengthened short-range connections (top) and weakened long-range connections (bottom). Only edges with FDR-corrected P-values $<0.05$ and $R^2 > 0.5$ were displayed. Edges were colored by the $R^2$ values of the linear correlations.

## 4 Discussion

The observed changes in fetal brain SCN suggested complicated development during the second-to-third trimester. On the whole-brain level, the significant increases in *Eglob* and *Eloc* reflected simultaneous integration and segregation of fetal brain SCN. The efficiency of information transfer was promoted on both global and local levels. The structural network presented adult-like small-world property as early as 26 weeks of gestation. *SW* increased significantly while $Lp_{norm}$ remained stable, indicating the increasing complexity of the network topology with a relatively unchanged wiring cost [14], enabling high information capacity of the network. The modularity of the fetal brain SCN increased significantly, which indicated that local communities emerged in the fetal brain to support the information specialization at regional modular structures. These findings agreed with previous dMRI studies based on postmortem fetuses and preterm neonates [3, 4].

Reversed trends of edge strength in long and short-range connections were observed (see Fig. 3), which might suggest distinct developmental events in these two kinds of fiber connections during this period. The cortical radial glial scaffolds gradually disappeared during the second-to-third trimester and more complex and anisotropic dendritic structures emerged [15]. The disappearance of glial fibers might cause the weakening of long-range connections. The high extracellular component and fast volume expansion of the unmyelinated long association fibers might also contribute to the decrease in fiber density [16]. Meanwhile, short-range cortico-cortical pathways such as the subcortical u-fibers emerged [17], enhancing the local integrity with the strengthened short-range connections, as observed in our results (see Fig. 3).

## 5 Conclusion

We studied the spatiotemporal development of fetal brain SCN, which displayed both integration and segregation patterns during the second-to-third trimester. Short-range cortico-cortical connections were strengthened while long-range connections were weakened, resulting in the complex topology of the fetal brain SCN. Small-world properties and modular structures emerged, indicating the adult-like brain network architecture started to take shape in early brain development.

## References

1. Takahashi, E., Hayashi, E., Schmahmann, J.D., et al.: Development of cerebellar connectivity in human fetal brains revealed by high angular resolution diffusion tractography. Neuroimage **96**, 326–333 (2014)
2. Brown, C.J., Miller, S.P., Booth, B.G., et al.: Structural network analysis of brain development in young preterm neonates. Neuroimage **101**, 667–680 (2014)
3. Song, L., Mishra, V., Ouyang, M., et al.: Human fetal brain connectome: structural network development from middle fetal stage to birth. Front. Neurosci. **11**, 561 (2017)
4. Zhao, T., Mishra, V., Jeon, T., et al.: Structural network maturation of the preterm human brain. Neuroimage **185**, 699–710 (2019)
5. Ball, G., Aljabar, P., Zebari, S., et al.: Rich-club organization of the newborn human brain. Proc. Natl. Acad. Sci. USA **111**(20), 7456–7461 (2014)
6. Tournier, J.D., Smith, R., Raffelt, D., et al.: MRtrix3: a fast, flexible and open software framework for medical image processing and visualisation. Neuroimage **202**, 116137 (2019)
7. Deprez, M., Price, A., Christiaens, D., et al.: Higher order spherical harmonics reconstruction of fetal diffusion MRI with intensity correction. IEEE Trans. Med. Imaging **39**(4), 1104–1113 (2020)
8. Tournier, J.D., Calamante, F., Connelly, A.: Robust determination of the fibre orientation distribution in diffusion MRI: non-negativity constrained super-resolved spherical deconvolution. Neuroimage **35**(4), 1459–1472 (2007)
9. Tournier, J.D.C., Calamante, F., Connelly, A.: Improved probabilistic streamlines tractography by 2nd order integration over fibre orientation distributions. In: Proceedings of the International Society for Magnetic Resonance in Medicine, vol. 1670 (2010)
10. Smith, R.E., Tournier, J.-D., Calamante, F., et al.: SIFT2: Enabling dense quantitative assessment of brain white matter connectivity using streamlines tractography. Neuroimage **119**, 338–351 (2015)
11. Gholipour, A., Limperopoulos, C., Clancy, S., et al.: Construction of a deformable spatiotemporal MRI atlas of the fetal brain: evaluation of similarity metrics and deformation models (2014)
12. Xu, X., Sun, C., Sun, J., et al.: Spatiotemporal atlas of the fetal brain depicts cortical developmental gradient in Chinese population. bioRxiv (2022)
13. Zhang, B., Horvath, S.: A general framework for weighted gene co-expression network analysis. Stat. Appl. Genet. Mol. Biol. **4**(1), 1–45 (2005)

14. Latora, V., Marchiori, M.: Efficient behavior of small-world networks. Phys. Rev. Lett. **87**(19), 198701 (2001)
15. Xu, G., Takahashi, E., Folkerth, R.D., et al.: Radial coherence of diffusion tractography in the cerebral white matter of the human fetus: neuroanatomic insights. Cereb. Cortex **24**(3), 579–592 (2014)
16. Chen, R., Sun, C., Liu, T., et al.: Deciphering the developmental order and microstructural patterns of early white matter pathways in a diffusion MRI based fetal brain atlas. NeuroImage 119700–119700 (2022)
17. Takahashi, E., Folkerth, R.D., Galaburda, A.M., et al.: Emerging cerebral connectivity in the human fetal brain: an MR tractography study. Cereb. Cortex **22**(2), 455–464 (2012)

# A Unified CNN-ViT Network with a Feature Distribution Strategy for Multi-modal Missing MRI Sequences Imputation

Yulin Wang and Qian Liu(✉)

School of Biomedical Engineering, Key Laboratory of Biomedical Engineering of Hainan Province, Hainan University, Haikou, China
qliu@hainanu.edu.cn

**Abstract.** Multi-modal magnetic resonance imaging (MRI) is of great clinical use for disease assessment and diagnosis, as it provides comprehensive and complementary information through multiple contrasts. However, due to potential obstacles of the scanning process and the patient's physical condition, the available scans of each subject may vary. Here, we propose a unified adversarial network based on the convolution neural network (CNN) and vision transformer (ViT) for missing MRI image synthesis in any input-output image configurations. The purpose of our network design is to develop a robust and efficient way to integrate the local information capturing ability of the convolutional operation and global contextual sensitivity of the multi-head self-attention (MSA) mechanism. Specifically, we employ a u-shape network as our generator and mix the convolutional path and the MSA path in a parallel manner at each network stage, the mixer is in place of the original MSA block of the canonical transformer, this design enables each layer to learn both global and local information simultaneously and takes advantage of the general ViT architecture. Furthermore, since these two branches have different frequency information preference, possessing all channels in each branch inevitably renders feature redundancy and introduces extra artifacts, accordingly, we adopt a channel splitting strategy that splits input features channel-wise and feed to each branch separately, meanwhile, considering each network stage has different desire of the high- and low-frequency information, we also explore various channel distribution ratios at each network stage. Our proposed method demonstrates reliable synthesis for healthy tissues and heterogeneous enhancement on BraTS2021 dataset. Furthermore, compare with four state-of-the-art methods including convolution-based, MSA-based and hybrid models in the MRI sequence synthesis field, our approach outperforms these methods quantitatively and qualitatively. Therefore, our method has the potential to be used as a candidate for medical image synthesis.

**Keywords:** Image synthesis · Multi-modal MRI · Visual transformer · Convolutional neural network · Deep learning


G. Wang et al. (Eds.): APCMBE 2023, IFMBE Proceedings 103, pp. 238–244, 2024.
https://doi.org/10.1007/978-3-031-51455-5_26

# 1 Introduction

Multi-modal magnetic resonance imaging (MRI) is widely used in the clinical practice since it can provide radiologists with various soft tissue contrasts information for disease diagnosis and treatment. However, the acquisition of multiple MRI scans is often hinder by scanning time and cost, potential scan corruptions, or patients' allergies to contrast agents [1].

With the rapid development of deep learning, multi-modal MRI image synthesis methods has been extensively proposed to alleviate the missing modality issue. Convolutional neural network (CNN) has first been applied as the fundamental backbone for several medical image synthesis methods [2–4]. However, the convolutional operation has limitations in modelling long-range dependency within images, which may cause the poor generalizability [5] and the loss of global (low-frequency) image information. Further improvement has provided by generative adversarial network (GAN) [6], although GAN-based synthesis approaches [7, 8] produce finer anatomical structures and image details, they are still convolution-based. In recent years, vision transformer (ViT) [9]-based models [10, 11] have been proposed to solved above problem through the multi-head self-attention (MSA) mechanism. However, these methods suffer from huge computation burden and insufficient high-frequency information distilling ability [14]. To combine the advantages of both CNNs and transformers, Dalmaz et al. [15] introduced ResViT to synthesis multi-modal medical images, but the serial combination of convolution and MSA block is unable to model global or local interactive relationships properly.

In this paper, we propose a unified hybrid network for multi-input multi-output MRI sequences imputation, which is capable of using any subset of available contrasts to synthesize missing modalities in one forward process. We incorporate the adversarial generative mechanism to guide the network to produce images with finer and more realistic detail. In each network stage of the generator, we replace the MSA operation in the general transformer network with a hybrid convolution-MSA module, specifically, the module contains a convolution path and a MSA path placed in a parallel manner, and we adopts a feature-splitting way to feed each of branch with a certain ratio of channels in different network stage to independently extract particular feature components, finally, two branches are fused by a merge module in each layer. Meanwhile, we apply separable discriminator for each modality to disentangle contrast representations.

# 2 Material and Methods

## 2.1 Overview

The overall architecture of our proposed method is presented in Fig. 1. Suppose the whole source image set across one patient has Z pulse sequences, where $Z = X + Y$. Firstly, we impute Y missing contrasts with zeros padding images and stack them with X available modalities as the input image of the generator. Secondly, we use the discriminator to classify the synthetic results.

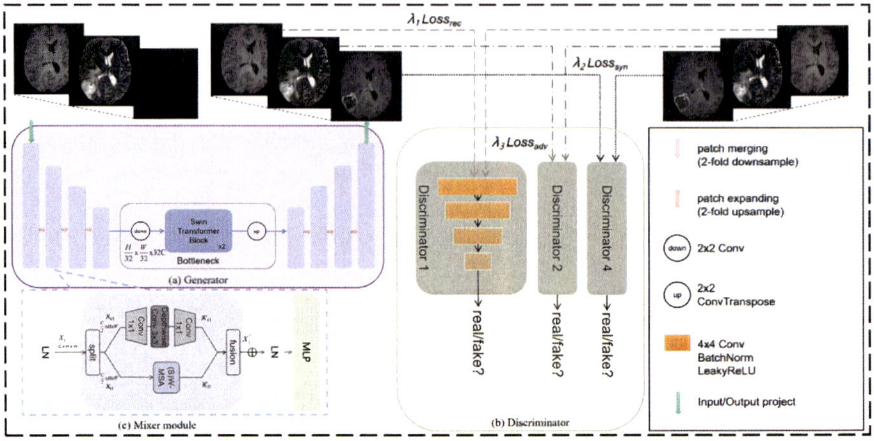


**Fig. 1.** Overview of the proposed unified framework for missing MRI sequences imputation and details of blocks.

## 2.2 Proposed Method

Our generator is depicted in Fig. 1a, it adopts a u-shape network architecture with skip connection between the encoder and decoder at each image scale. For each module of the encoder and decoder, we follow the general design in ViT [9] to maintain the deployment advantages and replace the MSA block with a hybrid convolution-MSA block, as shown in Fig. 1c.

The convolutional operation is notable for its strength of image detail perception. We adopt a combination of the 1x1 pointwise and the $3 \times 3$ depthwise convolution to generate features and exchange information between patches in a serial way, this mechanism has been proved in [17] to be more efficient than the traditional convolution. The output features of convolutional operation are residually connected with the input features for the final output.

Given our network design aims to synthesize reliable brain anatomic structure with diverse pathology, it is essential to apply the long-range dependencies modelling ability of the MSA operation. We follow the design proposed in [18], which introduces the shifting window MSA (SW-MSA) strategy to connect adjacent layers of windows and achieves excellent accuracy-speed trade-off.

To efficiently utilize the feature extracting abilities of two branches and avoid the computational burden and image noise caused by the redundant features, we apply a channel-splitting strategy to feed each branch with certain proportions of feature components in each layer of the encoder and decoder.

The bottleneck between the encoder and decoder is served to process encoding features at the smallest image scale, thus we first down-sample features to make the receptive field covers the whole feature map, and then we utilize pure MSA blocks to capture the global information within image. To empower our network to yield satisfying perceptual details, here, we follow the multi-scale discriminator proposed in [19] and apply separately for each contrast. This independent discriminator strategy is beneficial to disentangle each contrast representation and progressively generates realistic image contrast.

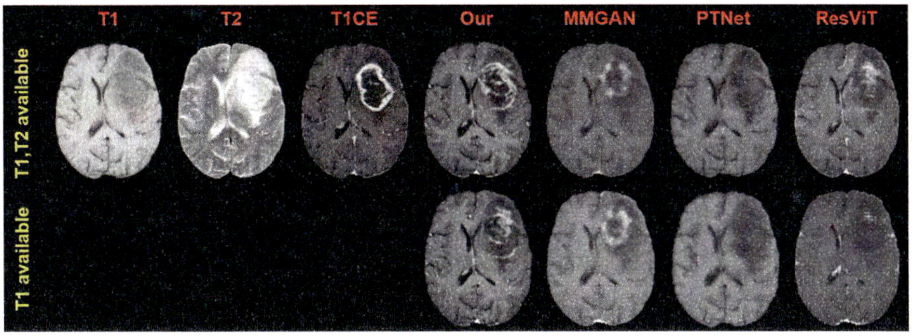


**Fig. 2.** Qualitative results of competing methods on two synthetic tasks

## 2.3 Loss Functions

First, we adopt the L1 loss to separably measure the pixel intensity difference for synthetic ($L_S$) and reconstruction ($L_R$) tasks with different weights. Second, we use the hinge loss as our adversarial loss ($L_A$), which adopts the idea of max-margin to classify the fake and real images.

The overall loss function is the linear combination of the above three loss terms, we set the weights of $L_S, L_R$ *and* $L_A$ as 50, 10, and 1 respectively.

## 2.4 Datasets

The BraTS 2021 dataset [20] consists of 1251 glioma patients scans. All images were skull-stripped and co-registered. We randomly selected 50, 10, and 20 cases for training, validation, and testing respectively with T1-weighted (T1), T1 contrast enhancement (T1CE), T2-weighted (T2) sequences.

## 2.5 Competing Methods and Evaluation Metrics

We evaluate the models using peak signal-to-noise (PSNR) and structure similarity index (SSIM). We conduct experiments on random missing contrasts settings and compare our methods with three state-of-the-art medical image models: MMGAN [7], PTNet [12], and ResViT [15], where MMGAN is a CNN-based adversarial network, PTNet is a pure transformer-based network and ResViT is a hybrid adversarial model.

# 3 Results

## 3.1 Missing Contrast Imputation

Table 1 presents the quantitative synthesis results of all methods based on PSNR and SSIM measurements for three input combination setups. Compared with all models, our method achieves higher PSNR and SSIM. To corroborate our method also has improved perceptual quality, in Fig. 2, we provide visual comparisons of T1CE sequence synthesis tasks with T1 and T2 contrasts available and single T1 contrast available respectively. As we can see, in comparison to all models, our method offers sharper and solid lesion and anatomies depiction due to its improved learning behavior.

## 3.2 Ablation Study

Considering the difference of frequency information preference between the convolution and MSA operator, as well as the lower layer often contains more high-frequency information while the higher layer includes more low-frequency, we perform a comparison of channel splitting ratio to verify the most suitable channel splitting manner at each network stage. In Table 2, we list the channel proportions of the convolutional branch from the bottom to top layers. The best result is achieved by the equally distribute the feature to both convolutional and MSA branches.

**Table 1.** Quantitative assessment between the proposed network and competing methods across the test dataset for three representative synthesis tasks

| | T1, T2 → T1CE | | T1, T1CE → T2 | | T1 → T2, T1CE | |
|---|---|---|---|---|---|---|
| | PSNR | SSIM | PSNR | SSIM | PSNR | SSIM |
| MMGAN | 32.08 | **0.961** | 28.99 | 0.952 | 29.78 | 0.950 |
| PTNet | 30.30 | 0.951 | 27.21 | 0.939 | 29.10 | 0.939 |
| ResViT | 31.39 | 0.956 | 28.50 | 0.945 | 29.31 | 0.943 |
| Ours | **32.19** | **0.961** | **29.07** | **0.954** | **29.96** | **0.952** |

**Table 2.** Ablation experiments on different feature distribution configurations

| | [1/2, 1/2, 1/2, 1/2] | [2/3, 1/2, 1/3, 1/12] | [3/4, 1/2, 1/4, 1/24] |
|---|---|---|---|
| PSNR | **29.41 ± 2.43** | 29.33 ± 2.40 | 29.37 ± 2.46 |
| SSIM | **0.954 ± 0.021** | 0.951 ± 0.020 | 0.953 ± 0.021 |

## 4 Discussion

In this work, we focus on the multi-modal MRI contrasts synthesis task and develop a unified model that is able to take in any available input sequences to synthesize missing contrasts without repetitive training. Our proposed method utilize a effective way to combine the MSA and convolutional operation. Extensive experiments on all possible source-target image configurations demonstrate that our method surpasses state-of-the-arts methods with various architecture design in medical image synthesis field. The ablation studies on multiple channel-splitting ratio show the best result is obtained by dividing the features equally in each scale of layer, this phenomenon could be explained as although different layers of the network contain different amounts of high and low frequency information, as well as different preferences for high and low frequency information in the two branches, the optimized rates of the two branches also need to be considered, while, unlike classification networks, the up-sampling process of generative networks also needs to extract enough high frequency information at the topper layer of the network. The merits of our channel-splitting parallel design are two-folds: (1) Combining the global modeling ability of MSA and the local information distilling ability of convolutional operation in a parallel manner in each network stage enable our network to simultaneously extracts and fuses adequate low- and high-frequency information within images. (2) The equal feature distribution strategy in channel dimension greatly alleviates the computing redundancy while guarantee the reliability of produced images by discarding features that may introduce extra noises.

## 5 Conclusions

Here we propose a unified network to infer any missing MRI images by leverage available sequences. For completing this tasks, we develop an efficient hybrid model to combine the convolutional and MSA operation, and we observe equally distribute features to two branches is the best way to balance them in our tasks. Results on extensive experiments show our proposed method has superior synthetic performance. Therefore, it has the potential to be used as a candidate for medical image synthesis.

## References


1. Gulani, V., Calamante, F., Shellock, F.G., et al.: Gadolinium deposition in the brain: summary of evidence and recommendations. Lancet Neurol. **16**(7), 564–570 (2017). https://doi.org/10.1016/S1474-4422(17)30158-8
2. Wang, Y., Wu, W., Yang, Y., et al.: Deep learning-based 3D MRI contrast-enhanced synthesis from a 2D noncontrast T2Flair sequence. Med. Phys. **49**(7), 4478–4493 (2022). https://doi.org/10.1002/mp.15636
3. Chartsias, A., Joyce, T., Giuffrida, M.V., et al.: Multimodal MR synthesis via modality-invariant latent representation. IEEE T Med Imaging **37**(3), 803–814 (2018). https://doi.org/10.1109/TMI.2017.2764326
4. Shen, L., Zhu, W., Wang, X., et al.: Multi-domain image completion for random missing input data. IEEE T Med Imaging **40**(4), 1113–1122 (2020). https://doi.org/10.1109/TMI.2020.3046444

5. Wang, X., Girshick, R., Gupta, A.: Non-local neural networks. In: Proceeding of the IEEE Conference on Computer Vision and Pattern Recognition, Salt Lake City, UT, USA, 2018, pp. 7794–7803 (2018)
6. Goodfellow, I.J., Pouget-Abadie, J., Mirza, M., et al.: Generative adversarial networks (2021). arXiv:1406.2661
7. Sharma, A., Hamarneh, G.: Missing MRI pulse sequence synthesis using multi-modal generative adversarial network. IEEE T Med. Imaging **39**(4), 1170–1183 (2020). https://doi.org/10.1109/TMI.2019.2945521
8. Dai, X., Yang, L., Yabo, F., et al.: Multimodal MRI synthesis using unified generative adversarial networks. Med. Phys. **47**(12), 6343–6354 (2020). https://doi.org/10.1002/mp.14539
9. Dosovitskiy, A., Beyer, L., Kolesnikov, A., et al.: An image is worth 16x16 words: transformers for image recognition at scale. ICLR (2021)
10. Liu, J., Pasumarthi, S., Duffy, B., et al.: One model to synthesize them all: multi-contrast multi-scale transformer for missing data imputation (2022). arXiv:2204.13738
11. Pan, K., Cheng, P., Huang, Z., et al.: Transformer-based T2-weighted MRI synthesis from T1-weighted images. In: 2022 44th Annual International Conference of the IEEE Engineering in Medicine & Biology Society (EMBC), Glasgow, Scotland, United Kingdom, 2022, pp 5062–5065 (2022)
12. Zhang, X., Xinzi, H., Jia, G. et al.: PTNet: a high-resolution infant MRI synthesizer based on transformer (2021) arXiv:2105.13993
13. Yan, S., Wang, C., Chen, W., et al.: Swin transformer-based GAN for multi-modal medical image translation. Front. Oncol. **12**, 942511 (2022)
14. Park, N., Kim, S.: How do vision transformers work? ICLR (2022)
15. Dalmaz, O., Yurt, M., Cukur, T.: ResViT: residual vision transformers for multi-modal medical image synthesis. IEEE T. Med. Imaging **41**(10), 2598–2614 (2022). https://doi.org/10.1109/TMI.2022.3167808
16. Si, C., Yu, W., Zhou, P., et al.: Inception transformer (2022). arXiv:2205.12956
17. Howard, A.G., Zhu, M., Chen, B., et al.: MobileNets: efficient convolutional neural networks for mobile vision applications (2017). arXiv:1704.04861
18. Liu, Z., Lin, Y., Cao, Y., et al.: Swin transformer: hierarchical vision transformer using shifted windows. In: IEEE Conference on Computer Vision and Pattern Recognition (CVPR), pp. 10012–10022 (2021)
19. Wang, T.C., Liu, M.Y., Zhu, J.Y., et al.: High-resolution image synthesis and semantic manipulation with conditional GANs. In: IEEE Conference on Computer Vision and Pattern Recognition (CVPR), pp. 8798–8807 (2018)
20. Baid, U., Ghodasara, S., Mohan, S., et al.: The RSNA-ASNR-MICCAI BraTS 2021 benchmark on brain tumor segmentation and radiogenomic classification (2021). arXiv:2107.02314

# Light-Sheet Laser Speckle Imaging for 3D Vascular Visualization

Kai Long[1], Keertana Vinod Ram[2], Shuhao Shen[3], E. Du[4], Ziheng Ren[5], Zhiyuan Gong[5], and Nanguang Chen[1,6](✉)

[1] Department of Biomedical Engineering, National University of Singapore, 4 Engineering Drive 3, Singapore S117583, Singapore
biecng@nus.edu.sg

[2] Institute of Bioengineering and Bioimaging, A*STAR, 31, Singapore S138669, Singapore

[3] Xidian University, Guangzhou Institute of Technology, Guangzhou 510555, China

[4] School of Microelectronics, Shenzhen Institute of Information Technology, Shenzhen 518172, China

[5] Department of Biological Sciences, National University of Singapore, 14 Science Drive 4, Singapore S117543, Singapore

[6] NUS (Suzhou) Research Institute, No. 377 Linquan Street, Suzhou Industrial Park, Suzhou, Jiangsu, China

**Abstract.** Laser speckle imaging (LSI) takes advantage of wide-field, non-invasive, label-free in blood flow imaging with high spatiotemporal resolution. The traditional laser speckle imaging is a 2D vasculature mapping method, while the vasculature virtually presents a spatial distribution *in vivo*. To bridge the gap of conventional laser speckle imaging in vascular structure, light-sheet laser speckle imaging (LSH-LSI) is proposed due to its inherent optical sectioning capability. In this research, two label-free imaging methods are implemented where both laser speckle images and bright-field transmitted images are collected by our optical system. Laser speckle images are processed by contrast algorithm, and the red cells in transmission images are traced by particle imaging velocimetry (PIV). The pretty intricate three-dimensional vasculature in the zebrafish head and heart region was simultaneously imaged for making cross-validation by LSI and PIV. The experimental results show that the vasculature in 15 layers presents both difference and continuity. The difference demonstrates that LSH-LSI definitely has optical sectioning capability among multilayers, and the continuity suggests that superposition between different layers enables 3D vascular visualization. The axial projection is acquired by aligning the LSH-LSI vasculatures in all layers, which is consistent with the transmission PIV mapping. The primary advantage of LSH-LSI is that it has better spatial resolution than PIV. LSH-LSI has great potential to enable 3D vasculature reconstruction.

**Keywords:** Laser speckle · 3D · Vasculature · Light sheet


G. Wang et al. (Eds.): APCMBE 2023, IFMBE Proceedings 103, pp. 245–253, 2024.
https://doi.org/10.1007/978-3-031-51455-5_27

# 1 Introduction

By catching the fluctuant pattern of scattering light, laser speckle imaging (LSI) is an emerging optical technology in detecting blood flow with label-free, non-destructive, full-filed, and cost-effective [1]. It has been widely used in the diagnosis and treatment of clinical diseases and basic scientific research of intracranial nerves [2]. LSI can monitor the changes in blood flow velocity through the statistical properties of the dynamic speckle pattern in real time [3]. There is no need for an additional injection of markers, so it is convenient and less harmful to the human body [4].

In raw data collection, the traditional wide-field illumination method has been used to evaluate the distribution of blood vessels and flow velocity in the mouse brain where illumination and acquisition are on the same side of the sample, and the objective lens collects reflected scattering [5]. For thick tissue, the traditional optical implementation has limitations in imaging penetration depth and signal-to-background ratio (SBR). To detect deep and small blood vessels, the line scan acquisition method is proposed. The principle is the same as confocal microscopy. Different from the traditional one, only the signal on the focal plane is collected, while the noise out of the focal plane is blocked [6–9]. However, each frame of the image is scanned line by line in the confocal acquisition method, so it has a lower temporal resolution even though it has a higher spatial resolution. To have a better SBR for the deep layer, a transmissive-detected laser speckle is proposed where the thick sample is illuminated at the bottom of the sample while the images are collected at the top of the sample [10–12]. While this method applies only to specific samples, such as the ear, hindlimb, and paw. While for the mouse brain vessels, only the top skull of the brain can be removed, so the sample can only be illuminated and collected on the top.

In laser speckle image analysis, models and algorithms are important factors in determining vascular morphology. Laser speckle contrast imaging (LSCI) [13], laser speckle auto-correlation imaging (LSAI) [14], and optical speckle image velocimetry (OSIV) [15] are the main laser speckle processing methods. Traditional laser speckle imaging methods are difficult to achieve a balance between data acquisition efficiency, spatiotemporal resolution and optical sectioning capabilities. LSI is very susceptible to noise, complex biological organization, and multiple scattering. At present, LSI can only quantify the surface movement of the sample. And for the thick sample, it still cannot quantify the velocity in the 3D model. What's more, traditional methods can only provide limited imaging depth.

In this paper, a novel light-sheet laser speckle imaging method is reported which can be used to visualize the three-dimensional blood flow distribution due to its instinctive optical sectioning capability. This method overcomes the poor visibility of the 3D vasculature in traditional laser speckle imaging methods.

# 2 Material and Method

## 2.1 Setup

As shown in Fig. 1a, the light-sheet laser speckle imaging system mainly included the illumination part below the dashed arrow line and the detection part above the dashed arrow line.

In the illumination light path, a 640nm coherent laser diode was collimated, and expanded by the beam expander. Then a cylindrical lens with a focal length of 50mm compressed the light beam to form a thin light sheet. At last, the sample was illuminated by the light sheet when the beam was focused by the objective lens (4 ×, NA0.1, Leica). In order to make a comparison with the laser speckle result, an LED light source with a central wavelength of 520nm was used for synchronous bright-field imaging.

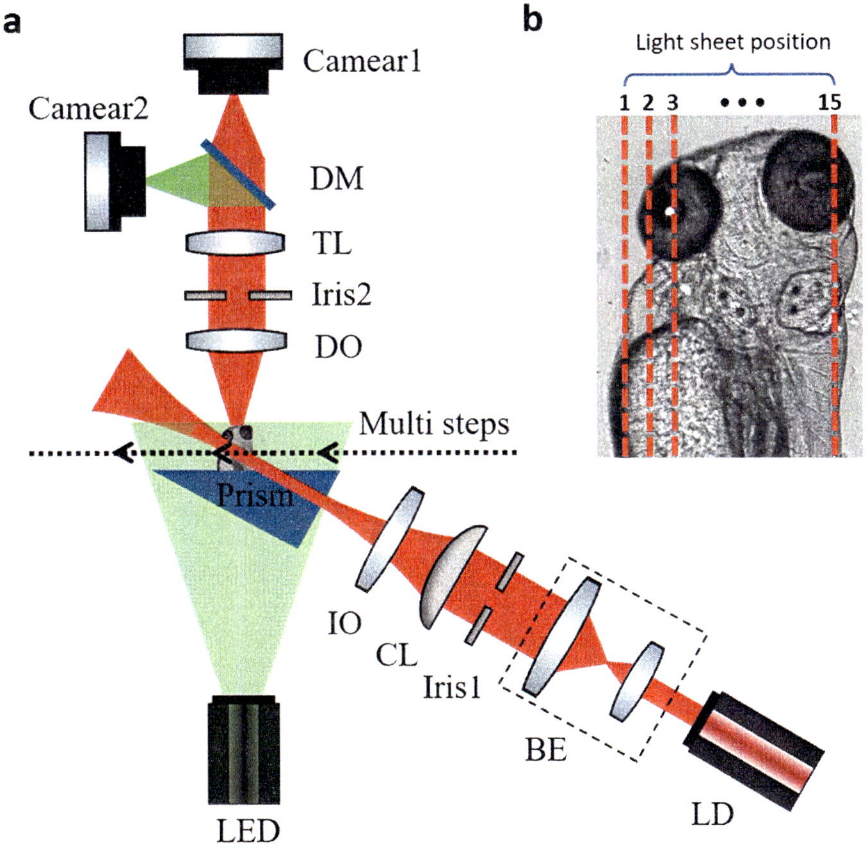


**Fig. 1.** Light-sheet laser speckle imaging configuration illustration. **a** The sample is illuminated by laser and LED below the sample stage. The laser speckle images and transmission images are detected above the sample stage. TL, tube lens; DM, dichroic mirror; DO, detection objective lens; IO, illumination objective lens; CL, cylindrical lens; BE, beam expander; LD, laser diode. **b** The shifted sample was illuminated by the fixed light sheet.

In the detection beam, both the laser speckle images and bright field images were acquired by the same detection objective lens (10 ×, NA0.25, Olympus) and tube lens (focal length: 100mm). Finally, the signal mixed with speckle and transmission images were separated by the dichroic mirror (DMLP605R, Thorlabs) and projected to the sCOMS (pco.dimax cs1, Excelitas Technologies® Corp, 3,086 fps at full-frame of 1296 × 1024 pixels) and CMOS (UI-3060CP-M-GL Rev.2, IDS, 166 fps at full-frame of 1936 × 1216 pixels).

The sample was fixed on the sample stage (not shown in Fig. 1) and the position of the sample can be transferred by an actuator (DMX3104SH-01, NTN) along the dashed arrow line for acquiring multi-layers of laser speckle images. The actuator was controlled by a single-channel data acquisition (DAQ) device (USB6008, National Instruments). The two cameras were synchronized by a dual-channel DAQ device (PCI6115, National Instruments).

### 2.2 Method

Raw laser speckle image stack with a 2-s duration was analyzed by the temporal LSCI method. When the raw speckle images are acquired with an ultra-high frame rate, and ultra-low exposure time, the instantaneous speckle intensity will be recorded. The faster the red blood cell moves, the faster the intensity value of the speckle changes. To quantify the degree of change, the K value is calculated,

$$K = \frac{\sigma}{I} \tag{1}$$

where $\sigma$ is the standard deviation of the pixel intensity values, and $I$ is the mean intensity in raw speckle images. The contrast value is calculated pixel by pixel in the same position of all frames. Then, combine all pixels to get a whole contrast image.

The transmission images are processed by the PIVlab for PIV results [16]. Firstly, the transmission image stack is imported into the tool. Secondly, we chose an ensemble algorithm, and the interrogation area is 8 pixels × 8 pixels with a step size of 4 pixels. Thirdly, calibration needs to be done after finishing the calculation. Then, we plot the blood vessel distribution in the full field of view.

### 2.3 Sample Preparation

The zebrafish is an ideal small animal model for imaging blood flow due to its innate transparency in the larval stage. In our experiment, the zebrafish embryos were cultivated in the incubator at 28 °C after fertilization. Before fixing the fish with 3.5% methylcellulose, zebrafish need to be anesthetized with 0.02% Tricaine. The sample is fixed in the petri dish where the bottom is the thin glass slide. All the experiments complied with the Institutional Animal Care and Use Committee (IACUC) of the National University of Singapore.

## 3 Result

### 3.1 Characteristics of Slanted Light-Sheet Laser Speckle System

In the traditional light-sheet fluorescence microscope, the detection light beam is orthogonal to the illumination plane (illumination beam). According to Mie Scattering theory, forward scattering has higher signal intensity than backscattering. In our laser speckle optical implementation, the angle between these two optical beams was maintained slanted at 120°. The effective thickness (t) and length (l) of the light sheet can be calculated by

$$t = \frac{2\lambda}{\pi * \mathrm{NA}} \tag{2}$$

$$l = \frac{t}{\mathrm{NA}} \tag{3}$$

where $\lambda$ is the illumination wavelength, and the numerical aperture (NA) of the illumination objective lens is related to the illumination beam size, which can be adjusted to match the thickness of the sample by the iris1 between CL and BE (Fig. 1a). A prism was fixed on the sample bottom plane for preventing the diffraction and deformation of the illumination beam where the beam axis was perpendicular to the incident plane of the prism. The iris2 in the detection beam was placed between the detection objective lens and the tube lens for adjusting the depth of field (DOF) of the detection objective lens due to the oblique light sheet [16].

### 3.2 Vascular Morphology in Different Layers

speckle imaging has optical sectioning capability in vascular morphology, the head and heart region of a 4-dpf zebrafish larva was scanned. Figure 1 shows the LSH-LSI scanning process, in which the zebrafish laid lateral position on the sample stage. The head-tail central axis of the larva and the shift direction (dashed arrow line) were kept orthogonal. The sample stage was shifted from right to left with a step size of 50 $\mu m$. Consequently, the sample was scanned from left to right on the contrary (Fig. 1b). Displayed the locations of the light sheet on the zebrafish larva bright field image. In each step, the raw speckle images were collected at 1500 frames per second (fps) and the duration was 2 s (3000 frames total in each step). The field of view of the image was 645μm × 1165 μm (264 x 476 pixels each frame). For acquiring morphological information on the head and heart region vasculature, the 3000 frames of each step were simply processed by calculating the contrast value K in Method part [9].

Vascular structures in 15 layers are displayed in Fig. 2. We found that the heart of the zebrafish larva was mainly in #1 to #5. The aorta and main vein mainly appeared in #6 to #10, and the dorsal blood vessels were distributed at #11 to #15. Light-sheet laser speckle imaging can detect not only the structure of the heart region but also the capillaries of the brain and eye regions. The distinction of the mapping between different layers reveals that our proposed LSH-LSI has excellent optical sectioning capability in imaging zebrafish larvae vasculature.

### 3.3 Comparison of LSH-LSI and PIV

To account for 3D vascular visibility with laser speckle imaging, transmission images were processed by PIV to enable comparison. As shown in Fig. 3a, the transmission images were collected at 200fps over 2 s, which is synchronized with the acquisition of raw laser speckle images. When these 400 transmission images were processed simply

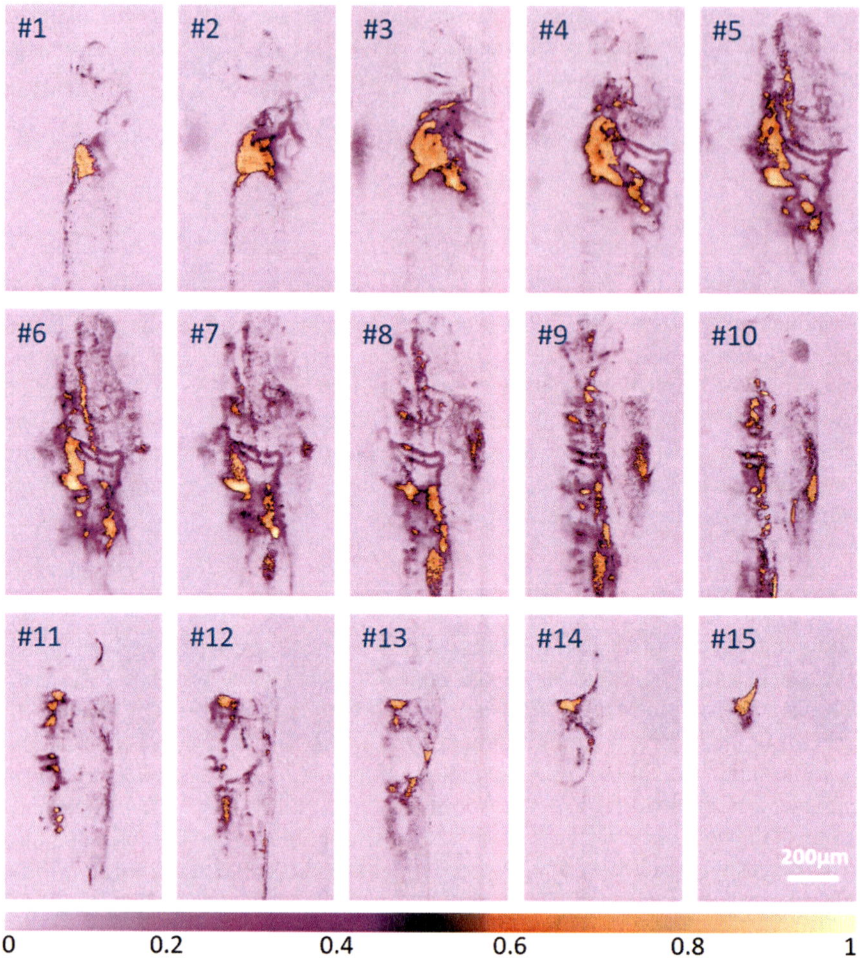


**Fig. 2.** Vascular structure in 15 layers corresponding to the positions of the light sheet in Fig. 1b. Scalar bar: 200 μm

by calculating the standard deviation of each pixel, the morphology of vasculature in the head and trunk region was displayed (Fig. 3b). The transmission stack was also processed by PIV, and the structure of the blood flow can also be seen, such as atrium (A), ventricle (V), bulbous arteriosus (BA), first branchial arch (AA3), second branchial arch (AA4), third branchial arch (AA5), fourth branchial arch (AA6), posterior cardinal vein (PCV), dorsal aorta (DA), Dorsal longitudinal vein (DLV), and so on, as shown in Fig. 3c.

For light-sheet laser speckle imaging, the morphological maps in 15 layers were projected into one complete 2D image, as shown in Fig. 3d. In addition to the vessels marked in Fig. 3c, prosencephalic artery (PrA), optic vein (OV), and posterior cerebral vein (PCeV) can also be visualized. When Fig. 3c and d were compared, we found that

LSH-LSI had better visualization than the transmission PIV imaging method, especially in the eye region, which resulted from LSH-LSI having an excellent optical sectioning capability and high spatial resolution. The 15 aligned 2D images can be used to render the 3D vasculature where the distance between two adjacent 2D images is 25 μm.

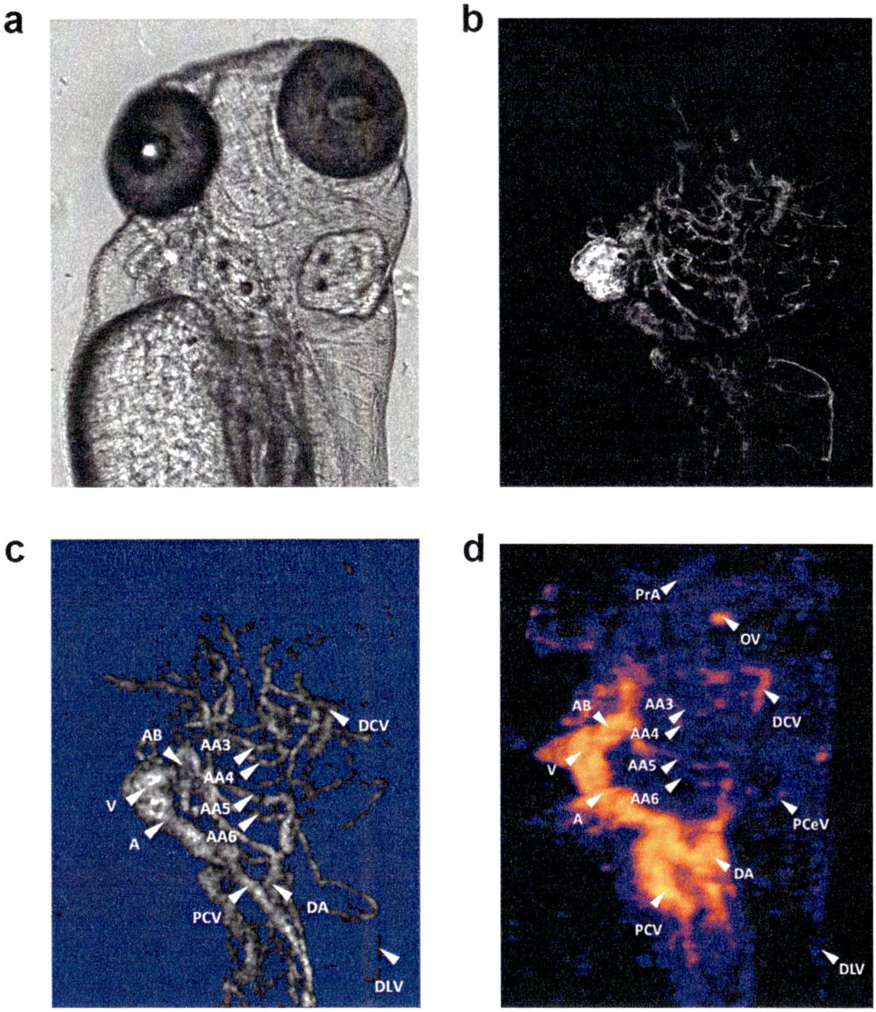


**Fig. 3.** Axial projection of zebrafish larva vasculature. **a** Transmission image. **b** The standard deviation of transmission stack. **c** Transmission PIV. **d** LSH-LSI axial projection.

## 4 Discussion

Compared with the traditional surface illumination laser speckle imaging, light-sheet illumination has inherently excellent optical sectioning performance, which provides critical support for the reconstruction of the 3D vasculature. In our experiment, the sample was scanned only by 15 steps, which resulted in a much lower axial resolution than lateral resolution.

The image segmentation and fitting algorithm between adjacent layers should be optimized so that the 3D rendering is smoother in the axial direction. For the capillary vessels in the eye region, a thinner light sheet can be achieved at the expense of reducing the effective length of the light sheet. Then much more layers can be acquired with a smaller scanning step size to improve the axial resolution. In addition, the synchronized transmission image can be fused with the speckle image, which helps to more accurately align the multi-layer 2D speckle images and contributes to 3D reconstruction furtherly.

## 5 Conclusion

In conclusion, we have developed an emerging light-sheet laser speckle imaging system that has excellent optical sectioning ability. The sample can be scanned by the light sheet for acquiring multilayers. The comparison between the PIV analysis and LSH-LSI axial projection demonstrates that LSH-LSI has a better lateral resolution. Better axial resolution can be achieved if the zebrafish head region could be scanned by a thinner light sheet and smaller step size, which enables the LSH-LSI to have great potential for 3D vasculature reconstruction.

**Acknowledgment.** Thanks for the Ministry of Education—Singapore (MOE2019-T2-2-094, MOE440 Tier I R-397-000-327-114) supporting this work.

## References

1. Jafari, C.Z., et al.: Effect of vascular structure on laser speckle contrast imaging. Biomed. Opt. Express **11**(10), 5826–5841 (2020)
2. Zhang, Y., et al.: Speckle illumination microscopy enables slide-free and non-destructive pathology of human lung adenocarcinoma. bioRxiv (2021). 10.11.464016
3. Bender, N., et al.: Customizing speckle intensity statistics. Optica **5**(5), 595–600 (2018)
4. Golberg, M., et al.: Assessment of tissue perfusion in the lower limbs using laser speckle analysis. In: Dynamics and Fluctuations in Biomedical Photonics XVIII. 2021. SPIE
5. Postnov, D.D., et al.: Dynamic light scattering imaging. Sci. Adv. **6**(45), eabc4628 (2020)
6. Du, E., et al.: Depth-dependent microscopic flow imaging with line scan laser speckle acquisition and analysis. In: Optics in Health Care and Biomedical Optics XI. 2021. SPIE
7. Du, E., et al.: Multifunctional laser speckle imaging. Biomed. Opt. Express **11**(4), 2007–2016 (2020)
8. Du, E., et al.: Line scan spatial speckle contrast imaging and its application in blood flow imaging. Appl. Sci. **11**(22), 10969 (2021)
9. Du, E., et al.: Confocal laser speckle autocorrelation imaging of dynamic flow in microvasculature. Opto-Electron. Adv. **5**(2), 210045–1–210045–11 (2022)

10. Li, D.-Y., et al.: Transmissive-detected laser speckle contrast imaging for blood flow monitoring in thick tissue: from Monte Carlo simulation to experimental demonstration. Light.: Sci. Appl. **10**(1), 241 (2021)
11. Dunn, J., et al.: A transmissive laser speckle imaging technique for measuring deep tissue blood flow: an example application in finger joints. Lasers Surg. Med. **43**(1), 21–28 (2011)
12. Meisner, J.K., et al.: Trans-illuminated laser speckle imaging of collateral artery blood flow in ischemic mouse hindlimb. J. Biomed. Opt. **18**(9), 096011 (2013)
13. Boas, D.A., Dunn, A.K.: Laser speckle contrast imaging in biomedical optics. J. Biomed. Opt. **15**(1), 011109–12 (2010)
14. Hou, J., et al.: Laser speckle correlation imaging with optical clearance for blood flows. In: Optics in Health Care and Biomedical Optics IX. 2019. SPIE
15. Qureshi, M.M., et al.: Quantitative blood flow estimation in vivo by optical speckle image velocimetry. Optica **8**(8), 1092–1101 (2021)
16. Long, K., et al.: Light-Sheet Laser Speckle Imaging (2022)

# A Framework for Diagnosis of Major Depressive Disorder

Jinyuan Wang[1], Cyrus Su Hui Ho[2,3], Roger Chun-Man Ho[2,3,4], Zhifei Li[1,4], and Nanguang Chen[1,5](✉)

[1] Department of Biomedical Engineering, National University of Singapore, Singapore, Singapore
biecng@nus.edu.sg
[2] Department of Psychological Medicine, Yong Loo Lin School of Medicine, National University of Singapore, Singapore, Singapore
[3] Department of Psychological Medicine, National University Hospital, Singapore, Singapore
[4] Institute of Health Innovation and Technology (iHealthtech), National University of Singapore, Singapore, Singapore
[5] NUS (Suzhou) Research Institute, Suzhou, China

**Abstract.** Early detection of Major Depressive Disorder (MDD) remains a significant challenge in the field of mental health. This work proposed an end-to-end deep learning framework designed to extract features from 52 channels of functional near-infrared spectroscopy (fNIRS) and aid in the diagnosis of MDD. We began by investigating the performance of multiple deep learning models as the core of our framework. Next, we implemented our novel deep learning framework, which employs an optimized model for MDD classification. We compared the performance of deep learning models both with and without our framework. In addition, we leveraged a traditional machine learning model, Support Vector Machine (SVM), to analyze single fNIRS channels to gain a deeper understanding of the impact areas of MDD. Our proposed framework, with a convolutional neural network (CNN) as the core model, achieved a highest classification rate of 82.4% on the test set of a large dataset of 374 subjects (including 181 MDD subjects and 193 healthy controls). Moreover, our framework improved the performance of deep learning models by 3.7%. Furthermore, the results from our classification of single channels revealed the crucial role of the dorsolateral prefrontal cortex and primary somatosensory cortex in MDD identification. Our study suggests that this framework may provide a promising methodology to facilitate the diagnosis of MDD. With the potential to help detect MDD at an earlier stage, the implementation of deep learning approaches in clinical practice could prove invaluable for the treatment of MDD.

**Keywords:** Major depressive disorder · Deep learning · Functional near-infrared spectroscopy · Convolutional neural network


G. Wang et al. (Eds.): APCMBE 2023, IFMBE Proceedings 103, pp. 254–261, 2024.
https://doi.org/10.1007/978-3-031-51455-5_28

## 1 Introduction

With the growing prevalence in contemporary societies, Major Depressive Disorder (MDD) is a widespread mental disorder that leads to significant morbidity, mortality, cost, and an elevated risk of suicide. MDD is typified by anhedonia, depressed mood, reduced interest, diminished energy, memory difficulties, feelings of worthlessness and guilt, impaired cognitive function, and vegetative symptoms such as disturbed sleep or appetite [1]. Depression may lead to the onset of psychotic symptoms, suicidal thoughts, and an increased risk of unnatural death [2]. According to a large-scale survey of one billion people, 5% of adults experience depression, causing MDD to emerge as a primary cause of disability and a significant contributor to the global burden of disease [3]. However, no established mechanism could fully account for all aspects of the disease.

Developing an objective methodology for the accurate diagnosis of the initial stage of MDD is crucial for clinicians to intervene more promptly, thus eliminating the bias of self-reporting of patients that is based on clinical interviews. Recently, neuroimaging approaches are being widely applied in the research of brain illness by providing biomarkers to distinguish the subtle differences of patients and healthy subjects. Functional near-infrared spectroscopy (fNIRS), as a non-invasive neuroimaging modality, is increasingly adopted in psychiatry for its ability to discriminate psychiatric disorders [4, 5]. Compared to other modalities, fNIRS has highlighted the neurophysiological abnormalities of MDD patients [6], providing hemodynamic changes in cerebral activity [7].

There is existing evidence that the abnormal function of frontal and temporal lobes was found in subjects with MDD during the paradigm of verbal fluency tests (VFT) [8]. The response of hemoglobin signals in MDD patients is weaker than in healthy subjects because of the decreased brain activity. Currently, more and more machine learning methods are being applied in the field of psychiatric illness for their ability to provide individual level analysis, in comparison to the traditional approach that utilized discriminant analysis [9]. Deep learning nowadays has been gaining popularity for its applications in various kinds of fields. Based on raw data, manual features, as well as channel correlations, Wang et al. [10] applied the Alex model to achieve an accuracy rate of 90% in depression detection with a dataset of 79 patients with depression and 17 healthy subjects using fNIRS. Besides, using an electroencephalography (EEG) signal, Uyulan et al. [11] employed a MobileNet architecture in MDD classification, which generated 92.66% classification accuracy within 92 data set. Although deep learning architecture has achieved success in MDD prediction, current research suffers from a limited amount of subjects, less than a hundred participants, which may lead to the issue of overfitting. Therefore, it is significantly necessary to analyze the feasibility of deep learning architecture based on a large dataset of depression subjects.

In this study, we aimed to investigate the feasibility of deep learning techniques in diagnosing MDD patients and the performance of a novel framework for deep learning models.

## 2 Materials and Methods

### 2.1 Participants

This study included 181 patients with MDD and 193 matched healthy controls (HCs). All individuals involved satisfied the criteria of being between 21 and 65 years old, English-speaking, and right-handed. Patients were recruited from the outpatient psychiatric clinic, diagnosed by a psychiatrist according to the fifth edition of the Diagnostic and Statistical Manual of Mental Disorders (DSM-5) [12] at the National University Hospital, Singapore. Age- and gender-matched HCs were recruited from the community and evaluated by a psychiatrist to certify that they were healthy. Participants were excluded if they had any neurological disorders, a history of head injury, unstable medical conditions, intellectual disability, or substance addiction. Each individual underwent an assessment of their depressive symptoms on the participation day using the 17-item Hamilton Rating Scale for Depression (HAM-D) and Global Assessment of Functioning (GAF), while the HCs had a HAM-D score of 8 or lower. All participants were fully informed of the study details and gave written informed consent. This study was conducted according to the Declaration of Helsinki and the ethical principles in the Belmont Report. It was approved by the Domain Specific Review Board of the National Healthcare Group, Singapore (protocol number 2017/00509).

### 2.2 Data Acquisition and Preprocessing

The NIRS signals were detected by a 52-channel system (ETG-4000; Hitachi Medical Co., Tokyo, Japan) during the verbal fluency task (VFT), which was adopted in previous studies to activate functional abnormalities [8, 13, 14]. The details of the measurement procedure were described in our earlier research [8, 14]. The hemoglobin concentration changes of oxy-hemoglobin (HbO) and deoxy-hemoglobin (HbR) were converted from NIRS signals according to the modified Beer-Lambert law [15].

### 2.3 Deep Learning Framework

In this study, we developed a deep learning framework to fully evaluate the discriminative signals of a single fNIRS channel as the neuroimaging biomarkers of MDD. This framework, shown in Fig. 1, utilized an individual core model to discriminate an fNIRS channel. The input of the deep learning model was the hemoglobin signals. Different deep learning models were analyzed as the core model, the outputs of which were concatenated and fed to a fully connected layer with 32 units and a softmax layer with two units. Adam optimization was utilized during training with a learning rate and batch size of 0.001 and 256.

In the experiment, 80% of subjects were used as the training set, while the other 20% of the dataset was adopted as the test set randomly. The hemoglobin data of all subjects were normalized using Z-normalization method. This study compared the Convolutional Neural Network (CNN) consisting of three one-dimensional convolutional layers, with convolution lengths and filter amounts of 8, 3, 3 and 32, 32, 1 separately; Fully Convolutional Neural Network (FCN) [16], the convolution layer of which was followed by a

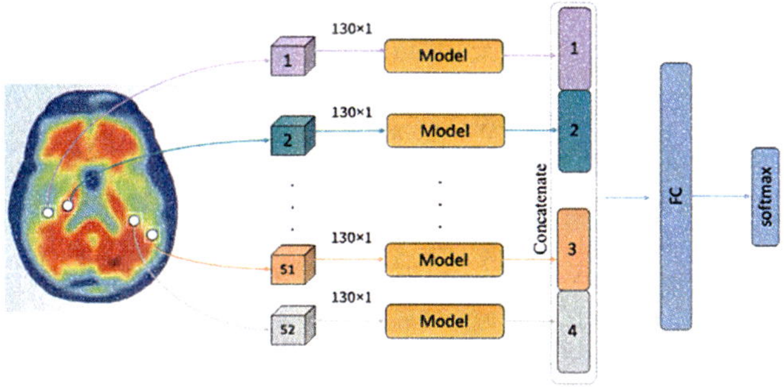


**Fig. 1.** Deep learning framework for 52 fNIRS channels

batch process and ReLU activation; Long Short-term Memory (LSTM) network with 64 units and dropout rate of 0.5; Attention Long Short-term Memory (ALSTM); Residual Neural Network (ResNet) [16] with convolution lengths and filter amounts of 8, 5, 3 and 64, 128, 128; Inception neural network with 6 Inception modules.

To take full advantage of different hemoglobin data, we concatenated the HbO, HbR, and HbT signal in the time domain and derived HbO+HbR, which is the concatenation of HbO and HbR along the time domain. Following the same procedure, HbO+HbT, HbR+HbT, as well as HbO+HbR+HbT can be derived.

Lastly, we adopted SVM with different kernel functions such as linear kernel, polynomial kernel, and Gaussian kernel to predict patients with MDD, in order to learn the discriminating ability of each channel when diagnosing MDD.

## 3 Results

### 3.1 Classification Accuracies of the Deep Learning Framework

The classification results of the framework were displayed in Table 1. In the study, several deep learning models were tested as the core of the framework. The average accuracy rates for the input of HbO, HbR, and HbT were 75.3%, 70.7%, and 71.6% respectively. These rates were higher than the accuracy rates for concatenated hemoglobin data HbO+HbT, HbO+HbR, HbR+HbT, and HbO+HbR+HbT, which resulted in 72.6%, 70.1%, 74.3%, and 69.5%. The results indicated that HbO was the best hemoglobin input data for diagnosing MDD using deep learning models.

In our work, we studied a variety of deep learning networks, including bi-kernel neural networks such as ALSTM+CNN, ALSTM+ResNet, ALSTM+Inception, and ALSTM+FCN, the classification accuracies of which were 74.7%, 73.4%, 72.6%, and 71.0% individually, slightly superior to the single-kernel neural networks CNN, LSTM, ALSTM, ResNet, FCN, and Inception, with the classification accuracies of 74.3%, 73.2%, 71.6%, 71.0%, 69.7%, and 68.5%. Bi-kernel networks exhibited an outstanding performance of generalization for the proposed network.

At last, we utilized CNN as the core of the framework, achieving the highest classification accuracy of 82.4% with the input hemoglobin data of HbO.

### 3.2 The Comparison of Framework-Based and Non-framework Based Deep Learning Architecture

To investigate the performance of the framework, we compared the classification accuracy of non-framework-based and framework-based deep learning models in predicting MDD, the average classification accuracies of which were 68.3 and 72.0%, respectively, which exhibited that the framework improved 3.7% ($p < 0.001$) classification accuracy rate of the deep learning models, shown in Fig. 2.

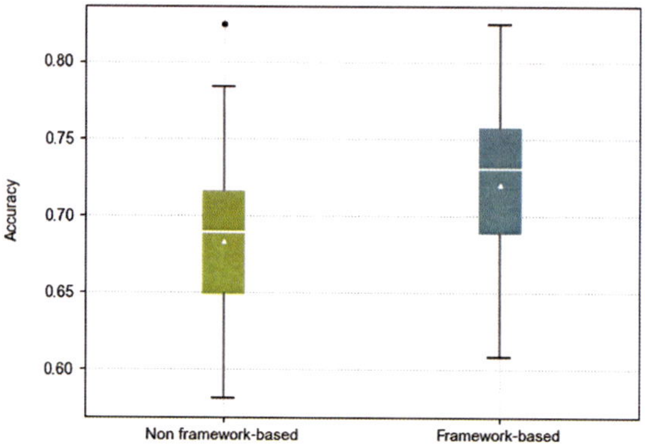


**Fig. 2.** Comparison of framework-based and non-framework-based models.

### 3.3 Single Channel Classification

From Fig. 3, the classification accuracy of individual channels differed from each other. Among the channels, channel 40 achieved the highest classification accuracy rate of 75.1%, located in primary somatosensory cortex. Besides, the channels of 4, 5, 12, 19, 22, 40, 45, 47, and 48 used to differentiate the patients with MDD achieved the classification accuracy over 70%. Channels 4 and 49 had the second and third precise discriminating performance, located in the dorsolateral prefrontal cortex area and frontopolar area. However, the average classification accuracy of channel 23 was only 50%, unable to perform the diagnosis task of MDD, which indicated the inability of some fNIRS channels in discriminating the patients with MDD from HCs.

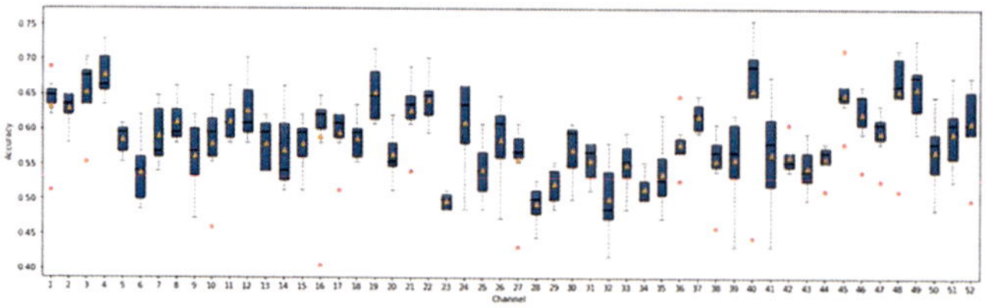

**Fig. 3.** Single channel classification accuracy of SVM

## 4 Discussion

The proposed deep learning framework with CNN as the core model and HbO as the input hemoglobin data reached the highest classification accuracy of 82.4%, which demonstrated a robust approach for differentiating the patients with MDD.

In the traditional deep learning model without the framework, the features of 52 channels were averaged as the input of the architecture, while the framework enabled the deep learning model to extract the features of each fNIRS channel, thus achieving outstanding performance and improving the classification accuracy by 3.7%. Besides, as shown in Fig. 3, there were some channels that may play a non-important role in discriminating the MDD patients due to the insufficient signals. The framework offered an approach to select and ignore the features of channel signals.

Through the single channel classification results, we found that the brain area of the dorsolateral prefrontal cortex was significantly sensitive in the discrimination of patients with MDD. These findings were consistent with the existing functional neuroimaging methods to study depression. The sensitive performance of dorsolateral prefrontal cortex demonstrated that VFT could activate working memory-related areas of brain, thus providing an objective biomarker to distinguish MDD.

Although the time domain concatenation methodology provided more features for the neural network in the prediction of MDD, it failed to achieve a better classification accuracy, which was beyond our expectations. The reason behind this may be the roughness of simple concatenation of two or three signals without a careful processing method, which led to the inability of discriminating the concatenated hemoglobin data.

The bi-kernel neural network as the core model proved to be helpful in improving the classification performance, owing to the network consisting of two deep learning neural networks. While one network, such as ALSTM, is appropriate in extracting long-term features, another network like Inception is skilled at deriving the short-term features.

## 5 Conclusion

In conclusion, our framework-based deep learning model using hemoglobin data demonstrated superior diagnostic accuracy in MDD compared to traditional models without the framework. It could potentially improve the accuracy of MDD classification, contributing to the application of deep learning in depression diagnosis based on fNIRS.

**Table 1.** Classification accuracy of different deep learning models and hemoglobin signals

| | CNN | FCN | Inception | LSTM | ResNet | ALSTM | ALSTM+CNN | ALSTM+FCN | ALSTM+ResNet | ALSTM+Inception | Average |
|---|---|---|---|---|---|---|---|---|---|---|---|
| HbO | 0.824 | 0.676 | 0.77 | 0.77 | 0.73 | 0.743 | 0.77 | 0.716 | 0.77 | 0.757 | 0.753 |
| HbR | 0.703 | 0.689 | 0.635 | 0.757 | 0.649 | 0.757 | 0.73 | 0.716 | 0.703 | 0.73 | 0.707 |
| HbT | 0.757 | 0.689 | 0.676 | 0.757 | 0.689 | 0.689 | 0.757 | 0.703 | 0.757 | 0.689 | 0.716 |
| HbO+HbT | 0.77 | 0.73 | 0.649 | 0.689 | 0.743 | 0.676 | 0.77 | 0.73 | 0.743 | 0.757 | 0.726 |
| HbOx+HbR | 0.716 | 0.716 | 0.689 | 0.689 | 0.743 | 0.676 | 0.716 | 0.676 | 0.662 | 0.73 | 0.701 |
| HbR+HbT | 0.743 | 0.73 | 0.77 | 0.784 | 0.716 | 0.73 | 0.743 | 0.77 | 0.77 | 0.676 | 0.743 |
| HbO+HbR+HbT | 0.689 | 0.649 | 0.608 | 0.676 | 0.703 | 0.743 | 0.743 | 0.662 | 0.73 | 0.743 | 0.695 |
| Average | 0.743 | 0.697 | 0.685 | 0.732 | 0.71 | 0.716 | 0.747 | 0.71 | 0.734 | 0.726 | |

**Acknowledgements.** This work was supported by the Ministry of Education—Singapore (MOE2019-T2-2-094, MOE440 Tier I R-397-000-327-114).

## References

1. Lim, G.Y., Tam, W.W., Lu, Y., Ho, C.S., Zhang, M.W., Ho, R.C.: Prevalence of depression in the community from 30 countries between 1994 and 2014. Sci. Rep. **8**(1), 2861 (2018)
2. Choo, C.C., Harris, K.M., Ho, R.C.: Prediction of lethality in suicide attempts: gender matters. OMEGA-J. Death Dying **80**(1), 87–103 (2019)
3. Lancet, T.: Ensuring care for people with depression. Lancet (London, England) **399**(10328), 885 (2022)
4. Fukuda, M.: Near-infrared spectroscopy in psychiatry. Brain nerve Shinkei kenkyu no shinpo **64**(2), 175–183 (2012)
5. Ho, C.S., Chan, Y.L., Tan, T.W., Tay, G.W., Tang, T.B.: Improving the diagnostic accuracy for major depressive disorder using machine learning algorithms integrating clinical and near-infrared spectroscopy data. J. Psychiatr. Res. **147**, 194–202 (2022)
6. Gao, S., Calhoun, V.D., Sui, J.: Machine learning in major depression: from classification to treatment outcome prediction. CNS Neurosci. Ther. **24**(11), 1037–1052 (2018)
7. Rupawala, M., Dehghani, H., Lucas, S. J., Tino, P., Cruse, D.: Shining a light on awareness: a review of functional near-infrared spectroscopy for prolonged disorders of consciousness. Front. Neurol. 350 (2018)
8. Husain, S.F., et al.: Validating a functional near-infrared spectroscopy diagnostic paradigm for major depressive disorder. Sci. Rep. **10**(1), 1–9 (2020)
9. Tak, S., Ye, J.C.: Statistical analysis of fNIRS data: a comprehensive review. Neuroimage **85**, 72–91 (2014)
10. Wang, R., Hao, Y., Yu, Q., Chen, M., Humar, I., Fortino, G.: Depression analysis and recognition based on functional near-infrared spectroscopy. IEEE J. Biomed. Health Inform. **25**(12), 4289–4299 (2021)
11. Uyulan, C., Ergüzel, T.T., Unubol, H., Cebi, M., Sayar, G.H., Nezhad Asad, M., Tarhan, N.: Major depressive disorder classification based on different convolutional neural network models: deep learning approach. Clin. EEG Neurosci. **52**(1), 38–51 (2021)
12. American Psychiatric Association: American psychiatric association: diagnostic and statistical manual of mental disorders, arlington (2013)
13. Zanelli, J., et al.: Specific and generalized neuropsychological deficits: a comparison of patients with various first-episode psychosis presentations. Am. J. Psychiatry **167**(1), 78–85 (2010)
14. Zhifei, L., et al.: Identifying neuroimaging biomarkers of major depressive disorder from cortical hemodynamic responses using machine learning approaches. EBioMedicine **79**, 104027 (2022)
15. Kocsis, L., Herman, P., Eke, A.: The modified beer-lambert law revisited. Phys. Med. Biol. **51**(5), N91 (2006)
16. Wang, Z., Yan, W., Oates, T.: Time series classification from scratch with deep neural networks: a strong baseline. In: 2017 International Joint Conference on Neural Networks (IJCNN), pp. 1578–1585. IEEE

# Neural Engineering

# Effect of Age-Related Hearing Loss on Mice Cochlear Structures Based on Optical Coherence Tomography

Shu Zheng[1,3], Yanru Bai[1,3], and Guangjian Ni[1,2,3](✉)

[1] Academy of Medical Engineering and Translational Medicine, Tianjin University, Tian Jin, China
niguangjian@tju.edu.cn
[2] Department of Biomedical Engineering, College of Precision Instruments and Optoelectronics 6 Engineering, Tianjin University, Tianjin, China
[3] Tianjin Key Laboratory of Brain Science and Neuroengineering, Tianjin, China

**Abstract.** With the increasing proportion of the elderly in the population, age-related hearing loss (ARHL) impacts the daily life of seniors and increases society's economic and medical burden. However, the change in the cochlear structures with age is still unknown. The emergency of Optical Coherence Tomography (OCT) makes it possible to observe the cochlea in vivo, which can provide high-resolution and high-imaging speed. In this article, we obtained the cochlear OCT image from mice of different ages, acquired the changes in the thickness of cochlear bone and modiolus, and analyzed the signal intensity of the round window and stria vascularis. We found that the thickness of the cochlear bone became thicker while the signal intensity became lower with the growth of age and the degeneration of hearing. These results not only prove the feasibility of OCT which can observe the structural changes of the cochlea but also indicate that age may affect the overall structure of the cochlea, especially stria vascularis, which may deepen our understanding of ARHL.

**Keywords:** Age-related hearing loss · Optical coherence tomography · Cochlear structure · In vivo imaging

## 1 Introduction

According to the《World Report on Hearing》published by World Health Organization, over 1.5 billion people suffer from varying degrees of hearing loss, which may reach 2.5 billion in 2050. Among this, more than 65% of adults above 60 are troubled by hearing loss [1]. Thus, age-related hearing loss (ARHL), also known as presbycusis, is caused by the accumulation of aging in the hearing system, which is affected by genetic predispositions, physiological stressors, and lifestyle behaviors. It is defined as progressive, bilateral, symmetrical sensorineural hearing loss and has become the main reason that adults older than 70 live with disability [2, 3]. Additionally, it will affect the patients' social communication and cognitive ability and increase the social burden [4, 5].


G. Wang et al. (Eds.): APCMBE 2023, IFMBE Proceedings 103, pp. 265–272, 2024.
https://doi.org/10.1007/978-3-031-51455-5_29

With the development of ARHL, the hearing threshold will gradually worsen, resulting in the degeneration of the cochlea and nervous system. However, it is still challenging to observe and quantify the structural changes of the cochlea *in vivo* at different ages. The emergence and evolution of Optical Coherence Tomography (OCT) technology make it possible to handle this problem.

OCT based on low-coherence interference is a novel imaging technology that can obtain a noninvasive three-dimensional image with high resolution and high speed [6]. The earliest use of OCT to observe the cochlea can be traced back to 2007, Steven L. Jacques et al. obtained the image of the Organ of Corti (Ooc) at the apex of the cochlea and successfully measured the vibration of BM at 14-kHz based on time-domain OCT [7]. In 2011, John S. Oghalai et al. proved that OCT could observe the soft tissue structures and anatomical changes of the cochlea during growth and development [8]. After that, more and more researchers take advantage of OCT to observe the auditory response of the cochlea [9–11]. However, the structural changes of the cochlea during ARHL are still unclear. The cochlear function of mice is similar to that of human beings, and C57BL/6N mice are born with genetic ARHL. In this article, we used OCT to obtain a cochlear image at the apex of mice with different ages *in vivo*, calculated and qualified the thickness of cochlear bone and modiolus, analyzed the signal intensity of round window (RM) and stria vascularis, hoping to enhance our comprehension of ARHL.

## 2 Materials and Methods

### 2.1 OCT System Description

The schematic of the swept-source OCT (SS-OCT) system is shown in Fig. 1. This system uses swept laser source (MEMS-VCSEL, Thorlabs, USA) with 1300 nm center wavelength and 100 nm bandwidth. The axial and transverse resolution was 9.8 $\mu m$ and 9.84 $\mu m$ in air, respectively. The sweep rate of this system is 200 kHz, and the three-dimensional image of 500 $\times$ 1000 $\times$ 1024 pixels can be obtained in five seconds. The maximum depth and width of this system are 5 mm and 3.8 mm, respectively. The average output power of the laser is 25 mw, while the power focused on the sample is 18 mw.

### 2.2 Animals

All experimental protocols were approved by the Institutional Animal Care and Use Committee of Tianjin University, Tian Jin, China. A total of ten C57BL/6N mice were used, and all of them were male. The age of five mice was 8 weeks (young group), and the others were 8 months (old group). All of them were fed routinely in low noisy environments.

### 2.3 Surgery Preparation

The mice were anesthetized with urethane first and positioned on a heating pad to maintain the temperature of 37 °C. . The additional overdose was supplemented every

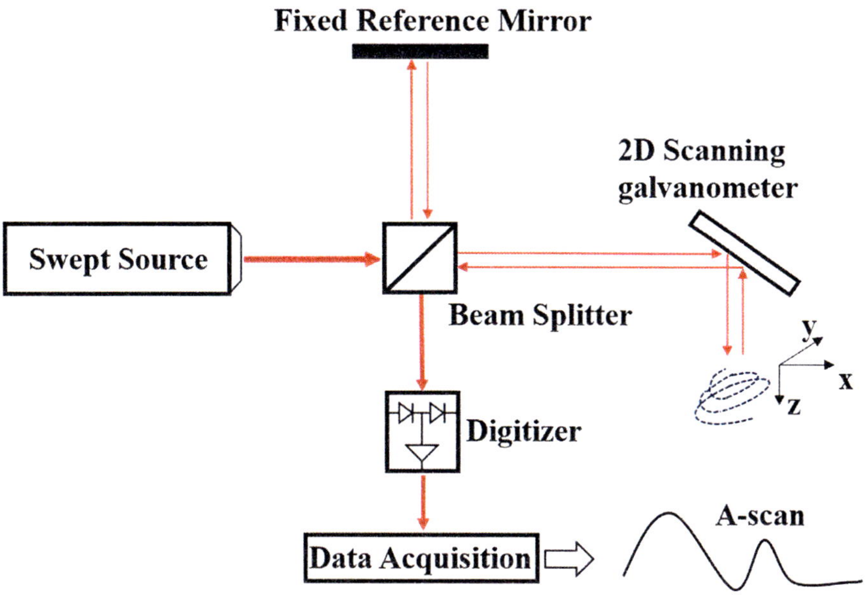


**Fig. 1.** The schematic of the swept-source OCT system.

half hour. The skins and muscles that covered the bulla were removed. Part of the masseter muscle was removed to create an ideal imaging angle, while the bleeding must be controlled strictly. Then the bulla was opened carefully, resulting in the exposure of the apex of the cochlea. The whole surgery was operated under the microscope (Stemi 508, Zeiss, Germany) and followed the article written by John S. Oghalai [12]. Finally, the mice were fixed in the hold header and placed on the platform below the sweep light source. The mice were killed after all experiments.

### 2.4 Image Analysis

The OCT image was analyzed using ImageJ and MATLAB. No adjustments were made. We measured the thickness of the modiolus, the bone in the apex of the cochlea, the average signal intensity of the round window, and stria vascularis.

### 2.5 Hearing Threshold

Auditory brain response (ABR) and distortion product otoacoustic emission (DPOAE) were used to evaluate the hearing level of mice. We applied click-stimulus to obtain the threshold of ABR while using tone stimulus ranging from 10 kHz to 20 kHz to measure DPOAE. All of the stimuli generated by BioSigRZ software (Tucker-Davis Technologies, Gainesville, FL) were swept from 90 to 10 dB SPL, and stepped in 5 dB when the intensity was below 60 dB SPL.

### 2.6 Statistical Analysis

Statistical analysis and data plotting was performed using GraphPad Prism (version 9.5.0, GraphPad Software Inc., La Jolla, CA). All data sets were tested by Student *t* test, and a $p < 0.05$ was considered statistically significant. The results were represented in mean ± standard error mean (SEM).

## 3 Results

### 3.1 Hearing Threshold

Compared with the young group, the ABR threshold of old mice apparently increased, as shown in Fig. 2a. Besides, the latency of ABR wave I of old mice under 60 dB SPL shown in Fig. 2b was prolonged significantly. Both threshold and latency had a statistical difference which proved the influence of age on hearing. The result of DPOAE is shown in Fig. 2c, which indicates that the threshold of DPOAE in the young group is better than in the old group under different frequencies. Furthermore, when the frequency exceeded 14 kHz, the difference between the two groups gradually became obvious with the increasing frequency. However, the threshold of DPOAE had no significant difference, which may be due to individual differences in hearing loss in older mice.

### 3.2 Cochlear Structure

Through SS-OCT system, we acquired the cochlea image of mice. A representative result of X-Z cross-section and A-line is shown in Fig. 3. In the cross-section, the different scales of the cochlea can be identified clearly, and there are visible correlations between the cross-section and reflectivity in the A-line. The marker we made was based on the previous plastic-embedded section and OCT image [13, 14].

- Thickness of bone

To analyze the effect of ARHL on cochlear structure, we first calculate the thickness of the cochlear bone and modiolus. The results indicated that the thickness of cochlear bone in old mice became thicker compared with young mice. The thickness is 111.58 ± 8.45 $\mu m$ in the young group and 97.98 ± 6.64 $\mu m$ in the old group, as shown in Fig. 4a. In addition, in Fig. 4b, the difference between the thickness of the modiolus was greater. The thickness of modiolus is 129.83 ± 13.11 $\mu m$ and 99.66 ± 8.77 $\mu m$, respectively. The thicker bone of the cochlea and modiolus probably demonstrated the degeneration of the cochlear structure with the growth of age and the occurrence of ARHL.

- Reflection intensity of soft tissue in the cochlea

Then we analyze the signal intensity of soft tissue in the cochlea. As shown in Fig. 3, the round window and stria vascularis can be identified clearly. Thus, we calculated the average intensity of these two parts. The results are expressed in Fig. 5. Compared with young mice, the average intensity of round window and stria vascularis from old mice both decreased.

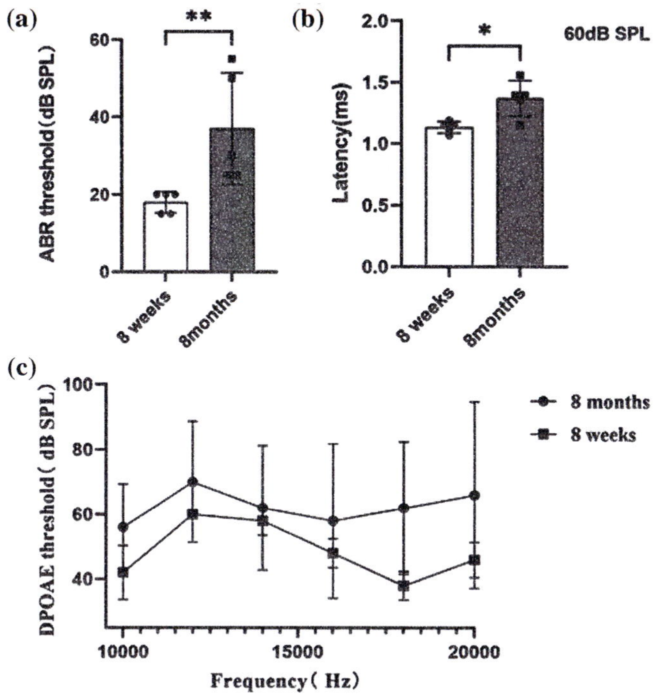


**Fig. 2.** ABR and DPOAE results of two groups (n = 5). **a** ABR threshold. **b** The latency of the ABR wave I is under 60 dB SPL. **c** DPOAE threshold at different frequencies. The results were expressed as mean ± SEM; n = 5 for each bar; * $P < 0.05$; ** $P < 0.01$.

## 4 Discussion

ARHL in older people is very common, however, our understanding of it is limited. C57BL/6N mice have the characteristics of ARHL. The related characteristics gradually appear after 16 weeks of born, and with increasing age, their ABR threshold gradually increases, and wave I latency is significantly prolonged, which has been reported many times [15]. In our study, we found the degeneration of cochlear bone. This degeneration not only involves the damage of outer hair cells and auditory nerve [16], which may make an impact on the whole cochlea. Apart from the auditory system, bone mass and strength decline due to age-related changes, such as oxidative stress, may also play a crucial role in this change [17]. Besides, previous studies show that the aged animals' cells become sparse, the vascular density in stria vascularis decreases, and the permeability of the blood–the labyrinth barrier increases [18, 19]. Based on the principle of the OCT system, the signal intensity reflects tissues' reflective properties, which depend on the composition and structure of tissues. Therefore, the reduced signal intensity can explain the sparsity of cells and blood vessels to a certain extent. Recently, many studies also have shown that oxidative stress, inflammation, and autophagy stress in the cochlea are the key mechanisms of ARHL [20, 21]. The research also stressed that the stria vascularis is an early site corresponding to the degeneration of the cochlea [22]. *In vivo*

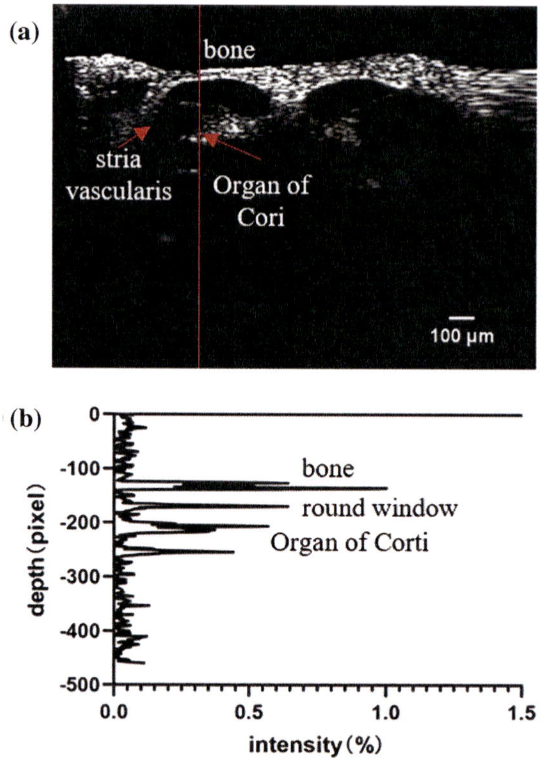


**Fig. 3.** **a** OCT image of 8 weeks mice. **b** The reflection intensity along the Z direction of the red line in **a**.

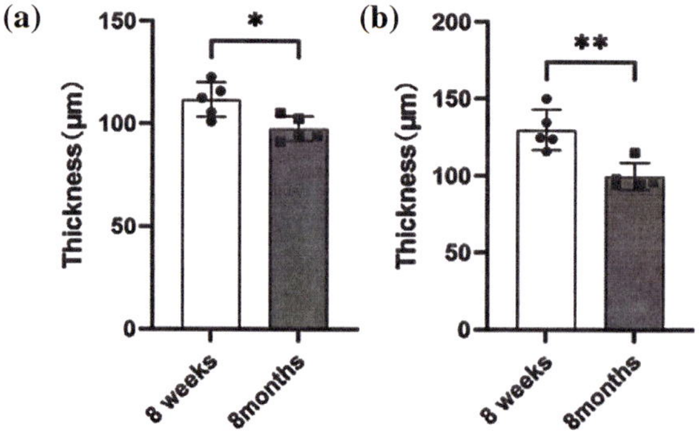


**Fig. 4.** The thickness of bone **a** and modiolus **b**.

imaging of stria vascularis is helpful for further comprehending the change progress of stria vascularis under different ages, thereby clarifying its mechanisms. Additionally, gender also affects the degree of ARHL, such as the high-frequency threshold shift is more evident in female mice [23].

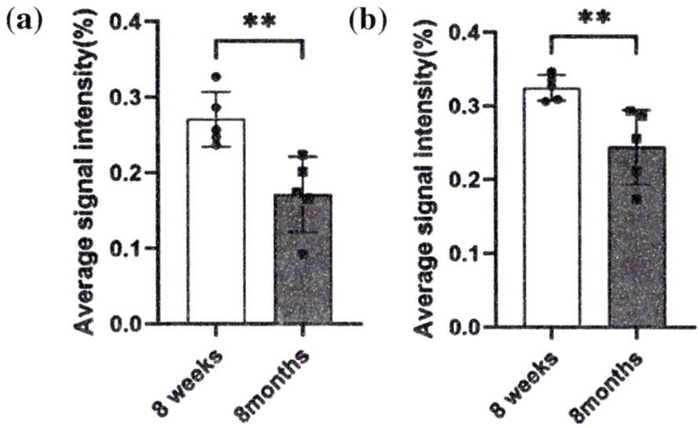


**Fig. 5.** The average signal intensity of RM (**a**) and stria vascularis (**b**).

Furthermore, the observation of cochlear structure was previously based on the technology of histological sections, which requires the animals to be killed before the operation. OCT avoids image artifacts caused by complicated histological progress and overcomes dehydration-induced shrinkage [8]. Angiography based on OCT may also create new vitality for the cochlea, which can evaluate blood vessel density and blood flow velocity. Moreover, the vibrometry with OCT can measure the vibration of the OoC, which may reveal the cochlear response mechanism with ARHL.

## 5 Conclusion

OCT can observe the cochlea structure of mice at different ages, which can provide sufficient resolution to quantitatively measure the soft tissue in the cochlea. Based on OCT, we observed the changes in the thickness of the cochlear bone and signal intensity of the round window and stria vascularis, which reveals the influence of ARHL on the cochlea and may provide guidance for exploring its underlying mechanisms.

**Acknowledgment.** This work was supported by grants from the Key Technologies Research and Development Program of China (No.2022YFF1202400) and the National Natural Science Foundation of China (No.81971698).

## References

1. W. H. Organization (2021) World report on hearing
2. Bowl, M.R., Dawson, S.J.: Age-related hearing loss. Cold Spring Harb. Perspect. Med. **9**(8), a033217 (2019). https://doi.org/10.1101/cshperspect.a033217
3. Carpena, N.T., Lee, M.Y.: Genetic hearing loss and gene therapy. Genomics Inform. **16**(4) 2018
4. Huddle, M.G., et al.: The economic impact of adult hearing loss: a systematic review. JAMA Otolaryngol. Neck Surg. **143**(10), 1040–1048 (2017). https://doi.org/10.1001/jamaoto.2017.1243

5. Thomson, R.S., Auduong, P., Miller, A.T., Gurgel, R.K.: Hearing loss as a risk factor for dementia: a systematic review. Laryngoscope Investig. Otolaryngol. **2**(2), 69–79 (2017)
6. Drexler, W.: Optical Coherence Tomography: Technology and Applications Conference on Lasers and Electro-Optics Europe and International Quantum Electronics Conference (2013)
7. Chen, F., Choudhury, N., Zheng, J., Matthews, S.K., Nuttall, A.L., Jacques, S.L.: In vivo imaging and low-coherence interferometry of organ of Corti vibration. J. Biomed. Opt. **12**(2), 021006 (2007). https://doi.org/10.1117/1.2717134
8. Gao, S.S., et al.: Quantitative imaging of cochlear soft tissues in wild-type and hearing-impaired transgenic mice by spectral domain optical coherence tomography. Opt. Express **19**(16), 15415–15428 (2011). https://doi.org/10.1364/OE.19.015415
9. Frost, B.L., Strimbu, C.E., Olson, E.S.: Using volumetric optical coherence tomography to achieve spatially resolved organ of Corti vibration measurements. J. Acoust. Soc. Am. **151**(2), 1115–1124 (2022). https://doi.org/10.1121/10.0009576
10. Cooper, N.P., Vavakou, A., van der Heijden, M.: Vibration hotspots reveal longitudinal funneling of sound-evoked motion in the mammalian cochlea. Nat. Commun. **9**(1), 1–12 (2018)
11. Lee, H.Y., Raphael, P.D., Park, J., Ellerbee, A.K., Applegate, B.E., Oghalai, J.S.: Noninvasive in vivo imaging reveals differences between tectorial membrane and basilar membrane traveling waves in the mouse cochlea. Proc. Natl. Acad. Sci. **112**(10), 3128–3133 (2015). https://doi.org/10.1073/pnas.1500038112
12. Jawadi, Z., Applegate, B.E., Oghalai, J.S.: Optical coherence tomography to measure sound-induced motions within the mouse organ of Corti in vivo. In: Auditory and Vestibular Research, pp. 449–462. Springer (2016). https://doi.org/10.1007/978-1-4939-3615-1_24
13. Johns, J.D., Adadey, S.M., Hoa, M.: The role of the stria vascularis in neglected otologic disease. Hear. Res. 108682 (2022).https://doi.org/10.1016/j.heares.2022.108682
14. Gao, S.S., et al.: Vibration of the organ of Corti within the cochlear apex in mice. J. Neurophysiol. **112**(5), 1192–1204 (2014). https://doi.org/10.1152/jn.00306.2014
15. Cai, R., Montgomery, S.C., Graves, K.A., Caspary, D.M., Cox, B.C.: The FBN rat model of aging: investigation of ABR waveforms and ribbon synapse changes. Neurobiol. Aging **62**, 53–63 (2018). https://doi.org/10.1016/j.neurobiolaging.2017.09.034
16. Jeng, J.Y., et al.: Age-related changes in the biophysical and morphological characteristics of mouse cochlear outer hair cells. J. Physiol. **598**(18), 3891–3910 (2020)
17. Manolagas, S.C., Parfitt, A.M.: What old means to bone (in eng). Trends Endocrinol Metab **21**(6), 369–374 (2010). https://doi.org/10.1016/j.tem.2010.01.010
18. Neng, L., et al.: Structural changes in thestrial blood–labyrinth barrier of aged C57BL/6 mice. Cell Tissue Res. **361**(3), 685–696 (2015). https://doi.org/10.1007/s00441-015-2147-2
19. Gratton, M., Schmiedt, R., Schulte, B.: Age-related decreases in endocochlear potential are associated with vascular abnormalities in the stria vascularis. Hear. Res. **102**(1–2), 181–190 (1996)
20. Kalinec, G.M., Lomberk, G., Urrutia, R.A., Kalinec, F.: Resolution of cochlear inflammation: novel target for preventing or ameliorating drug-, noise-and age-related hearing loss. Front. Cell. Neurosci. **11**, 192 (2017). https://doi.org/10.3389/fncel.2017.00192
21. Menardo, J., et al.: Oxidative stress, inflammation, and autophagic stress as the key mechanisms of premature age-related hearing loss in SAMP8 mouse Cochlea. Antioxid. Redox Signal. **16**(3), 263–274 (2012). https://doi.org/10.1089/ars.2011.4037
22. Lang, H., et al.: The stria vascularis in mice and humans is an early site of age-related cochlear degeneration, macrophage dysfunction, and inflammation. Macrophage Dysfunct. Inflamm.
23. Henry, K.R.: Males lose hearing earlier in mouse models of late-onset age-related hearing loss; females lose hearing earlier in mouse models of early-onset hearing loss. Hear. Res. **190**(1–2), 141–148 (2004). https://doi.org/10.1016/S0378-5955(03)00401-5

# An Improved Canonical Correlation Analysis for EEG Inter-Band Correlation Extraction

Zishan Wang[1,2], Ruqiang Huang[1,3], Lei Zhang[1,2], Shaokai Zhao[1,3](✉), Bei Wang[2], Jing Jin[2], Ye Yan[1,3], and Erwei Yin[1,3]

[1] Tianjin Artificial Intelligence Innovation Center (TAIIC), Tianjin, China
lnkzsk@126.com
[2] East China University of Science and Technology, Shanghai, China
[3] Defense Innovation Institute, Academy of Military Sciences (AMS), Beijing, China

**Abstract.** As the most active and promising research fields of affective computing, emotion recognition based on EEG signal has attracted much attention. Traditional methods usually pay their attention on single-channel features which reflect time-domain, or frequency-domain of EEG and bi-channel features which reflecting channel-wise relationship across brain regions. However, emotional features which capturing the coupling between the EEG frequency bands was seldom to discuss. In this paper, we proposed a method to extract the inter-bands correlation (IBC) features based on canonical correlation analysis (CCA). Firstly, we verified the validity of the IBC features through several experiments and found that the more correlated features between the EEG frequency bands contribute more to emotion classification. Then, the IBC features and traditional differential entropy (DE) were fused at the decision-level, which significantly improves the accuracy of emotion recognition on SEED dataset and local CUMULATE dataset. Our results show that IBC features is a promising method to promote the emotion recognition accuracy.

**Keywords:** EEG · IBC · CCA · DE · Decision-level fusion

## 1 Introduction

With the rapid development of human-computer interaction (HCI), affective computing has become a research hotspot in recent years. Affective computing aims to empower computers with the ability to perceive, understand and express human emotions so that it has higher intelligence to interact with mankind. As the most active and promising research field of affective computing, emotion recognition is becoming more and more critical. It is of great significance in the diagnosis of emotion-related diseases and the construction of harmonious and friendly human-computer interaction systems.

Generally speaking, two kinds of signals are always adopted by current emotion recognition methods as their system input. One is based on non-physiological signals, such as facial expressions [1], body movements, and speech signals. The other type is based on physiological signals, such as Electroencephalography (EEG) [2], Electrocardiogram (ECG), Electromyography (EMG), and galvanic skin response (GSR).


G. Wang et al. (Eds.): APCMBE 2023, IFMBE Proceedings 103, pp. 273–280, 2024.
https://doi.org/10.1007/978-3-031-51455-5_30

Compared with non-physiological signals, physiological signals have the advantage of being difficult to camouflage, so they can reflect the underlying emotional states of humans. Among the numerous physiological signals, EEG is the most used signal for emotion recognition because it can dynamically reflect changes in the central nervous system and contains rich emotional information [3].

In the emotion recognition task, the quality of feature extraction [4] affects its performance directly. For EEG signals, the features commonly used for emotion recognition mainly include time domain, frequency domain, and time-frequency domain features. Duan proposed a feature called differential entropy (DE) [5]. The experimental results on 6 subjects show that differential entropy is an effective feature to identify emotions and outperforms traditional power spectral density (PSD) features. In addition, some studies suggest that the relationship between EEG channels is also a feature that needs to be considered. Moon [6] identified emotions by extracting the connectivity features between different brain channels, including Pearson correlation coefficient (PCC), phase lock value (PLV), and phase lag index (PLI). They constructed a connectivity matrix as the input of the convolutional neural network (CNN) by calculating the connectivity coefficient between any two EEG channels. The results showed that connectivity between the EEG channels is indeed an important feature of emotion, reflecting the synergy between different brain regions as emotions arise and change.

At present, lots of studies have considered the relationship between EEG channels but seldom concentrate on the relationship between EEG frequency bands. Theoretically, the production of emotion is accompanied by the common activity of multiple frequency bands. Therefore, in this paper, we consider the synergy between EEG frequency bands. First, we extracted the DE features of each frequency band of the multi-channel EEG signals. Then the correlation features between EEG frequency bands were extracted by canonical correlation analysis (CCA) [7] based on DE features(inter-band-DE). Finally, the cross-band DE features was integrated with traditional DE feature to train a classifier to identify emotions through decision-level fusion, which significantly improves the accuracy of emotion recognition.

The other parts of this paper are arranged as follows: In Sect. 2, we describe in detail the dataset we used, and methods employed in analyzing the data. In Sect. 3, the experimental results are presented and some analysis and discussion are carried out. Section 4 summarizes the main conclusions and contributions of our study.

## 2 Methods and Materials

### 2.1 Datasets and Preprocessing

Two datasets, the SJTU Emotion EEG Dataset (SEED) [8] and our local Continuous Upgrading Multi-Model Affect Elicitation (CUMULATE) dataset [9] were adopted in this research to evaluate the efficiency of our methods.

The SEED dataset consists of 15 participants (7 males and 8 females, mean age 23.27 years, variance 2.37). Each subject participated in three experiments and in each experiment, they were required to watch 15 emotional film clips to elicit three emotions: positive, neutral, and negative. This dataset recorded EEG signals from 62 electrodes with ESI NeuroScan System. To filter out noise and artifacts, the signals were processed using a bandpass filter from 0.3 to 50 Hz, followed by down sampling the sampling rate from 1000 Hz to 200 Hz. Afterward the EEG signal corresponding to the video clip was segmented and the data of each channel is divided into 5s lengths without overlap.

The CUMULATE dataset is our local dataset, containing a three-classes sub-dataset of calm, fear, and happy(CUMULATE3), a four-classes sub-dataset of calm, fear, happy(CUMULATE4), and sad, and a five-classes sub-dataset of calm, fear, happy, sad, and angry(CUMULATE5). Each sub-dataset contained 15 subjects, five of whom participated in both rounds of the experiment, so a total of 40 subjects participated in the experiment (30 males and 10 females, mean age 26.20 years, variance 4.74). In each type of sub-dataset, there are five video clips for each emotion. Thus 15, 20, and 25 video clips were viewed by subjects in the three-classes, four-classes, and five-classes sub-dataset, respectively. A total of 60 EEG channels were recorded with ESI NeuroScan System. After that, the same bandpass filtering process of 0.3–50 Hz is performed on the original EEG signal to remove the high-frequency noise, and a notch filter of 50 Hz is used to remove power line interference. The signal is then down-sampled to 200 Hz for subsequent processing. To avoid the interference of eye movement artifacts, the eye movement artifacts were removed by independent component analysis (ICA). Similarly, the pre-processed EEG signal was segmented. The data of each channel was divided into 5s lengths without overlap.

## 2.2 Differential Entropy

Differential entropy is a generalized form of Shannon's information entropy on continuous variables, which is often used as a feature of EEG-based emotion recognition, and its defining equation is shown as follows:

$$DE = -\int_X p(x)\log(p(x))dx\# \qquad (1)$$

where $p(x)$ is the probability density function of the random variable $X$.

Studies have shown that for a fixed-length EEG signal, the differential entropy of the EEG signal in a frequency band is equivalent to the logarithm of the energy spectrum in the frequency band [10]. Thus, we can calculate the differential entropy of five frequency bands ($\delta$:1–4 Hz, $\theta$:4–8 Hz, $\alpha$:8–13 Hz, $\beta$:13–30 Hz, $\gamma$:30–50 Hz) per channel for each sample. For the SEED dataset, we can extract 310 dimensional features (62 channels*5 bands) for each sample, and for the CUMULATE dataset, we can extract 300 dimensional features (60 channels * 5 bands) for each sample.

## 2.3 Inter-Band Correlation Features Based on CCA

CCA is usually used to obtain the maximum correlation coefficient between two sets of random variables by reducing both sets of data to one dimension The solution of the problem is finally transformed into the maximum singular value problem of matrix M. In fact, the two sets of data can be reduced to k dimension by CCA to solve the first k maximum correlation coefficient which is transformed into the first k singular values of the matrix M.

The generation and changes of emotions usually involve multiple bands of brain activity, and there are synergies between these bands, so the inter-bands correlation (IBC) features can be extracted using CCA. Figure 1 shows the framework for IBC feature extraction based on original DE features.

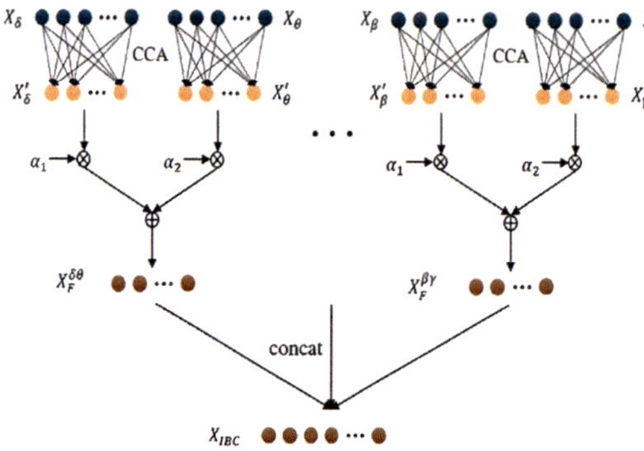


**Fig. 1.** IBC Feature Extraction Based on Original DE Features

Any two frequency bands of DE features $X$ and $Y$ can be linearly transformed by CCA, so that the correlation coefficients of the two groups of random variables after transformation are the first k of the maximum, and the linearly transformed random variables reflects the correlation features between the two frequency bands:

$$X_1^{'} = W_1^T X_1\#$$

$$X_2^{'} = W_2^T X_2\# \tag{3}$$

According to [11], two parameters $\alpha_1$ and $\alpha_2$ is set to satisfying $\alpha_1 + \alpha_2 = 1$. After that, a weighted summation of the correlation features between the two frequency-band obtained above was performed, as shown in Eq. (4), to get the IBC features $X_F$ between the two frequency bands:

$$X_F = \alpha_1 X^{'} + \alpha_2 X_2^{'}\# \tag{4}$$

For the 5 frequency bands of the EEG, features like $X_F$ can be obtained between any two frequency bands, so we can obtain 10 sets of features like $X_F$. Finally, we concatenate 10 sets of features, which is the final inter-band correlation feature $X_{IBC}$, as shown in Eq. (5):

$$X_C = \left[X_F^{\delta\theta}, X_F^{\delta\alpha}, X_F^{\delta\beta}, \ldots, X_F^{\beta\gamma}\right]\# \tag{5}$$

### 2.4 Decision-Level Fusion

Considering that some of the original information may be lost when the IBC features are obtained from the original DE features, a decision-level fusion method is adopted for the original DE features and the IBC features to classify emotions. For each of these two features, a classifier is trained using a linear kernel SVM. Let $\omega_k (k = 1, 2, \ldots, c)$ to represent the category of emotions, $y_{DE}$ and $y_{IBC}$ to represent the labels of emotions predicted by the classifier, respectively. The result of decision-level fusion is shown as follow:

$$y_{Fusion} = \underset{w_k}{\text{argmax}}\left[p(w_k|y_{DE}) + p(w_k|y_{IBC})\right](k = 1, 2, \ldots, c)\# \tag{6}$$

where $p(w_k|y_{DE})$ and $p(w_k|y_{IBC})$ represent the confidence of the classifiers trained by DE features and trained by IBC features to identify the $k$-th emotion, respectively. We take the labels corresponding to the highest sum of confidence of the two classifier outputs as the final prediction label.

## 3 Result and Discussion

### 3.1 Validity of IBC Features

To verify the validity of the IBC features, that is, whether the extracted IBC features are really correlated with emotions, the singular values of the matrix $M$ were sorted in descending order. Then, we select the IBC features corresponding to the largest half of the singular values and the IBC features corresponding to the other half of the singular values to classify emotions, respectively. When the weighted summation is performed on the correlation features of two frequency bands, we assumed that the importance of each frequency band is the same, so that letting $\alpha_1 = 0.5$ and $\alpha_2 = 0.5$. The classification results are shown in Fig. 2.

Figure 2 illustrates the comparison of classification accuracy between the first 30/31 IBC features and the last 30/31 IBC features on CUMULATE and SEED datasets. A paired sample t-test is performed on the classification accuracy respectively. The result shows that, whether for the local CUMULATE dataset or SEED dataset, the classification accuracy of the first 30/31 IBC features is significantly higher than the last 30/31 IBC features. For the CUMULATE3, the average classification accuracy of the first 30 IBC features is 78.34%, 60.77% and 53.23%, respectively, which is much higher than the average classification accuracy of the last 30 IBC features corresponding to 58.70% ($p < 0.001$), 46.61% ($p < 0.001$) and 41.27% ($p < 0.001$). On the SEED dataset, the average classification accuracy of the first 31 IBC features is 70.00%, which is significantly higher than the other half of the features corresponding to 58.83% ($p < 0.001$).

In fact, a larger singular value corresponds to a more correlated feature between the frequency bands. Therefore, the first 30/31 IBC features better reflect the correlation between the two frequency bands than the last 30/31 IBC features. The more correlated features between the frequency bands are more beneficial to the recognition of emotions, therefore the features that are correlated between bands may be the features that are embedded in emotions.

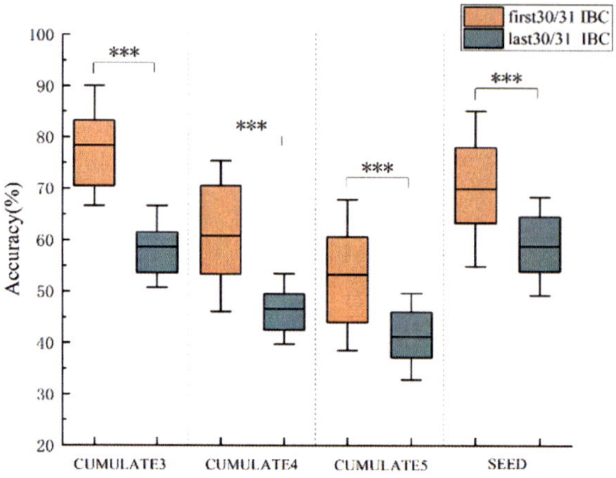


**Fig. 2.** Comparison of classification accuracy between the first 30/31 IBC features and the last 30/31 IBC features on CUMULATE and SEED datasets which demonstrate the effectiveness of IBC.

## 3.2 Classification Results

Based on the results in the previous subsection, the IBC features corresponding to the first 30/31 feature were selected to train a classifier. Then, another classifier was trained using the original DE features. Both are adopted and combined into a decision-level fusion classifier with sum rule.

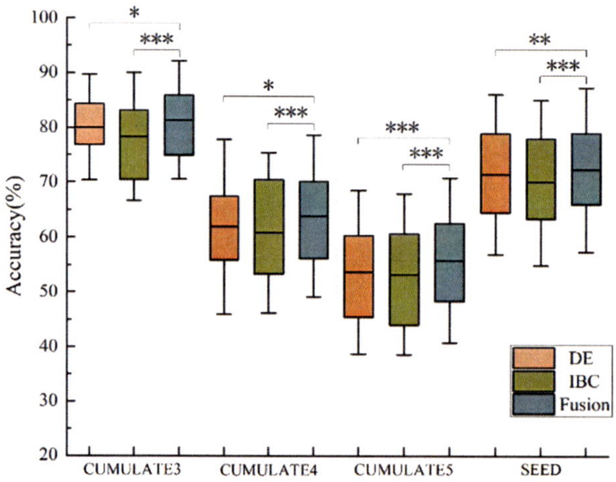


**Fig. 3.** Emotion recognition accuracy using DE features, IBC features and their decision-level fusion on local CUMULATE dataset and SEED dataset. Paired T-test is adopted in this experiment. '*' represents $p \leq 0.05$; '***' represents $p \leq 0.001$.

Figure 3 shows the emotion recognition accuracy using DE, IBC features and their decision-level fusion. There is no significant difference on the classification results between using the DE feature alone and using the IBC feature alone. However, the fusion of DE and IBC features can significantly improve the classification accuracy compared with that of a single feature. For the three sub-datasets of CUMULATE, the average classification accuracies after fusion are 81.36%, 63.88% and 55.77%, respectively, which are significantly higher than the average classification accuracies of 80.02% ($p < 0.05$, paired t-test), 61.86% ($p < 0.05$, paired t-test) and 53.61% ($p < 0.001$, paired t-test) using DE features alone as well as significantly higher than the average classification accuracies of mean classification accuracy of 78.34% ($p < 0.001$, paired t-test), 60.77% ($p < 0.001$, paired t-test), and 53.23% ($p < 0.001$, paired t-test) using IBC features alone. The same results are obtained on the SEED dataset. The average classification accuracy after fusion is 72.35%, which is significantly higher than the average classification accuracy of 71.49% ($p < 0.01$, paired t-test) using the DE features alone as well as higher than the average classification accuracy of 70.00% ($p < 0.001$, paired t-test) using IBC features alone. This result shows that some information is lost when IBC features are obtained by CCA on DE features, but some new information is added that is not contained in the DE features. There is complementary information between DE features and IBC features.

## 4 Conclusions

In this paper, we propose a novel method to extract emotional cross-band features based on widely used differential entropy. Compared with traditional inter-band feature extraction, such as PAC(phase-amplitude coupling), our method is based on machine learning and avoids surrogate test, which is a time-consuming method, thus improving the real-time ability of our model. The validity of the IBC features is evaluated on the public SEED dataset and the local CUMULATE dataset, respectively. Our results show that, compared with two single features, combining cross-band DE features with traditional DE features can effectively improve the accuracy of emotion recognition, which proves the effectiveness of this method.

## References


1. Yan, J., et al.: Integrating facial expression and body gesture in videos for emotion recognition. IEICE Trans. Inf. Syst. **97**(3), 610–613 (2014)
2. Wang, X.-W., Nie, D., Lu, B.-L.: Emotional state classification from EEG data using machine learning approach. Neurocomputing **129**, 94–106 (2014)
3. Heller, W.: Neuropsychological mechanisms of individual differences in emotion, personality, and arousal. Neuropsychology **7**(4), 476 (1993)
4. Jenke, R., Peer, A., Buss, M.: Feature extraction and selection for emotion recognition from EEG. IEEE Trans. Affect. Comput. **5**(3), 327–339 (2014)
5. Duan, R.-N., Zhu, J.-Y., Lu, B.-L.: Differential entropy feature for EEG-based emotion classification. In: International IEEE/EMBS Conference on Neural Engineering (NER), 2013, pp. 81–84 (2013)
6. Moon, S.-E., Jang, S., Lee, J.-S.: Convolutional neural network approach for EEG-based emotion recognition using brain connectivity and its spatial information. In: IEEE International Conference on Acoustics, Speech and Signal Processing (ICASSP), 2018, pp. 2556–2560 (2018)

7. Liu, Q., et al.: Efficient representations of EEG signals for SSVEP frequency recognition based on deep multiset CCA. Neurocomputing **378**, 36–44 (2020)
8. Zheng, W.-L., Lu, B.-L.: Investigating critical frequency bands and channels for EEG-based emotion recognition with deep neural networks. IEEE Trans. Auton. Ment. Dev. **7**(3), 162–175 (2015)
9. Wang, X., et al: The increasing types of negative emotion impose an extra pressure on the accuracy of emotion recognition. In: International Conference on CAICE, 2022, pp. 259–266 (2022)
10. Shi, L.-C., Jiao, Y.-Y., Lu, B.-L.: Differential entropy feature for EEG-based vigilance estimation. In: 35th Annual International Conference of the IEEE Engineering in Medicine and Biology Society (EMBC), 2013, pp. 6627–6630 (2013)
11. Liu, W., et al.: Comparing recognition performance and robustness of multimodal deep learning models for multimodal emotion recognition. IEEE Trans. Cogn. Dev. Syst. **14**(2), 715–729 (2021)

# Gender Modulates Visual Attention to Emotional Faces: An Eye-Tracking Study

Ludan Zhang, Junling Wang, Huiqin Xue, Shuang Liu(✉), and Dong Ming

Academy of Medical Engineering and Translational Medicine, Tianjin University, Tianjin, China
shuangliu@tju.edu.cn

**Abstract.** Autism spectrum disorder (ASD) is a neurodevelopmental disorder with a high prevalence in males. Most studies are based on the sample of male ASD individuals, which may lead to a bias in understanding female ASD individuals. Not only in the diagnostic characteristics but also the social cognitive performance, gender differences have been found in the ASD population, but the reason is still unclear. To explore whether gender differences are due to specific pathology of ASD or the different social attention between males and females, we collected behavioral and eye movement data from 48 typically developing (TD) adults during a facial emotion discrimination task. We analyzed the behavioral performance, gaze patterns, and pupillary responses during the emotional face processing between males and females. Results showed that the two groups had similar accuracy for facial emotion discrimination, but males spent more time. In addition, males preferred the mouth region while processing emotional faces. In contrast, females preferred to fixate on the eye region and had greater pupillary responses to this region than males. These findings suggest that males and females differ in their visual processing strategies and sensitivity to emotional faces, which may extend to the ASD population.

**Keywords:** Gender · Facial emotion · Eye movement · Visual attention · Autism spectrum disorder

## 1 Introduction

Autism spectrum disorder (ASD) is a neurodevelopmental disorder more common in males. It is likely four times more prevalent than in females [1]. Because of this, the number of female ASD individuals included in the existing studies is insufficient, so that difficult to accurately evaluate the potential gender effect on symptom presentation. To date, we remain puzzled about the nature of gender differences in ASD, and thus, it is warranted to continue the research.

Gender differences are not only reflected in the diagnostic characteristics of ASD. Regarding social cognition, individuals with ASD generally have impaired attention to social stimuli, especially face stimuli, which has been well demonstrated by eye-tracking technology [2]. Individuals with ASD fixate less on the core features of the emotional face, especially the eye region [3, 4], leading researchers to speculate that


G. Wang et al. (Eds.): APCMBE 2023, IFMBE Proceedings 103, pp. 281–288, 2024.
https://doi.org/10.1007/978-3-031-51455-5_31

abnormal visual processing may be a major reason for poor emotional discrimination in ASD, which in turn aggravates their difficulty in interpreting facial expressions. Existing research found that visual attention to faces is also modulated by gender in ASD: females focus more on faces in the social scene than males [5]. Also, the gender effects are found in typically developing (TD) individuals: females are more sensitive to emotional faces than males, and as age increases, they still perform better in emotional recognition [6, 7]. Therefore, it remains to be studied whether the gender differences in the visual processing of emotional faces are due to the pathology of ASD or to differences in social attention between males and females.

Based on the above points, to provide intuitional evidence, we employed eye-tracking technology, designed a dynamic facial emotion discrimination task, and recruited TD adults as participants. We compared and analyzed behavioral performance, visual fixation patterns, and the pupillary response of emotional faces between genders, exploring whether the visual processing of emotional faces is modulated by gender.

# 2 Method

## 2.1 Participants

Fifty-one TD university students participated in our study, of whom three participants were excluded due to poor data quality, and finally, 48 participants were included in further analysis. All participants have normal or corrected-to-normal vision. Of the participants, 24 were male, ranging in age from 19 to 29 years (M = 22.65, SD = 2.27), and 24 were female, ranging in age from 19 to 28 years (M = 22.74, SD = 2.29). No significant difference in age was found between males and females by the two-sample t-test. This research was approved by the Ethics Committee of Tianjin Children's Hospital, and all participants provided written informed consent.

## 2.2 Stimuli and Experimental Paradigm

Face stimuli were chosen from the Karolinska Directed Emotional Faces (KDEF) database [8], containing the emotional facial photo of 10 male and 10 female actors.

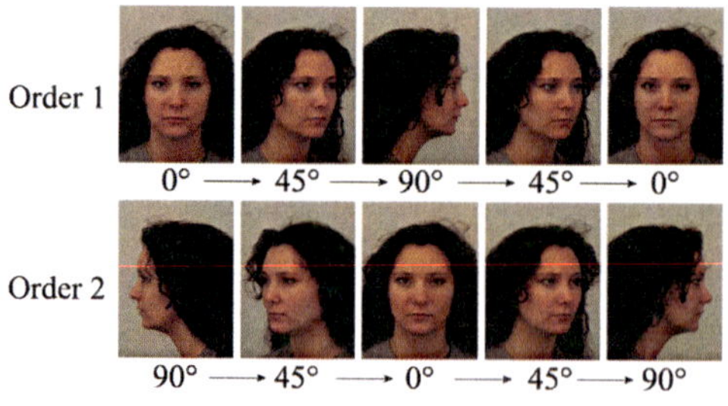


**Fig. 1.** Examples of face stimuli presentation

The stimuli presented four emotions: neutral, happy, sad, and angry, and included three angles: 0° (left or right), 45° (left or right), and 90°. All photos were the same size (width: 17° visual angle, height: 23° visual angle), and the critical face features were standardized to the same location. We designed two orders of stimuli presentation, as shown in Fig. 1. Among them, order 1 presents face photos from angle 0° to 90° to 0°, and order 2 presents from 90° to 0° to 90°. This dynamic stimulus presentation imitated the pattern of viewing faces in daily life, improving the ecological validity of the experiment.

### 2.3 Procedure

The experiment was conducted in a quiet, soft lightroom. Participants were guided to sit approximately 60cm away from a 27-inch monitor comfortably, which resolution is 1920*1080 pixels. Eye movement data were recorded by Tobii Pro Spectrum eye tracker; the sampling rate is 1200 Hz. Before the experiment, participants conducted a 5-point calibration with the Tobii Pro Lab software. After participants were fully aware of the emotion-discrimination task, the experiment was started by the experimenter pressing the space key.

The experiment consisted of 5 blocks, a total of 80 trials. A cartoon character was first presented in each trial to attract participants' visual attention to the centre of the screen, lasting for 3s. Then five photos of the same actor, the same emotion, but different angles of the faces were presented in a specific order (as shown in Fig. 1), each lasting for 2s, a total of 10s. The participants were required to discriminate the emotion shown by the actor within 10s of the presentation and give feedback with the mouse by clicking the corresponding icon on the screen at the moment of recognition. The response time and whether correct were recorded, and the participants themselves would not get the result. Across the 80 trials, the two orders of presentation and the four emotional conditions were balanced in number and presented in random order. The eye movement data were recorded throughout the whole process for each block.

### 2.4 Data Analysis

Data were exported for offline analysis with MATLAB. For behavioral data, the average accuracy and average response time (in the case of correct discrimination) of 48 participants were calculated in two orders of presentation and four emotional conditions, respectively.

For the eye movement data, we calculated the preference index and pupil diameter variation as features. First, taking the nose as the boundary, we divided the face stimuli into eye and mouth ROI. Then we calculated the proportional fixation time for each ROI. And we subtracted the proportional fixation time of the mouth from that of the eye, which is the preference index. If positive, the participant is fixated more on the eyes; if negative, the participant is fixated more on the mouth. For the pupil diameter variation, we filtrated the pupil data during the fixation of the eye ROI. Subsequently, the pupil diameter of the first 3s was used as the baseline, and the baseline was subtracted from the diameter of the facial photos, obtaining the pupil diameter variation. We averaged the two features according to the corresponding presented order and emotional conditions.

In this article, we used behavioral characteristics and eye-movement characteristics as dependent variables, gender as between-group variables, order (1 and 2), and emotion conditions (neutral, happy, sad, angry) as within-group variables. As the dependent variables did not follow the normal distribution, statistical analysis was performed using the generalized estimating equation (GEE) with a significance level of 0.05, adjusting for multiple comparisons using the Bonferroni method.

# 3 Results

## 3.1 Behavioral Results

For accuracy, after statistical testing, only the main effect of emotion was significant ($p < 0.001$). There was no significant difference in accuracy between males (M = 93.45, SD = 3.89) and females (M = 93.55, SD = 3.79). Figure 2 shows that the happy condition has the highest accuracy (M = 98.07, SD = 3.88), followed by the neutral condition (M = 96.61, SD = 4.20). Angry was third (M = 91.92, SD = 7.67) and significantly less accurate than happy ($p < 0.001$) and neutral ($p = 0.001$) conditions. The sad condition (M = 87.06, SD = 8.95) was the lowest and significantly lower than happy ($p < 0.001$), neutral ($p < 0.001$), and angry ($p = 0.001$) conditions.

The response time is influenced by order, emotion, and gender, as shown in Fig. 3. The statistical analysis showed that the main effect of order ($p < 0.001$), emotion.

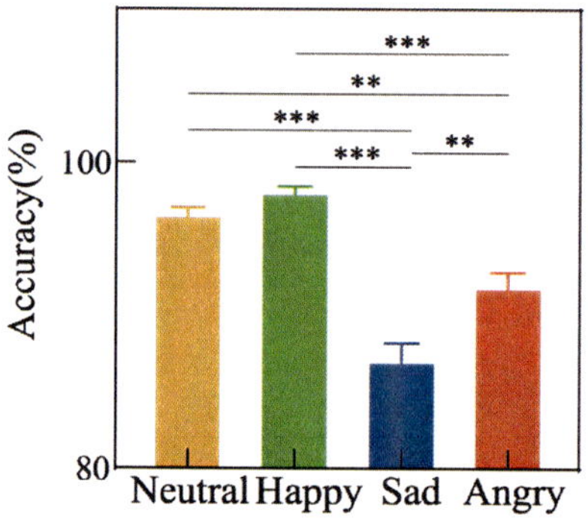


**Fig. 2.** Comparison of response accuracy under four emotion conditions (*** $p < 0.001$)

($p < 0.001$), gender ($p = 0.034$), and the interaction effect of order*emotion ($p < 0.001$) were significant. Further analysis found that males took more time to discriminate emotions than females, regardless of the stimuli. While for emotion, we found that when the stimuli were presented in order 1, the response time of happy (M = 1.57, SD = 0.42) was the lowest, followed by neutral (M = 2.00, SD = 0.97), angry (M = 2.26, SD = 0.80), and sad (M = 2.51, SD = 0.74) was the highest. There were significant differences between each two of these four emotions. When the stimuli were presented in order 2, the happy condition (M = 2.19, SD = 0.82) was the lowest, which was significantly lower than the neutral ($p < 0.001$), sad ($p < 0.001$), and angry ($p < 0.001$). But there

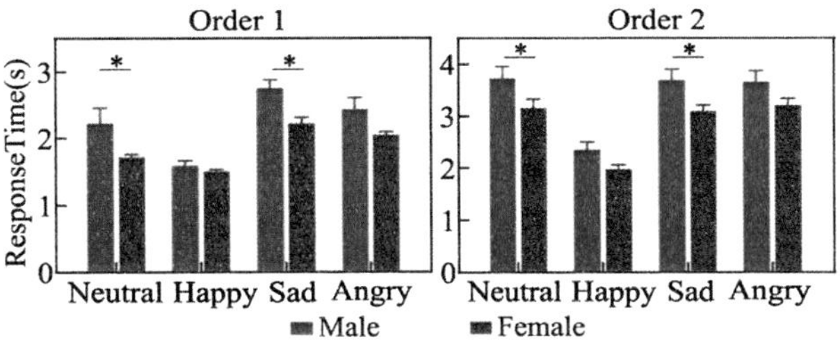


**Fig. 3.** Comparison of male and female response times under different presented order and emotion conditions (* p < 0.05)

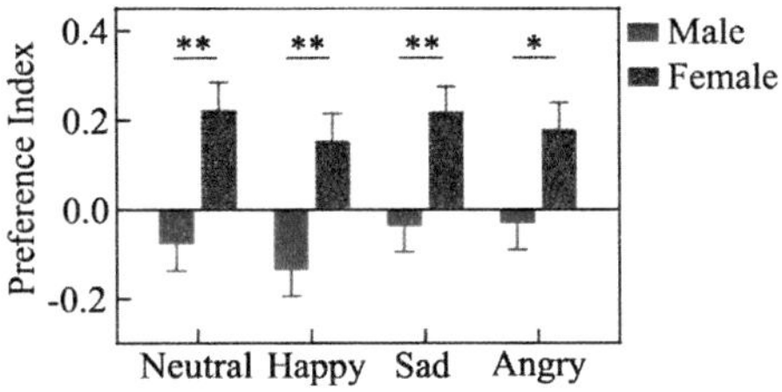


**Fig. 4.** Gender contrast of the preference index under different emotion conditions (*** p < 0.001, ** p < 0.01, * p < 0.05)

were no significant differences between the remaining three emotions (neutral: M = 3.47, SD = 1.23; sad: M = 3.42, SD = 1.05; angry: M = 3.47, SD = 1.08).

Unexpectedly, we found that response times were significantly lower in order 1 than in order 2, regardless of emotions. This may be due to the 0° faces presented first, providing more emotional information and helping participants quickly discriminate.

Overall, males and females have similar discriminated accuracy for the task, but males spent more time. In addition, they both discriminate happy emotions accurately and quickly, while two negative emotions, especially sad, were discriminated less accurately and slower.

### 3.2 Preference Index Results

To explore the fixation patterns of males and females to emotional faces, we calculated the preference index to reflect the difference in fixation preference between the two groups, and the results are shown in Fig. 4. Statistical analysis showed that the main effects of gender ($p = 0.002$), order ($p < 0.001$), and emotion ($p < 0.001$) were all significant, and there was a significant interaction effect of gender*emotion ($p = 0.006$). From Fig. 4, we can clearly see that the preference index of males was significantly lower than that of females (neutral: $p = 0.001$; happy: $p = 0.001$; sad: $p = 0.002$; angry: $p = 0.012$). This result indicates that during visual scanning of emotional faces, males tend to focus on the mouth region and females tend to focus on the eye region. Both males and females tended to focus more on the mouth region for happy faces and more on the eye region for negative emotional faces. In addition, we were surprised to find

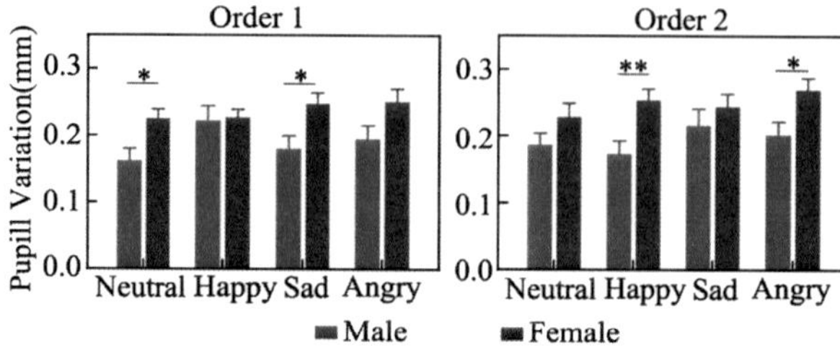


**Fig. 5.** Comparison of male and female pupil diameter variation under different presented order and emotion conditions (** $p < 0.01$, * $p < 0.05$)

out that the preference index in order 1 was significantly higher ($p < 0.001$), suggesting that viewing the 0° face first may increase subsequent attention to the eye region.

### 3.3 Pupil Diameter Variation Results

Pupil diameter can reflect participants' physiological responses to emotional faces. To further investigate gender differences, we calculated the pupil diameter variation of the eye region, as shown in Fig. 5. Statistical analysis found that the main effect of gender ($p = 0.026$) and emotion ($p = 0.021$) was significant, and the interaction effect of order*emotion*gender ($p = 0.003$) was significant. The further specific analysis found that the pupil variation of males was less than that of females. In order 1, the male pupil diameter variation in the eye region of neutral and sad faces was significantly lower than that of females (neutral: $p = 0.017$; sad: $p = 0.019$). And in order 2, the male pupil diameter variation in the eye region of happy and angry faces was significantly lower than that of females (happy: $p = 0.006$; angry: $p = 0.026$). Overall, females responded greater to emotional faces than males, suggesting more sensitivity to the emotional information conveyed by eyes.

## 4 Discussion

This study verifies the behavioral and visual performance differences when TD males and females in the facial emotion discrimination task. Specifically, we find that males required more time to achieve similar discrimination accuracy as females. Further, males were more preferred to focus on the mouth region and showed a weaker pupillary response to the eye region. On the other hand, females are more preferred to view the eye region and respond greater.

Attention to the eye region shows salient importance to face processing. In our study, females paid more attention to the eyes than males, suggesting that females are more efficient in capturing facial information. According to neuroimaging studies, in the facial perception stage, females have greater limbic system activation, facilitating primary emotion processing. But males' emotion processing style tends to be analytical, which may potentially be slower in perception [9]. Meanwhile, the limbic system structurally overlaps with the central autonomic network (CAN), which can modulate the pupillary response through the noradrenergic sympathetic pathway [10]. Therefore, females may experience emotions with greater intensity when viewing emotional faces, have higher emotional arousal, and eventually show larger pupil dilation.

Overall, we found apparent gender effects on visual processing strategies for emotional faces and the sensitivity to emotional information conveyed by the eyes. In the subsequent studies, we will include clinical data to verify whether the gender effect can be extended in the ASD population.

## 5 Conclusions

The current work focused on gender effects on emotional face processing. In general, we have three main findings: (A). Males required more time to achieve similar emotional discrimination accuracy as females. (B). Males preferred to fixate on the mouth region during processing of emotional faces, while females preferred the eye region. (C). Females had greater pupillary responses to eye region than males. These findings prove that TD females have stronger social attention for emotional faces and are more sensitive to emotional information conveyed by the eyes. In the future, we will verify these results in the ASD group and make a comparison between the ASD and TD groups.

**Acknowledgment.** This research was supported by the Tianjin Key Technology R&D 21JCYBJC00360.

## References

1. Maenner, M.J., Shaw, K.A., Bakian, A.V., et al.: Prevalence and characteristics of autism spectrum disorder among children aged 8 Years—autism and developmental disabilities monitoring network, 11 sites, United States, 2018. MMWR Surveill. Summ. **70**(11), 1–16 (2021). https://doi.org/10.15585/MMWR.SS7011A1
2. Chita-Tegmark, M.: Social attention in ASD: A review and meta-analysis of eye-tracking studies. Res. Dev. Disabil. **48**, 79–93 (2016). https://doi.org/10.1016/j.ridd.2015.10.011
3. Wieckowski, A.T., White, S.W.: Eye-gaze analysis of facial emotion recognition and expression in adolescents with ASD. J. Clin. Child Adolesc. Psychol. **46**(1), 110–124 (2017). https://doi.org/10.1080/15374416.2016.1204924
4. Bochet, A., Franchini, M., Kojovic, N., et al.: Emotional versus neutral face exploration and habituation: An eye-tracking study of preschoolers with autism spectrum disorders. Front. Psychiatry **11**(January), 1–13 (2021). https://doi.org/10.3389/fpsyt.2020.568997
5. Harrop, C., Jones, D., Zheng, S., et al.: Visual attention to faces in children with autism spectrum disorder: Are there sex differences? Mol. Autism **10**(1), 1 (2019). https://doi.org/10.1186/s13229-019-0276-2
6. Kraines, M.A., Kelberer, L.J.A., Wells, T.T.: Sex differences in attention to disgust facial expressions. Cogn. Emot. **31**(8), 1692–1697 (2017). https://doi.org/10.1080/02699931.2016.1244044
7. Abbruzzese, L., Magnani, N., Robertson, I.H., et al.: Age and gender differences in emotion recognition. Front. Psychol. **10**(OCT), (2019). https://doi.org/10.3389/fpsyg.2019.02371
8. Lundqvist, D., Flykt, A., Öhman, A.: The Karolinska directed emotional faces−KDEF, CD ROM from Department of clinical neuroscience, Psychology section. Karolinska Inst. (1998)

9. Whittle, S., Yücel, M., Yap, M.B.H., et al.: Sex differences in the neural correlates of emotion: Evidence from neuroimaging, 87(3). Biol. Psychol. (2011). https://doi.org/10.1016/j.biopsycho.2011.05.003
10. Ferencová, N., Višňovcová, Z., Bona Olexová, L., et al.: Eye pupil—a window into central autonomic regulation via emotional/cognitive processing. Physiol. Res. **70**, S669–S682 (2021). https://doi.org/10.33549/physiolres.934749

# EEG Studies of the Effects of Music Training on Rhythm, Music Phrases and Syntax Perception

Jiacheng Nie[1,2], Yanru Bai[1], Qi Zheng[3], and Guangjian Ni[1,3(✉)]

[1] Academy of Medical Engineering and Translational Medicine, Tianjin University, Tianjin, China
niguangjian@tju.edu.cn
[2] Tianjin International Engineering Institute, Tianjin University, Tianjin, China
[3] College of Precision Instruments and Optoelectronics Engineering, Tianjin University, Tianjin, China

**Abstract.** The effects of music training are reflected in auditory perception. Behavioral, brain structural and functional changes were found in musicians and nonmusician controls, demonstrating the effects of music training. Rhythm, music phrases and syntax are complex music elements, which involve higher level of auditory processing. EEG studies of the perception of these music elements and the effects of music training were summarized and discussed in this review. The ERP early and mid-latency components, P3a, P3, N5, ERAN (early right anterior negativity), CPS (closure positive shift) and neural entrainment to beat frequencies were EEG features to study complex music perception between musicians who received music training and nonmusician controls. Musicians showed more complex ERP components related to rhythm, music phrases and syntax features and stronger neural entrainment to music beats. These results showed different cortical processing of rhythm, music phrases and syntax in musicians and nonmusicians and explained the effects of music training on auditory perception on a deeper level.

**Keywords:** EEG · Music training · Rhythm · Music phrases · Music syntax

## 1 Introduction

Studies have found that musicians outperform nonmusicians on the behavioral level in many aspects, probably due to advanced perceptual skills and working memory through years of musical training [1, 2]. Changes in brain functions and structures explain the effects of music training. Evidence was found on the neurobiological level, where musicians showed better information encoding and stronger cross-modal auditory-motor integration, supporting the musician's advantage on corresponding perception [3, 4].

Music perception involves cognition, emotion, and other underlying brain mechanisms [5]. Studies of music perception explained musician advantage over nonmusicians in a more underpinning way. Various neuroimaging techniques have been used in studies


G. Wang et al. (Eds.): APCMBE 2023, IFMBE Proceedings 103, pp. 289–295, 2024.
https://doi.org/10.1007/978-3-031-51455-5_32

of music perception for the different properties of cortical responses to musical stimuli [6]. Electroencephalography (EEG), a powerful tool in the field of neuroscience and brain science, allows for the analysis of continuous processes in time, frequency, and other domains, therefore, has been frequently used in studies of music perception. EEG provides researchers with various methods and evidence helping to understand music perception profoundly. Here, we focus on EEG methods and findings of music perception in musicians and non-musicians.

The EEG studies of music perception is conditioned by the interested musical contents and the form of stimulus. EEG features that we usually discovered, which reveals the cortical decoding of music, depend on experiment tasks and paradigms. The perception of basic musical elements, such as pitch, timbre, etc., has been widely studied in recent years, whereas the effects of systematic music training have not been adequately embodied [7]. Rhythm, music phrases, and syntax are complex musical materials for which the EEG paradigms should be carefully designed. The investigation of these musical materials involves more complex brain activities. Cortical processing of the perception of these music elements would explain the differences between musicians and nonmusicians on a deeper level. EEG studies of the effects of music expertise are summarized in this review according to the three forms of musical stimulus.

## 2 Effects of Music Training on Music Perception

### 2.1 Perception of Rhythm

Temporal pattern or structure is essential to the perception of music. A rhythm is a sequence of musical sound groups temporally patterned by duration or stress [8]. In studies of rhythm perception, subjects perceive repeating rhythmic units or beats. Subjects' responses to violations of rhythmic patterns or durations are analyzed using EEG or behavioral measures [9]. Most EEG studies of rhythm perception investigated (1) the ERP out of EEG recordings or (2) the neural entrainment to steady beats stimulus [10]. The study of rhythm perception requires high temporal resolution, and ERP enables a close examination of the time course of the changing rhythmic pattern. ERP P3 components were found to correlate with the performance of detection of speeding up or slowing down target beats after a four-beat sequence [11]. Subcomponents of P3 can further recognize the two kinds of rhythm violations.

Geiser et al. discovered the perception of meter and rhythm under two attention modes in musicians and nonmusicians utilizing early ERPs components within 300 ms [12]. Subjects were to detect and distinguish changes in meter (the number of beats in a loop) and rhythm (temporal pattern in the fixed loop) in repeating standard 3-beat rhythmic units. The musicians showed significantly better behavioral performance. The early negative deflection was elicited by rhythm and meter deviants in the attended condition, while in the unattended condition, only rhythm deviants elicited negative deflection. No group effects were found across all experimental conditions concerning ERP results, indicating that rhythm and meter are processed similarly in the early stage attentively or inattentively for both musicians and non-musicians. The effects of musicianship were found in a more complicated experiment revealed by P3a component [13]. Two rhythm processing modes were introduced: a sequential processing hypothesis that individuals expect incoming beats in a fixed position and a hierarchical processing hypothesis that individuals expect incoming beats in all possible positions. Target beat appears on one of six positions where few of them fit the meter. Subjects were to determine if there was a meter violation. Musicians showed significantly longer P3a latency than non-musicians. Moreover, the correlation coefficients of P3a, which express the resemblance of two P3a from different conditions, of nonmusicians could be compared fairly well with the correlation coefficients as predicted by the sequential hypothesis. In contrast, musicians' results fit the hierarchical hypothesis more. All the P3a results discovered in this study suggest that temporal patterns are processed sequentially in nonmusicians and processed hirarchically in musicians.

The neural oscillations entrain to a stimulus of fixed time period [14]. These neural entrainments in music perception are usually synchronizations of neural excitability and underlying music rhythms [15]. It is analyzed similarly to steady-state evoked potentials (SSEP) where amplitude peaks of signals' frequency spectra are plotted and compared. The differences between musicians and nonmusicians in rhythm perception are revealed by neural entrainment to musical rhythms [16]. Stupacher et al. designed a complex experiment in which subjects listened to a quadruple rhythm and a quadruple-triple combined polyrhythm. Then after a silent, subjects were asked to determine if the upcoming stimulus was early, on time or late. EEG signals were recorded through whole process. The normalized frequency spectrum amplitudes of EEG responses during silent periods before the target stimulus showed a significant effect of music expertise. The neural entrainment of 3-beat frequencies (1.5 Hz and 3 Hz) were significantly larger in musician group. The observed difference during silent period indicated that the beat-related top-down controlled neural oscillations can exist without continuous stimulus and the endogenous oscillations were enhanced by music expertise. Another study of rhythm perception found a stronger neural entrainment to 3-beat rhythm in musicians than in nonmusicians [17]. The rhythmic cues from different spatial angular positions induced a sense of 3-beat rhythm. The stronger responses to 3-beat rhythm in musicians were only observed under attentive condition, suggesting that top-down attentional mechanisms were in play for rhythm perception and the neural entrainment to spatial cue rhythms were strengthened by music expertise.

## 2.2 Perception of Music Phrase and Syntax

Music develops based on phrases like language. Melodies and harmony series are composed into musical phrases and may have different functions in the corresponding phrase according to music theory. The perception of musical phrases and syntax has been studied [18–20]. The perception of musical phrases or syntax may correlate with music experience and be reflected in EEG responses. Influences of long-term musical experience on the processing of musical phrases or syntax are summarized below.

A commonly used experimental paradigm of music syntax perception is a chord sequence that includes violations against the expectations of the chord progression [21]. By changing the ending chord, the music syntactic appropriateness and expectancy are violated, which elicits ERP components related to music syntax perception. An early right anterior negativity (ERAN) ERP component was found specifically sensitive to the violation of musical regularities. ERAN has a latency of 200 ms, which is similar to MMN and is usually followed by an N5. The ERAN evoked by harmonically inappropriate chords in a sequence was larger in musicians than non-musicians [22]. Their results indicate that the automatic neural mechanisms that process musical syntax irregularities reflected by ERAN can be modulated by music expertise. Portabella et al. discovered the dissonance perception in a chord progression of the two groups. Chords that violate the regularities in the middle or end of the sequence evoked P3 and N5 components. The amplitude of these components varied between musicians and non-musicians. Moreover, they found that the predictability of dissonant chords did not modulate the ERP responses [23].

More complex phrases were used as musical syntax stimuli. James et al. studied the brain process of music syntax perception in different populations using spatial-temporal ERP, Microstate, and ERP source imaging [24]. Subjects listened to ten-second expressive string quartet pieces, which ended in one regular version or two transgressed versions, after which the subjects had to respond if they appraised the stimulus as satisfactory or not. The effects of musical expertise on the neural processing revealed by ERP response and microstate lay in a 300–500 ms window after the onset of the target stimulus. The P3b-like components and characteristic microstates differentiated nonmusicians, amateur pianists, and expert pianists from each other. The underlying sources for these microstates were localized in the right middle temporal gyrus, anterior cingulate, and right parahippocampal areas. Ma et al. discovered the neural responses of subjects with different musical experiences to musical syntax that follows finite state grammar (FSG) and phrase structure grammar (PSG) [25]. In the FSG condition, different final chord types were not reflected in ERP responses in non-musician group. Irregular final chords evoked ERAN-N5 responses in medium− and pro-musician groups. In terms of PSG condition, only in the pro-musician group were observed ERAN-N5 responses evoked by irregular final chords. Their results suggested that the effects of musical expertise on the perception of musical phrases were reflected in syntactic complexity and early ERAN and late N5 components. EEG responses were also studied during the aesthetic judgment of the chord sequences with different closures [26]. Musicians showed negative potentials during the beauty judgment task compared to the correctness judgment task, while this phenomenon was not seen in non-muscian group. However, during the listening stage in non-musician group, differences were observed between the correctness and aesthetic judgment tasks. The neural correlates of aesthetic music processing were modulated by musical expertise.

Another subject of music phrase perception that has been studied is the perception of phrase boundaries [27]. An ERP positive wave of approximately 550 ms latency after the phrase boundary offset was found. The observed peak was similar to a positive component in respond to prosodic phrase boundaries in speech perception [28]. It was termed as closure positive shift (CPS) for correlating with prosodic phrase closure. The musical CSP was studied and found to be modulated by music expertise [27]. Nuehaus et al. used EEG and MEG methods and musical melody stimulus with phrase boundaries in the middle. Musicians showed an electric CPS and a magnetic CPS (CPSm) evoked by phrased melody versions, while nonmusicians showed an early negativity and a smaller

**Table 1.** EEG features to study complex music perception between musicians and nonmusician

| EEG features | Results |
|---|---|
| ERP early components | Early negative deflection elicited in different conditions with no group effects |
| ERP P3a | The longer latency of P3a in musicians |
| Neural entrainment to beat frequencies | The stronger neural entrainment in musicians |
| ERAN | Larger ERAN evoked by dissonant chords in musicians |
| P3 and N5 | Larger P3 and smaller N5 evoked by dissonant chords in musicians |
| Mid-latency ERP components and Microstate | Characteristic ERP responses of musicians in 300–500 ms with corresponding activated areas |
| CPS | More complex CPS in musicians |

CPSm. Zhang et al. designed a complex musical stimulus which contains boundaries at three hierarchical levels. All three boundaries evoked CPS in musician group and their amplitudes were modulated by hierarchical levels. Only period boundary (most obvious one) elicited CPS in nonmusicians and an undistinguishable negativity was induced at the three boundaries. These findings of music phrase perception suggest that the musical phrasing ability could be enhanced by music expertise or the phrasing perceptual strategies are different between the two groups.

## 3 Summary

In this paper, we reviewed EEG studies of music perception on rhythm, music phrases, and syntax perception between musicians and nonmusicians to show the effect of music training from the perspective of behavioral and cortical levels.

In summary, the perception of rhythm was usually studied using ERP or neural entrainment. Neural responses of musicians and nonmusicians were similar in the early stage and different in the later stage of rhythm processing. The P3a component evoked by a meter violation in the beats expectation task demonstrated the effects of music expertise, where musicians showed later P3a. The neural oscillations entrain to a rhythmic beat, where this entrainment was stronger in musicians than in non-musicians. Moreover, the endogenous beat-related top-down controlled neural oscillations were modulated by music expertise. These findings suggest that musicians and nonmusicians process complex rhythmic temporal patterns differently.

Moreover, neural entrainment is strengthened in musicians. In addition, musicians and nonmusicians process music phrases and syntax differently, revealed by evoked responses (ERAN, P3, and N5) to violations of chord sequences. Microstate and ERP source imaging also revealed the different mechanisms in the mid-latency period and involved cortical areas of musicians and nonmusicians in the perception of music syntax. The prosodic phrase boundaries-related CPS showed better musical phrasing ability in musicians.

The above studies revealed that cortical processing of rhythm, music phrases, and syntax differs between musicians and nonmusicians, reflecting the effects of music training on the perception of complex music elements. The mentioned EEG features and corresponding results are listed in Table 1. It should be mentioned that the discovered results are strictly conditioned by the experiment paradigm due to the complexity of the stimulus. Further EEG studies of music perception are recommended to investigate the interplay of these mechanisms, for example, in attentive and inattentive conditions.

**Acknowledgment.** This work was supported by grants from the Key Technologies Research and Development Program of China (No.2022YFF1202400) and the National Natural Science Foundation of China (No.81971698&No.82202290).

## References

1. Parbery-Clark, A., Skoe, E., Lam, C., et al.: Musician enhancement for Speech-In-Noise. Ear Hear. **30**(6), 653–661 (2009)
2. Miendlarzewska, E.A., Trost, W.J.: How musical training affects cognitive development: rhythm reward and other modulating variables. Front. Neurosci.,**7**, (2014). https://doi.org/10.3389/fnins.2013.00279
3. Du, Y., Zatorre, R.J.: Musical training sharpens and bonds ears and tongue to hear speech better. Proc. Natl. Acad. Sci. U.S.A. **114**(51), 13579–13854 (2017). https://doi.org/10.1073/pnas.1712223114
4. Bosnyak, D.J., Eaton, R.A., Roberts, L.E.: Distributed auditory cortical representations are modified when non-musicians are trained at pitch discrimination with 40 Hz amplitude modulated tones. Cereb. Cortex **14**(10), 1088–1099 (2004). https://doi.org/10.1093/cercor/bhh068
5. Koelsch, S.: Neural substrates of processing syntax and semantics in music. Curr. Opin. Neurobiol. **15**(2), 207–212 (2005)
6. González, A., Santapau, M., González Julián, J., et al.: EEG analysis during music Perception. In: Hideki, N (Ed.) Electroencephalography, pp. Ch. 2. IntechOpen, Rijeka (2020)
7. Koelsch, S.: Toward a neural basis of music perception–a review and updated model. Front. Psychol., **2**, (2011)
8. Krumhansl, C.L.: Rhythm and pitch in music cognition. Psychol. Bull. **126**(1), 159–179 (2000)
9. Phillips-Silver, J., Trainor, L.J.: Feeling the beat: Movement influences infant rhythm perception. Science **308**(5727), 1430 (2005)
10. Nozaradan, S.: Exploring how musical rhythm entrains brain activity with electroencephalogram frequency-tagging. Philos. Trans. R. Soc. B-Biol. Sci., **369**(1658), (2014)
11. Jongsma, M.L.A., Meeuwissen, E., Vos, P.G., et al.: Rhythm perception: Speeding up or slowing down affects different subcomponents of the ERP P3 complex. Biol. Psychol. **75**(3), 219–228 (2007). https://doi.org/10.1016/j.biopsycho.2007.02.003
12. Geiser, E., Ziegler, E., Jancke, L., et al.: Early electrophysiological correlates of meter and rhythm processing in music perception. Cortex **45**(1), 93–102 (2009)
13. Jongsma, M.L.A., Desain, P., Honing, H.: Rhythmic context influences the auditory evoked potentials of musicians and nonmusicians. Biol. Psychol. **66**(2), 129–152 (2004)

14. Winkler, I., Denham, S.L., Nelken, I.: Modeling the auditory scene: predictive regularity representations and perceptual objects. Trends Cogn. Sci. **13**(12), 532–540 (2009)
15. Schroeder, C.E., Lakatos, P.: Low-frequency neuronal oscillations as instruments of sensory selection. Trends Neurosci. **32**(1), 9–18 (2009). https://doi.org/10.1016/j.tins.2008.09.012
16. Stupacher, J., Wood, G., Witte, M.: Neural entrainment to polyrhythms: A comparison of musicians and Non-musicians. Front. Neurosci. **11**, 1–17 (2017). https://doi.org/10.3389/fnins.2017.00208
17. Celma-Miralles, A., Toro, J.M.: Ternary meter from spatial sounds: Differences in neural entrainment between musicians and non-musicians. Brain Cogn. **136**, (2019). Koelsch, S., Gunter, T., Friederici, A.D., et al.: Brain indices of music processing: "Non-musicians" are musical. J. Cogn. Neurosci., **12**(3), 520–541 (2000). https://doi.org/10.1162/089892900562183
18. Koelsch, S., Gunter, T.C., Schroger, E., et al.: Differentiating ERAN and MMN: An ERP study. NeuroReport **12**(7), 1385–1389 (2001)
19. Sun, L.J., Feng, C., Yang, Y.F.: Tension experience induced by nested structures in music. Front. Hum. Neurosci., **14**, (2020)
20. Koelsch, S., Grossmann, T., Gunter, T.C., et al.: Children processing music: electric brain responses reveal musical competence and gender differences. J. Cogn. Neurosci. **15**(5), 683–693 (2003). https://doi.org/10.1162/jocn.2003.15.5.683
21. Koelsch, S., Schmidt, B.H., Kansok, J.: Effects of musical expertise on the early right anterior negativity: An event-related brain potential study. Psychophysiology **39**(5), 657–663 (2002)
22. Pages-Portabella, C, Bertolo, M, Toro, J.M.: Neural correlates of acoustic dissonance in music: The role of musicianship, schematic and veridical expectations. Plos One, **16**(12), (2021)
23. James, C.E., Oechslin, M.S., Michel, C.M., et al.: Electrical neuroimaging of music processing reveals mid-latency changes with level of musical expertise. Front. Neurosci., **11**, (2017)
24. Ma, X., Ding, N., Tao, Y., et al.: Syntactic complexity and musical proficiency modulate neural processing of non-native music. Neuropsychologia **121**, 164–174 (2018)
25. Muller, M., Hofel, L., Brattico, E., et al.: Electrophysiological correlates of aesthetic music processing comparing experts with laypersons. In: DallaBella, S., Kraus, N., Overy, K., Pantev, C., Snyder, J. S., Tervaniemi, M., Tillmann, B., Schlaug, G., (Eds.), Neurosciences and Music Iii: Disorders and Plasticity, vol. 1169, pp. 355–358. (2009)
26. Neuhaus, C., Knosche, T.R., Friederici, A.D.: Effects of musical expertise and boundary markers on phrase perception in music. J. Cogn. Neurosci. **18**(3), 472–493 (2006)
27. Steinhauer, K., Friederici, A.D.: Prosodic boundaries, comma rules, and brain responses: the closure positive shift in ERPs as a universal marker for prosodic phrasing in listeners and readers. J. Psycholinguist. Res. **30**(3), 267–295 (2001)
28. Zhang, J.J., Jiang, C.M., Zhou, L.S., et al.: Perception of hierarchical boundaries in music and its modulation by expertise. Neuropsychologia **91**, 490–498 (2016)

# Virtual Reality Game-Based Adaptive Neurofeedback Training for Motor Imagery

Kun Wang[1], Feifan Tian[1], Lincong Pan[2], Minpeng Xu[1,2(✉)], Minglun Li[2], Bowen Dong[1], and Dong Ming[1,2]

[1] Academy of Medical Engineering and Translational Medicine, Tianjin University, Tianjin, China
xmp52637@tju.edu.cn

[2] College of Precision Instruments and Optoelectronics Engineering, Tianjin University, Tianjin, China

**Abstract.** Motor imagery-based brain-computer interfaces (MI-BCIs) are promising tools for motor rehabilitation applications. However, neurofeedback training (NFT) of traditional MI is boring and takes a long time. This study aimed to investigate whether adaptive NFT in virtual reality (VR) scenes could improve MI-BCI performance. In this study, we proposed a VR game-based MI-BCI paradigm that contained left and right upper limbs MI tasks. In the course of training, the system could adaptively adjust the game difficulty and dynamic output decoding result according to the training performance of individuals. Six subjects participated in the experiments. After three days of NFT, the activation of the motor cortex was enhanced. The average accuracy of MI tasks reached 83.52%, with an increase of 10.46%, compared with before training. The results demonstrate that the adaptive NFT system based on VR games proposed in this study has a good effect on MI performance and is expected to be used in rehabilitation training and treatment for stroke.

**Keywords:** Motor imagery · Virtual reality game · Electroencephalogram · Event-related De-synchronization · Neurofeedback training

## 1 Introduction

Recently, brain-computer interfaces (BCIs) have attracted wide attention for their great potential in clinical applications. As one of the most important BCI paradigms, motor imagery-based BCI (MI-BCI) is usually applied in stroke rehabilitation [1]. For the study of BCIs, electroencephalogram (EEG) is one popular brain signal recording method due to its high time resolution, low cost, and non-invasive. MI tasks could induce event-related de-synchronization/synchronization (ERD/ERS) patterns in alpha (8~13 Hz) and beta (13~30 Hz) frequency bands over the brain region corresponding to the motor cortex.

Wang and Tian: These authors contributed equally to this work and should be considered co-first authors


G. Wang et al. (Eds.): APCMBE 2023, IFMBE Proceedings 103, pp. 296–303, 2024.
https://doi.org/10.1007/978-3-031-51455-5_33

In fact, the principle of rehabilitation based on MI-BCI is to enhance neuroplasticity through neurofeedback training (NFT) which offers online feedback to users to facilitate neural self-regulation [2]. For stroke rehabilitation studies, researchers focused on whether the ERD features were enhanced and whether the accuracy of motor intention decoding was improved after NFT based on MI-BCI [3]. However, the training process of the traditional MI-BCI paradigm was boring and took a long time, which reduced the effect of NFT. Hence, researchers explored multi-modal sensory feedback methods such as vision, hearing, and touch, and combined them with MI-BCI to induce the reconstruction and enhancement of motor functions [4–6].

In recent years, many studies have added virtual reality (VR) technology and game scenarios into the design of MI paradigms, which has made MI training more efficient and interesting. For instance, Vourvopoulos et al. allowed stroke patients to practice observation and drive the virtual incarnation arm in VR, which showed the clinical practicality of the BCI-VR system [7]. Karácsony et al. further indicated that the MI-BCI-VR system can be used for real-time game applications [8]. Miao et al. showed that stroke patients who used virtual limb and FES feedback had better medical rehabilitation outcomes than those who used FES feedback alone [9].

Although the existing research has proven the feasibility of the MI-BCI-VR system, few studies focused on optimizing the length of training time and difficulty. In this work, we proposed a real-time MI-BCI paradigm based on a VR "fruit-cutting" game. The NFT training time and difficulty can be adjusted adaptively according to different training individuals and training effects. This study aimed to investigate the effects of VR game-based adaptive NFT on MI performance.

## 2 Materials and Methods

### 2.1 Participants

Six subjects participated in this experiment (all right-handed, 20~25 years old, 3 men). All subjects were healthy without any limb motor disorders or neurological diseases. They were all beginners in MI experiments. Before the experiment, we obtained the consent of the subjects and the approval of the Ethics Committee of Tianjin University.

### 2.2 Procedure of Experiment

All experiments were conducted in a quiet laboratory and subject sat comfortably in a chair during the experiment. When performing MI tasks, they uniformly imagined the movement of bent and stretched-out elbows in kinesthetic imagery. In this study, each subject performed the same experiment 3 times on days 1, 3, and 5. The experiment of each time was divided into 4 sessions. The main purpose of session 1 was to collect the subject's resting state EEG, consisting of 30 trials. Session 2 and Session 4 were identical paradigms based on the classic MI-BCI paradigm Graz to compare the training effects of the VR-based adaptive NFT paradigm. Session 3 was the MI-BCI-VR "fruit-cutting" game paradigm designed by Unity3D software and used for NFT. Sessions 2, 3, and 4 each had 3 blocks. Each block included 20 trials (10 trials for left MI tasks, and 10

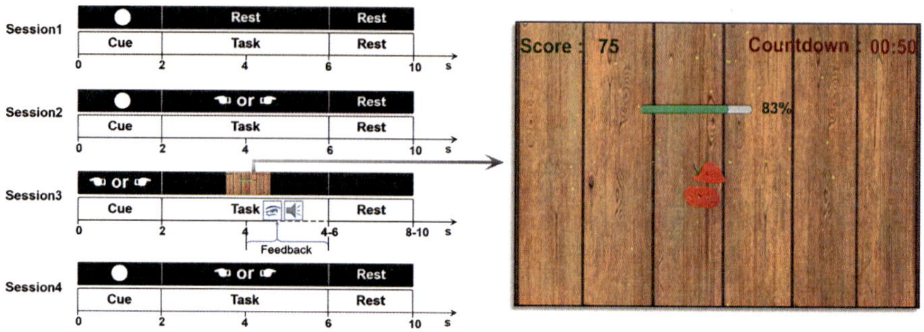


**Fig. 1.** The timeline of one trial of the experimental paradigm

trials for right MI tasks, randomly sorted). It was worth noting that only session 3 was an adaptive online experiment, and the other three sessions were offline experiments.

The timeline of a single trial for each session is presented in Fig. 1. In the offline sessions, every trial commenced with a white circle appearing in the center of the display screen for a duration of 2 s. Then a symbol or words of instruction lasting for 4s were presented to the subjects, during which they were instructed to perform the specified MI task or relax. The trial concluded with a 4s period of rest. In session 3, the subjects wore the VR headset display device throughout the process and completed the experiment in a virtual scene. At 0~2 s of a trial, the direction cue appeared in the center of the visual field. Then, a fruit randomly popped up from the lower left or lower right of the screen (to prevent brain lateralization [10], the range of fruit appeared near the center of the screen), during which, the subjects performed their MI tasks. In 4~6 s, if the system decoded the subject's motor intention correctly, released the game scene in which the fruit was cut, if it incorrectly, the fruit disappeared. Then the maximum decision value of the trial was fed in the form of the progress bar, and the 4s rest state followed.

During EEG signal collection, a Neuroscan Synamps2 amplifier was utilized to record signals from 60 electrodes, which were positioned according to the international 10–20 system, with the reference electrode placed above the head and the prefrontal lobe serving as ground. To eliminate frequency interference, a 50 Hz trap filter was also employed.

## 2.3 EEG Signals Analysis

First of all, we resampled the original sampling frequency from 1000 Hz to 200 Hz. Then we conducted a 1~40 Hz bandpass filtering and Common average reference (CAR) processing. In order to analyze the ERD patterns generated by different limb movements, we calculated the event-related spectral perturbation (ERSP) value of left and right MI tasks in session 2 and session 4 (hereinafter referred to as Graz1 and Graz2). The frequency range was 5~30 Hz, and the time range was 1.5~6 s. The ERSP average value of 1.5~2 s was used as the baseline. The typical channels C3 and C4 were selected for the time-frequency analysis. In addition, we also calculated the average ERSP of alpha and beta rhythm within 2~6s, which was used to characterize brain topographical distribution containing the spatial characteristics of 60 channels.

## 2.4 Feature Extraction and Pattern Classification

For the feature extraction of offline data in session 1 and session 2, we selected 36 channels (FT7, FC5, FC3, FC1, FCz, FC2, FC4, FC6, FT8, T7, C5, C3, C1, CZ, C2, C4, C6, T8, TP7, CP5, CP3, CP1, CPz, CP2, CP4, CP6, TP8, P7, P5, P3, P1, Pz, P2, P4, P6, P8) for data processing. The study used the integrated frequency band Common Spatial Pattern (CSP) algorithm to optimize the CSP frequency band parameter. We divided 4~36 Hz into 46 sub-frequency bands with overlapping and different widths using different 5-order Butterworth filters. After that, Multiclass CSP was used to extract the features of 3 task categories (resting state, left MI, right MI) in each sub-band signal. We employed the Multiclass Support Vector Machine (SVM) algorithm for classification by Libsvm software package [11]. And then selected the 30 sub-frequency bands with the highest accuracy by grid search method to establish their SVM models for online decisions of session 3.

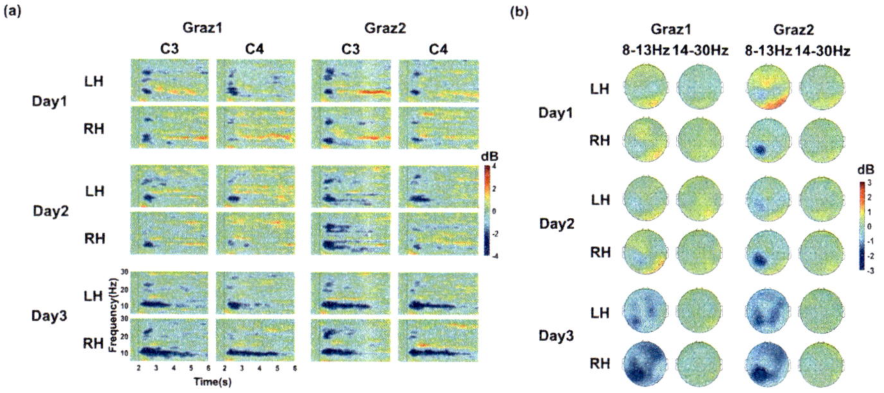


**Fig. 2.** **a** The average time-frequency diagram of the Graz paradigm; **b** The average ERSP topography of the Graz paradigm

Session 3 was a scoring game, with the difficulty of each block determined by the user's performance in the previous experiment. The subjects completed the game interaction of brain-controlled fruit cutting through the MI task. In a block of 100 points, they scored 5 points for cutting one fruit. In each trial of session 3, the system calculated 2 ~ 4, 2~4.4, 2 ~ 4.8, 2~5.2s, 2~5.6 s, 5 time periods' decision results and fed back in real-time. During each time online decision, the percentage of correct prediction of 30 SVM models established in the offline stage was taken as the decision value. In addition, we set a fixed decision threshold for each block. When the decision value above was greater than this threshold, the fruit would be cut. Hence, the fruit can be cut or not adaptively within 4~6 s depending on the subject's MI performance. We set the first block threshold to 50%, changed the threshold of the latter block according to the previous block game score, then the "game difficulty" would be changed.

Due to observing the impact of adaptive NFT on classification accuracy, we used the integrated frequency band CSP algorithm and SVM algorithm to perform feature extraction and pattern recognition on the data of Graz1 and Graz2 (left MI and right MI categories), respectively.

# 3 Results

## 3.1 EEG Patterns of Motor Imagery

Figure 2a is the average time-frequency diagram of the traditional paradigm Graz before and after VR game-based adaptively NFT under channels C3 and C4. When the subject began to perform the MI task after 2 s, the ERSP decreased significantly, which is an ERD phenomenon. The improvement in ERD intensity of Graz2 was not improved after the first day of NFT. On both the second and third days, the subjects' ERD pattern performance in Graz2 after the online fruit-cutting training was superior to that of Graz1 before the training. Moreover, the intensity, duration, and frequency band distribution of ERD activation in Graz2 increased gradually with the number of training days, especially in alpha rhythm. But Graz1 did not show this pattern of improvement. This meant that NFT was effective on the day, but the durability of the improvement needs further evaluation.

Figure 2b is the average ERSP topographical distribution of the Graz paradigm in the alpha and beta rhythm. As can be seen from the figure, the ERD in the alpha rhythm is more pronounced than in the beta rhythm. In addition, we found that the ERSP values in the right MI are lower than that in the left MI, and showed a better contralateral ERD dominance, possibly due to the subjects being right-handed. With an increase in the number of training days, the intensity of ERD in both left and right MI was enhanced, and the range of ERD distribution in brain regions was gradually expanded. However, similar to the time-frequency diagram, the effect of daily training could be observed in the brain topographic map of Graz2, but this improvement was not continuously enhanced across days in Graz1.

## 3.2 Classification Performance

To evaluate the effectiveness of NFT, classification accuracy is a crucial metric. The average accuracies (left MI and right MI categories) of 6 subjects in the Graz, paradigm are displayed in Fig. 3. The results are generated by the integrated band CSP feature extraction algorithm and SVM classification recognition algorithm above. As can be seen from the results of a single day, although each NFT improved the classification accuracy rate differently, Graz2 outperformed Graz1 in terms of accuracy rate, with a maximum increase of 12.59% ($p < 0.05$, paired T-test) on the third day. Despite the growth trend of a single day not extending to the entire cross-day experiment process, the classification accuracy rate of Graz2 on the third day was the highest within three days which reached 83.52% and increasing 10.46% compared to Graz1's on the first day. Therefore, the upper limb MI-BCI paradigm based on the VR "fruit-cutting" game has been used for NFT with positive effects on MI performance.

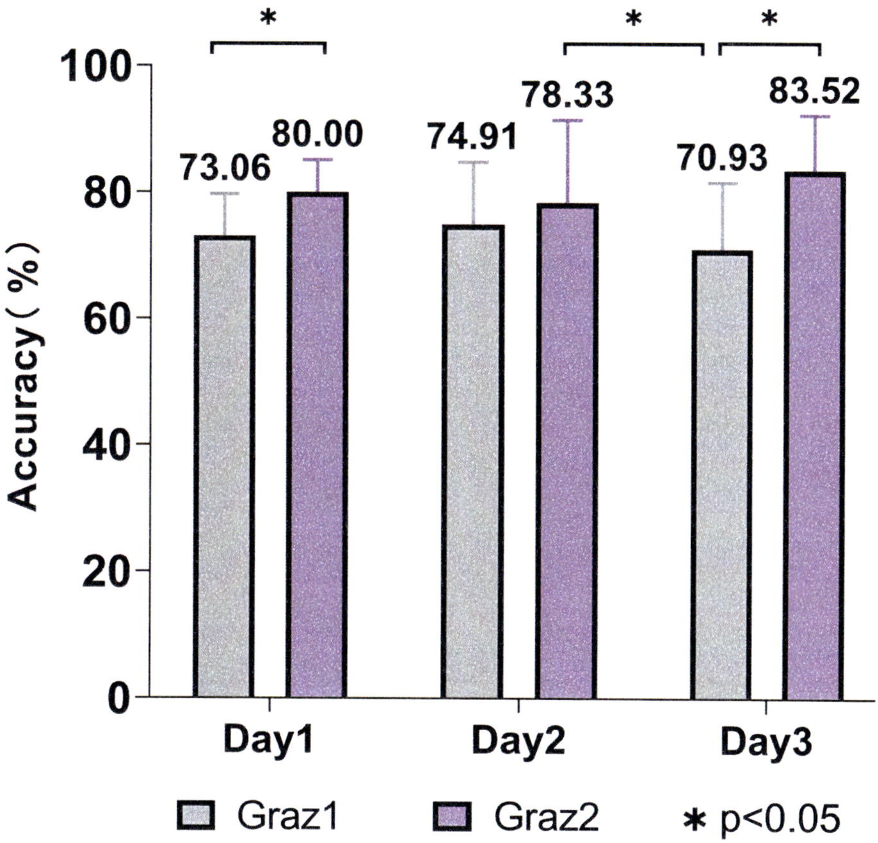


**Fig. 3.** The average accuracy of the subjects in the Graz paradigm

## 4 Discussion

This study demonstrated that the day's adaptive NFT based on the VR game could not only enhance the intensity, duration, and channel distribution range of ERD induced by MI but also improve the classification accuracies of upper limbs MI tasks (Figs. 2 and 3). Nonetheless, with an increase in the number of training days, we did not observe a consistent enhancement in MI performance across the training days. This indicates that the improvement was only effective on the day of training and did not carry over to the beginning of the subsequent training session. Which was inconsistent with existing research [1]. Despite this, it is still worthwhile to investigate cross-day neurofeedback training since the MI performance of the subjects showed significant improvement after the final day of training compared to their performance before the initial day of training in this study. The EEG signal is nonstationary, which leads to the difference across time, and fluctuations in MI performance. The limited number of subjects in this paper may be another reason for the inconsistent results. In addition, the immersion and vividness of the VR game in this paper need to be further improved. In future research, we will optimize the experimental scheme, add the control experiments of the traditional NFT, and analyze the effect of the VR game-based NFT on MI performance from multiple perspectives.

## 5 Conclusions

In this study, we proposed a novel MI-BCI paradigm based on a VR game for adaptive NFT and used the traditional Graz paradigm to analyze the effects of NFT. Experimental results showed that both ERD activations classification accuracies were noticeably improved after the VR game-based adaptive NFT. These findings verified the effectiveness of the proposed paradigm in enhancing the activation of the motor cortex and improving MI-BCI performance. It is expected to be further used in the rehabilitation treatment of stroke patients and real-time game applications of MI-BCI in the future.

**Acknowledgment.** We express our sincere gratitude to all participants for their invaluable contributions to this study. Additionally, we acknowledge the support of STI 2030—Major Projects 2022ZD0208900, National Natural Science Foundation of China (62206198, 62122059, 81925020).

## References

1. Wang, Z., Cao, C., Chen, L., et al.: Multimodal neural response and effect assessment during a BCI-based neurofeedback training after stroke. Front. Neurosci. **16**, 884420 (2022). https://doi.org/10.3389/fnins.2022.884420
2. Sitaram, R., Ros, T., Stoeckel, L., et al.: Closed-loop brain training: the science of neurofeedback. Nat. Rev. Neurosci. **18**(2), 86–100 (2017). https://doi.org/10.1038/nrn.2016.164
3. Biasiucci, A., Leeb, R., Iturrate, I., et al.: Brain-actuated functional electrical stimulation elicits lasting arm motor recovery after stroke. Nat. Commun. **9**(1), 2421 (2018). https://doi.org/10.1038/s41467-018-04673-z
4. Hecht, D., Reiner, M., & A, K.: Enhancement of response times to bi- and tri-modal sensory stimuli during active movements. Exp. Brain. Res. **185**(4), 655-665 (2008). https://doi.org/10.1007/s00221-007-1191-x
5. Shams, L., AR, S.: Benefits of multisensory learning. Trends Cogn. Sci. **12**(11), 411-417 (2008). https://doi.org/10.1016/j.tics.2008.07.006
6. Wang, Z., Zhou, Y., Chen, L., et al.: A BCI based visual-haptic neurofeedback training improves cortical activations and classification performance during motor imagery. J. Neural Eng. **16**(6), 066012 (2019). https://doi.org/10.1088/1741-2552/ab377d
7. Vourvopoulos, A., Marin-Pardo, O., Neureither, M., et al.: Multimodal head-mounted virtual-reality brain-computer interface for stroke rehabilitation, virtual, augmented and mixed reality, vol. 11574. Multimodal Interaction, FL, USA **2019**, 165–179 (2019)
8. Karácsony, T., Hansen, J.P., Iversen, H.K., et al.: Brain computer interface for neuro-rehabilitation with deep learning classification and virtual reality feedback, the 10th Augmented Human International Conference, Reims, France, 2019. pp 1-8 (2019)
9. Miao, Y., Chen, S., Zhang, X., et al.: BCI-Based Rehabilitation on the Stroke in Sequela Stage. Neural Plast. **2020**, 8882764 (2020). https://doi.org/10.1155/2020/8882764

10. Wu, X., Kong, X., Vatansever, D., et al.: Dynamic changes in brain lateralization correlate with human cognitive performance. PLoS Biol. **20**(3), e3001560 (2022). https://doi.org/10.1371/journal.pbio.3001560
11. Chang, C.C., Lin, C.J.: LIBSVM: a library for support vector machines. ACM Trans. Intell. Syst. Technol. (TIST) **2**(3), 1–27 (2011). https://doi.org/10.1145/1961189.1961199

# Effects of Sequence Order on Motor Imagery Based on Observing and Delayed Matching Task

Mengfan Li[1,2,3,4(✉)], Enming Qi[1,2,3,4], Qi Zhao[1,2,3,4], and Guizhi Xu[1,2,3,4]

[1] State Key Laboratory of Reliability and Intelligence of Electrical Equipment, Tianjin 300132, China
mfli@hebut.edu.cn

[2] School of Health Sciences and Biomedical Engineering, Hebei University of Technology, Tianjin 300132, China

[3] Hebei Key Laboratory of Bioelectromagnetics and Neuroengineering, Tianjin 300132, China

[4] Tianjin Key Laboratory of Bioelectromagnetic Technology and Intelligent Health, Tianjin 300132, China

**Abstract.** Motor Imagery (MI) is one of the widely used paradigms for BCI, and its signal is an endogenous EEG signal that is not dependent on external stimuli. The performance of brain-computer interfaces (BCI) based on motor imagery is influenced by the way people imagine. Action sequences are the basic units for imitating, learning, and remembering motor behaviors, and it is unclear whether action sequences affect MI-BCI. This study proposes a task paradigm with different sequence order to investigate the effect of sequence order on MI by guiding people through images and videos for action observation (AO) and MI. The MI performance of four subjects is analyzed under different sequence order. The test results show that different sequence order leads to different MI classification accuracy, with positive sequence acting with 9.69% higher MI classification accuracy than negative sequence ($p < 0.05$). The study shows that the sequence order has a significant effect on MI. It is expected that the study in this paper may provide a new perspective for improving MI—BCI imaging.

**Keywords:** Action observation · Sequence order · Brain-computer interfaces · Motor imagery

## 1 Introduction

Brain-computer interfaces (BCI) can translate brain activity directly into commands, establishing a communication path between the brain and external devices independent of peripheral nerves and muscles [1]. Motor imagery (MI) [2, 3], steady-state evoked potentials (SSVEP) [4], and event-related potentials (ERP) [5] are all common approaches to EEG-based BCI. The MI-based BCI system (MI-BCI) is a BCI system that does not require external stimuli and can reflect the user's voluntary motor awareness [6]. When people only imagine limb movement, event-related desynchronization (ERD) and event-related synchronization (ERS) phenomena occur in the sensorimotor areas of


G. Wang et al. (Eds.): APCMBE 2023, IFMBE Proceedings 103, pp. 304–310, 2024.
https://doi.org/10.1007/978-3-031-51455-5_34

the contralateral and ipsilateral hemispheres, respectively [7]. And the performance of ERD directly affects MI classification accuracy. In many cases, subjects have difficulty completing abstract MI processes, which leads to a low level of sensorimotor cortical activation and thus limiting the effective recognition of motor intention. Therefore, how to train subjects to perform MI effectively is important to improve MI-BCI performance.

Action observation (AO) can be defined as "the perception of another person's movement", and it is a simulation of motor behavior, as is MI [8]. Research has shown that there is a functional association between AO and MI: they both activate motor neural networks, and the cortical areas activated for the same movement pattern overlap [9]. Furthermore, studies have shown that task-complexity has a significant effect on the MI performance. Specifically, complex imagery task induces a stronger activation of sensorimotor cortical, which increases a stronger ERD phenomenon and further improves the classification accuracy of the MI-BCI. Researches have shown that both increasing task complexity and adopting a fusion paradigm help to modulate brain sensorimotor rhythms and optimize subjects' MI performance. However, task complexity is defined by setting imaginary task difficulty gradients in most studies. Few reports have shown how the sequence order of actions in the MI paradigm affects MI performance, and sequence order is also an important factor affecting action difficulty. The literature first proposed the use of positive sequences instead of random sequences for yield augmentation, which reduced workload and improved comfort [10]. Another similar study found that positive sequences performed better for memory learning compared to random sequences [11]. However, there are few reports on how action sequences affect MI performance. We hypothesize that sequence order has an effect on MI and attempt to explore this by using the MI paradigm of sequence order.

In this paper, we propose a novel fusion paradigm with additional action sequence sequences to investigate the effects of sequence order on MI. The paradigm combines AO images and video guidance to verify the differences in subjects' motor imagery effects for different sequence order. The effect of sequence order on MI-BCI found in this study not only provides a new approach to explore the MI-BCI process, but also provides a guide to improve MI-BCI performance through action sequence order in the future.

# 2 Material and Method

## 2.1 Experimental Paradigm

(1) Order of the Action sequences

As shown in Fig. 1, two types of sequence order are applied to explore the influence of action sequences on the MI performance: the positive sequence of actions (P) and the negative sequence of actions (N). In this study, the discrete sequences are arranged in chronological order according to people's habits, and the sequence is defined as a positive sequence, and the order of discrete sequences in the negative sequence is exactly opposite to the order of positive sequences in terms of chronological order. In this study, sketches were used as experimental materials, and videos and images of sketching on white paper with a pen in hand were used as visual materials.

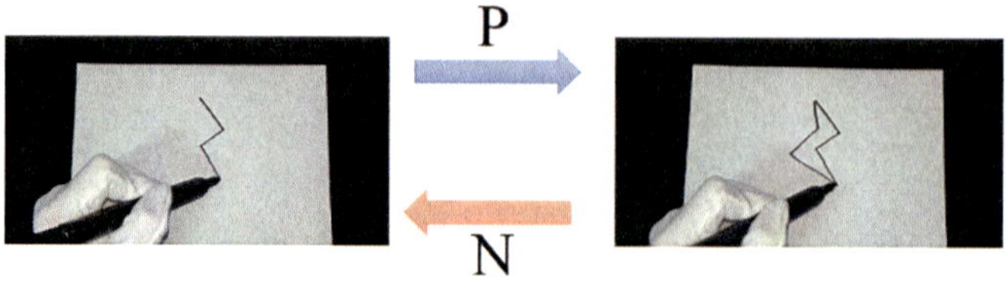


**Fig. 1.** Order of the Action sequences. P: the positive sequence of actions. N: the negative sequence of actions.

(2) The Paradigm Processes

Our MI paradigm with different sequence order in time is shown in Fig. 2. In one trial, subjects performed the corresponding task time sequences according to the trial as shown in Fig. 2. Each subject performs two trials.

First, a total of six sequential videos are played for the subjects to memorize, with each group spaced 3 s apart. And then, subjects match 25 visual image stimuli to the video of the action sequence from memory by pressing keys. At the beginning (t = 0 s), a white cross is displayed in the center of the screen for 3 s (t = 0–3 s) to remind the subject to prepare. Then, a visual image stimulus is presented in the next 6s (t = 3–9 s) to allow the subject to make a judgment. A total of 25 trials constitute this phase. Finally, subjects performed MI while performing AO. First, 0–1 s is the cueing phase, 1–7 s is the MI phase, where arrows indicate which hand to imagine, and the video provides dynamic guidance for the subject's specific imagery actions. Each subject performed two sets of sequence order MI of P and N, each with a total of 160 trials can be collected from a single subject in a single experiment.

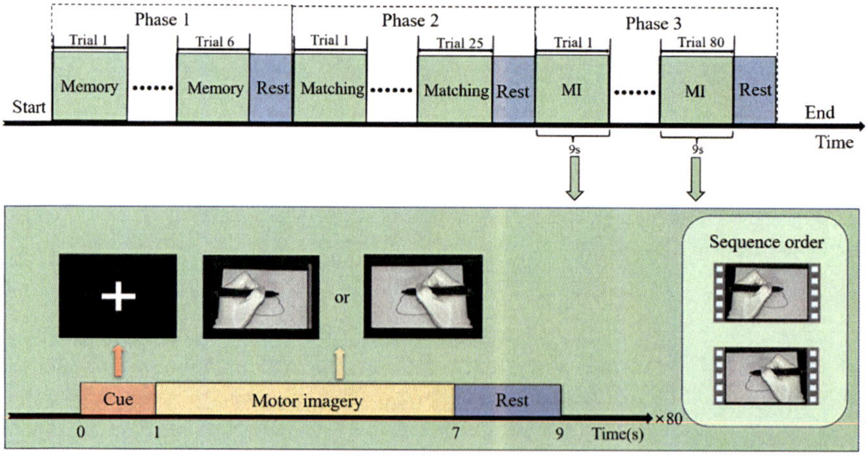


**Fig. 2.** Timing of our subject-specific MI paradigm with different sequence order.

### 2.2 Data Collection and Preprocessing

Subjects were asked to sit 80 cm from the screen with their eyes at the same level as the screen. The visualization interface is located in the center of a 19–inch LED monitor with a refresh rate of 60 Hz and a screen resolution of 1920 × 1080. 64 channels of EEG data from the whole brain were acquired using Neuroscan SynAmps2 amplifiers at a sampling rate of 1000 Hz. The channels are arranged according to the 10–20 international system. Twenty-one channels located near the supplementary motor area are selected for analysis of the subject's MI. Reference channels are located in the binaural mastoids A1 and A2. All impedances are below 5 kΩ.

Common spatial pattern (CSP) is a widely used spatial filtering feature extraction algorithm for MI-BCI for extracting the spatial distribution components [12, 13]. The specific formulation can be found in the paper [14]. Support vector machine (SVM) is used to classify the left and right hands [15]. In this paper, a support vector machine is used to classify the features extracted by the CSP with a linear kernel function and a regularization parameter set to 1.

## 3 Result

### 3.1 EEG Results Analysis

To illustrate the impact of the sequence order on the MI, Fig. 3 uses the power spectral densities (PSD) to evaluate four subjects' ERD/ERS in the P and N. For the P task, the energy from right-hand motor imagery is lower than left-hand motor imagery at C3, and the energy from left-hand motor imagery is lower than right-hand motor imagery at C4. For the N task, there was no significant difference of two classes of MI tasks at C3. This PSD analysis implies that the paradigm designed in this paper can activate the MI activity in the main frequency, and the P evokes a larger ERD/ERS difference than the N.

### 3.2 Classification Accuracy of the MI-BCI

To more visually represent the differences in subjects' MI performance in different sequence orders, the average offline classification accuracy of the four subjects is given in Table 1 and Fig. 4. The results show that the sequence order of actions has a significant effect on classification accuracy. The average classification accuracy of positive sequence is 70.94%, 9.69% higher than that of negative sequence ($P < 0.05$). Among the 4 subjects, S3 have the best classification performance, and the classification accuracy of positive sequence was 88.75%, 13.75% higher than that of negative sequence ($P < 0.05$). This indicates that sequence order can significantly affect the classification precision of MI and thus affect the performance of MI-BCI.

## 4 Discussion

The results show that the average classification accuracy of the positive sequences of the four subjects is 70.94%, and the average classification accuracy of the negative sequences is 61.25%, and the positive sequences are 9.69% higher than the negative sequences.

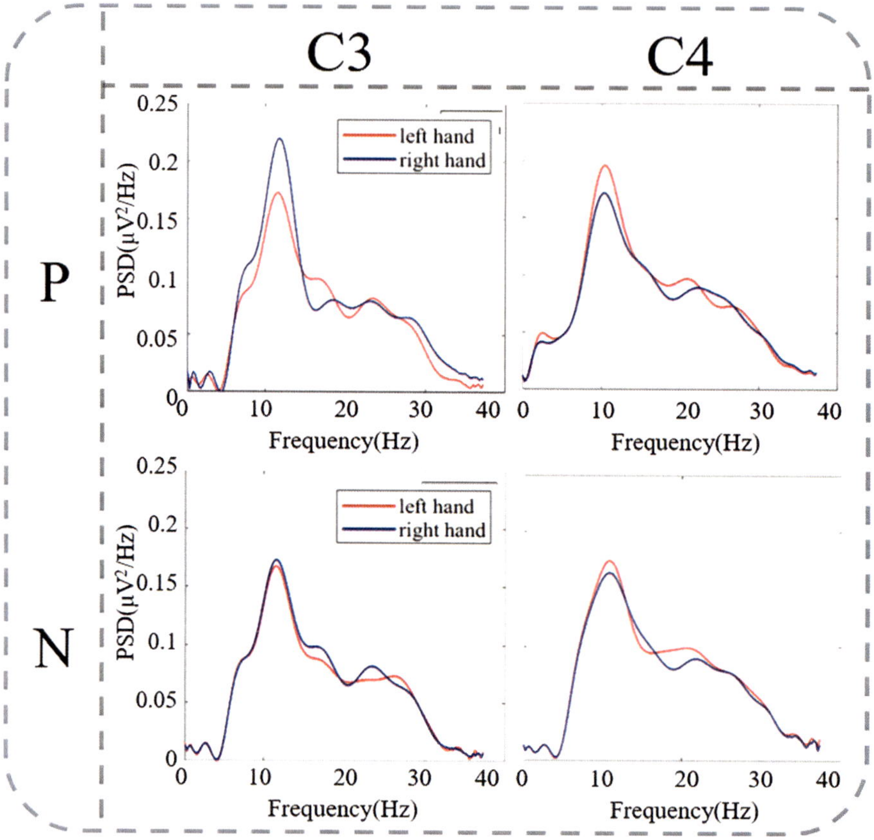


**Fig. 3.** This Fig displays the averaged PSD of P and N at C3 and C4 (blue: right hand, red: left hand).

**Table 1.** Accuracy in different sequence order

| Subject | Positive sequence | Negative sequence |
|---|---|---|
| S1 | 75.00 | 62.50 |
| S2 | 61.25 | 56.25 |
| S3 | 88.75 | 75.00 |
| S4 | 58.75 | 51.25 |
| Average | 70.94 | 61.25 |

The average accuracy of positive sequences is higher than that of negative sequences for all four subjects. According to the above results, it can be seen that the sequence order has a significant impact on MI, and the positive sequence can produce higher accuracy in MI classification.

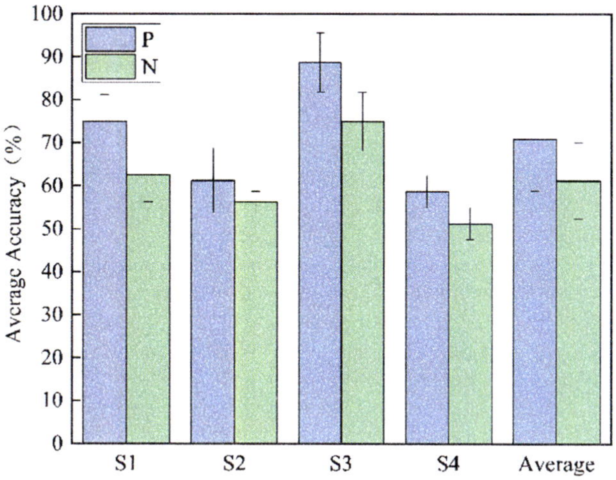


**Fig. 4.** Average accuracy of different sequence order

The major possible reason is that the degree of familiarity may be the main reason for the difference. Many studies have shown that familiar actions and scenes help to improve subjects' imagery effects. Due to familiarity, The P seems to be more suitable for most subjects, People are approaching almost all tasks in a positive order. In most cases, subjects tend to feel simpler with things they are more familiar with, and familiar actions and scenes help improve subjects' image effects. Those with high proficiency have significantly higher MI effects when imagining actions than those with low proficiency. Positive sequences are more widely known, and therefore subjects obtain better MI performance in P. The PSD curves shown in Fig. 3 also validate this belief. For channels C3 and C4, the PSD of P at the main frequency is significantly higher than that of N where fatigue is higher. This indicates that stronger fatigue inhibits activation of the subject's sensorimotor areas, thereby attenuating the signal provided for categorization, and therefore subjects obtain worse MI performance in N.

## 5 Conclusion

This study proposes a new task paradigm, which demonstrates the effect of sequence order on MI through positive sequences and negative sequences of actions. The results show that sequence order significantly affects MI-BCI performance, and that positive sequence yields higher MI classification accuracy. This study provides an insight into the factors affecting MI and BCI performance and has the potential to further improve the BCI system. Theoretically, the factors that cause differences in BCI control performance can all be used as predictors of BCI manipulation ability. If a method can be used in the future to identify an individual's preferred action sequence before the subject undergoes MI training, the training efficiency of MI can be effectively improved.

## References

1. Ju, J., Feleke, A.G., Luo, L., Fan, X.: Recognition of drivers' hard and soft braking intentions based on hybrid brain-computer interfaces. Cyborg and Bionic Systems **2022**, 1–13 (2022). https://doi.org/10.34133/2022/9847652
2. Zhu, Y., Li, C., Jin, H., Sun, L.: Classifying motion intention of step length and synchronous walking speed by functional near-infrared spectroscopy. Cyborg and Bionic Systems **2021**, 1–11 (2021). https://doi.org/10.34133/2021/9821787
3. Achanccaray, D., Izumi, S.-I., Hayashibe, M.: Visual-electrotactile stimulation feedback to improve immersive brain-computer interface based on hand motor imagery. Comput. Intell. Neurosci. **2021**, 1–13 (2021). https://doi.org/10.1155/2021/8832686
4. Wang, M., et al.: A new hybrid BCI paradigm based on P300 and SSVEP. J. Neurosci. Methods **244**, 16–25 (2015). https://doi.org/10.1016/j.jneumeth.2014.06.003
5. Jin, J., Daly, I., Zhang, Y., Wang, X., Cichocki, A.: An optimized ERP brain–computer interface based on facial expression changes. J. Neural Eng. **11**(3), 036004 (2014). https://doi.org/10.1088/1741-2560/11/3/036004
6. Bufalari, I., Sforza, A., Cesari, P., Aglioti, S.M., Fourkas, A.D.: Motor imagery beyond the joint limits: A transcranial magnetic stimulation study. Biol. Psychol. **85**(2), 283–290 (2010). https://doi.org/10.1016/j.biopsycho.2010.07.015
7. Boiten, F., Sergeant, J., Geuze, R.: Event-related desynchronization: the effects of energetic and computational demands. Electroencephalogr. Clin. Neurophysiol. **82**(4), 302–309 (1992). https://doi.org/10.1016/0013-4694(92)90110-4
8. Kaneko, N., Yokoyama, H., Masugi, Y., Watanabe, K., Nakazawa, K.: Phase dependent modulation of cortical activity during action observation and motor imagery of walking: An EEG study. Neuroimage **225**, 117486 (2021). https://doi.org/10.1016/j.neuroimage.2020.117486
9. Kaneko, N., Yokoyama, H., Masugi, Y., Watanabe, K., Nakazawa, K.: Phase dependent modulation of cortical activity during action observation and motor imagery of walking: An EEG study. NeuroImage, **225**, 117486
10. Höhne, J., Tangermann, M.: Towards user-friendly spelling with an auditory brain-computer interface: The CharStreamer Paradigm. PLoS ONE, **9**(6), e98322
11. Garr, E.: Contributions of the basal ganglia to action sequence learning and performance. Neurosci. Biobehav. Rev. **107**, 279–295 (2019). https://doi.org/10.1016/j.neubiorev.2019.09.017
12. Ang, K.K., Chin, Z.Y., Zhang, H., Guan, C.: Robust filter bank common spatial pattern (RFBCSP) in motor-imagery-based brain-computer interface. In: 2009 Annual international conference of the IEEE engineering in medicine and biology society, minneapolis, MN, pp. 578–581. https://doi.org/10.1109/IEMBS.2009.5332817
13. Qiu, Z., et al.: Optimized motor imagery paradigm based on imagining chinese characters writing movement. IEEE Trans. Neural Syst. Rehabil. Eng., **25**(7), 1009–1017
14. Lotte, F., Guan, C.: Regularizing common spatial patterns to improve BCI designs: unified theory and new algorithms. IEEE Trans. Biomed. Eng., **58**(2), 355–362 (2011). https://doi.org/10.1109/TBME.2010.2082539
15. Ahn, S., Ahn, M., Cho, H., Chan Jun, S.: Achieving a hybrid brain–computer interface with tactile selective attention and motor imagery. J. Neural Eng., **11**(6), 066004

# Hand Movement Recognition Using Dynamical Graph Convolutional Neural Network in EEG Source Space

Yi Tao[1,2], Weiwei Xu[1,2], Jialin Zhu[1,2], Maode Wang[3], and Gang Wang[1,2](✉)

[1] Key Laboratory of Biomedical Information Engineering of Ministry of Education, School of Life Science and Technology, Institute of Health and Rehabilitation Sciences, Xi'an Jiaotong University, Xi'an, China
ggwang@xjtu.edu.cn

[2] Key Laboratory of Neuro-Informatics and Rehabilitation Engineering of Ministry of Civil Affairs, Xi'an, China

[3] Department of Neurosurgery, The First Affiliated Hospital of Xi'an Jiaotong University, Xi'an, China

**Abstract.** Brain-computer interface (BCI) has been widely used in the field of medical rehabilitation related to hand movement. However, the single-handed multi-class movement recognition has remained mostly unexplored. In order to improve the accuracy of hand movement classification, an algorithm using dynamical graph convolutional neural network (DGCNN) in electroencephalogram (EEG) source space (sDGCNN) was proposed in this paper. The algorithm firstly maps EEG signals to source space by spatial source localization method. Secondly, time-domain features are extracted from each brain region. Finally, the graphs with brain regions as nodes and extracted features as node values are input into DGCNN for four-classification. The signals in $\gamma$ band (30–100 Hz) reached the highest accuracy of $90.16 \pm 6.8\%$, which indicates that the high-frequency components of brain may have important significance for hand movement decoding. The result shows that the sDGCNN method significantly improves the accuracy of hand movement classification. The high accuracy also proves the effectiveness of the method in hand movement recognition.

**Keywords:** Brain-computer interface · Source space · Dynamical graph convolution neural network · Hand movement intent recognition

## 1 Introduction

Brain computer interface (BCI) [1] is able to predict movement by analyzing changes in brain activity before the movement is performed, enabling the device to identify and execute the corresponding command earlier. BCI has been widely used in the field of medical rehabilitation related to hand function movement [2, 3]. By extracting and analyzing features related to hand movements from brain signals, the movement intention of subjects can be obtained. The output command from the BCI can then control the


G. Wang et al. (Eds.): APCMBE 2023, IFMBE Proceedings 103, pp. 311–322, 2024.
https://doi.org/10.1007/978-3-031-51455-5_35

intelligent prosthesis [4] or help patients complete rehabilitation training [5]. At present, some studies have achieved good results in binary classification of single hand [6–9]. However, there are still many problems to be solved in the research of one-handed multi-class movement classification [10–12].

Electroencephalogram (EEG) is a signal transmitted to the scalp after the discharge of neurons, which is detected and recorded by electrodes on the scalp. Due to its non-invasive and high safety [13, 14], EEG has been analyzed in many studies. However, the signal amplitude will be diminished to a certain extent during the propagation. In addition, the electrical signals of neurons in the adjacent areas also interfere. These bring great challenges to hand movement decoding. Therefore, some studies used EEG source localization technology to project scalp EEG into source space, which manifest the geometric structure of the brain, to distinguish single-handed multi-class hand movements [15].

With the popularity of deep learning, an accumulating body of research applies convolutional neural network (CNN) to extract features from signals and then classify [16]. The traditional CNN uses convolution kernel to extract local features, which is suitable for 1D, 2D and 3D data. However, EEG signals of different channels are distributed in different regions of the brain, which can be regarded as irregular non-Euclidean structural data. In this case, CNN is inappropriate because it results in the loss of information about the spatial distribution of EEG. Inspired by the graph theory [17], Defferrard et al. [18] designed graph convolution neural network (GCNN) for non-Euclidean data analysis. Song et al. [19] proposed dynamic graph convolution neural network (DGCNN) on the basis of GCNN. By dynamically learning the internal relationship between different channels, EEG graph features related to brain structure can be extracted, and the performance of the model can be improved.

Based on the above research status, the algorithm using DGCNN in EEG source space (sDGCNN) was proposed in this paper. The method firstly transforms the recorded EEG signals to the source space by EEG source localization. Secondly, the source data is divided into 79 brain regions according to Brodmann area, and time-domain features are extracted from each region. Finally, the graphs with brain regions as nodes and extracted features as node values are input into DGCNN for four-kind hand movement classification.

## 2 Methods

### 2.1 Experimental Protocol and Data Acquisition

Thirteen healthy male subjects aged 20−32 were recruited for the experiment, and they were sequentially identified as S1−S13. All subjects were right-handed, visual acuity or corrected visual acuity met the experimental requirements. All subjects accepted the written description of the study and signed an informed consent form.

The experiment was conducted in a quiet room away from electrical equipment and high-frequency radiation. The subjects were required to minimize body movements.

EEG and EMG signals were recorded by Neuroscan (Neuroscan Systems, Compumedics, Charlotte, NC, 145 USA). The ground electrode was located in the prefrontal area between Fz and FCz, and the reference electrode was placed on right mastoid. Thirty channels of FP1, FP2, F7, F3, FZ, F4, F8, FT7, FC3, FCZ, FC4, FT8, T7, C3,

CZ, C4, T8, TP7, CP3, CPZ, CP4, TP8, P7, P3, PZ, P4, P8, O1, OZ, O2 were recorded in accordance with the international 10–20 standard electrode placement method. EMG signals were acquired simultaneously from the extensor digitorum, extensor carpi radialis, flexor carpi ulnaris, and palmaris longus using four pairs of disposable Ag/AgCl differential electrodes. We set the elbow as the reference and the sampling frequency was set at 1000 Hz for both EEG and EMG.

Signals were collected when each subject prepared to perform the four kinds of movements of tip pinch, multiple tip pinch, hand close, and hand open. With each movement performed 60 trails, a total of 240 samples were collected from each subject. To reduce the impact of fatigue during the experiment, every 20 trials were divided into one group and 5-min rest was set between each group. A single trial consists of a 4-s preparation phase, a 4-s movement execution and a 3-s rest. The flow of one trial is shown in Fig. 1.

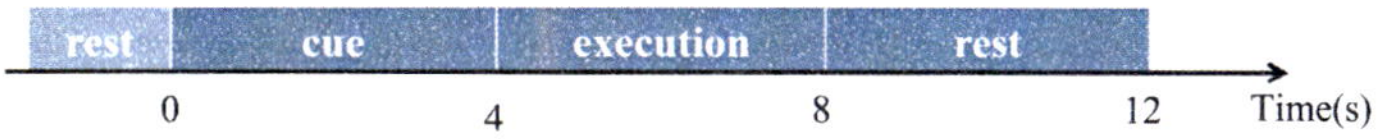


**Fig. 1.** Sequence diagram of single trial

The recorded data were filtered with a band-pass from 0.1 to 100 Hz and notch filtered at 50 Hz to remove the power-line artifacts. The moving time window method [20] was used to analyze the EMG signals to determine the real starting point of the movement, and the 2 s pre-movement data were extracted for the subsequent analysis.

### 2.2 sDGCNN Algorithm

The sDGCNN algorithm proposed in this paper first maps the EEG in sensor space to the source space after spatial source localization, and then extracts the standard deviation (STD), square root amplitude (SRA) and root mean square (RMS) of the source space signal as features to input into DGCNN for classification. The specific algorithm flowchart is shown in Fig. 2.

1. EEG source localization

EEG source localization, also known as the EEG inverse problem, is the reverse estimation of information on the location, direction and intensity of neural activity source in the brain based on the EEG signal recorded from the scalp. The mathematical model is as follows:

$$b = AX + n \tag{1}$$

where $b$ represents the recorded scalp data, which is a matrix of size 30*1000 in this paper, where 30 is the number of EEG channels in sensor space and 1000 is the length of time sampling for each sample after cropping; $X$ denotes the information of source activity within the brain, with the size of 15002*1000, where 15002 is the number of brain sources in the selected model and 1000 is the length of time series after mapping to

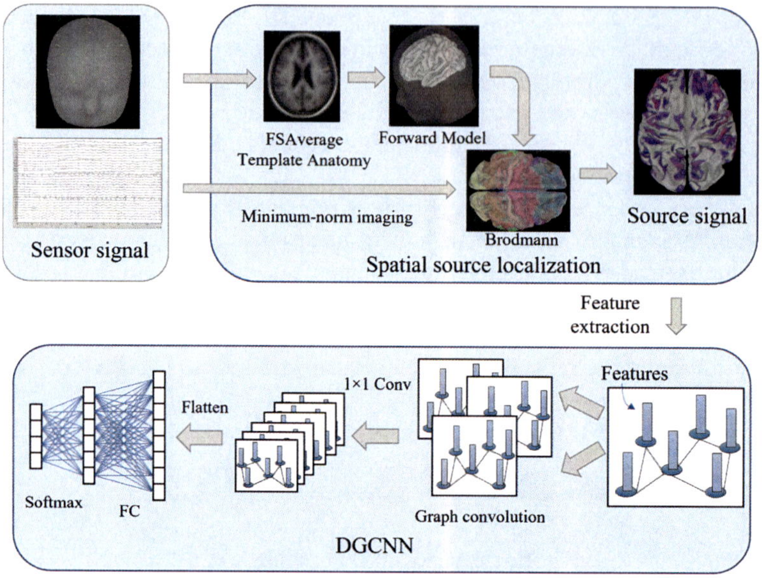


**Fig. 2.** Flowchart of the proposed algorithm

source space; $A$ is the transfer matrix, which reflects the contribution of each source in the brain to EEG channel; $n$ is the measurement noise. The inverse problem is to calculate $X$ when $b$ is known. Before that, it is necessary to solve the EEG positive problem. That is to build a head model of the brain which can elaborate how cortical neuronal activity is projected onto the scalp through brain volume effects and cranial conduction, i.e., matrix $A$. The main parts of the head model include the geometry of the brain and the different tissues through which neuroelectric activity propagates (gray matter, white matter, cerebrospinal fluid, skull, and skin). In this paper, a three-shell conduction model representing the scalp, skull and internal brain tissues with a conductivity of 1:1/8:1 was developed using the boundary element method based on a real head model with FSAverage template.

Theoretically, the solution of the EEG inverse problem is the process that minimizes the residual between the recorded scalp EEG and the corresponding potential calculated from a known dipole. But in general, the solution of the inverse problem is not unique. It's necessary to obtain a unique brain source solution by determining a source model that is both anatomically meaningful and mathematically convenient to compute.

Source models are generally divided into equivalent current dipole model (ECD) and distributed source model (DS). The former equates the brain source activity in a region by a single or a small number of dipoles, which is only suitable for accurate estimation of local regions and cannot be accurately reconstructed for the source activity of the whole brain. Therefore, in this paper, we chose DS model in which the signal sources are uniformly distributed in the cerebral cortex. Since the number of sources in the brain (15002) is much larger than the number of channels in the scalp EEG (30), EEG inverse problem exists infinite solutions. It's required to have an additional suitable constraint. In this paper, the minimum norm estimate (MNE) [21] method is used to solve the inverse problem, and its solution formula is as follows:

$$\min_{X} ||AX - b||^2 + \eta||WX||^2 \tag{2}$$

The optimal solution for $X$ will be the solution with the smallest residual between the estimated and recorded scalp EEG in the L2 parametric least squares sense, where $\eta \geq 0$ is the regularization parameter, and $W$ is a weight matrix.

After the signals in the source space are obtained, the dipoles in the same brain region are summed according to the Brodmann area. The accumulated data of brain regions are prepared for the subsequent processing. There are 79 brain areas in total, as shown in Fig. 3, so the data has shape of 79 * 1000.

2. DGCNN

Source signals can be modeled as graphic signals. In this case, the brain region is set as the node of the graph, and the features extracted from one brain region are the value of the node. The graph can be defined as $G = \{N, E\}$, where $N$ represents the node set with the number of $|N| = R$, and $E$ represents the edge set connecting nodes. Define $M \in \mathbb{R}^{R \times R}$ as adjacency matrix that describes the relationship between any two nodes in $N$. $R$ is the number of brain region. The items of $M$ in row $i$ and column $j$ are marked as $m_{ij}$, indicating the importance of the connection between the $i$th and $j$th nodes. Define $D \in \mathbb{R}^{R \times R}$ as degree matrix and $D_{ij} = \sum_j M_{ij}$.

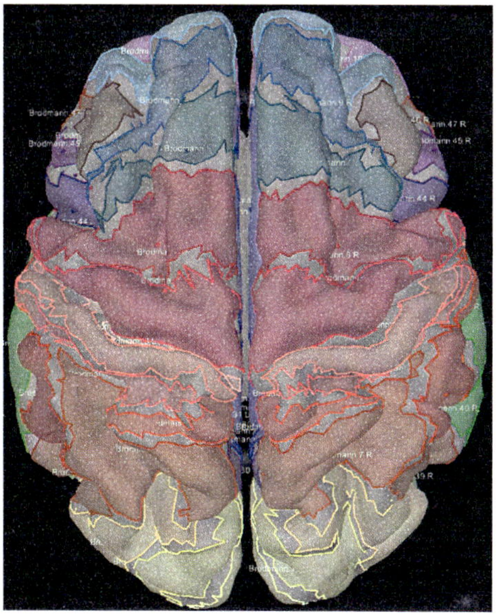

**Fig. 3.** Spatial source localization—Brodmann area

Graph convolution is a common graphics data processing method that can be calculated using the Graph Fourier Transform [22]:

$$g * s = g(L)s = g(U \wedge U^T)s = Ug(\wedge)U^T s \tag{3}$$

The graph convolution of signals $s \in \mathbb{R}^R$ and $g$, can be expressed as $s$ filtered by $g$ in the Fourier domain. In formula 1, $g$ can be interpreted as a filter function. $U$ is an orthonormal matrix, which can be calculated from the graph Laplacian matrix $L = I_R - D^{-\frac{1}{2}}AD^{-\frac{1}{2}} = U \wedge U^T$ of the singular value decomposition, where $I_R$ is the $R \times R$ identity matrix. $\Lambda = diag([\lambda_o, ..., \lambda_{N-1}])$ is a diagonal matrix. $g(\Lambda)$ is difficult to calculate directly, so Defferrard et al. [18] proposed to use the $K$-order Chebyshev polynomials to simplify the calculation process by:

$$g(\wedge) = \sum_{k=0}^{K-1} \theta_k T_k(\widetilde{\wedge}) \tag{4}$$

where $\theta_k$ is the coefficient of Chebyshev polynomials $T_k(\widetilde{\wedge})$ and $T_k\left(\widetilde{\wedge}\right) = 2\ \widetilde{\wedge}\ T_{k-1}\left(\widetilde{\wedge}\right) - T_{k-2}(\widetilde{\wedge})$,with $T_0(\widetilde{\wedge}) = 1$ and $T_1(\widetilde{\wedge}) = \widetilde{\wedge}$.

According to Eq. (4), the graph convolution defined in Eq. (3) can be rewritten by:

$$g * s = \sum\nolimits_{k=0}^{K-1} \theta_k T_k(\tilde{L})s \tag{5}$$

where $\tilde{L} = 2L/\lambda R_{max}$.

The DGCNN used in this paper consists of four main layers, that it, input layer, graph convolution layer, convolution layer, full connection layer, and the output layer. Specifically, the input of the DGCNN model corresponds to features extracted from multiple brain regions in source space, in which each region is represented as a node in the model. The following is a convolution layer with a 1 × 1 kernel [19]. In addition, in order to achieve the non-linear mapping ability of the network, the Relu activation function is used to ensure that the output of the graph data filter layer is non-negative. Then, the output of the activation function is flattened and sent to a fully connected layer, which sets 32 nodes. Finally, the softmax function is used for four classifications of hand movements.

For DGCNN, adjacency matrix $M$ can be dynamically learned during training. The optimal network parameters are iteratively optimized using back propagation (BP) method, cross-entropy is used as the loss function, Adam optimizer [23] is used to learn adjacency matrix, the learning rate $\rho = 0.001$, $\beta_1 = 0.9$, and $\beta_2 = 0.999$.

## 2.3 Setting of Experiments

In the experiment, a six-fold cross-validation method was used to randomly divide all samples into six groups. For each fold, four groups were selected as the training set, one groups as the validation set, and one group as the test set. The average accuracy of six-fold cross-validation is used to evaluate the performance of the model.

Since deep learning requires a large number of samples for training, we used a time window of one second to crop the data. The moving step was set to 50 ms. Through this operation, the 2-s EEG data can be expanded into twenty-one 1-s EEG segments. On the other hand, since the training set, validation set and test set were divided before cropping, the crops with overlapping information would not affect the classification results. In the end, a total of 240 samples of 2-s long for a single subject became 5040 samples of 1-s long after the augmentation operation.

# 3 Results

In this paper, the decoding performance of the proposed algorithm was evaluated usi ng classification accuracy. The classification accuracy is defined as the ratio of the number of all correctly classified samples to the total number of samples, and the average accuracy of the six-fold cross-validation is taken as the final result to verify the effectiveness of this algorithm. The significance analysis of data was realized by Wilcoxon signed-rank tests.

## 3.1 Decoding Effects of Different Features

Table 1 presents the average accuracy of 13 subjects using sDGCNN method with 11 different features. The feature extraction in this part was based on $1-100$ Hz signal. It can be observed that the three features standard deviation, root mean square, and square root amplitude achieved the best three results. Thus, the three features are extracted as DGCNN node values in the following research.

**Table 1.** Average classification accuracy of all su bject based on different features

| Feature | Mean | Standard deviation | Kurtosis |
|---|---|---|---|
| Accuracy | 34.97% | 60.40% | 34.81% |
| Feature | ***Skewness*** | ***Root mean square*** | ***Kurtosis factor*** |
| Accuracy | 38.17% | 60.09% | 37.03% |
| Feature | ***Margin factor*** | ***Waveform factor*** | ***Pulse factor*** |
| Accuracy | 36.95% | 35.67% | 36.87% |
| Feature | ***Square root amplitude*** | | |
| Accuracy | 56.91% | | |

## 3.2 Decoding Effect of Algorithms Under Different Frequency Bands

Table 2 shows the average accuracy under the three features of STD, RMS, and SRA for 13 subjects in different frequency bands. The frequency ranges were divided according to common EEG rhythms, and *all band* means using data with frequency 1 to 100 Hz. It can be observed that the sDGCNN method had the highest accuracy in $\gamma$-band with $90.16 \pm 6.8\%$, which represents the good performance of the algorithm.

**Table 2.** Classification accuracies in different frequency ranges

| Subject | δ band 1−3 Hz (%) | θ band 4–7 Hz (%) | α band 8−13 Hz (%) | β band 14−30 Hz (%) | γ band 30−100 Hz (%) | all band 1−100 Hz (%) |
|---|---|---|---|---|---|---|
| S1 | 26.47 | 32.54 | 41.79 | 86.15 | 95.44 | 68.41 |
| S2 | 32.02 | 33.95 | 39.33 | 53.47 | 96.11 | 48.49 |
| S3 | 38.51 | 38.99 | 34.25 | 53.23 | 77.28 | 60.20 |
| S4 | 39.98 | 38.49 | 43.71 | 74.68 | 83.43 | 60.50 |
| S5 | 34.98 | 29.90 | 33.27 | 41.69 | 81.49 | 42.54 |
| S6 | 41.51 | 37.68 | 50.65 | 74.50 | 97.38 | 76.75 |
| S7 | 30.54 | 30.36 | 34.48 | 40.34 | 82.18 | 46.92 |
| S8 | 28.71 | 22.98 | 36.71 | 71.53 | 89.66 | 64.25 |
| S9 | 32.14 | 33.04 | 52.28 | 79.38 | 95.38 | 67.16 |
| S10 | 27.20 | 32.26 | 37.00 | 63.81 | 86.88 | 59.13 |
| S11 | 35.04 | 39.98 | 54.27 | 75.40 | 95.85 | 62.36 |
| S12 | 40.99 | 48.51 | 37.18 | 62.16 | 97.48 | 72.74 |
| S13 | 27.58 | 27.92 | 32.18 | 64.90 | 93.51 | 64.07 |
| Mean | 33.51 | 34.35 | 40.55 | 64.71 | 90.16 | 61.04 |
| Std | 5.20 | 6.19 | 7.23 | 13.65 | 6.80 | 9.61 |

## 4 Discussion

In this paper, sDGCNN was proposed to classify hand movement. The sensor signals were mapped to source space and then input to DGCNN. The extracted features and suitable frequency band were compared, and the accuracy are shown in part III. It's obvious that the γ-band data achieved the best result, indicating that the signal in the high frequency band is more closely related to hand movement recognition, which is also consistent with the results of some recent literatures [24, 25].

In the past, many studies improved the classification accuracy by increasing the number of EEG channels. However, high-density EEG sensor arrays for data acquisition are expensive and time-consuming. In this study, the EEG source localization method mapped the sensor space data to source space, which increased the spatial information in EEG recordings and improved the spatial resolution of the signal. In order to prove the validity of the source space data, we performed the same calculation using sensor space data. The specific comparison results are shown in Fig. 4. It can be seen that the source-space data outperforms the sensor-space data in all frequency band, and there are significant differences ($p < 0.05$) except all frequency band (1−100 Hz). The result well confirms the effectiveness of the source space signal.

Furthermore, in order to evaluate the proposed method in this paper more objectively, the article compares the classification accuracy of the proposed method with other advanced methods, including MECN [25], GCB Net [26], EEGNet [27], DeepNetConv [28], deepCNN [29], Filter bank common spatial pattern (FBCSP) [30] and MEMD-CSP [31]. The results are shown in Fig. 5. MECN is our previously proposed algorithm. In this method, data is decomposed by Multivariate Empirical Mode Decomposition (MEMD) and then input into CNN by forward sequence search to find the optimal multiple multivariate intrinsic mode functions (MIMF) combination. The specific steps can be referred to the literature [25]. For the four deep learning networks, GCB Net, EEGNet, DeepNetConv, and deepCNN, the input data was only simply preprocessed and no other features were extracted manually. The average accuracies of the seven methods were $81.14 \pm 6.76$, $56.34 \pm 11.05$, $68.02 \pm 10.93$, $67.06 \pm 9.78$, $55.67 \pm 8.92$, $66.86 \pm 10.17$, and $60.35 \pm 10.08\%$, respectively, all of which were significantly lower than that of the proposed method sDGCNN in this paper ($p < 0.05$). These results indicate that, compared with the state-of-the-art deep learning methods and traditional MEMD-CSP and FBCSP methods, the proposed method sDGCNN performed better.

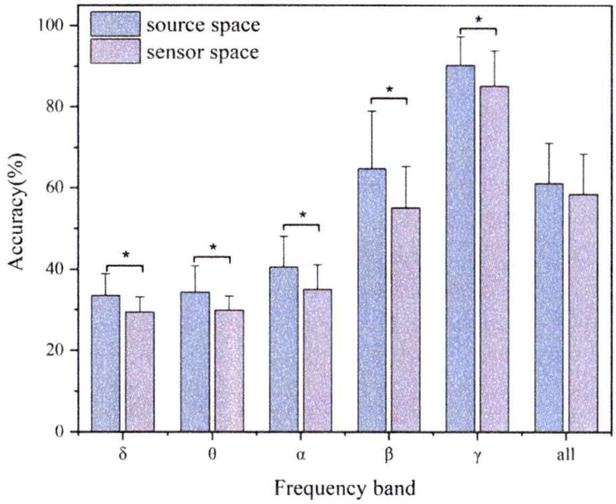


**Fig. 4.** Classification accuracies of all subjects using data from source space and sensor space

Additionally, compared with the conventional CNN, the adjacency matrix in DGCNN is special. The non-diagonal values of the adjacency matrix can be used to analyze the connectivity between brain regions, and the diagonal elements indicate the importance of different brain regions to the hand movement recognition, which provide a potential way to improve the performance of hand movement decoding. This topic will be our future work.

Another issue of concern is the node features of DGCNN. The features used in this paper were determined by the accuracy of each listed time-domain feature. But frequency domain, time-frequency domain, and nonlinear features are not involved. Besides, the appropriate features cannot be determined conveniently, which is also an area for future exploration.

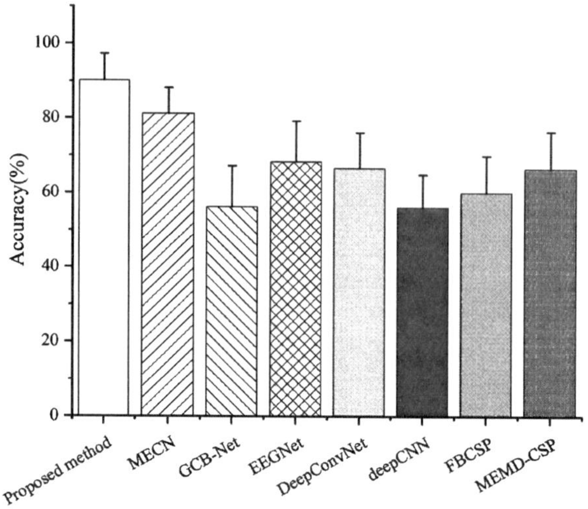


**Fig. 5.** Comparison results with other algorithms

## 5 Conclusion

The sDGCNN algorithm proposed in this paper used the EEG source localization method to map the EEG signals acquired in sensor space to the source space, followed by calculating the STD, RMS and SMA of each brain region as features. Then features were input to DGCNN for classification. The highest average classification accuracy achieved $90.16 \pm 6.8\%$, which was calculated with the data in $\gamma$-band. It indicates that the high-frequency components of the brain may have important significance for hand movement decoding.

**Acknowledgment.** This work was supported in part by the National Natural Science Foundation of China under Grant 32071372 and Grant 62271385; in part by the Science and Technology Project of Sichuan under Grant 2022YFS0030. The authors also acknowledge the support by the HPC platform of Xi'an Jiaotong University.

## References

1. Choi, W., Yeom, H.: Studies to overcome brain-computer interface challenges. Appl. Sci. **12**, 2598 (2022). https://doi.org/10.3390/app12052598
2. Frolov, A.A., Mokienko, O., Lyukmanov, R., et al.: Post-stroke rehabilitation training with a motor-imagery-based brain-computer interface (BCI)-controlled hand exoskeleton: a randomized controlled multicenter trial. Front Neurosci-Switz., **11**, (2017). https://doi.org/10.3389/fnins.2017.00400
3. Ramos-Murguialday, A., Curado, M.R., Broetz, D., et al.: Brain-machine interface in chronic stroke: randomized trial long-term follow-up. Neurorehab Neural Re **33**, 188–198 (2019). https://doi.org/10.1177/1545968319827573

4. Cantillo-Negrete, J., Carino-Escobar, R.I., Carrillo-Mora, P., et al.: Brain-computer interface coupled to a robotic hand orthosis for stroke patients' neurorehabilitation: a crossover feasibility study. Front. Hum. Neurosci, **15**, (2021). https://doi.org/10.3389/fnhum.2021.656975
5. Hu, Y., Gao, T., Li, J., et al.: Motor imagery-based brain-computer interface combined with multimodal feedback to promote upper limb motor function after stroke: a preliminary study. Evid-Based Compl ALT **2021**, 1 (2021). https://doi.org/10.1155/2021/1116126
6. Lou, X., Xiao, S., Qi, Y., et al.: Corticomuscular coherence analysis on hand movement distinction for active rehabilitation. Comput Math Method M **2013**, 1 (2013). https://doi.org/10.1155/2013/908591
7. Liao, K., Xiao, R., Gonzalez, J., et al.: Decoding individual finger movements from one hand using human EEG signals. PLoS ONE **9**, e85192 (2014). https://doi.org/10.1371/journal.pone.0085192
8. Chouhan, T., Robinson, N., Vinod, A.P., et al.: Wavlet phase-locking based binary classification of hand movement directions from EEG. J Neural Eng **15**, 66008 (2018). https://doi.org/10.1088/1741-2552/aadeed
9. Wang, J., Bi, L., Fei, W., et al.: Decoding single-hand and both-hand movement directions from noninvasive neural signals. IEEE T Bio-Med Eng **68**, 1932–1940 (2021). https://doi.org/10.1109/TBME.2020.3034112
10. Hajipour, S.S., Shamsollahi, M.B.: Selection of efficient features for discrimination of hand movements from MEG using a BCI competition IV data set. Front Neurosci-Switz **6**, 42 (2012). https://doi.org/10.3389/fnins.2012.00042
11. Jochumsen, M., Niazi, I.K., Dremstrup, K., et al.: Detecting and classifying three different hand movement types through electroencephalography recordings for neurorehabilitation. Med Biol Eng Comput **54**, 1491–1501 (2016). https://doi.org/10.1007/s11517-015-1421-5
12. Alazrai, R., Alwanni, H., Daoud, M.I.: EEG-based BCI system for decoding finger movements within the same hand. Neurosci Lett **698**, 113–120 (2019). https://doi.org/10.1016/j.neulet.2018.12.045
13. Shafiul, H.S., Siddiquee, M.R., Atri, R., et al.: Prediction of gait intention from pre-movement EEG signals: a feasibility study. J Neuroeng Rehabil **17**, 50 (2020). https://doi.org/10.1186/s12984-020-00675-5
14. Huang, C., Xiao, Y., Xu, G.: Predicting human intention-behavior through EEG signal analysis using multi-scale CNN. IEEE ACM T Comput BI **18**, 1722–1729 (2021). https://doi.org/10.1109/TCBB.2020.3039834
15. Mammone, N., Ieracitano, C., Morabito, F.C.: A deep CNN approach to decode motor preparation of upper limbs from time-frequency maps of EEG signals at source level. Neural Netw. **124**, 357–372 (2020). https://doi.org/10.1016/j.neunet.2020.01.027
16. Al-Saegh, A., Dawwd, S.A., Jassim, M.A.: Deep learning for motor imagery EEG-based classification: A review. Biomed. Signal Process. Control. **63**, (2021). https://doi.org/10.1016/j.bspc.2020.102172
17. Chung, F.R.K.: Spectral graph theory. American Mathematical Society (1997)
18. Defferrard, M., Bresson, X., Vandergheynst, P.: Convolutional neural networks on graphs with fast localized spectral filtering. In: 30th conference on neural information processing systems (NIPS), Barcelona, SPAIN (2016)
19. Song, T., Zheng, W., Song, P., et al.: EEG emotion recognition using dynamical graph convolutional neural networks. IEEE T Affect Comput **11**, 532–541 (2020). https://doi.org/10.1109/TAFFC.2018.2817622
20. Wang, G., Ren, D.: Classification of surface electromyographic signals by means of multifractal singularity spectrum. Med Biol Eng Comput **51**, 277–284 (2013). https://doi.org/10.1007/s11517-012-0990-9

21. Hamalainen, M.S., Ilmoniemi, R.J.: Interpreting magnetic fields of the brain: minimum norm estimates. Med Biol Eng Comput, 35–42 (1994)
22. Shuman, D.I., Narang, S.K., Frossard, P., et al.: The emerging field of signal processing on graphs. IEEE Signal Proc Mag, 83–98 (2013). https://doi.org/10.1109/MSP.2012.2235192
23. Kingma, D.P., Ba, J.L.: Adam: A method for Stochastic Optimization. Computer Science, (2014)
24. Mohseni, M., Shalchyan, V., Jochumsen, M., et al.: Upper limb complex movements decoding from pre-movement EEG signals using wavelet common spatial patterns. Comput Meth Prog Bio **183**, 105076 (2020). https://doi.org/10.1016/j.cmpb.2019.105076
25. Tao, Y., Xu, W., Wang, G., et al.: Decoding multi-class eeg signals of hand movement using multivariate empirical mode decomposition and convolutional neural network. IEEE T Neur Sys REH **30**, 2754–2763 (2022). https://doi.org/10.1109/TNSRE.2022.3208710
26. Zhang, T., Wang, X., Xu, X., et al.: GCB-Net: Graph convolutional broad network and its application in emotion recognition. IEEE T Affect Comput **13**, 379–388 (2022). https://doi.org/10.1109/TAFFC.2019.2937768
27. Lawhern, V.J., Solon, A.J., Waytowich, N.R., et al.: EEGNet: a compact convolutional neural network for EEG-based brain-computer interfaces. J Neural Eng **15**, 56013 (2018). https://doi.org/10.1088/1741-2552/aace8c
28. Schirrmeister, R.T., Springenberg, J.T., Fiederer, L.D.J., et al.: Deep learning with convolutional neural networks for EEG decoding and visualization. HUM BRAIN MAPP **38**, 5391–5420 (2017). https://doi.org/10.1002/hbm.23730
29. Tang, Z., Li, C., Sun, S.: Single-trial EEG classification of motor imagery using deep convolutional neural networks. Optik **130**, 11–18 (2017). https://doi.org/10.1016/j.ijleo.2016.10.117
30. Ang, K.K., Zhang, Y.C., Zhang, H., et al.: Filter bank common spatial pattern (FBCSP) in brain-computer interface. In: IEEE International Joint Conference on Neural Networks, vol. 10. IEEE, pp 2390–2397 (2008)
31. Pramod, G., Bilas, P.R., Hui, W., et al.: An automatic subject specific intrinsic mode function selection for enhancing two-class EEG-based motor imagery-brain computer interface. IEEE SENS J **19**, 6938–6947 (2019). https://doi.org/10.1109/JSEN.2019.2912790

# Rehabilitation Engineering

# Sensorimotor Cortical Activities Induced by NMES During INB

Yun Zhao[1,2], Guanghui Xie[1], Renqiang Yang[1], Haiyan Qin[1], Xiaoying Wu[2,3,4], and Wensheng Hou[2,3,4](✉)

[1] School of Smart Health, Chongqing College of Electronic Engineering, Chongqing, China
zyyy90@163.com

[2] The Key Laboratory of Biorheological Science and Technology, Ministry of Education, Chongqing University, Chongqing, China
w.s.hou@cqu.edu.cn

[3] The Chongqing Medical Electronics Engineering Technology Research Center, Chongqing, China

[4] The Chongqing Key Laboratory of Artificial Intelligence and Service Robot Control Technology, Chongqing, China

**Abstract.** Ischemic nerve block (INB) can successfully separate muscle spindle afferents from sensory afferents evoked by neuromuscular electrical stimulation (NMES) above motor threshold. The purpose of this study is to explore how the sensorimotor cortex perceives the incoming muscle spindle afferents evoked by NMES above motor threshold during INB. An experimental protocol was composed by four tasks conceived according to a $2 \times 2$ factorial design. In particular, the first factor was the INB state (Before INB and during INB) and the second factor was the NMES intensity (Sup− and sub−motor threshold). During the tasks, 64-channel EEG signals from 11 healthy subjects were record and analyzed to detect beta event-related desynchronization (Beta ERD) for quantizing the activation level of sensorimotor cortex. The psychophysical test was used to assess changes in sensation and movement of the right hand when the right wrist was blocked by the blood pressure cuff. At the same time, active and passive index finger flexion and extension tasks were set before and during INB. The statistical results showed that during INB, beta ERD on the contralateral sensorimotor cortex induced by NMES with the sup-motor threshold was significantly decreased, and the difference of Beta ERD values on the contralateral sensorimotor cortex induced by NMES with sup− and sub motor threshold was significant. In addition, contralateral dominance of beta ERD on the sensorimotor cortex induced by NMES was transferred to ipsilateral during INB. INB significantly reduced sensorimotor cortical activity induced by NMES with the sup-motor threshold and decreased its perception on the stimulus intensity, which may result from the rapid functional reorganization of the sensorimotor cortex induced by INB.

**Keywords:** Ischemic nerve block · Neuromuscular electrical stimulation · Sensorimotor cortex · Muscle spindle afferents


G. Wang et al. (Eds.): APCMBE 2023, IFMBE Proceedings 103, pp. 325–335, 2024.
https://doi.org/10.1007/978-3-031-51455-5_36

# 1 Introduction

After hand amputation, neuromuscular electrical stimulation (NMES)-evoked somatic sensations of phantom finger have been used to restore sensory feedback of hand amputees and then improve the control of a hand prosthesis through stimulating the skin or muscle at the end of the stump. Proprioceptive feedback plays a key role in various daily flexible movements of human hands [1]. NMES-evoked sensory feedback is mostly electrotactile sensation using stimulation amplitude with below motor threshold [2], and rarely involves the electric proprioception activated by the current intensity above motion threshold. Exploring artificial proprioception evoked by NMES is important to improve the precise and dexterous control of hand prosthesis.

To facilitate performing the experiment of NMES-evoked sensation, able-bodied subjects are usually recruited for the experiment. However, due to the differences of distal joint movements in able-bodies subjects, and the neural changes caused by hand amputation [3], most sensory feedback schemes are often unable to be applied to amputees. Therefore, it is necessary to explore how to improve the effectiveness of sensory feedback schemes with NMES above motor threshold applied to hand amputees through able-bodies.

Therefore, some studies have modelled acute functional hand loss through a variety of techniques, such as restricting the hand and wrist movements, and ischemic nerve block (INB). The use of a blood pressure cuff to induce INB by blocking sensory afferent from the limb, and has been used in studies on rehabilitation of amputees, such as changes in phantom hand sensations and cortical activities [4–10]. Recent INB studies mainly focused on sensory degeneration and phantom limb sensation during the procedure of INB [11], and the changes of cortical activities during INB [12–15].

NMES-evoked sensations during INB are mostly activated using the current intensity below motor threshold [16], which is also used in sensory feedback of hand prosthesis through activates skin receptors to generate electrotactile sensation [17]. However, few studies focused to investigate the artificial proprioception evoked by NMES above motor threshold through activating muscle spindle to generate proprioceptive afferent signals [18]. Studies have shown that limb movements evoked by NMES above motor threshold can induce sensorimotor cortical activities similar to those caused by active [19] and passive limb movements [20], and the task-related cortical activities are related to proprioceptive information of the limb movements [21]. Therefore, evoking muscle activities at the end of the limb stump using NMES above motor threshold may provide proprioceptive feedback for hand prosthesis, which is also the key to the flexible control of objects for the human hand.

To address the above issues, this paper selected INB technique to model acute functional hand loss, and then delivered the stimulation currents with two intensities (above and below motor threshold) to forearm extensor muscle respectively. During NMES, EEG data were recorded. Beta-band event-related desynchronization (Beta ERD) was used to quantify sensorimotor cortical activities induced by the evoked proximal muscle contraction before and during INB because of its ability to characterize cortical activity caused by limb movements.

# 2 Materials and Methods

## 2.1 Subjects

Data was collected from 11 healthy right-handed subjects (4 females and 7 males, 25 $\pm$ 4 years old). Inclusion criteria for the subjects included: no history of former cardiovascular disease, neurological disorders or orthopedic problems in arms, the dominant right hand, free of upper limb resistance training in the past 6 months. All protocols and recruitment procedures were approved by the ethical committee of Chongqing Cancer Hospital. All subjects signed the informed consent before the experiments.

## 2.2 Experimental Setup

A commercial blood pressure cuff (Yuwell hemopiezometer, Yuwell Medicine, China) applying to right forearm near the wrist was used to achieve INB of the whole right hand. Above the cuff, the stimulation electrodes were placed on the top of index finger extensor to evoke extension movement or the sensation of index finger. The stimulation current was delivered using Programmable Stimulator (Master-9, AMPI, Jerusalem, Israel) with isolated cables (ISO-Flex, AMPI, Jerusalem, Israel). The stimulation parameters were set with the stimulation frequency of 40 Hz and the bipolar pulse width of 1 ms, while the stimulation intensity included two levels: one was set as the intensity to evoke fully extension of index finger with 1.5 s, another was set as the amplitude to evoke maximal sensation of index finger without extension movement. For the task of active index finger extension, bipolar Ag/AgCl electromyography (EMG) electrodes were placed between the two stimulation electrodes which were not used in this task to record muscle activity from index finger extensor for detecting the onset of active movements. EMG signals were amplified and conditioned using a data acquisition card (NI USB-6008) with a low-pass filter of 500 Hz and sampling at 1 kHz. For the passive movement, a special finger cap made by white medical tape was placed on the index fingertip and marked with a blue marker pen to detect finger movement trajectory. The finger cap was connected with a white nylon rope with the diameter of 2 mm using for the experimenter to control the index finger movement. A camera of commercial smartphone, supported by a professional camera tripod, was placed at 40 cm directly above subjects' right hand. The camera was used to record the video of the index finger extension during passive task for detecting the movement onset, and the video data was sampled at 30 Hz. Scalp EEG was recorded by a 62-sensor cap according to the International 10–20 system with the reference electrode placed at the middle between Cz and CPz. Electro-oculograms (EOG) were recorded via two electrodes of them: horizontal EOG was recorded by placing an electrode to the outer canthus of subjects' right eye, and vertical EOG by an electrode below subjects' left eye. Both EEG and EOG signals were recorded by a multichannel neural data acquisition system (Cerebus 128; Cyberkinetics Neurotechnology Systems, Inc., Foxborough, MA, USA) with a low-pass of 500 Hz, sampled at 1 kHz and grounded with an electrode placed over the middle between FPz and AFz. Impedance for all electrodes was $<50$ k$\Omega$. In addition, another channel of the system was used to synchronously record trial marker signals from with a sampling frequency of 1 kHz. EMG data or the video data were synchronized by the trial marker signal. The experimental setup is shown in Fig. 1A.

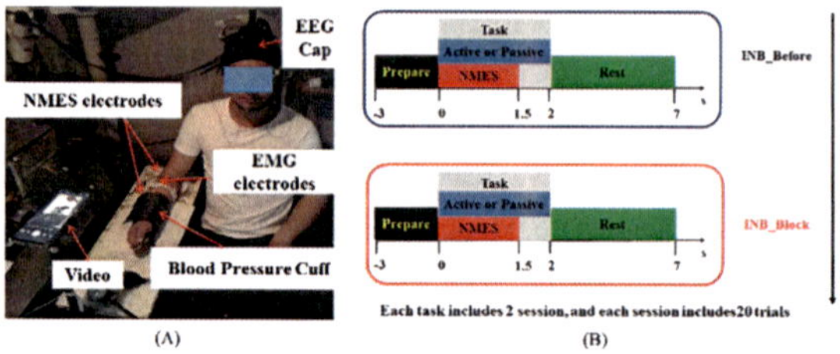


**Fig. 1.** **A** The experimental setup, **B** The experimental protocol

### 2.3 Experimental Protocol

Subjects sat comfortably in a chair with their right arm placed at a customized wood platform on the right side of the chair. The elbow joint was constrained with a bandage to immobilize the forearm.

Each subject was asked to perform 4 tasks: NMES-evoked movement of index finger extension (NMES-aMT), passive index finger extension movement (Passive movement), NMES-evoked somatic sensation of index finger (NMES-bMT) and active index finger extension movement (Active movement). Due to the restricted ischemic time, four tasks were divided into two groups and separately performed in two different days with a time interval of at least one week for all subjects. The first two performed tasks were NMES-aMT and Passive movement while the remaining two tasks were completed later. Each subject performed each task with two conditions in the following order: before INB (INB_Before) and during fully INB (INB_Block), as shown in Fig. 1B. Each trial commenced with a waring cue shown in a computer screen with a black shape "+", followed 3 s later by a trigger to open electrical stimulator to delivery stimulation current to the finger extensor for 1.5 s (NMES-aMT or NMES-bMT) or a word "GO" indicated to perform index finger extension movement for 1.5s (Passive or Active movement), and then 0.5 s for index finger returning back to home place voluntarily. For Passive movement, the experimenter dragged subjects' index finger to perform extension movement by controlling the finger cap with the nylon rope. Before the experiment, the experimenter was trained to perform the passive task reliably and consistently. During Active movement, subjects were required to voluntarily perform index finger extension similar to passive task according the "GO" cue in the computer screen, while in the INB_Block condition, subjects were instructed to try to perform the movements as in the INB_Block condition. Finally, there was a 5s rest for subjects before the next trail. Each condition of all tasks included 20 trials. Between two conditions, a 5 min rest was set for subject to avoid muscle fatigue. All tasks were firstly performed in the INB_Before condition.

After the INB_Before condition, subjects' hand was kept extension naturally and then fully flexed when the blood pressure cuff across the wrist was rapidly inflated to a pressure of 260 mm Hg. Cuff pressure was maintained constant through this whole experimental condition. Before achieving complete block of large fiber sensory afferents, the experimenter conducted psychophysical evaluation every 5 min for the first 20 min and then did every 2 min. The evaluation was performed to test the light touch position, sensation intensity of hand using a cotton swab. The movement sensation of fingers was measured with a plastic rod to pull certain finger, and subjects were required to rate the sensation of finger movement and position, and the effort to extend fingers voluntarily by a numerical rating scale (NRS), with the left end '0' representing 'not affected' and '7' represening 'inability to extend fingers'.

Once subjects cannot correctly report their sensations of light touch and finger movement, the hand was completely blocked, and then the tasks in INB_Block condition were performed right away. Immediately after task completion, the cuff was gradually deflated and then removed, limiting the maximum total ischemic time no more than 45 min.

## 3 Data Analysis

Video data was firstly processed using image processing methods to extract movement trajectory of index finger during passive task, which was then used to detect the onset and offset of passive index finger movements. EMG data were also used to detect the onset and offset of active index finger movement through the processing procedures of high-pass filtering of 20 Hz, rectification, and low-pass filtering of 4 Hz.

The EEG preprocessing was done in EEGLAB: EEG was firstly resampled to 200 Hz, and filtered using a zero phase-shift Butterworth bandpass filter (2~40 Hz). Then EEG data of the bad channels were interpolated using the CleanLine plugin. After that, we applied independent component analysis (ICA) method to EEG data for removing power line interferences and electrooculogram artifacts. EEG data were segmented from −3 to 7 s, with 0 s aligned to the onset of active, passive, or NMES tasks, and then corrected using the baseline of −2.5 to−0.5 s.

Event-Related Spectral Perturbation (ERSP) was utilized to inspect the spectral power changes of the preprocessed EEG data in time-frequency domain for ERD evaluation [22], as follows:

$$ERSP(f,t) = \frac{1}{N}\sum\nolimits_{n=1}^{N}(F_n(f,t))^2 \tag{1}$$

where, $F_n(f,t)$ is the spectral estimation of trial n at frequency f and time t, and $ERSP(f,t)$ is the power spectrum averaging across N trials at frequency f and time t. The ERSP maps for Electrode C3 of all tasks were computed using wavelet transform with Morlet wavelets of 7 cycles applied in EEGLAB.

And then, Beta ERD values were calculated during the experiment tasks:

$$ERD_{mean} = \frac{1}{M}\sum_{f=k}^{K}\sum_{t=t_1}^{t_2} ERSP(f,t) \tag{2}$$

where, $M$ is the number of time-frequency bins in beta band at time $t$ segment ($t_1 \le t \le t_2$; $t_1$=0, $t_2$=1.5). $k$ and $K$ are the minimal frequency (13 Hz) and maximal frequency (30 Hz) in Beta band respectively.

$ERD_{mean}$ values of EEG data in 21 channels (FC5, FC3, FC1, FCz, FC2, FC4, FC6, C5, C3, C1, Cz, C2, C4, C6, CP5, CP3, CP1, CPz, CP2, CP4, CP6) associated with the sensorimotor cortex were used to draw the topographic map of the brain. The averaged $ERD_{mean}$ values at the electrodes of FC3, C3 and CP3 were used as the activity level of the contralateral sensorimotor cortex corresponding to the right hand for quantifying cortical activities during the tasks.

### 3.1 Statistical Analysis

A two-way ANOVA with repeated measures was performed on $ERD_{mean}$ values during the tasks, with the factors of INB state (2: INB_Before and INB_Block) and stimulation intensity (2: NMES_aMT and NMES_bMT). Paired t test was used to compare the differences of $ERD_{mean}$ values during INB_Before or INB_Block between during active task and during passive task respectively. IBM SPSS, version 22 was used for statistical analysis, and the significance level was set at $p < 0.05$ for all procedures.

## 4 Results

### 4.1 Evaluation of the Model of Acute Hand Loss

*Psychophysical evaluation:* The statistical results of psychophysical tests showed that: for the touch sensation of the hand position, the finger touch was the first to be completely blocked, which occurred at 25.50 ± 3.61 min after the blood pressure cuff compression, followed by the palm touch and the back touch, which occurred at 27.75 ± 2.82 min and 28.25 ± 2.52 min respectively. After 27.38 ± 2.70 min, subjects could not feel finger movement at all, that is, finger motor sensation was completely blocked. In addition, after 25.25 ± 3.17 min, the maximum effort (7 points) of subjects was unable to perform finger extension, that is, the subjects' finger motor ability was completely lost.

*Beta ERD during active and passive tasks:* Fig. 2 shows the statistical results of $ERD_{mean}$ values in the sensorimotor cortex between INB_Before and INB_Block during passive and active tasks respectively. During the passive task, $ERD_{mean}$ values of the contralateral sensorimotor cortex increased significantly during INB_Block compared with that during INB_Before ($p < 0.05$), seen in Fig. 2A; During the active task, there was no significant difference of $ERD_{mean}$ values in the contralateral sensorimotor cortex between INB_Before and INB_Block ($p < 0.05$), as shown in Fig. 2B.

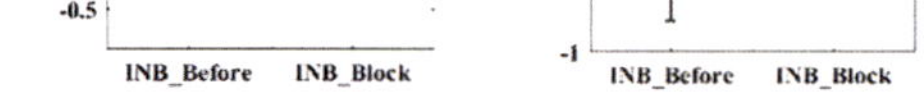


**Fig. 2.** The comparation of beta ERD values ($ERD_{mean}$: Mean ± STD) of contralateral sensorimotor cortex between INB_Before and INB_Block during passive task (**A**) and active task (**B**). *Notes* *indicates $p < 0.05$

### 4.2 Effect of INB on Beta ERD Values In Contralateral Sensorimotor Cortex Induced By NMES

Figure 3 showed that INB significantly influenced $ERD_{mean}$ values induced by NMES_aMT (Fig. 3A), that is, NMES_aMT-induced $ERD_{mean}$ values during INB_Before were significantly lower than that during INB_Block ($p < 0.01$); but no significant difference of $ERD_{mean}$ values induced by NMES_bMT (Fig. 3B) was found between during INB_Before and during INB_Block ($p > 0.05$).

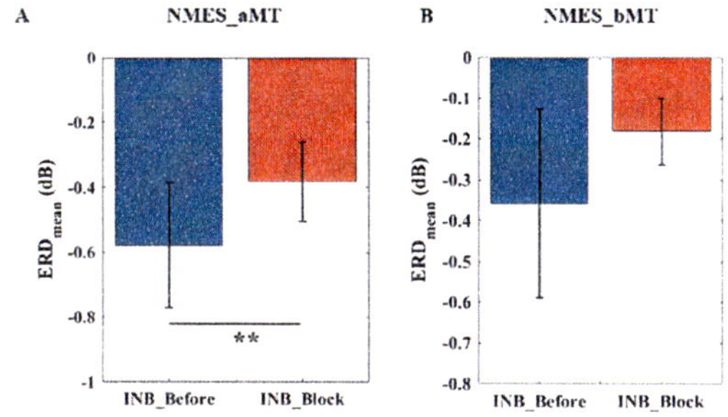


**Fig. 3.** The comparation of beta ERD values ($ERD_{mean}$: Mean ± STD) of contralateral sensorimotor cortex induced by NMES_aMT (**A**) and NMES_bMT (**B**) between before and during INB during. *Notes* ** indicates $p < 0.01$

The statistical results of $ERD_{mean}$ values between two NMES tasks during INB_Before or INB_Block were shown in Fig. 4. For INB_Before (Fig. 4A), $ERD_{mean}$ values during NMES_aMT were significantly lower than that during NMES_bMT ($p < 0.05$), but no significant difference ($p > 0.05$) of $ERD_{mean}$ values between the two NMES tasks were observed for INB_Block (Fig. 4B).

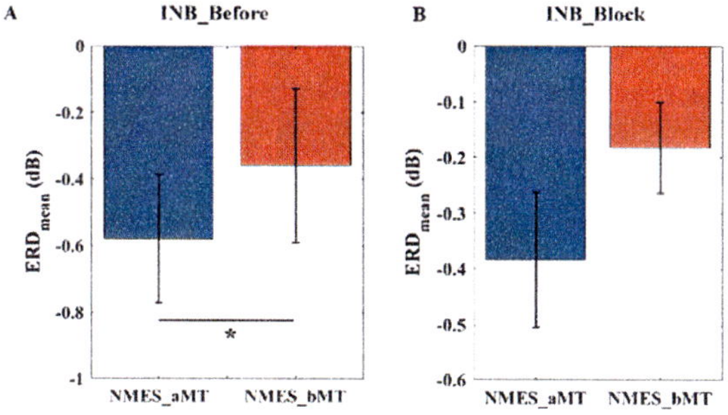


**Fig. 4.** The difference of beta ERD values ($ERD_{mean}$: Mean ± STD) of contralateral sensorimotor cortex between NMES_aMT and NMES_bMT during INB_Before (**A**) and during INB_Block (**B**): * denotes significant difference ($p < 0.05$).

## 5 Discussion

This study investigated sensorimotor cortex perception changes during INB in response to NMES-evoked proximal forearm extensor muscle (relative to the block position) activities, and the differences in NMES-evoked somatic perception between above and below motor threshold. The resulted showed that (1) Building a model of acute hand loss successfully; (2) During INB, Beta ERD in contralateral sensorimotor cortex induced by NMES_aMT significantly decreased (higher $ERD_{mean}$ values), but no significant changes during NMES_bMT; (3) NMES_aMT induced stronger Beta ERD (lower $ERD_{mean}$ values) than NMES_bMT before INB, but no significant difference between two NMES intensities during INB.

The model of acute hand loss established by INB is effective. We firstly assessed sensory degradation in the right hand using a psychophysical test [11], a common method for evaluating the effect of ischemic nerve block. The results showed that the sensations of fingertips, palms and backs of right hands gradually disappeared after 25 min of the pressure cuff compression, which was consistent with literature reports [11]. The physiological mechanism was that the cuff pressure blocked the blood flow of hands. With the blocking time increases, the conduction function of neural activities in afferent fibers gradually weakened until it could not do it. In addition, the degradation of the conduction function of large-diameter fibers is preferred to that of small-diameter fibers [23]. Sensory fibers belong to large diameter afferent fibers, so the hand sensation degraded firstly. And then, the fingers could not be extended due to muscle paralysis, and finally the finger motor sensation disappeared due to the block of afferent fibers of the finger proprioception (muscle spindle, tendon Golgi apparatus and afferent fibers corresponding to the joint capsule, etc.). Those results indicated that INB used in this study was successful. Further, we analyzed Beta ERD in contralateral sensorimotor cortex during active and passive index extension movements before and during INB. The results revealed that Beta ERD of the sensorimotor cortex induced by passive finger extension movements was significantly decreased during INB, indicating that the successful block of sensory feedback of the hand resulted in the decrease of sensorimotor cortical activities. This was consistent with the results of literature studies, namely, after the block, fMRI showed that the activation of the somatosensory cortex was significantly decreased during the passive ankle movement. While the sensorimotor cortical activities induced by active tasks were not affected by INB, because after the degeneration of sensory feedback of hand movements, active movement execution relied more on the prediction and estimation of limb behavior to supplement the reduced proprioceptive input of somatosensory cortex [18]. Therefore, combined with the results of psychophysical test and Beta ERD in sensorimotor cortex, it is further proved that the INB technique can successfully model the acute hand loss.

INB attenuated the cortical activities in contralateral sensorimotor cortex induced by NMES_aMT. Before INB, the sensory afferent information of forearm muscle contraction evoked by NMES_aMT included sensory afferent information of hand joint movements, skin touch and muscle spindle at the stimulation site. However, the sensory afferent information that NMES_bMT stimulated forearm muscle only included the cutaneous tactile information [24, 25]. During INB, cortical activities in the contralateral sensorimotor cortex induced by NMES_aMT was correspondingly weakened due to the absence of sensory feedback of the hand movement; However, INB did not affect the skin tactile afferent information activated by NMES_bMT, so cortical activities in the contralateral sensorimotor cortex induced by NMES_bMT were not significantly different than that before INB. Therefore, the attenuated NMES_aMT-induced cortical activites mainly derived from the loss of proprioceptional information caused by the acute hand "loss".

What's more, INB attenuated the perception of contralateral sensorimotor cortex' on the NMES intensity. Relevant studies have reported that the sensorimotor cortex can perceive the changes of the NMES intensity [26], which was also verified before INB in this paper, that is, there are significant differences of Beta ERD in the contralateral sensorimotor cortex between two NMES tasks with different current intensities (above and below motor threshold). This is because NMES above motor threshold not only activates tactile afferent fibers in the skin (tactile receptors) that can be also activated by NMES below motor threshold, but also depolarises proprioceptive afferent fibers (receptors such as muscle spindles, tendon Golgi apparatus, joint capsules and skin extension) [18], and then generates more sensory afferent information to induce stronger activities in the sensorimotor cortex. However, there was no significant difference of Beta ERD in contralateral sensorimotor cortex induced by between the NMES tasks with two current intensities during INB_Block, one of the reasons being that INB prevented proprioceptive afference of the hand. However, this did not fully explain the huge reduction of Beta ERD in contralateral sensorimotor cortex induced by NMES above motor intensity. Because even without the proprioceptive information of the hand movements, the afferent information from the skin and muscle spindle during NMES above motor threshold should be higher than that induced by the NMES below motor threshold. Based on previous findings that INB could induce acute functional reorganization in the cerebral cortex [7], we believe that INB alters the perception of contralateral sensorimotor cortex on NMES intensity.

## 6 Conclusions

This paper utilized INB to model the amputation state of the hand, and then explored the perception changes of sensorimotor cortex on NMES intensity under this state. The results revealed that the absence of proprioception and cortical reorganization after hand "loss" weakened the perception of sensorimotor cortex on NMES intensity. Artificial evoked proprioception feedback is a key factor to improve the control performance of hand prosthesis. Recent studies on the NMES-evoked sensory feedback in hand prosthesis mainly focus on the skin tactile evoked by NMES below motor threshold, rather than proprioception evoked by NMES above motor threshold. Therefore, the results of this study may provide some references for the sensorimotor cortex to perceive the current intensity of NMES above motor threshold inducing hand proprioception, which show a potential value in investigating the sensory feedback of hand prosthesis.

**Acknowledgment.** The authors sincerely thank all subjects for their support of the experiment voluntarily. This work was supported by Key-Area Research and Development Program of Guangdong Province (2020B0909020004), National Natural Science Foundation of China (NSFC31771069, NSFC82272117), and the Science & Technology Program of Chongqing Municipal Education Commission (KJZD-K202303103, KJZD-K202203104, KJQN202103112).

## References

1. Delhaye, B.P., Long, K.H., Bensmaia, S.J.: Neural basis of touch and proprioception in primate cortex. Compr. Physiol. **8**(4), 1575–1602 (2011)
2. Stephens-Fripp, B., Alici, G., Mutlu, R.: A review of non-invasive sensory feedback methods for transradial prosthetic hands. IEEE Access, **2018**, 1–1
3. Simoes, E.L., et al.: Functional expansion of sensorimotor representation and structural reorganization of callosal connections in lower limb amputees. J. Neurosci. **32**(9), 3211–3220 (2012)
4. Schlee, G., Milani, T.L., Sterzing, T., Oriwol, D.: Short-time lower leg ischemia reduces plantar foot sensitivity. Neurosci. Lett. **462**(3), 286–288 (2009)
5. Lundborg, G., Bjorkman, A., Hansson, T., Nylander, L., Nyman, T., Rosen, B.: Artificial sensibility of the hand based on cortical audiotactile interaction: a study using functional magnetic resonance imaging. Scand. J. Plast. Reconstr. Surg. Hand Surg. **39**(6), 370–372 (2005)
6. Bjorkman, A., Rosen, B., Lundborg, G.: Enhanced function in nerve-injured hands after contralateral deafferentation. NeuroReport **16**(5), 517–519 (2005)
7. Bjorkman, A., Rosen, B., Lundborg, G.: Acute improvement of hand sensibility after selective ipsilateral cutaneous forearm anaesthesia. Eur. J. Neurosci. **20**(10), 2733–2736 (2004)
8. Baron, G.C., Irving, G.A.: Effects of tourniquet ischemia on current perception thresholds in healthy volunteers. Pain Pract. **2**(2), 129–133 (2002)
9. Pluto, C.P., Lane, R.D., Rhoades, R.W.: Local GABA receptor blockade reveals hindlimb responses in the SI forelimb-stump representation of neonatally amputated rats. J. Neurophysiol. **92**(1), 372–379 (2004)
10. Ziemann, U., Hallett, M., Cohen, L.G.: Mechanisms of deafferentation-induced plasticity in human motor cortex. J. Neurosci. **18**(17), 7000–7007 (1998)
11. Inui, N., Walsh, L.D., Taylor, J.L., Gandevia, S.C.: Dynamic changes in the perceived posture of the hand during ischaemic anaesthesia of the arm. J. Physiol. **589**(Pt 23), 5775–5784 (2011)
12. Werhahn, K.J., Mortensen, J., Kaelin-Lang, A., Boroojerdi, B., Cohen, L.G.: Cortical excitability changes induced by deafferentation of the contralateral hemisphere. Brain **125**(Pt 6), 1402–1413 (2002)
13. Brasil-Neto, J.P., et al.: Rapid modulation of human cortical motor outputs following ischaemic nerve block. Brain **116**(Pt 3), 511–525 (1993)
14. McNulty, P.A., Macefield, V.G., Taylor, J.L., Hallett, M.: Cortically evoked neural volleys to the human hand are increased during ischaemic block of the forearm. J. Physiol. **538**(Pt 1), 279–288 (2002)
15. Vallence, A.M., Hammond, G.R., Reilly, K.T.: Increase in flexor but not extensor corticospinal motor outputs following ischemic nerve block. J. Neurophysiol. **107**(12), 3417–3427 (2012)
16. Hayashi, R., Ogata, K., Nakazono, H., Tobimatsu, S.: Modified ischaemic nerve block of the forearm: use for the induction of cortical plasticity in distal hand muscles, (in English). J. Phys-London **597**(13), 3457–3471 (2019)
17. Stephens-Fripp, B., Alici, G., Mutlu, R.J.I.A.: A review of non-invasive sensory feedback methods for transradial prosthetic hands. **6**, 6878–6899 (2018)

18. Carson, R.G., Buick, A.R.: Neuromuscular electrical stimulation-promoted plasticity of the human brain. J. Physiol, (2019)
19. Qiu, S., et al.: Event-related beta EEG changes during active, passive movement and functional electrical stimulation of the lower limb. IEEE Trans. Neural Syst. Rehabil. Eng. **24**(2), 283–290 (2016)
20. Alegre, M., Labarga, A., Gurtubay, I.G., Iriarte, J., Malanda, A., Artieda, J.: Beta electroencephalograph changes during passive movements: sensory afferences contribute to beta event-related desynchronization in humans. Neurosci. Lett. **331**(1), 29–32 (2002)
21. Muller, G.R., Neuper, C., Rupp, R., Keinrath, C., Gerner, H.J., Pfurtscheller, G.: Event-related beta EEG changes during wrist movements induced by functional electrical stimulation of forearm muscles in man. Neurosci. Lett. **340**(2), 143–147 (2003)
22. Delorme, A., Makeig, S.: EEGLAB: An open source toolbox for analysis of single-trial EEG dynamics including independent component analysis. J. Neurosci. Methods **134**(1), 9–21 (2004)
23. Walsh, L.D., Gandevia, S.C., Taylor, J.L.: Illusory movements of a phantom hand grade with the duration and magnitude of motor commands. J. Physiol. **588**(Pt 8), 1269–1280 (2010)
24. Maffiuletti, N.A., Herrero, A.J., Jubeau, M., Impellizzeri, F.M., Bizzini, M.: Differences in electrical stimulation thresholds between men and women, (in English). Ann. Neurol. **63**(4), 507–512 (2008)
25. Golaszewski, S.M., et al.: Modulation of motor cortex excitability by different levels of whole-hand afferent electrical stimulation, (in English). Clin. Neurophysiol. **123**(1), 193–199 (2012)
26. Muthalib, M., et al.: Effects of increasing neuromuscular electrical stimulation current intensity on cortical sensorimotor network activation: A time domain fNIRS study, (in English). Plos One, **10**(7), (2015)

# Optimal Design of Rocker-Profile Footwear: How Does Forefoot Rocker Radius Affect Walking Economy in Healthy Individuals?

Hao Chen[1], Xin Ma[1,3], and Wen-Ming Chen[1,2,3](✉)

[1] Academy for Engineering & Technology, Fudan University, 220 Handan Rd., Shanghai, China
chenwm@fudan.edu.cn

[2] Institute of Biomedical Engineering & Technology, Fudan University, 220 Handan Rd., Shanghai, China

[3] Department of Orthopedics, Huashan Hospital Affiliated to Fudan University, Shanghai, China

**Abstract.** While there have been some studies on the effects of rocker shoes on lower extremity biomechanics, potential efficacies on metabolic costs, in particular to walking economy, have not been fully understood. The purpose of this study is to examine the energy expenditure of healthy individuals when walking with shoes designed with different forefoot rocker radius, to determine whether certain rocker-profile would provide an energy benefit. Sixteen subjects participated in the study. The cumulative energy expenditure ($J$) is calculated from the oxygen uptake and respiration quotient at steady state, with a wearable oxygen consumption device. The cumulative energy expenditure values and average oxygen consumption rates ($VO_2$: $mlkg^{-1}min^{-1}$) under four different forefoot rocker conditions were compared using repeated measures ANOVA, and $\alpha < 0.05$ was considered statistically significant. The cumulative energy expenditures were reduced under rocker shoe conditions, and R18.5 with rocker radius at 185 mm was found to be optimal. The results of average oxygen consumption rate in most subjects showed the oxygen consumption rate when wearing rocker shoes was reduced, and mean differences between Flat and R21, R18.5, and R16 were 2.123%, 3.0671, and 3.7761%, respectively. It is suggested that the forefoot rocker-profile footwear design affects walking mechanics from an energy expenditure perspective. Further investigations on sole material compositions and stiffness characteristics are needed to consolidate the rocker-profile designs that are more economic under walking conditions, which may benefit the elderly with reduced walking capacities.

**Keywords:** Biomechanics · Energy expenditure · Rocker radius · Rocker-profile · Footwear design


G. Wang et al. (Eds.): APCMBE 2023, IFMBE Proceedings 103, pp. 336–344, 2024.
https://doi.org/10.1007/978-3-031-51455-5_37

# 1 Introduction

Shoes designed with rocker radius may affect gait stability and walking economy. In particular, increasing the rocker radius may improve the stability of subjects to withstand external disturbances, suggesting that rocker radius affects walking stability [1]. In addition, the use of rigid sole with rocker radius close to 1/3 leg length in healthy people reduced energy expenditure compared to those with smaller or larger rocker radius [2], suggesting an optimal rocker radius may exist for walking economy.

A study comparing metabolic costs in healthy people [3] found that metabolic costs were higher when wearing commercial MBT shoes with rocker soles. Shane R. Wurdeman et al. suggested that the increased metabolic cost may be due to the soft heel area of MBT shoes, which may lead to increased muscle activity in the lower extremities. They also noted that the weight gain of MBT shoes compared to regular shoes is a potential factor that could lead to an increase in metabolic energy costs.

While there have been some studies on the effects of the rocker-profile on the biomechanics of lower extremity joints, potential efficacies on energy expenditure when wearing such shoes have not been understood [4]. Some studies on energy expenditure haven been conducted, but conflicting results were reported. Santo et al. (2012) found no differences in metabolic costs of rocker- versus flat-bottom shoes [5]. In contrast, others have reported either increased [6] or decreased [7] energy expenditure when walking in rocker- versus flat-bottom shoes.

Therefore, the purpose of this study is to experimentally examine the energy expenditure of healthy individuals when walking with four forefoot rocker radius conditions, and the goal was to determine whether there exists a forefoot rocker-profile that would provide an optimal energy benefit during walking conditions.

# 2 Methods

## 2.1 Rocker-Profile Footwear Design

To limit the number of experimental shoes, only one size of high-top leather shoe (shoe length 270 mm) was selected for this study. Subjects walked on a flat-bottom and three shoes with a modified forefoot rocker radius. The radius chosen were: 160 mm, 185 mm and 210 mm (referred to as R16, R18.5 and R21, respectively), and all rocker shoes had the apex position placed in the proximal position (65% of the shoe length with reference to the heel) and had a neutral apex angle of 90° [8–11]. Although rocker shoes with larger radius should be configured with smaller sole forefoot thicknesses, in order to keep all rocker parameters (including outsole thickness) unchanged except radius, the toe portion of R18.5 and R21 was thicker in this study (depicted as forefoot thickness d in Fig. 1). The relative radius (R/L) of R16, R18.5 and R21 are 0.59, 0.69 and 0.78, respectively. However, the size of R/L alone is not sufficient to optimize the biomechanical effect of the rocker shoe in gait. Combined with the forefoot apex position, the arc length of the rocker curve can be determined, and thus the tangent angle of the rocker curve at the end of the sole ($\alpha$). This relationship can be summarized in the following equation:

$$R*\sin\alpha = L*(1 - apex) \tag{1}$$

$$h = R - R * \cos\alpha \tag{2}$$

According to (2), we obtain $\cos\alpha$ :

$$\cos\alpha = \sqrt{1 - \left(\frac{L * (1 - apex)}{R}\right)^2} \tag{3}$$

Then (3) is brought into (2) to obtain h,

$$h = R\left(1 - \sqrt{1 - \left(\frac{L * (1 - apex)}{R}\right)^2}\right) \tag{4}$$

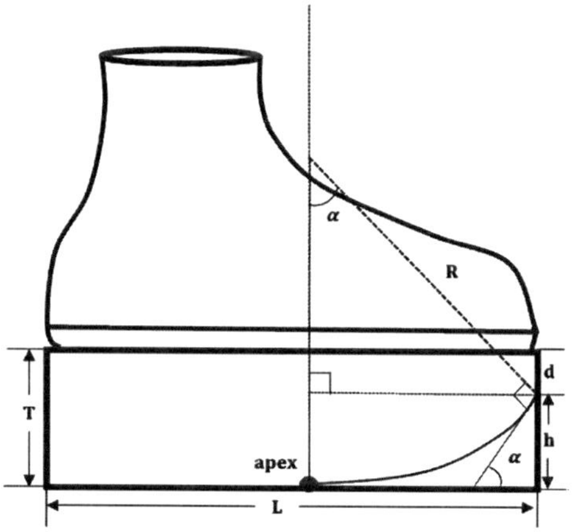


**Fig. 1.** Rocker-profile footwear design parameters. R: the radius of the arc length that defines the forefoot rocker; L: shoe length; apex: expressed as a percentage of the length of the shoe starting from the heel that defines the beginning of the forefoot arc; T: heel thickness; h: forefoot allowance; d: thickness of the toe section; $\alpha$: the angle of tangency of the rocker curve at the end of the sole. The fabricated rocker shoes with a controlled forefoot rocker radius.

To make the sole with rocker-profile, we first calculated the parameters of rocker angle ($\alpha$), forefoot allowance (h) and forefoot thickness (d) corresponding to different rocker radius by using the theoretical model in Fig. 1. In this study, the $\alpha$ of R16, R18.5 and R21 were 36.20°, 30.72° and 26.74°, respectively (Table 1). After cutting off the excess material and sanding, the rocker shoes were ready for use (Fig. 2).

## 2.2 Subjects and Data Acquisition

Sixteen subjects participated in this study (12 males and 4 females), who were primarily master's students at Fudan University. Subjects first went through a consent process approved by the Institutional Review Board of Fudan University and provided written consent at the end of the process.

**Table 1.** Shoe parameters with different forefoot rocker radius.

| Shoe | R (mm) | Rocker angle (°) | h (mm) | d (mm) |
|---|---|---|---|---|
| Flat | ∞ | 0 | 0 | 30.89 |
| R21 | 210 | 36.20 | 22.46 | 8.42 |
| R18.5 | 185 | 30.72 | 25.96 | 4.93 |
| R16 | 160 | 26.74 | 30..89 | 0 |

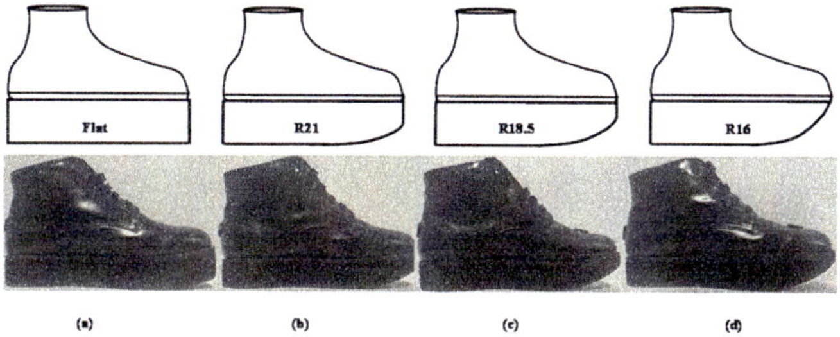


**Fig. 2.** The rocker-profile designs: **a** control shoe: Flat shoe, **b** experimental shoe R21, **c** R18.5, and **d** R16. The experimental shoe soles were made of foam to reduce weight. The thickness of all experimental outsoles was kept at 35 mm.

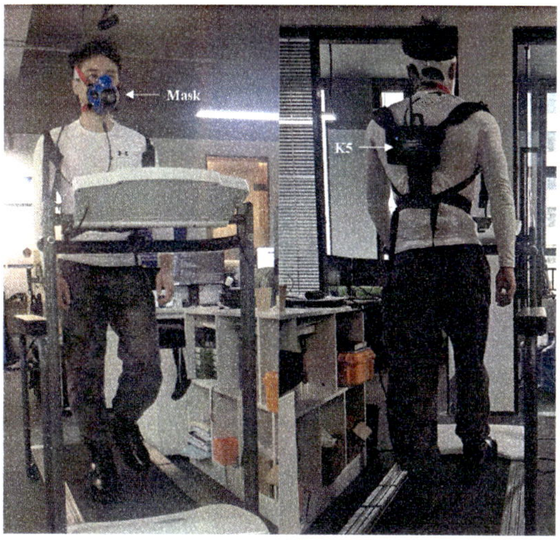


**Fig. 3.** Energy expenditure experiments with subjects walking on a treadmill at a constant speed. Measurements were taken using the wearable spirometer.

## 2.3 Experimental Procedures

The energy expenditure of different forefoot rocker radius (Flat, R21, R18.5, and R16) was tested in a random order. For different rocker radius conditions, subjects walked at a speed of 2.5 km/h chosen during their gait experiments (Fig. 3). Measurements were performed using a wearable spirometer (COSMED K5, Italy) with an open-circuit continuous respiratory gas analysis system. The system allows continuous recording and monitoring of oxygen consumption ($VO_2$) and carbon dioxide production ($VCO_2$) through a mask that does not restrict breathing or vision. Prior to data collection, the gas collection system was calibrated using known concentrations of gas and desiccant according to the K5 system instructions.

Before starting the experiment, subjects sat quietly for 10 min to establish an initial baseline state for the experimental test. Then, for four pairs of shoes, they randomly chose one pair to walk on the treadmill at 2.5 km/h for 6 min. To reduce the interaction between the forefoot rocker radius conditions, subjects sat quietly for 10 min between the two pairs of shoes to re-establish an initial baseline state. In total, there were four walking trials and five rest periods.

### 2.4 Data Analysis

The metabolic energy expenditures were analyzed using dedicated software (OMNIA, COSMED) and custom MATLAB code (MathWorks, Inc., Natick, MA). The $VO_2$ and $VCO_2$ values were normalized to the participant's body mass (kg). Data for the 6 min of each shoe condition are averaged to calculate the average $VO_2$ (mlkg$^{-1}$min$^{-1}$) and respiratory entropy for analysis. The cumulative energy expenditure (J) is calculated from oxygen uptake and respiratory quotient at steady-state conditions.

## 3 Results

Figure 4 showed the cumulative metabolic energy expenditure curve of the subjects walking at a speed of 2.5 km/h in four rocker radius conditions. It was observed that the cumulative curve of energy expenditure was approximately straight, indicating that the subjects were basically in a steady state during the six-minute test.

Figure 5 showed the differences in the average oxygen consumption rate between the Flat shoe and three types of rocker shoes with different forefoot rocker-profiles. The X-axis represents the oxygen consumption of each subject walking in Flat shoe; Y-axis, showing the percentage difference between flat- and rocker-bottom shoes, i.e., $[(\mathrm{mean}(VO_{2\mathrm{Flat})}\mathrm{mean}(VO_{2_{\mathrm{Rocker}}}))/VO_{2\mathrm{Flat}}] \times 100$, where the values above zero indicated improved walking economy as compared to Flat shoe conditions.

Figure 5a, R21 vs. Flat, seven subjects showed walking economy while wearing R21 and the other four subjects showed walking economy while wearing Flat; Fig. 5b, R18.5 vs. Flat, nine subjects showed walking economy while wearing R18.5 and other two subjects showed walking economy while wearing Flat; Fig. 5c, R16 vs Flat, eight subjects showed walking economy in wearing R16 and other three subjects showed walking economy in wearing Flat. The mean differences between Flat and R21, R18.5, and R16 were 2.123%, 3.0671%, and 3.7761%, respectively.

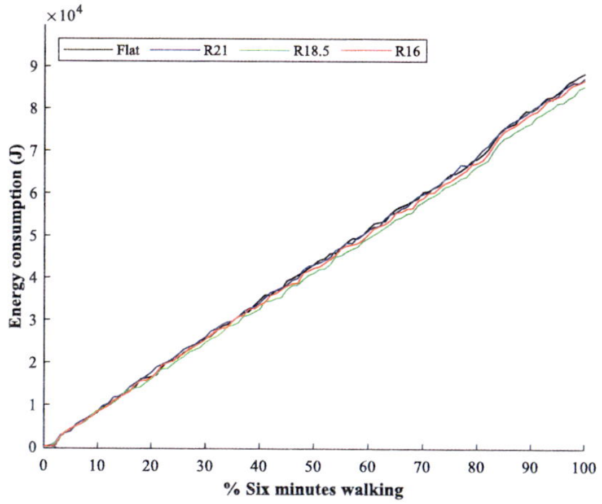


**Fig. 4.** Subjects had a 6-min cumulative metabolic energy expenditure while walking at a speed of 2.5 km/h for four rocker radius conditions.

## 4 Disscussion

The current study experimentally examined the walking economy in young subjects when walking with shoes at different rocker radius. The rocker shoes were improved by designing rocker-profiles with different radius in the forefoot area of the shoes. In general, walking with rocker shoes, in particular to the R18.5 design, resulted in a lower cumulative metabolic energy expenditure as compared with Flat shoe conditions, suggesting different forefoot rocker-profile affect walking mechanics from an energy expenditure perspective.

Previous studies have shown that adding 100 g of mass to shoes increases oxygen consumption by approximately 1% [12–14]. However, our findings showed that the mean difference between flat- and rocker-bottom shoes could reach up to 2.123%, 3.0671%, and 3.7761%, respectively. This result suggests that factors other than the quality of the shoe may play an important role in energy expenditure. We believe that rocker shoes have unique biomechanical characteristics compared to ordinary flat-bottom shoes, which may be an important factor influencing the energy expenditure pair.

In previous biomechanical studies [15], commercial MBT rocker shoes can greatly alter biomechanics of lower extremity joints, especially in the ankle joint. Since our rocker shoe design and the MBT shoe in the above study share a similar forefoot rocker radius feature, it can be inferred that similar changes in treadmill walking energy consumption would occur.

In addition, it has been reported that there is a correlation between energy expenditure and some spatiotemporal gait variables such as step length and cadence [16, 17]. These variables can potentially be influenced by rocker shoe designs, resulting in less energy costs while walking. However, this study does not focus on the biomechanical mechanisms underlying these differences; our goal is to gain a preliminary understanding of the biomechanical characteristics of walking with rocker shoes, particularly the energy expenditure.

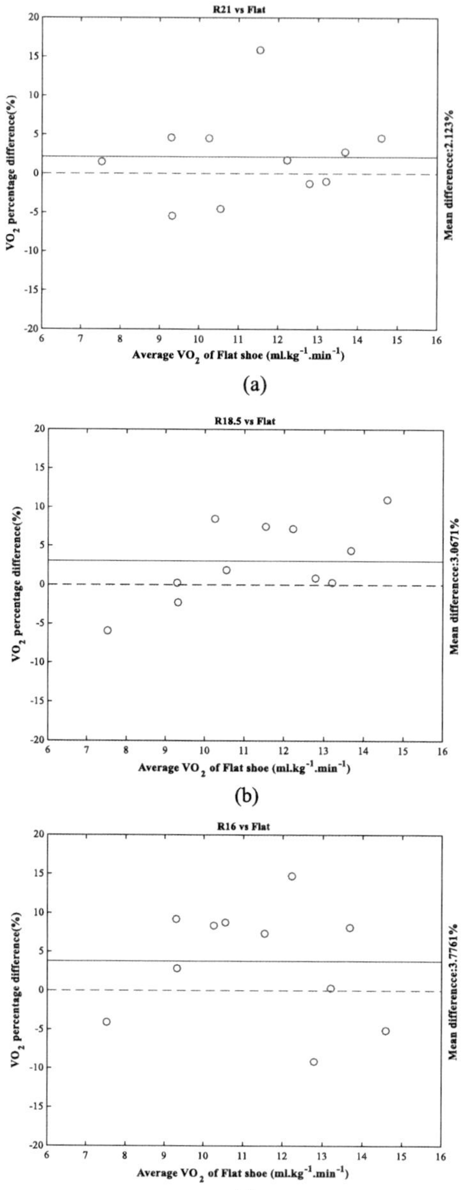


(c)

**Fig. 5.** The average oxygen consumption rate measured on a breath-by-breath basis for three types of rocker shoes as compared to the flat shoe condition.

The weight of the shoe might be a potential confounding factor, but the difference should be negligible for the customized shoes. Also, due to limited number of subjects recruited in the study, it may be not statistically powerful enough to detect small differences between Flat, R21, R18.5 and R16. Generalization of the results to other populations may be compromised since all experiments were only performed in healthy young individuals. Cautious should be exercised when extrapolation of the findings from this study to other population, such as elderly with reduced walking capacities.

## 5 Conclusions

To conclude, this study suggests that the metabolic costs while walking with the designed forefoot rocker-profiles could be lower than those with Flat shoes, and certain rocker-profile may provide an extra energy benefit in walking. We found that the rocker-profile with a curvature of R18.5 had the best energy consumption compared to Flat shoe. Although the underlying mechanisms are not completely known, further investigations on other sole material compositions and stiffness characteristics are needed to consolidate the optimal rocker-profile designs that are more walking economic under walking conditions, than conventional rocker shoes.

**Acknowledgment.** This study was funded by the National Key R&D Program of China (2022YFC2009500), National Natural Science Foundation of China (NSFC, No. 12372322), the Shanghai Science and Technology Development Funds (No. 20S31901000 & No. 21511102200), Medical Engineering Fund of Fudan University (No. yg2021-019 & yg2022-5).

## References

1. Wisse, M., van Frankenhuyzen, J.: Design and construction of MIKE: a 2Dautonomous biped based on passive dynamic walking. In: Kimura, H., Tsuchiya, K. (eds.) Adaptive Motion of Animals and Machines. Springer-Verlag, Tokyo (2006)
2. Adamczyk, P.G., Collins, S.H., Kuo, A.D.: The advantages of a rolling foot in human walking. J. Exp. Biol. **209**(Pt 20), 3953–3963 (2006)
3. Wurdeman, S.R. et al.: An unstable shoe with a rocker bottom redistributes external work. Footwear Sci. **4**(2), 153–158 (2012). IFMBE at http://www.ifmbe.org
4. Greve, C., Schuitema, D., Otten, B., van Kouwenhove, L., Verhaar, E., Postema, K., Dekker, R., Hijmans, J.M.: Biomechanical effects of rocker shoes on plantar aponeurosis strain in patients with plantar fasciitis and healthy controls. PLoS One. **14**(10), e0222388 (2019). https://doi.org/10.1371/journal.pone.0222388. PMID: 31600227; PMCID: PMC6786540
5. Nigg, B., Hintzen, S., Ferber, R.: Effect of an unstable shoe construction on lower extremity gait characteristics. Clin. Biomech. **21**(1), 82–88 (2006). ISSN 0268-0033, https://doi.org/10.1016/j.clinbiomech.2005.08.013
6. Houdijk, H., Brown, S.E., van Dieën, J.H.: Relation between postural sway magnitude and metabolic energy cost during upright standing on a compliant surface. J. Appl. Physiol. (1985). **119**(6), 696–703 (2015). https://doi.org/10.1152/japplphysiol.00907.2014. Epub 2015 Jul 9. PMID: 26159762
7. Maffiuletti, N.A., Malatesta, D., Agosti, F., Sartorio, A.: Unstable shoes increase energy expenditure of obese patients. Am. J. Med. **125**(5), 513–516 (2012). ISSN 0002-9343, https://doi.org/10.1016/j.amjmed.2012.01.001
8. Arazpour, M., Hutchins, S.W., Ghomshe, F.T., Shaky, F., Karami, M.V., Aksenov, A.Y.: Effects of the heel-to-toe rocker sole on walking in able-bodied persons. Prosthet. Orthot. Int. **37**(6), 429–435 (2013). https://doi.org/10.1177/0309364612474920

9. Lockhart, T.E., Smith, J.L., Woldstad, J.C.: Effects of aging on the biomechanics of slips and falls. Hum Factors. Winter **47**(4), 708–729 (2005). https://doi.org/10.1518/001872005775571014. PMID: 16553061; PMCID: PMC2895260
10. Daryabor, A., Arazpour, M., Aminian, G.: Effect of different designs of ankle-foot orthoses on gait in patients with stroke: a systematic review. Gait Posture **62**, 268–279 (2018). ISSN 0966-6362, https://doi.org/10.1016/j.gaitpost.2018.03.026
11. Pijnappels, M., Bobbert, M.F., van Dieën, J.H.: Push-off reactions in recovery after tripping discriminate young subjects, older non-fallers and older fallers.Gait Posture **21**(4), 388–394 (2005). ISSN 0966-6362, https://doi.org/10.1016/j.gaitpost.2004.04.009
12. Choi, H.S., Kim, H.S., Kim, Y.H.: Effects on foot/ankle roll-over characteristics according to different heel heights during walking. Key Eng. Mater. **321–323 II**, 1022–1027 (2006). https://doi.org/10.4028/0-87849-412-x.1022
13. Effective rocker shapes used by able-bodied persons for walking and fore-aft swaying: implications for design of ankle–foot prostheses. Gait Posture **32**(2), 181–184 (2010). ISSN 0966-6362, https://doi.org/10.1016/j.gaitpost.2010.04.014
14. Chapman, J.D., Preece, S.J., Nester, C.J., Braunstein, B., Höhne, A., Brüggermann, G.-P.: What is the best Rocker Shoe design? J. Foot Ankle Res. **5**, O6–O6 (2012)
15. Forghany, S., Nester, C.J., Richards, B., Hatton, A.L., Liu, A.: Rollover footwear affects lower limb biomechanics during walking. Gait Posture 39(1), 205–212 (2014). ISSN 0966-6362, https://doi.org/10.1016/j.gaitpost.2013.07.009. https://www.sciencedirect.com/science/article/pii/S0966636213003172
16. Taniguchi, M., Tateuchi, H., Takeoka, T., Ichihashi, N.: Kinematic and kinetic characteristics of Masai Barefoot Technology footwear. Gait Posture **35**(4), 567–572 (2012). ISSN 0966-6362, https://doi.org/10.1016/j.gaitpost.2011.11.025
17. Schwartz, M.H.: Protocol changes can improve the reliability of net oxygen cost data. Gait Posture **26**(4), 494–500 (2007). ISSN 0966-6362, https://doi.org/10.1016/j.gaitpost.2007.07.014

# Effects of Visual-Vestibular Conflicts Caused by Visual Input on Out-of-Body Experience Induced by Visual-Tactile Stimulation in Virtual Reality

Zhe Song[1], Xiaoya Fan[2], Jiaoyang Dong[1], Xiting Zhang[1], Xiaotian Xu[1], Shuyu Li[3], and Fang Pu[1,4](✉)

[1] State Key Laboratory of Virtual Reality Technology and System, School of Biological Science and Medical Engineering, Beihang University, HaiDian District, XueYuan Road No. 37, Beijing 100083, China
pufangbme@buaa.edu.cn

[2] Key Laboratory for Ubiquitous Network and Service Software of Liaoning Province, School of Software, Dalian University of Technology, Dalian 116620, Liaoning, China

[3] State Key Laboratory of Cognitive Neuroscience, Beijing Normal University, Beijing 100875, China

[4] Research Unit of Virtual Body and Virtual Surgery Technologies, Chinese Academy of Medical Sciences, Beijing 2019RU004, China

**Abstract.** Out-of-body experience (OBE) is a feeling that people observe and feel his/her own body from somewhere outside the physical body. In this paper, we examined the effects of visual-vestibular conflict caused by visual input on OBE induced by visual-tactile stimulation in 15 healthy young participants with virtual reality (VR). We fabricated the visual-vestibular conflict by giving rotating VR scene to the participants. Four experimental conditions were designed. Each participant completed a questionnaire and a proprioceptive drift test in VR. Results showed that the participants experienced subjective alteration of body ownership under conditions with synchronous visual-tactile stimulation, regardless of the presence of rotation VR scene, also revealed a significantly larger drift with rotation VR scene, compared to without, when synchronous visual-tactile stimulation was applied. But such elevation disappeared under conditions without visual-tactile stimulation. We concluded that the OBE induced by synchronous visual-tactile stimulation is modulated by visual-vestibular conflict.

**Keywords:** Out-of-body experience · Virtual reality · Visual-vestibular conflict · Visual-tactile stimulation

## 1 Introduction

Visual-guided motor training with virtual reality (VR) is commonly used in motor rehabilitation [1]. However, the clinical effects of some trainings in third-person-perspective (3PP) are not well performed, and may attributed to the absence of sense of ownership


G. Wang et al. (Eds.): APCMBE 2023, IFMBE Proceedings 103, pp. 345–352, 2024.
https://doi.org/10.1007/978-3-031-51455-5_38

(SOO, i.e., the feeling that a body or a limb belongs to himself/herself) over virtual body [2]. Fortunately, out-of-body experience (OBE) [3] may provide a novel way to solve this problem. Under the synchronous visual-tactile stimulation [4] or visual-motor stimulation [5] on both the physical body and the virtual body at 2 m in front of the participant, participant produced SOO over virtual body. The effect of visual-vestibular conflict on OBE has also been reported [6]. Visual-vestibular conflict could be induced either by disturbed vestibular signals or visual input [7, 8]. When coming to disturbed vestibular signals, it has been shown that vestibular signal is involved in bodily self-consciousness [9–12] and further affects OBE induction. Hence, we speculate that visual-vestibular conflict due to visual input will also affect OBE induction as that caused by vestibular input.

This paper aims to study the effect of visual-vestibular conflict caused by visual input on OBE induced by visual-tactile stimulation. We expect that the visual-vestibular conflict caused by visual input may have an effect on OBE induced by visual-tactile stimulation. In order to create vivid multisensory stimulations, we used virtual reality (VR). VR is essentially the re-input and re-integration of the sensory information that a person percept, and finally forms a cognition of the virtual world in the brain [13]. Research on OBE is of great significance for understanding the mechanisms underlying bodily self-consciousness, and may provide benefits to clinical VR rehabilitation through SOO in 3PP.

## 2 Materials and Methods

### 2.1 Participants

Fifteen college students participated in the present study (8 males and 7 females, aged between 20 and 35 years old). All participants gave written informed consent. The current study adhered to the tenets of the Declaration of Helsinki, and ethical approval was approved by Beihang University (BM20200064).

### 2.2 Procedure

A head-mounted display (HMD; Valve Index, Valve Corporation, Seattle, State of Washington, USA) was used. The participant held a Valve Index Controller with a trigger button on, through which the participant's response could be received. A physical bar was tracked by an HTC Vive Tracker. The VR scene is developed using Unity 3D (Unity Technologies, San Francisco, CA) and the SteamVR SDK.

Four conditions were carried out (Fig. 1b and e).

*Condition 1*: Non-Rotation VR scene without stimulation (NR-NS). Participant was instructed to pay attention to the virtual body for 2 min.

*Condition 2*: Non-Rotation VR scene with synchronous visual-tactile simulation (NR-VT). The experimenter held a physical bar touched the participant's back while a virtual bar synchronously touching the virtual body for 2 min. The physical bar was tracked by an HTC Vive Tracker to keep synchrony.

*Condition 3*: Rotation VR scene without stimulation (R-NS). Participant was instructed to perform as in Condition 1, but with the VR scene rotating around the vertical axis of the virtual body.

*Condition 4*: Rotation VR scene with synchronous visual-tactile simulation (R-VT). Participant was given the same VT stimulus as in Condition 2, but with the VR scene rotating around the vertical axis of virtual body.

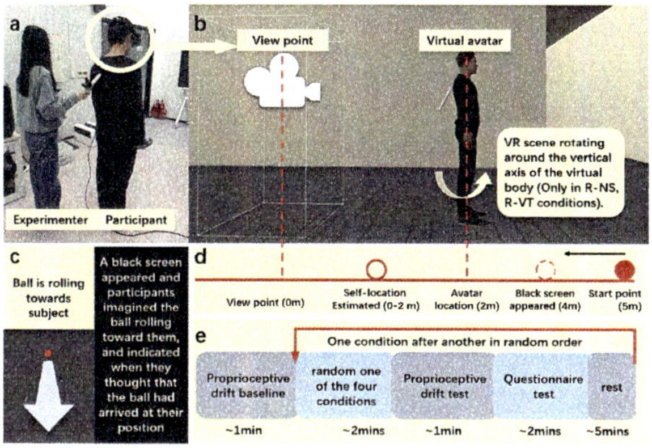


**Fig. 1.** **a** The participant is standing still with the HMD on and Valve Index Controller in hand. The experimenter is holding a white bar touching the participant's back. **b** The virtual scene. The virtual body is standing still. The position of the camera icon represents the view point of the participant. **c** Participant's view in proprioceptive drift task. **d** Illustration of the process in proprioceptive drift test. **e** The flowchart of whole experiment.

## 2.3 Measurements and Data Analysis

*Self-location*: Proprioceptive drift test [14] was carried out before four conditions to measure the baseline of self-location. A red test ball appeared on the floor 5 m in front in the VR scene (Fig. 1c and d), and later the test ball began to roll to the participant at a speed of 0.5 m/s. After 2 s, the participant's view was covered by black scene. The participant was asked to press the trigger button when he/she thought that the test ball arrived at his/her own position. The distance between the ball and the participant's view point position, i.e., the proprioceptive drift, was analyzed using 2 × 2 repeated-measures ANOVA. Paired-samples t-tests were also conducted for post hoc analysis.

*Subjective self-reports of SOO*: Following the proprioceptive drift test of Condition 2 and Condition 4, the scores of questionnaires were recorded. The questionnaire (Table 1) consists of 7 questions, of which Q1-Q3 are OBE-related, Q4-Q7 are control questions. The questions were asked verbally in random order. A score of −3 meant "totally disagree", +3 meant "totally agree", and 0 meant "uncertain". The questionnaire in this study refers to previous studies [3, 14, 15]. The scores of questionnaires were compared through paired-samples t-tests. All statistical tests were performed in IBM SPSS Statistics Version 26 (IBM Corporation).

**Table 1.** Questionnaire to measure SOO to the virtual body in out-of-body experience [14]

| Num | Question |
|---|---|
| Q1 (Touch referral) | It seemed as if I were feeling the touch of the white bar in the location where I saw the virtual body touched |
| Q2 (Touch referral) | It seemed as though the touch I felt was caused by the white bar touching the virtual body |
| Q3 (Out-of-Body) | It felt as if the virtual body was my body |
| Q4 (Control) | It seemed as if I might have had more than one body |
| Q5 (Control) | It seemed as if the touch I was feeling came from somewhere between my own body and the virtual body |
| Q6 (Control) | It appeared (visually) as if the virtual body were drifting backwards (towards the real body) |
| Q7 (Control) | It felt as if my (real) body was drifting towards the front (towards the virtual body) |

# 3 Results

## 3.1 Self-reports of SOO

Figure 2a shows results of questionnaire scores analysis. The scores were significantly higher [$t(14) = 9.505$, ***$p < 0.001$] for OBE-related questions (Q1-Q3, M = 2.04, SD = 0.59, SE = 0.15) compared to control questions (Q4-Q7, M = -0.75, SD = 1.30, SE = 0.34) under NR-VT condition. The scores also differ significantly [$t(14) = 7.575$, ***$p < 0.001$] under R-VT condition between OBE-related questions (Q1-Q3, M = 2.09, SD = 0.68, SE = 0.18) compared to control questions (Q4-Q7, M = −0.32, SD = 1.05, SE = 0.27). Significant difference was found between NR-VT and R-VT conditions neither in OBE-related questions [Q1-Q3, $t(14) = -0.24$, $p = 0.818$] nor OBE-independent control questions [Q4-Q7, $t(14) = -1.36$, $p = 0.194$], although R-VT is slightly higher than NR-VT.

## 3.2 Self-location

A main effect of rotation [$F(1,14) = 6.327$, *$p = 0.025$, $\eta_p^2 = 0.311$] was revealed, but not found in stimulation mode [$F(1,14) = 0.003$, $p = 0.958$, $\eta_p^2 = 0.000$]. There was no significant interaction effect of visual-vestibular state × stimulation mode [$F(1,14) = 1.169$, $p = 0.298$, $\eta_p^2 = 0.077$]. However, paired-samples t-tests showed different results. No significant difference was found in mean drifts [$t(14) = -1.008$, $p = 0.331$] between NR-NS (M = 0.25, SD = 0.69, SE = 0.18) and R-NS (M = 0.38, SD = 0.72, SE = 0.19). But the drift under R-VT (M = 0.50, SD = 0.67, SE = 0.17) condition is significantly higher [$t(14) = -2.414$, *$p = 0.030$] than that under NR-VT (M = 0.14, SD = 0.46, SE = 0.12) condition. No significant difference was found in drifts between two stimulation modes, regardless of the visual-vestibular state, whether rotate [$t(14) = 1.214$, $p = 0.245$] or not [$t(14) = -0.537$, $p = 0.599$]. Figure 2b illustrates the Proprioceptive drift of 4 conditions.

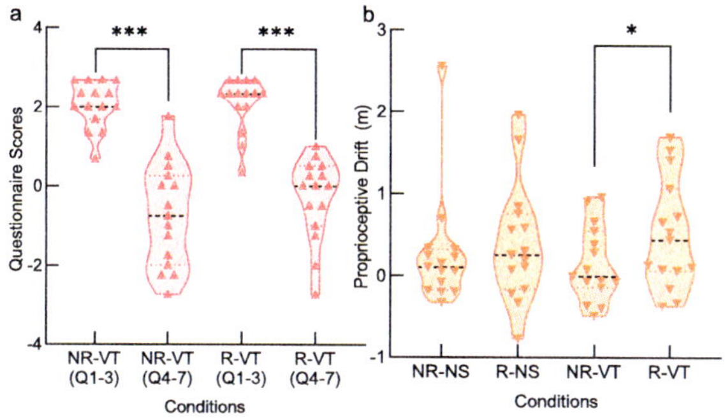


**Fig. 2.** Questionnaire scores **a** for NR-VT and R-VT conditions and comparison of proprioceptive drifts **b** under different conditions (*$p < 0.05$, ***$p < 0.001$).

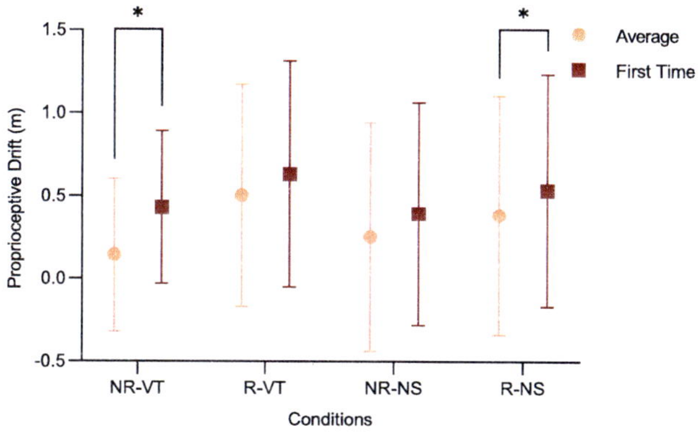


**Fig. 3.** Result of time effect on proprioception drift for four experimental conditions (*$p < 0.05$).

In addition, there was a significant difference (Fig. 3) between the first measure of proprioception drift and the average of five measures under NR-VT and R-NS conditions ($t_{NR\text{-}VT}(14) = -2.476$, *$p = 0.027$; $t_{R\text{-}VT}(14) = -1.773$, $p = 0.098$; $t_{NR\text{-}NS}(14) = -1.407$, $p = 0.181$; $t_{R\text{-}NS}(14) = -2.66$, *$p = 0.019$). The drift measured the first time was significantly higher than the average of the five consecutive repetitions under both NR-VT and R-NS conditions (differences range from 0.13 to 0.28 m).

## 4 Discussion

In this study, we aim to investigate the effect of visual-vestibular conflict caused by visual input on OBE induced by visual-tactile stimulation. Firstly, significant higher scores of OBE-related questions were reported compared to control questions, when conducting synchronous visual-tactile stimulation, regardless of whether the VR scene rotates or not. No significant difference was found in questionnaire scores between R-VT and NR-VT conditions (Fig. 2a). Therefore, we conclude that the newly formed SOO (i.e., subjective cognition of own body) was mainly attributed to the synchronous visual-tactile stimulation, rather than the visual-vestibular conflict. Secondly, visual rotation of VR scene had no significant effect on proprioception drift, when no visual-tactile stimulation was applied. But under the premise of abnormal SOO (newly formed over virtual body) caused by visual-tactile integration, visual rotation significantly strengthened abnormal self-location (Fig. 2b). This is consistent with previous findings that visual-vestibular conflict could affect bodily self-consciousness in the process of multisensory integration and had a modulation effect on OBE. Therefore, formation of new SOO to the virtual body caused by synchronous visual-tactile stimulation seems necessary for visual rotation to disrupt self-location. Without newly formed SOO, visual-vestibular conflict due to visual input is not sufficient to interfere self-location.

Based on these results, we argue that in this scenario, the mistake of visual-tactile integration causes an abnormal SOO, while the visual-vestibular conflict disrupts self-location (drifts to the virtual body), which further confirms the SOO over the virtual body and enhances the OBE. Previous study has demonstrated a modulation effect of visual-vestibular disintegration on OBE [6]. The failure of visual (external space) and vestibular (personal space) integration leads to the disintegration between the personal and the extra personal space, resulting in the experience of seeing his/her own body from other position [16]. These OBE models emphasize the contradiction between vestibular perception and visual information, known as *the visuo-vestibular splitting of somatosensory body image.* A study also proposed [17] that visual-vestibular conflict was one of the factors in distorted bodily self-consciousness. The results of present study complement these OBE models and provide more details.

In addition, our results also showed a time effect on proprioceptive drift. More specifically, the drift is significantly larger for the first proprioceptive test immediately after stimulation, compared to the average of five consecutive tests (Fig. 3), indicating a degenerating effect of stimulation after removal. Such a rapid degenerating could be attributed to the short period of stimulation, which is insufficient to alter the top-down prior of the bodily self-consciousness established from daily experience (i.e., a stable body image from top to bottom). Body image refers to the stable top-down representation formed in long term and is not susceptible to temporal sensory input. The functional representation formed after receiving real-time sensory input and motor feedback (i.e., when using tools, the hand temporarily has the function of the tool) is known as body schema, which is susceptible to temporal sensory input [18, 19]. The time effect revealed in this study could be explained by the process that stable body image corrects the representation of body schema affected by the transient stimulation.

## 5 Conclusions

This paper investigated the effects of visual-vestibular conflict on OBE induced by synchronous visual-tactile stimulation. Our results showed that with visual-vestibular conflict, OBE induced by visual-tactile stimulation could be strengthened. Results also revealed a time effect of stimulation which is in support of the theory of body image and body schema. Research on OBE inducing mechanism can promote better understanding on human self-consciousness and may provide benefits to clinical VR rehabilitation through SOO in 3PP.

**Acknowledgment.** *Conflict of Interest*: The authors declare that they have no conflict of interest.

*Consent to participate:* We obtained written informed consent from all individual participants included in the study.

*Consent for publication:* All the authors contributed to this article and consent to the publication of this research work.

*Data availability statement*: All the data and materials in the current study are available from the corresponding author on reasonable request.

Funding: This research was funded by the National Natural Science Foundation of China (Grant No. 12072019), and CAMS Innovation Fund for Medical Sciences (CIFMS) under Grant 2019-I2M-5-016.

## References

1. Sevcenko, K., Lindgren, I.: The effects of virtual reality training in stroke and Parkinson's disease rehabilitation: a systematic review and a perspective on usability. Eur. Rev. Aging Phys. Act. **19**(1), 4 (2022)
2. Tambone, R., et al.: Using body ownership to modulate the motor system in stroke patients. Psychol. Sci. **32**(5), 655–667 (2021)
3. Lenggenhager, B., et al.: Video ergo sum: manipulating bodily self-consciousness. Science **317**(5841), 1096–1099 (2007)
4. Droit-Volet, S., et al.: Embodied time and the out-of-body experience of the self. PeerJ **8**, e8565 (2020)
5. Bourdin, P., et al.: A virtual out-of-body experience reduces fear of death. PLoS One **12**(1), e0169343 (2017)
6. Blanke, O.: Multisensory brain mechanisms of bodily self-consciousness. Nat. Rev. Neurosci. **13**(8), 556–571 (2012)
7. Tanahashi, S., Ujike, H., Ukai, K.: Visual rotation axis and body position relative to the gravitational direction: effects on circular vection. Iperception **3**(10), 804–819 (2012)
8. Butler, J.S., et al.: Bayesian integration of visual and vestibular signals for heading. J. Vis. **10**(11), 23 (2010)
9. Sedda, A., et al.: Left caloric vestibular stimulation as a tool to reveal implicit and explicit parameters of body representation. Conscious. Cogn. **41**, 1–9 (2016)
10. Pfeiffer, C., Serino, A., Blanke, O.: The vestibular system: a spatial reference for bodily self-consciousness. Front. Integr. Neurosci. **8**, 31 (2014)
11. Lopez, C., et al.: Vestibular stimulation modifies the body schema. Neuropsychologia **50**(8), 1830–1837 (2012)
12. Lopez, C., Blanke, O., Mast, F.W.: The human vestibular cortex revealed by coordinate-based activation likelihood estimation meta-analysis. Neuroscience **212**, 159–179 (2012)
13. Slater, M., Sanchez-Vives, M.V.: Enhancing our lives with immersive virtual reality. Front. Rob. AI **3** (2016)
14. Nakul, E., et al.: Measuring perceived self-location in virtual reality. Sci. Rep. **10**(1), 6802 (2020)

15. Ehrsson, H.H.: The experimental induction of out-of-body experiences. Science **317**(5841), 1048 (2007)
16. Blanke, O., et al.: Out-of-body experience and autoscopy of neurological origin. Brain **127**(Pt 2), 243–258 (2004)
17. Lopez, C.: A neuroscientific account of how vestibular disorders impair bodily self-consciousness. Front. Integr. Neurosci. **7**, 91 (2013)
18. Mann, J.: The medical avatar and its role in neurorehabilitation and neuroplasticity: a review. NeuroRehabilitation **46**(4), 467–482 (2020)
19. Schettler, A., Raja, V., Anderson, M.L.: The embodiment of objects: review, analysis, and future directions. Front. Neurosci. **13**, 1332 (2019)

# A Convolutional Neural Network with Narrow Kernel and Dual-View Feature Fusion for sEMG-Based Gesture Recognition

Hao Wu[1], Bin Jiang[1](✉), Qingling Xia[1], Hanguang Xiao[1], Fudai Ren[1], and Yun Zhao[2](✉)

[1] School of Artificial Intelligence, Chongqing University of Technology, Yubei District, No. 459, Pufu Avenue, Longxing Town, Chongqing, China
jb20200132@cqut.edu.cn

[2] School of Smart Health, Chongqing College of Electronic Engineering, Shapingba District, No. 76, University City East Road, Chongqing, China
zyyy90@163.com

**Abstract.** For gesture recognition based on surface Electromyography (sEMG), Convolutional Neural Network (CNN)-based techniques have made prominent progress to gesture features extract for motor rehabilitation or bionic hand control. However, the performance of traditional CNN algorithms shows limited capability to characterize the time-varying properties and channel independence of sEMG. In this paper, a Narrow Kernel and Dual-view Feature Fusion Convolutional Neural Network (NKDFF-CNN) is proposed. The Narrow Kernel was firstly used to fully extract the temporal features of each channel to protect the channel independence of sEMG. Feature fusion between two views to effectively reduce the number of the model parameters and avoid the overfitting phenomenon. Then, shallow and deep features were fused in the decision phase to improve the multi-dimensional characterization of sEMG. Finally, a more powerful Arcface loss function replaced Softmax for gesture classification. The algorithm was validated experimentally on the Ninapro DB2 dataset using a 200 ms window length. The results showed that NKDFF-CNN achieved an average recognition accuracy of 87.96% for 40 subjects, which is 0.94% higher than the best result using other methods. This algorithm presented in this paper effectively improved the performance of gesture recognition based sEMG and provided a new idea for this research direction.

**Keywords:** Surface electromyography (sEMG) · Gesture recognition · Narrow kernel · Dual-view · Feature fusion

## 1 Introduction

Human hand is one of the most important tools of the human workforce and a reliable means of interaction between humans and the outside world [1]. Surface electromyography (sEMG) in upper limb with collected non-invasive and convenient collection contains large information of hand motion intention, and is a reliable signal for human-computer


G. Wang et al. (Eds.): APCMBE 2023, IFMBE Proceedings 103, pp. 353–362, 2024.
https://doi.org/10.1007/978-3-031-51455-5_39

interaction systems such as prosthetic control and motor rehabilitation [2]. Gesture recognition algorithms play a key role in extracting and decoding sEMG features to achieve accurate, flexible and stable motion pattern recognition in upper limb. Therefore, how to optimize those techniques for gesture recognition has become a research hotspot in the fields of rehabilitation medicine, intelligent bionic hand, exoskeleton robotics, etc. [3].

The traditional sEMG-based gesture recognition algorithms have already showed good recognition performance in classification tasks with a small number of gesture types, while exist deficiency in performing tasks with a high number of gesture types [4]. Therefore, researchers have focused on deep learning to feature extraction and classification of sEMG so as to achieve more stable and accurate myoelectric control [5]. In previous studies, Wang et al. [6] used deformable convolution to automatically learn the offset of the convolution kernel to adaptively adjust the receptive field, significantly improving the gesture recognition accuracy on the Ninapro DB1 dataset. Sun et al. [7] used inflated Long Short-Term Memory (LSTM) to achieve better memory for historical information without increasing the number of layers and units. Although the accuracy on Ninapro DB2 was only 82%, the number of model parameters was extremely small. Peng et al. [8] used a divide-and-conquer three-view learning strategy to divide the sEMG into three inputs to separate convolutional streams, performed multi-view feature fusion, and achieved a gesture recognition accuracy of 82% on Ninapro DB2. Recently, Fatayer et al. [9] developed a label noise processing algorithm to re-delineate active segments in real-time during Convolutional Neural Network (CNN) training, which effectively eliminated mislabeling and achieved an accuracy of 87.9% for 41-class gesture recognition.

Although the above studies effectively used different CNN means to improve the performance of sEMG gesture recognition, the network structures of those CNN methods did not fully consider the time-varying properties and channel independence of sEMG, which should be improved in feature extraction ability. To further improve the gesture recognition performance, the contributions in this paper can be summarized as follows:

1. Since sEMG are a multi-channel time-varying signals with strong independence among each channel, this paper utilized a narrow convolutional kernel to fully extract the temporal correlation of sEMG in each channel.
2. Feature fusion between two views by add, the model volume and the possibility of overfitting are reduced.
3. The model's deep features and shallow features are fused in the decision phase by concat to enhance further the extracted features' expressiveness.
4. The Arcface loss function is used instead of Softmax to further improve the performance of the classification.

## 2 Materials and Methods

### 2.1 Data and Pre-processing

In this paper, we utilized the subset DB2 of the NinaPro dataset (https://paperswithcode.com/dataset/ninapro-db2) [10, 11] to verify the proposed algorithm. The 12-channel sEMG from 40 healthy subjects were recorded with the sampling frequency of 2 kHz. Each subject performed 49 gestures, repeated six times in every gesture task within 5 s, and then had a short rest of 3 s.

Data pre-processing procedures showed as the following:

1. Noise reduction was performed on the raw data by using a bandpass filter of 10–500 Hz [12], and then a notch filter of 50 Hz to eliminate the power-line interference. Wavelet decomposition with a sym mother wavelet was applied to the sEMG signals [13] to remove the stubborn noise.
2. Eliminating the resting state data with label 0, taking the 2nd and 5th of 6 repetitions of each gesture as the testing set and the rest as the training set, and normalizing the data sets by the Z-score method (as in Eq. 1).
3. Using the sliding window method to expand the data size while slicing the data. Previous studies showed that the window length below or above a threshold will adversely affect the performance of the system [14]. Therefore, this paper used a window length of 200 ms and chose a sliding step length of 10 ms. The sampling points of the window $L$ is calculated as Eq. 2. Finally, the N pieces of 400*12 data obtained from the division were dimensioned into 1*400*12 data for model training.

$$x^* = \frac{x-\mu}{\sigma} \tag{1}$$

where $x^*$ is the normalized value, $x$ is the original value, $\mu$ is the mean value, and $\sigma$ is the standard deviation.

$$L = f * T \tag{2}$$

where $f$ is the sampling frequency, $T$ is the window length.

## 2.2 Methodology

The structure of the NKDFF-CNN proposed in this paper is shown in Fig. 1; Part 1 is the convolutional part, Part 2 is the fully connected part, and the specific composition and specific parameters of Part 1 and Part 2 are shown in Tables 1 and 2, the blank data in the tables are the default values.

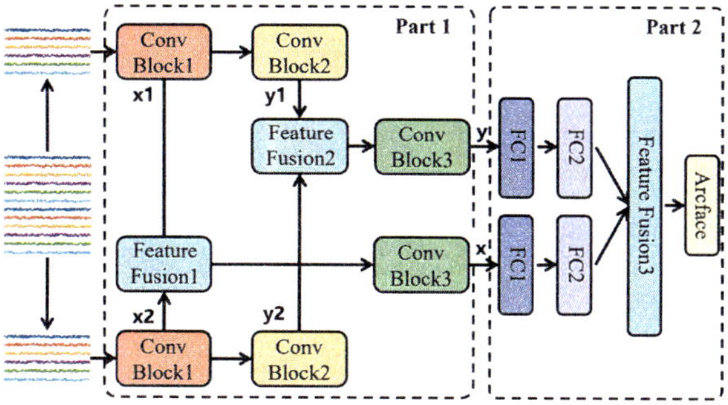


**Fig. 1.** Schematic diagram of the structure of NKDFF-CNN

The input of NKDFF-CNN, sEMG data of 400*12*1, is divided into two inputs with the size of 400*6*1 to feed into two convolutional paths with the same structure for Dual-view learning.

In Part 1, each view (i.e., each convolutional path) contains two parts: Convblock1 is used to extract shallow feature maps x1 and x2, and ConvBlock2 is used to extract deep feature maps y1 and y2. Feature Fusion1 can fuse shallow features on x1 and x2, and Feature Fusion2 can fuse deep features on y1 and y2. The nature of feature fusion1 and feature fusion2 is add, i.e., which reduces the size of the feature map by half compared with the traditional single-view structure, significantly decreasing the total number of parameters and effectively avoiding overfitting.

The feature fusion1 and feature fusion2 are connected to ConvBlock3 for further extraction of the features correlated among the channels to obtain the shallow feature map x and the deep feature map y. The calculation is shown in Eqs. 3 and 4.

$$x = ConvBlock3 \quad (x1 + x2) \tag{3}$$

$$y = ConvBlock3 \quad (y1 + y2) \tag{4}$$

**Table 1.** NKDFF-CNN Part 1 structure and parameter settings

| Block name | Layer name | Number of kernels | Kernel size | Kernel stride | Padding |
|---|---|---|---|---|---|
| Convblock1 | Conv1 | 8 | 5*1 | (2,1) | |
| | Avgpool1 | | 2*1 | (2,1) | |
| | Conv2 | 16 | 5*1 | (2,1) | |
| | Avgpool2 | | 2*1 | (2,1) | |
| Convblock2 | Conv3 | 24 | 3*1 | | |
| | Conv4 | 32 | 3*1 | | |
| | Conv5 | 32 | 1*6 | | (0,3) |
| Convblock3 | Conv6 | 32 | 5*1 | | |
| | Avgpool3 | | 2*1 | (2,1) | |
| | Conv7 | 32 | 1*6 | | (0,3) |

In Part 1, since sEMG data in each channel is independent from that in other channels and time-varying, the standard N*N convolution kernel mainly focuses on the inter-channel spatial features and then dilutes the intra-channel temporal features, which will destroy the channel independence of the sEMG data in each channel. Therefore, a narrow convolutional kernel of size N*1 along the time direction is firstly used to prioritize the full learning of temporal features of the sEMG data within each channel. After that, a narrow convolutional kernel of size 1*N along the channel direction is used to learn the spatially correlated features among channels.

All the convolutional layers in Part 1 are followed by a Batch Normalization [15] (BN) layer and a Leaky-Relu [16] nonlinear activation layer. The BN makes the distribution of the output of the convolutional layers relatively stable and accelerates the model learning

**Table 2.** NKDFF-CNN Part 2 cell number setting

| Layer name | Units |
|---|---|
| FC1 | 512 |
| FC1 | 128 |
| Arcface | 49 |

speed. The Leaky-Relu is used to enhance the nonlinear fitting ability of the network. Meanwhile, the Convolutional Block Attention Module [17] (CBAM) is added at the end of each ConvBlock to enhance model attention to high contribution features from a global perspective.

For feature maps x and y, shallow feature vectors and deep feature vectors with the length of 128 are obtained using two Fully Connected (FC) layers after Flatten, respectively, and then a fused feature vector with the length of 256 is obtained by decision-level feature fusion of feature fusion3. The nature of feature fusion3 is concat. By shallow features to assist deep features for classification, the extracted features are richer and more expressive, improving the recognition effect. With Relu nonlinear activation layers, FC1 and FC2 use Dropout with a ratio of 0.5 to mitigate overfitting.

Arcface [18] is a new loss function with trainable parameters used in face recognition. This method can aggregate the scores of the features in the same class and differentiate the scores of the features among different classes, which is better for classification than traditional Softmax. Therefore, Arcface is selected in this paper, and the calculation includes: The feature vector with the length of 256 output by feature fusion3 is first fully connected to a feature vector with the length of 49. The components of the vector are mapped by the inverse trigonometric function to $\theta_{y_i}$, where $i \in (1, 49)$, and then the angular $\theta_{y_i}$ are transformed similarly to Softmax by Eq. 5 ($m$ and $s$ are hyperparameters), and the final output is a vector with the length of 49, i.e., the scores belong to each gesture $Score_i$.

$$Score_i = -log\frac{e^{s\cos\left(\theta_{y_i}+m\right)}}{e^{s\cos\left(\theta_{y_i}+m\right)}+\sum_{j=1,j\neq y_i}^{N}e^{s\cos\theta_j}} \tag{5}$$

## 2.3 Experiment

After the pre-processing in the part of Data and pre-processing above, sEMG data can be input into the algorithm model in the part of Methodology for training, and the accuracy of the testing set is recorded, and the formula is defined as Eq. 6, and finally, the average accuracy of all subjects is calculated as the evaluation index.

$$\text{Accuracy} = \frac{\text{Number of correct classification}}{\text{Total number of test samples}} \times 100\% \tag{6}$$

In this paper, Arcface is used as the loss function, and the Adam optimizer is used to update the network parameters during backpropagation, and the initial learning rate is determined to be 0.001, and the learning rate is dynamically adjusted by cosine annealing strategy during training, with a total of 50 epochs trained and 256 batch size.

All experiments were performed on workstations equipped with NVIDIA GEFORCE RTX 3080ti and i5-10600KF and using the Pytorch 1.11.0 framework.

To verify whether the proposed NKDFF-CNN employs the correct choice of dual views and feature fusion scheme, the experiments of A and B are conducted on subjects 5, 10, 15, 20, 25, 30, 35, and 40. Experiment A was based on the NKDFF-CNN structure by changed the number of views from 1 to 4, where the input of each view was the sEMG data of 400*C*1, and the C was 12, 6, 4 and 3. The structure of each view was the same, and the structure of each block was referred to in Fig. 1, Table 1 and Table 2(where the kernels size of conv5 and conv7 are changed to 1*C and the padding is changed to 1*0.5C), the average accuracy of the model obtained by the four view segmentation methods is recorded to get Fig. 2. Experiment B constructs two models based on the NKDFF-CNN structure: Model 1 used only the shallow features for classification and masked the deep features, Model 2 used only the deep features for classification and masked the shallow features, and Model 3 is NKDFF-CNN, which used a decision-level fusion of shallow and deep features for classification. The average accuracy of the three models is then recorded to obtain Fig. 3.

To further understand the practical effects of the optimization schemes such as dual-view structure, feature fusion, narrow kernel and Arcface used in this paper, we conducted gesture classification experiments with Ninapro DB2 of 40 subjects to investigate the performance of NKDFF-CNN and following five models. Model A is created using a single-view structure based on NKDFF-CNN (same method as above); Model B is created by masking out shallow features and then using only deep features for classification based on NKDFF-CNN; Model C is created using standard convolution kernel instead of narrow convolutional kernels based on NKDFF-CNN. Model C changes the kernel size of all convolution layers of NKDFF-CNN to 3*3, padding to (1, 1), and all the rest of the network structure is the same as Fig. 1, Table 1 and Table 2; instead of Arcface based on NKDFF-CNN, Softmax is used for classification to created Model D. Model E is created only by the deep features based on a single-view structure of NKDFF-CNN with standard kernel and traditional Softmax. The results are shown in Table 3.

## 3 Results and Discussion

Figure 2 shows that the Dual-view is the most accurate among the four view segmentation methods. Among them, the performance of single-view decreases, probably due to the larger feature map size making overfitting by increased parameters, which negatively affects the algorithm performance. In contrast, the performance of three and four views becomes lower and lower, which may derive from too many view divisions resulting in a too small feature map after feature fusion by add. In summary, Dual-view is the best choice.

From Fig. 3, it can be found that the highest gesture recognition accuracy rate can be obtained by merging shallow features and deep features for decision-level fusion. The accuracy rate is reduced using only deep features or shallow features. The lowest performance is obtained using shallow features, indicating that deep features involve

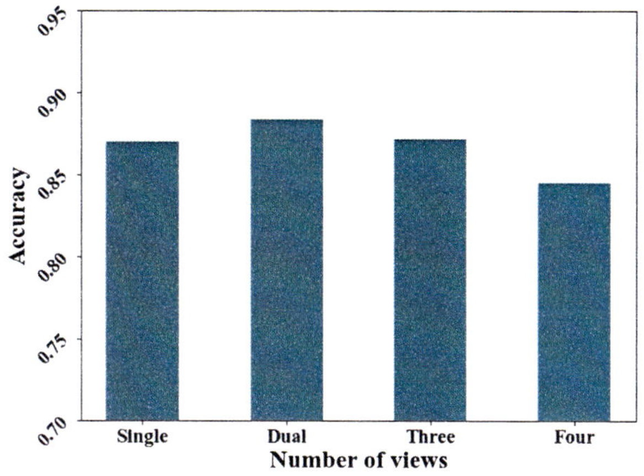


**Fig. 2.** Accuracy of gesture recognition using four view segmentation methods

more powerful feature expression capability than shallow features. Also, the results fully demonstrate the effectiveness of the proposed method for gesture classification based on sEMG data.

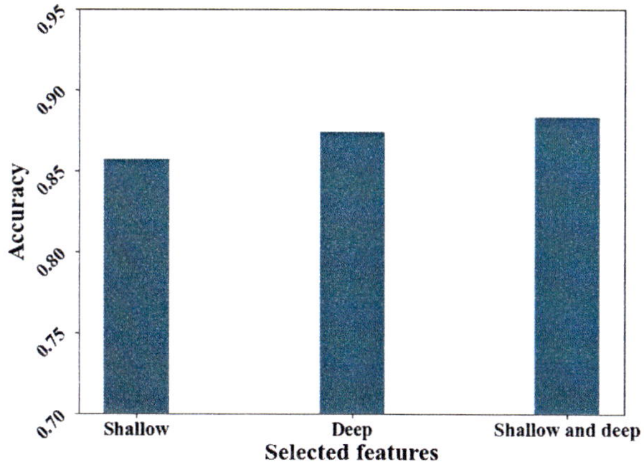


**Fig. 3.** Accuracy of gesture recognition with different features selected for classification

As shown in Table 3, based on the results of the experimental data of NKDFF-CNN, we can conclude: (1) When the dual-view strategy is eliminated, the number of the parameters in Model A inflates significantly from 2.39 M to 4.17 M, and the accuracy rate decreases by 0.92%, indicating that the feature fusion strategy by add operation between two views does effectively reduce the number of parameters. (2) When the shallow features are masked out, although the number of parameters in Model B is reduced, the accuracy rate decreases significantly by 1.11% due to the absence of the shallow features, indicating that the shallow features compensate for the lower dimensional information missing from the deep features mainly focusing on higher dimensional

**Table 3.** Number of parameters and recognition accuracy of each model constructed in this paper, where M is in millions

| Model name | Params | Accuracy |
|---|---|---|
| Model A | 4.17 M | 87.04% |
| Model B | 1.72 M | 86.85% |
| Model C | 2.79 M | 86.43% |
| Model D | 2.40 M | 86.93% |
| Model E | 3.91 M | 82.46% |
| NKDFF-CNN | **2.39 M** | **87.96%** |

information, which can effectively enhance the expression ability of the features and the classification performance. (3) When using the standard convolution kernel, the number of parameters of Model C increases slightly, and the fitting ability of the model seems to be enhanced, but the accuracy rate drops significantly by 1.53%, which is the lowest performance except Model E. It indicates that the standard convolution kernel destroys the independence of sEMG in each channel, resulting in overly extracting the spatial correlation among channels rather than the temporal correlation features within each channel. This is not in line with the own characteristics of sEMG data, which can be effectively improved by the narrow kernel. (4) The number of parameters of Model D is not significantly changed after replacing Arcface with Softmax, but the recognition accuracy decreases by 1.03%, effectively proving that Arcface can improve the performance of sEMG-based gesture recognition. (5) For Model E, after eliminating all the optimization strategies, the number of the model parameters will increase, but more importantly, the recognition accuracy decreases by 7.5%, and the model performance is much lower than the other five models, while NKDFF-CNN obtains the best accuracy with only more parameters than Model B. Those results strongly proof that the algorithm proposed in this paper significantly improves the performance of convolutional neural networks in sEMG gesture recognition.

We compare the NKDFF-CNN proposed in this paper with the gesture recognition algorithms in recent years on the Ninapro BD2. From Table 4, Our method performs well in the recognition accuracy when the window length matches the mainstream selection and the number of gestures classified is high.

## 4 Conclusions

This paper proposes NKDFF-CNN to improve the performance of deep learning in sEMG gesture recognition. The NKDFF-CNN algorithm utilizes a narrow convolutional kernel to extract temporal features in each independent channel preferentially, and features fusion of two views by an add operation to mitigate overfitting, and fuses shallow and deep features in the decision phase to enhance the representation of the features, and finally introduce an Arcface loss function instead of Softmax to improve the classification performance. The experimental results show that the NKDFF-CNN algorithm performs

**Table 4.** Comparison of NKDFF-CNN with other studies

| Method | Window length | Classes | Accuracy |
|---|---|---|---|
| Attention-CNN-RNN [19] | 200 ms | 49 | 82.2% |
| Dilation-LSTM [7] | 300 ms | 49 | 82% |
| CNN-LSTM [20] | 200 ms | 17 | 83.91% |
| DVMSCNN [21] | 640 ms | 49 | 83.29% |
| CNN [22] | 100 ms | 49 | 83.23% |
| MvCNN [23] | 200 ms | 49 | 85.8% |
| Transformer [24] | 200 ms | 49 | 86.18% |
| MSFF-net [8] | 200 ms | 49 | 87.02% |
| NKDFF-CNN | **200 ms** | **49** | **87.96%** |

the recognition accuracy of 87.96% for 49 gesture recognition on the Ninapro DB2 dataset, which is 0.94% higher than the current state-of-the-art results, and reach the various functions as expected. Therefore, it can be concluded that the NKDFF-CNN algorithm constructed in this paper shows an excellent performance and provides a new effective idea for optimizing sEMG gesture recognition technologies.

**Acknowledgment.** The authors sincerely thank the institute of Information Systems Institute at the University of Applied Sciences Western Switzerland for sharing the sEMG data (https://paperswithcode.com/dataset/ninapro-db2). This work was supported by Scientific and Technological Research Program of Chongqing Municipal Education Commission (KJQN202201142), the Chongqing Research Program of Basic Research Frontier Technology (Grant No. CSTB2022BSXM-JCX0069CCCC), the Scientific Research Foundation of Chongqing University of Technology(2021ZDZ010) and Training Program of the National Natural Science Foundation of China and National Social Science Fund of China of Chongqing University of Technology(2022PYZ030).

## References

1. Liu, H., Dong, W., Li, Y., et al.: An epidermal sEMG tattoo-like patch as a new human–machine interface for patients with loss of voice. Microsyst. Nanoeng. **6**(1), 1–13 (2020)
2. Sun, Y., Xu, C., Li, G., et al.: Intelligent human computer interaction based on non redundant EMG signal. Alex. Eng. J. **59**(3), 1149–1157 (2020)
3. Brinton, M.R., Barcikowski, E., Davis, T., et al.: Portable take-home system enables proportional control and high-resolution data logging with a multi-degree-of-freedom bionic arm. Front. Rob. AI **7**, 559034 (2020)
4. Kuzborskij, I., Gijsberts, A., Caputo, B.: On the challenge of classifying 52 hand movements from surface electromyography. In: Proceedings of the Annual International Conference of the IEEE Engineering in Medicine and Biology Society, pp. 4931–4937 (2012)
5. Zia ur Rehman, M., Waris, A., Gilani, S.O., et al.: Multiday EMG-based classification of hand motions with deep learning techniques. Sensors **18**(8), 2497 (2018)

6. Wang, H., Zhang, Y., Liu, C., et al.: SEMG based hand gesture recognition with deformable convolutional network. Int. J. Mach. Learn. Cybern. **13**(6), 1729–1738 (2022)
7. Sun, T., Hu, Q., Gulati, P., et al.: Temporal dilation of deep LSTM for agile decoding of sEMG: application in prediction of Upper-Limb motor intention in NeuroRobotics. IEEE Rob. Autom. Lett. **6**(4), 6212–6219 (2021)
8. Peng, X., Zhou, X., Zhu, H., et al.: MSFF-Net: multi-stream feature fusion network for surface electromyography gesture recognition. PLoS One **17**(11), e0276436 (2022)
9. Fatayer, A., Gao, W., Fu, Y.: sEMG-based gesture recognition using deep learning from noisy labels. IEEE J. Biomed. Health Inf. (2022)
10. Atzori, M., Gijsberts, A., Castellini, C., et al.: Electromyography data for non-invasive naturally-controlled robotic hand prostheses. Sci. Data **1**(1), 1–13 (2014)
11. Atzori, M., Gijsberts, A., Kuzborskij, I., et al.: Characterization of a benchmark database for myoelectric movement classification. IEEE Trans. Neural Syst. Rehabil. Eng. **23**(1), 73–83 (2014)
12. Fan, Y., Yin, Y.: Active and progressive exoskeleton rehabilitation using multisource information fusion from EMG and force-position EPP. IEEE Trans. Biomed. Eng. **60**(12), 3314–3321 (2013)
13. Karnam, N.K., Dubey, S.R., Turlapaty, A.C., et al.: EMGHandNet: a hybrid CNN and Bi-LSTM architecture for hand activity classification using surface EMG signals. Biocybern. Biomed. Eng. **42**(1), 325–340 (2022)
14. Englehart, K., Hudgins, B.: A robust, real-time control scheme for multifunction myoelectric control. IEEE Trans. Biomed. Eng. **50**(7), 848–854 (2003)
15. Ioffe, S., Szegedy, C.: Batch normalization: accelerating deep network training by reducing internal covariate shift. In: International Conference on Machine Learning. PMLR, 448–456 (2015)
16. Xu, B., Wang, N., Chen, T., et al.: Empirical evaluation of rectified activations in convolutional network (2015). arXiv preprint arXiv:1505.00853
17. Woo, S., Park, J., Lee, J.Y., et al.: Cbam: convolutional block attention module. In: Proceedings of the European Conference on Computer Vision (ECCV), pp. 3–19 (2018)
18. Deng, J., Guo, J., Xue, N., et al.: Arcface: additive angular margin loss for deep face recognition. In: Proceedings of the IEEE/CVF Conference on Computer Vision and Pattern Recognition, pp. 4690–4699 (2019)
19. Hu, Y., Wong, Y., Wei, W., et al.: A novel attention-based hybrid CNN-RNN architecture for sEMG-based gesture recognition. PLoS One **13**(10), e0206049 (2018)
20. Kim, J.S., Kim, M.G., Pan, S.B.: Two-step biometrics using electromyogram signal based on convolutional neural network-long short-term memory networks. Appl. Sci. **11**(15), 6824 (2021)
21. Zhang, Y., Yang, F., Fan, Q., et al.: Research on sEMG-based gesture recognition by dual-view deep learning. IEEE Access **10**, 32928–32937 (2022)
22. Xing, K., Ding, Z., Jiang, S., et al.: Hand gesture recognition based on deep learning method. In: 2018 IEEE Third International Conference on Data Science in Cyberspace (DSC), pp. 542–546. IEEE (2018)
23. Wei, W., Hong, H., Wu, X.: A hierarchical view pooling network for multichannel surface electromyography-based gesture recognition. Comput. Intell. Neurosci. **2021** (2021)
24. Zabihi, S., Rahimian, E., Asif, A., et al.: TraHGR: transformer for hand gesture recognition via electromyography (2022). arXiv e-prints: arXiv: 2203.16336

# Tongue Visualization Model for Mandarin Pronunciation Based on MRI

S. C. Zhang[1], C. Liu[1], F. J. Li[1], L. Wang[1], and H. J. Niu[1,2(✉)]

[1] School of Biological Science and Medical Engineering, Beihang University, Haidian District, Zhichun Road, Beijing, China
hjniu@buaa.edu.cn

[2] Advanced Innovation Center for Biomedical Engineering, Haidian District, Zhichun Road, Beijing, China

**Abstract.** An improved tongue statistical model was presented. Volume images of tongue were acquired by MRI from one subject uttering a corpus representative of Chinese vowel-consonant articulations. Three-dimensional tongue surface outline was represented by a mesh obtained by the set of tongue contours traced from the volume images. The set of the 3D coordinates of all vertices of the tongue mesh constituted the variables on which linear component analysis was applied and subsequently six linearly independent components which has physiological significance were firstly extracted. Jaw parameter, the first of these six parameters, can control tongue rotation. Parameters of tongue body and tongue dorsal control respectively tongue forward and backward, flattening and bunching movements, and the last three tongue tip parameters control tongue tip up and down, anterior and posterior, and upward movements respectively. These six parameters can explain 87.4% of the variance of the tongue data, which has a good simulation effect and better than other research. The method proposed reduced the complexity of tongue modeling and can be effectively applied to the modeling of tongue for Chinese Mandarin pronunciation.

**Keywords:** Statistical model · MRI · Tongue · PCA · Articulation

## 1 Introduction

Studies have shown that speech organ visualization is of great significance for the understanding of pronunciation mechanisms, treatment of speech diseases, and development of human-computer interaction systems [1, 2]. As one of the most important vocal organs, the study of tongue articulatory visualization has attracted the attention of many researchers. Because it is not completely visible during the vocalization process, the articulatory visualization of the tongue requires special image acquisition techniques, including X-ray imaging, ultrasound imaging, and magnetic resonance imaging (MRI). X-ray imaging is fast, but is not sensitive to soft tissues and not suitable for the collection of large amounts of data during speech due to serious radiation [3, 4]; Ultrasound imaging can provide the dynamic surface data of tongue in real time, and it is easy to extract motion information, but it has drawbacks such as low image clarity, lack of information


G. Wang et al. (Eds.): APCMBE 2023, IFMBE Proceedings 103, pp. 363–370, 2024.
https://doi.org/10.1007/978-3-031-51455-5_40

of tongue tip and lateral margins, and complex model reconstruction algorithms [5, 6]. MRI imaging is suitable for constructing precise three-dimensional geometric models of tongue thanks to its high resolution for soft tissues, although the imaging speed is slow [7–9].

Tongue models can be classified into three typical types: parametric modeling, physiological modeling and statistical modeling. A statistical model is established by statistical analysis based on the assumption of the linear relationship between the control parameters and the motions of the speech organ. Because of the advantages of simple calculation, fewer control parameters, fast simulation speed and strong interpretability, the statistical modeling is especially suitable for describing the motion of tongue which changes fast during speech. At present, there is little research on statistical modeling for Chinese Mandarin. Only a few research teams in China have carried out this work. Wei's research team built a 3D tongue model controlled by five parameters with statistical modeling, and its simulation contribution rate is 85.1%, despite this, there is still room for improvement in model precision and these parameters has no any significance [10].

To improve the accuracy of tongue modeling, in this paper, an improved tongue statistical model based on MRI was presented by methods of linear component analysis and the control parameters which can control tongue shape are extracted. Contribution of each of control parameters to control overall tongue shape was evaluated.

# 2 Data

## 2.1 Corpus and Speaker

According to the shape change of tongue during Chinese Mandarin vowel-consonant pronunciation, as well as the articulatory way of forming, holding and removing obstruction for airflow, a corpus was designed as to cover the maximal range of Chinese allophones. The corpus included a set of 49 artificially sustained articulations: 8 vowels, 40 consonants in CV (consonant-vowel), and a rest position (Table 1). The corpus comes from a 25-year-old female Mandarin speaker who has no speech disorders or dysphonia. The speaker has been informed of all experiment procedures and signed the informed consent form.

## 2.2 Image Acquisition and Tongue Mesh

Tongue images were acquired from MRI based on the above corpus. While acquiring the MR images, for vowels, the speaker sustained artificially the articulation, either in full apnoea or breathing out very slowly in some sort of whispering mode. For consonants, the speaker produced the initial consonant transition, kept the occlusion during image acquisition, and finally produced the consonant-vowel sequence.

Supplementary images of hard palate, jaw, and hyoid bone were acquired by Computed Tomography (CT) and Jaw positions were also determined, because the parameter extraction process requires the height distance of the upper and lower incisors and the information of upper and lower jaws is missing in MR images. The specific equipment and parameter settings can be seen in Table 2.

**Table 1.** Corpus

| Vowels | | | | |
|---|---|---|---|---|
| ɑ[A] o[o] e[ɣ] ê[ɛ] i[i] u[u] ü[y] er | | | | |
| Consonants in CV sequences | | | | |
| | a | o | i | u |
| b | ba | bo | bi | bu |
| m | ma | mo | mi | mu |
| f | fa | fo | | fu |
| d | da | | di | du |
| n | na | | ni | nu |
| l | la | | li | lu |
| g | ga | | | gu |
| h | ha | | | hu |
| j | | | ji | |
| x | | | xi | |
| zh | zha | | zhi | zhu |
| sh | sha | | shi | shu |
| r | | | ri | ru |
| z | za | | zi | zu |
| s | sa | | si | su |

**Table 2.** Acquisition of MR and CT images

| | | |
|---|---|---|
| MRI | Equipment | GE (Signa HDXT1.5T) |
| | Layers | 15 lays |
| | Thickness | 3.6 mm |
| | Interval | 1.0 mm |
| | Size | 512*512 pixel |
| | Resolution | 0.4 mm/pixel |
| | Acquired time | 1.18 min |
| CT | Equipment | GE64 CT680 |
| | Size | 512*512*157 pixel |
| | Resolution | 0.4*0.4*0.6 mm/pixel |

The tongue contour points were extracted by manual marking to establish static tongue model, and the three-dimensional static tongue model was represented, for each of the 49 articulations of the corpus, by a mesh obtained by fitting a generic mesh to the set of tongue contours traced from the MR images.

# 3 Method

## 3.1 Modeling Principle

The procedure employed by [11] was modified to extract control parameters based on a controlled use of Principal component analysis (PCA) and multiple linear regression analysis (MLR). The statistical modeling is constructed based on Hypothesis 1 and Hypothesis 2.

Hypothesis 1: The control parameters are independent of each other;

Hypothesis 2: There is a linear relationship between the morphological changes of the organ and the control parameters.

Based on the above assumptions, the tongue shape data vectors DV (Data Vector) was decomposed into linear combinations of a set of associated coefficient AC (Associated coefficient) weighted by control factors CF (Control Factors), in addition to their average neutral shape DV. The calculation formula is shown in (1) [11].

$$DV = \overline{DV} + CF * AC \tag{1}$$

In the (1), $\overline{DV}$ is the average shape of all static tongue models of the 49 articulations of the corpus, while $CF$ and $AC$ are determined iteratively in the following way: (1) the control factor $CF$ is mainly determined using PCA, (2) the associated coefficient $AC$ is determined by the linear regression of the current residue data for the whole corpus over $CF$; and (3) the contribution of the $CF$ refers to its product with the associated matrix $AC$, and is finally subtracted from the current residue in order to provide the next residue for determining the next component, to ensure independence between control parameters.

## 3.2 Control Parameters and Motion Simulation

Based on the above modeling method, the control parameters are extracted from the coordinates of midsagittal tongue contour. Because of the physiological relationship between the tongue and the lower jaw, and it is difficult to separate the motion of the tongue caused by the jaw with the motion led by the active motion of the tongue muscle itself. Jaw height JH is defined as the first control parameter, which is the centered and normalized value of the height difference between the upper and lower incisors. After the contribution of Jaw Height (JH) is removed, PCA was applied on the tongue body and the tongue bottom part, and the first two principal components obtained were defined as the tongue body parameter (TB) and the tongue back parameter (TD). Continually, the contributions of TD and TB parameters are removed, PCA analysis was subsequently applied on the tongue tip to obtain the first three principal components as tongue tip parameters: Tongue Tip Vertical (TTV), Tongue Tip Horizontal (TTH), and Tongue Tip Upturned, (TTU).

The motion simulation of the model is realized by linear combination of the above 6 control parameters. Based on (1), the value of each control parameter can be adjusted to generate various tongue shapes according to its effect on the tongue motion. The associated coefficients were obtained by the MLD method between coordinates of tongue static models and the parameters. The simulation of two-dimensional and three-dimensional tongue models of 49 articulations in the corpus can be obtained through the linear combination between 6 control parameters and associated coefficients.

# 4 Results

The simulation effect was evaluated from two aspects: control contribution rate (known as Varex), cumulative control contribution rate (known as Varexcum) and simulation error (known as RMS). The contribution rate is the variance relative to the total variance of the tongue model, explained by each parameter. And the simulation error is the root mean square of the corresponding vertices between the simulated and the original static tongue models.

## 4.1 Simulation Results of All Articulations

From the findings of the simulation results of the 3D tongue model, the contribution rate of the six control parameters is 87.4% higher than other research [10] and the simulation error is 0.149 cm which is acceptable (Table 3). As demonstrated in Fig. 1, the main influence area and effect of each control parameter on the tongue is obvious when its value is adjusted linearly with all the other parameters being set to zero. Among them, the parameter JH controls the rotation angle of the tongue around one point of the tongue back region, the parameter TB controls the amplitude of the forward and backward contraction of the tongue body, the parameter TD controls the amplitude of the upward arch and downward depression of the tongue, and the parameters TTH and TTV control respectively the amplitude of up, down, and back and forth movement of the tongue tip. And the parameter TTU controls the amplitude of the tongue tip upturning around the one point of the tongue tip.

## 4.2 Simulation Results of Vowels and Consonants

The specific deformation of tongue can be obtained according to changing the value of specific parameter and setting other parameters to zero. From the perspective of vowels and consonants, as shown in Fig. 2, the overall change trend of the value of each parameter is consistent with the contribution rate of each parameter. The value of TB parameter (vowels: 2.83, consonant: 1.19) is the greatest in these six parameters', consistent with the contribution rate (48.4%), whatever vowels and consonants.

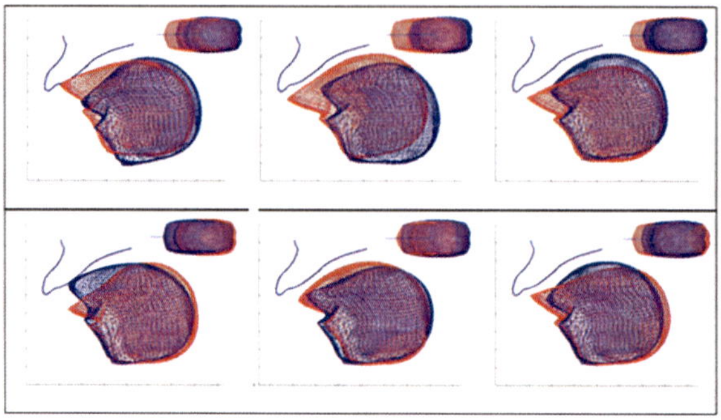

**Fig. 1.** From upper left to lower right represent the simulation effect of 3D motion with parameters JH, TB, TD, TTV, TTH, TTU varying (the unit of the horizontal and vertical coordinates of the grid is cm, corresponding to the true size of the tongue. Red line is the shape at the min parameter and green lines is the shape at max parameter).

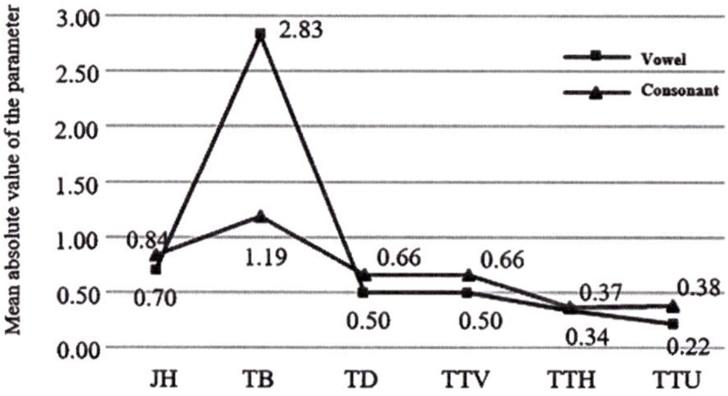


**Fig. 2.** The absolute-mean value of the control parameters corresponding to the vowel and consonant static tongue models.

**Table 3.** Evaluation result of the 3D tongue model motion simulation

| Guided PCA | | | |
|---|---|---|---|
| Parameter | Varex | Varexcum | RMS (cm) |
| JH | 15.1% | 15.1% | 0.386 |
| TB | 48.4% | 63.5% | 0.253 |
| TD | 10.9% | 74.4% | 0.212 |
| TTV | 7.5% | 81.9% | 0.178 |
| TTH | 2.7% | 84.6% | 0.164 |
| TTU | 2.8% | 87.4% | 0.149 |

## 5 Discussion

The method referred to [11], were modified and applied to Chinese Mandarin articulations. Considering that the tongue tip changes more complicated in Chinese Mandarin pronunciation than French, we analyzed the reconstruction error of the tongue tip independently, and added a new parameter TTU, which reduced the tongue tip error. The control parameter HY, the original parameter, extracted by [11] has little influence on the effect of Mandarin pronunciation, so we rejected this parameter. According to the results of simulation evaluation, the total contribution rate of TTV and TTH in Chinese Mandarin tongue model is 10.2%, which is higher than that of French (7.3%), indicating that the degree of change in tongue tip during Chinese pronunciation is more complicated. The contribution rate of TD is similar to that of French, but the contribution of TB is 7% higher than that of French. it is related to that the forward movement of tongue is larger than French's. The contribution rate of JH is slightly lower than that of French, which indicates that the jaw's opening degree of speaker is less than French.

Compared with other research [10], Our accuracy is slightly higher than theirs(2% higher). we found that directly calculating the overall simulation error weaken the simulation effect of the tongue tip because of its small volume ratio compared with entire tongue's.

Previous studies on the muscle movement of the tongue have proved that these control parameters are closely related to jaw and hyoid positions, and to the actions of tongue muscles such as the genioglossus, the hyoglossus or the styloglossus. Our research gets that JH can control the rotation movement of the tongue driven by the mandibular expansion, TB can control the anterior and posterior extension of the tongue associated with the posterior genioglossus and lingual muscles, TD is used to control the lingual and anterior tongue respectively muscle-related tongue arching and depression movements, TTV and TTU are used to control the upward movement of the tongue tip caused by the sublingual longitudinal muscle, and TTH can control the anterior and posterior movement of the tongue tip caused by the upper longitudinal muscle of the tongue. Although statistical modeling does not simulate the physiological structure of the tongue, the extracted parameters achieve similar effect to the tongue muscles, and this is also the advantage of statistical modeling.

The current study used only one subject, in future studies, we will consider the individual differentiation and try to use multiple subjects to build a more robust model.

**Acknowledgment.** The authors thank Beijing Friendship Hospital for providing equipment.

## References

1. Denby, B., Schultz, T., Honda, K., et al.: Silent speech interfaces. Speech Commun. **52**(4), 270–287 (2010)
2. Yu, J., Chen, C.: From talking head to singing head: a significant enhancement for more natural human computer interaction. In: 2017 IEEE International Conference on Multimedia and Expo (ICME), pp. 511–516. Hong Kong, China (2017)

3. Zhang, J., Wu, X., Kong, J.: Tongue shape variation model for simulating Mandarin Chinese articulation. In: 10th International Symposium on Chinese Spoken Language Processing (ISCSLP), pp. 1–5. Tianjin, China (2016)
4. Lindblom, B., Sundberg, J.: Acoustical consequences of lip, tongue, jaw, and larynx movement. J. Acoust. Soc. Am. **50**(4B), 1166–1179 (1971)
5. Maureen, S.: A guide to analysing tongue motion from ultrasound images. Clin. Linguist. Phon. **19**(6–7), 455–501 (2005)
6. Xu, K., Yang, Y., Jaumard, A., et al.: A 3D tongue motion visualization based on ultrasound image sequences. InterSpeech **2014**, 1482–1483 (2014)
7. Engwall, O.: Combining MRI, EMA and EPG measurements in a three-dimensional tongue model. Speech Commun. **41**(2–3), 303–329 (2003)
8. Parthasarathy, V., Prince, J., Stone, M.: Measuring tongue motion from tagged cine-MRI using harmonic phase (HARP) processing. J. Acoust. Soc. Am. **121**(1), 491–504 (2007)
9. Narayanan, S., Toutios, A., Ramanarayanan, V., et al.: Real-time magnetic resonance imaging and electromagnetic articulography database for speech production research (TC). J. Acoust. Soc. Am. **136**(3), 1307–1311 (2014)
10. Fang, Q., Chen, Y., Wei, J., et al.: An improved 3D geometric tongue model. InterSpeech **2016**, 1104–1107 (2016)
11. Badin, P., Serrurier, A.: Three-dimensional linear modeling of tongue: articulatory data and models. In: 7th International Seminar on Speech Production, ISSP7, pp. 395–402 (2006)

# A Convolutional Neural Network Based Classification Method for Mild to Moderate Parkinson's Disease at Turns

Xinge Li[1], Xiayu Huang[2], Jun Pang[1], Lin Meng[1(✉)], and Dong Ming[1,3]

[1] Academy of Medical Engineering and Translational Medicine, Tianjin University, No. 92 Weijin Road, Tianjin, China
linmeng@tju.edu.cn

[2] Tianjin International Engineering Institute, Tianjin University, Tianjin, China

[3] Department of Biomedical Engineering, School of Precision Instrument and Opto-Electronics Engineering, Tianjin University, Tianjin, China

**Abstract.** As the second most common neurodegenerative disease, more than 10 million people live with Parkinson's disease (PD) and suffer with non-motor and motor symptoms. It is essential to identify PD at early stage for timely treatment. Although early PD may exhibit various but subtle symptoms, they would show more deteriorated gait performance in complex gait tasks, such as turning. In this study, we proposed a convolutional neural network (CNN) based classification model at turns to identify mild and moderate PD from healthy controls. The data derived from sensors attached to the lower limb segments was segmented and normalized into two datasets based on gait cycles and gait tasks (straight walking and turning). Multidimensional data was visualized into RGB images as inputs of CNN which was built with the use of the leave-one-out methods. Results demonstrated that the CNN model at turns obtained a highest accuracy of 91.07% compared to that from straight walking indicating that PD patients exhibited more distinctive motor features during complex gait task. The CNN-based PD multiclassification model is more sensitive to mild and moderate PD patients than the machine learning based models. The proposed method provides a potential tool to identify mild to moderate PD patients in clinical practice.

**Keywords:** Parkinson's disease · Inertial measurement unit · Convolutional neural network · Turning · PD classification

## 1 Introduction

Parkinson's disease (PD) is a prevalent neurodegenerative disorder that has a high disease rate in elders and patients usually suffer from typical motor symptoms including bradykinesia, tremor, postural instability, and etc. [1]. Clinical scale methods, such as the Unified Parkinson's Disease Rating Scale (UPDRS) and Hoehn & Yahr Scale

Xinge Li and Xiayu Huang authors have contributed equally to this work and share first authorship.


G. Wang et al. (Eds.): APCMBE 2023, IFMBE Proceedings 103, pp. 371–378, 2024.
https://doi.org/10.1007/978-3-031-51455-5_41

(H&Y), are commonly applied for PD assessment [2], where the reliability and accuracy would dependent on observers' experience and subtle progression may be difficult to be detected. Therefore, it is essential to develop quantitative methods to precisely identify PD and its disease progression.

Patients with PD display motor fluctuations and different forms of gait disorders as the disease advances which may be hidden at early stage [3–5]. Studies have shown that patients with mild PD exhibited more severe motor impairments when performing complex motor activities (e.g., turning) including longer stride lengths, increased number of steps [4]. The change in gait performance at turning is significantly related to the severity of freezing of gait (FoG) [5]. It is envisaged that motor characteristics during turning would be potential new objective indicators for PD diagnosis.

The inertial measurement unit (IMU) can reflect motion acceleration and velocity of segments in real time with it unique advantages of low price, small size and high wearability. Elham Rastegari et al. found that features collected from an accelerometer attached to the ankle can effectively differentiate PD in the middle stage and healthy older adults [6, 7]. Naoya Hasegawa et al. investigated sensitive objective metrics in which subjects wore eight IMUs to perform experimental movement. The results demonstrated that turning speed contributed the most to the random forest dichotomous model (ICC = 0.95, Minimal Detectable Change = 23.26) with a recognition accuracy of 82.4% [8]. Features based on kinematic variables were also applied for PD classification in the study by Jochen et al. [9] 694 motion features were extracted from the recorded angular velocity and acceleration signals as input to the SVM classifier for a binary classification study between different groups, and the results showed that the model obtained an overall classification accuracy of 81%, with the highest binary classification recognition accuracy of 91% for the H&Y stage III and healthy control groups, but only 70% for the H&Y stage I group and the healthy control group. However, only a few studies investigated the methods for identifying PD at early-stage and the recognition rate was relatively low [6].

As inspired by the biological neural network, the deep learning method incorporates several hidden layer neural networks that can uncover details that humans cannot explain, which is superior to traditional machine learning algorithms. Yang et al. [10] compared the performance of machine learning and deep learning method for the PD 4 levels classification problem. The results demonstrated that the overall recognition accuracy of the PD classification model constructed based on Convolutional Neural Networks (CNN) reached 92.95% and the recognition accuracy for mild PD increased from 55 to 77% compared to the machine learning approach. However, the experimental paradigm is based on the generic scale normative action design, with simple and reproducible actions, which has strong limitations.

Taking strengths of deep learning method and complex gait task in PD detection, we proposed a novel CNN-based classification model for PD patients at mild to moderate stages where sample segmentation and normalization was based on gait cycles and gait tasks and a multiple channel data fusion method based on visualization. The model performance was compared to that from traditional machine learning methods.

## 2 Methods

### 2.1 Participants and Experiment Protocol

19 healthy older adults, 24 PD with a UPDRS Part III score of less than 30 or insufficient for DBS surgery at mild stage and 13 moderate PD with a UPDRS Part III score of higher than 30 or sufficient for DBS surgery were enrolled in the experiment. The experiment was approved by the Tianjin University and Tianjin Huanhu Hospital ethics committees, and data collection was conducted from October 2019 to October 2021 in the motor rehabilitation laboratory of Tianjin University and the neurology outpatient clinic of Tianjin Huanhu Hospital. All patients participated within four hours after the medication. Participants' basic information was detailed in Table 1.

**Table 1.** Basic information of participants

| | HE | PD-mild | PD-moderate |
|---|---|---|---|
| Year | 63.13(5.53) | 62.74 (7.11) | 67.14 (6.45) |
| Gender | 9 M, 10 F | 10 M, 14 F | 5 M, 8 F |
| Height (cm) | 167.58(5.02) | 166.22 (7.24) | 168.29(7.05) |
| Weight (kg) | 68.63(4.38) | 69.09 (10.62) | 69.57(6.23) |
| UPDRS Part III (score) | – | 13.91 (6.94) | 40.14 (12.32) |
| H&Y (stage) | – | 1.37 (0.55) | 2.42 (0.53) |
| MoCA (score) | 25.67(2.13) | 25.32(1.82) | 25.01(1.86) |

MoCA: Montreal Cognitive Assessment Scale
H&Y: Hoehn & Yahr Classification Scale

As shown in Fig. 1A, the participant wore seven IMU sensors (myoMOTION™, Noraxon, US) respectively on the upper trunk, thigh shank and feet of both legs. Three dimensional accelerations and three dimensional orientational angles from six sensors attached to the lower limb segments were used. It needs to mention that the upper trunk sensor was only used for gait task recognition in data preprocessing. In the experiment, the participant was required to complete five consecutive laps of "7 m straight path—180° left turn—7 m straight path—180° left turn" at a self-comfortable pace.

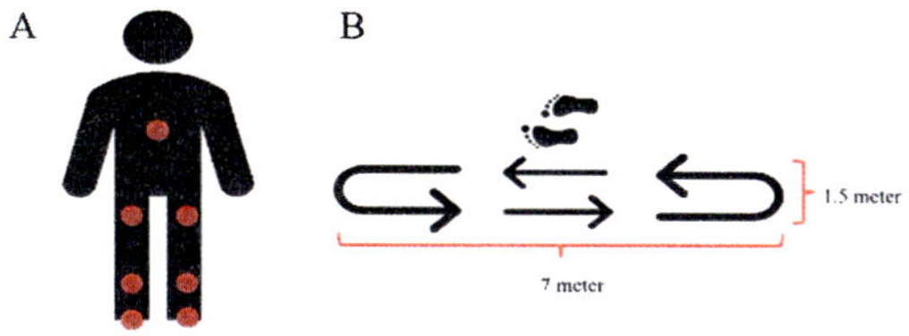


**Fig. 1.** **A** Locations of seven sensor **B** Experimental setup

## 2.2 Data Extraction

Gait event detection algorithm proposed in our previous study [11] was used to segment data record into gait cycle based samples while gait task detection algorithm was employed to categorized samples into straight walking and turning datasets. One gait cycle is regarded as one heel off (HO) to next HO. The sample length was further normalized into 100 points while amplitude was normalized to 0 ~ 1 to eliminate the effect of data type. The performance of the gait cycle based segmentation method was compared to a sliding window method in which the window length and step length were both set to 100 points. Samples of which encompassing straight walking and turning task were discarded. The total number of data samples derived based on the abovementioned segmentation methods is shown in Table 2.

**Table 2.** Number of data samples derived based on the two data segmentation methods

| Method | Dataset | HE | PD-mild | PD-moderate | Total |
|---|---|---|---|---|---|
| Gait cycle–based | Straight walking | 377 | 537 | 288 | 1202 |
| | Turning | 322 | 525 | 217 | 1064 |
| Sliding window–based | Straight walking | 701 | 898 | 344 | 1934 |
| | Turning | 606 | 825 | 314 | 1745 |

Because only knee flexion angle was calculated, the sensors at both calves had 7 data channels while the remaining 4 sensors contained 9 data channels each, resulting in a total of 50 channels of sensor data. The 50 channel temporal data samples were constructed into an image by considering of the geographical local dependence of multiple IMU data, as shown in Fig. 2A. The 'visualized' sample contains not only temporal data information but also spatial properties. A two-dimensional convolutional neural network was used to further extract the hidden properties of motion data between multiple IMUs and improve the model's recognition capabilities [12].

The visualization method transforms the standardized data samples into two-dimensional color images, in which the acceleration data, orientation angles, and joint angles respectively corresponding to the RGB channels of the color image. Each color channel was composited by 18 columns of temporal signals collected from six sensors. E.g., the R channel contains all 3-dimensional acceleration data samples from the both feet, shanks, and thighs. For consistency with the other two of channels, the knee flexion angle data were duplicated twice to fill the adjacent channels. Figure 2B showed typical image sample for each group during straight walking and turning.

## 2.3 Convolutional Neural Network Model

We referred to the University of Toronto's AlexNet network architecture to develop the multiclassification model for PD [13]. The network architectural parameters are listed in Table 3.

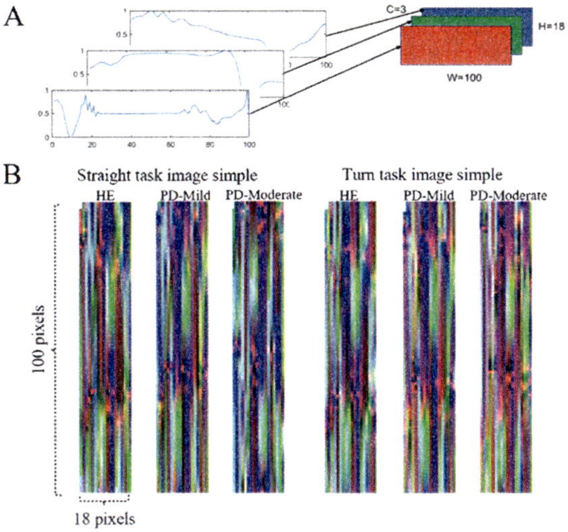


**Fig. 2.** **A** The image construction process for multiple data fusion. **B** Typical image samples for the three groups under straight walking and turning tasks.

**Table 3.** Parameters of CNN network architecture

| Network layer | Parameters | Number of kernels | Activation function | Padding | Stride |
|---|---|---|---|---|---|
| Convolution 1 | 3*3 | 6 | Relu | – | 1 |
| Max-pooling 1 | 2*2 | None | – | Same | 1 |
| Convolution 2 | 3*3 | 10 | Relu | – | 1 |
| Max-pooling 2 | 2*2 | None | – | Same | 1 |
| Dropout | – | – | – | – | – |
| Fully connected 1 | 30 | – | Relu | – | – |
| Fully connected 2 | 3 | – | Softmax | – | – |

A local search was carried out to find optimal hyperparameter set for the model. After a number of experimental validations, the CNN model's hyperparameters were determined as indicated in Table 4. This model used the Stochastic Gradient Descent (SGD) method with momentum to update the neural network parameters (weights and biases) and uses the Cross-Entropy Loss function to assess the performance of the PD multiclassification model. The model was trained and evaluated using "leave-one-out" on a 64-bit PC with an AMD Ryzen 7 5800H CPU, 16GB RAM, and a GTX1650 4GB graphics card. After 30 training rounds, the model reached saturation accuracy, and the loss function curve was smooth and not overfit. Each model training took approximately 20 min, 30 iterations with GPU acceleration.

Traditional machine learning methods, including support vector machine (SVM), K-nearest neighbor (KNN), and random forest (RF) were utilized to develop PD multi-classification models for performance comparison. It worths to be mentioned that a single participant was chosen as the minimum unit for model evaluation, rather than a single gait data sample.

**Table 4.** Hyper-parameters values

| Hyper-parameter | Optimal values |
|---|---|
| Activation function | Relu |
| Learning rate | 0.01 |
| Learning rate decay | 0.1 |
| Learning rate decline cycle | 10 |
| Optimizer | SGDM |
| Batch | 64 |
| Iterations | 40 |
| Random inactivation rate | 0.5 |

## 3 Results

As shown in Table 5, the model performance of data samples respectively derived by sliding window and gait cycle based data segmentation methods were compared. The model performance was more pronounced when the gait cycle-based data segmentation method used under both gait tasks. Compared to straight walking task, the recognition accuracy from the turning task was increased by 3.58 and 8.93%, respectively.

**Table 5.** Model performance comparison based on two data segmentation methods

| Segmentation | Gait task | Model training time (min) | Accuracy (%) |
|---|---|---|---|
| Based on gait cycle | Straight walking | 23 | 82.14 |
| | Turning | 20 | 91.07 |
| Based on sliding window | Straight walking | 36 | 73.21 |
| | Turning | 34 | 76.79 |

Figure 3 showed the recognition performance of the CNN-based PD multi-classification model compared to three machine learning models. We observed that the CNN-based PD classification model obtained the highest accuracy rates for both turning and straight walking tasks (91.07% and 82.14%). Compared to the models based on

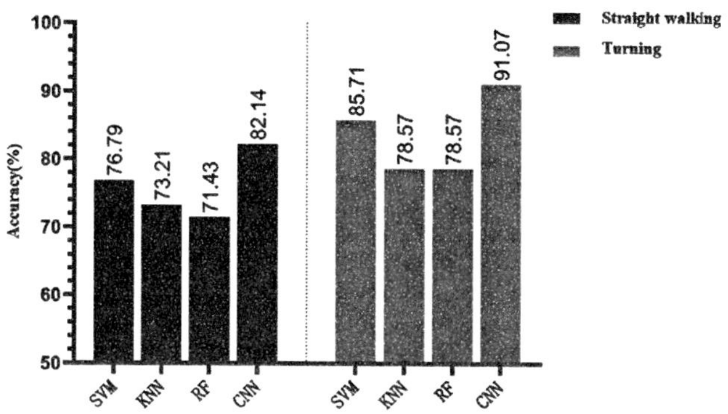


**Fig. 3.** Recognition accuracy comparison of CNN-based model and three machine learning based models

the three machine learning algorithms, the recognition accuracy was improved by an average of 8.33% and 10.12% for the straight walking and turn tasks, respectively.

Table 6 demonstrated the model performance for each classification group. When data samples of turning task were utilized as model input, the CNN model obtained the best classification performance where the HE group classification performance achieved 100% recognition accuracy and specificity with F1 score of 97.30%. The CNN-based model was sensitive to mild and moderate PD, with a sensitivity of 95.83% for the PD-Mild group, and F1 values of 90.20% and 83.33% for the PD-Mild and PD-Moderate groups, respectively. The turning task effectively improved the classification recognition performance of the model.

**Table 6.** Model performance under straight walking and turning tasks

| Gait task | Participants | Pre (%) | Sen (%) | Spe (%) | F1 (%) |
|---|---|---|---|---|---|
| Straight walk | HE | 94.44 | 89.47 | 97.30 | 91.89 |
| | PD-mild | 76.92 | 83.33 | 81.25 | 80.00 |
| | PD-moderate | 75.00 | 69.23 | 93.02 | 72.00 |
| Turning | HE | 100.00 | 94.74 | 100.00 | 97.30 |
| | PD-mild | 85.19 | 95.83 | 87.50 | 90.20 |
| | PD-moderate | 90.91 | 76.92 | 97.67 | 83.33 |

## 4 Conclusions

In this paper, we proposed a CNN-based multi-classification model for mild and moderate PD at turns. The model utilized a novel gait cycle-based sample segmentation and visualization method for multiple inertial temporal data fusion. The effect of data segmentation and gait task on model performance was investigated while the gait cycle-based segmentation method was compared to commonly used sliding window method. The results demonstrated that the gait cycle based segmentation method has a significant improvement in the model performance. The CNN-based PD multiclassification model is more sensitive to mild and moderate PD patients than the machine learning based models, and its best recognition accuracy is 90.17% at turning task which validated that PD patients exhibited more motor disorders during turning. The proposed method provides a potential tool to identify mild to moderate PD patients in clinical practice.

## References


1. Rizek, P., Kumar, N., Jog, M.S.: An update on the diagnosis and treatment of Parkinson disease. CMAJ **188**(16), 1157–1165 (2016)
2. Xu, S.: Research on the Quantitative Evaluation and Quantitative Classification Evaluation Method of Gait Disorder in Patients with Parkinson's Disease. University of Science and Technology of China (2017) (in Chinese)
3. Doná, F., et al.: The effects of dual task gait and balance training in Parkinson's disease: a systematic review. Physiother. Theory Pract. **36**(10), 1088–1096 (2020)
4. Shah, V.V., et al.: Digital biomarkers of mobility in Parkinson's disease during daily living. J. Parkinsons Dis. **10**(3), 1099–1111 (2020)
5. Bertoli, M., Della Croce, U., Cereatti, A., et al.: Objective measures to investigate turning impairments and freezing of gait in people with Parkinson's disease. Gait Posture **74**, 187–193 (2019)
6. Rastegari, E., Marmelat, V., Najjar, L., et al.: Using gait parameters to recognize various stages of Parkinson's disease. In: 2017 IEEE Int. Conf. Bioinform. Biomed., Kansas City, USA, 2017, pp. 1647–1651 (2017)
7. Bobić, V.N,, Đurić-Jovičić, M.D., Radovanović, S.M., et al.: Classification of Parkinsonism based on foot tapping test. In: 5th Int. Conf. Electr. Electron. Comput. Eng. (2018)
8. Hasegawa, N., Shah, V.V., Carlson-Kuhta, P., et al.: How to select balance measures sensitive to Parkinson's disease from body-worn inertial sensors—separating the trees from the forest. Sensors **19**(15), 3320 (2019)
9. Ongsulee, P.: Artificial intelligence, machine learning and deep learning. In: 15th International Conference on ICT and Knowledge Engineering (ICT&KE), pp. 1–6 (2017)
10. Yang, Y.: Automatic Classification of PD Based on Motion Parameters. Dongnan University (2018) (in Chinese)
11. Yang, Y., Chen, L., Pang, J., et al.: Validation of a spatiotemporal gait model using inertial measurement units for early Parkinson's disease detection during turns. IEEE Trans. Biomed. Eng. **69**(12), 3591–3600 (2022)
12. Long, Q.: Research on Human Behavior Recognition Based on Improved CNN-LSTM. University of Electronic Science and Technology of China (2020) (in Chinese)
13. Alom, M.Z., Taha, T.M., Yakopcic, C., et al.: The history began from AlexNet: a comprehensive survey on deep learning approaches (2018)

# Biomedical Sensing and Wearable Systems

# Microfluidic Chip-Based Analysis on the Biological Characterization of Medical Magnesium Alloy

Juan Su[1], Jie Liu[2], Jin Zhang[1], Xiran Jiang[1], and Xianzheng Sha[1](✉)

[1] School of Intelligent Medicine, China Medical University, No. 77 Puhe Road, Shenyang, China
xzsha@cmu.edu.cn

[2] Second Department of Prosthodontics, Affiliated Stomatological Hospital of China Medical University, Liaoning Institute of Dental Research, Shenyang, China

**Abstract.** Magnesium alloy (Mg alloy) has been widely used as medical implant material in recent years. The good biodegradable performance of the Mg alloy results in pH variation after implantation in human body because of high degradation rate and hydrogen evolution, affecting on cell growth, which has been rarely reported. This study fabricated a microfluidic chip and evaluated degradation characteristics of the Mg alloy and effects on vascular the endothelial cell and Schwann cell. Micro-arc oxidation (MAO) treated as well as untreated Mg alloy were co-cultured with the cells. Degradation characteristics of the Mg alloy were analyzed and discussed. The MAO-treated magnesium alloy slice was apparently slower than the untreated slice, and the ceramic oxidation film generated via MAO treatment was believed to distinctly increasing the corrosion resistance of the magnesium alloy material.

**Keywords:** Magnesium alloy · Micro-arc oxidation · Cell culture

## 1 Introduction

Metal materials exhibiting good mechanical properties were suitable for medical implant applications [1]. Recent studies have shown that the magnesium alloy presents similar density and modulus of elasticity with human tissues, comparing with traditional materials (e.g. titanium, copper and cobalt), which made the Mg alloy an ideal stent material especially using in load-bearing parts [2]. The good degradation performance of Mg alloy in vivo helped to avoid second surgery and reduce the suffering of patients. Considering the degradation products showed no harm to human body, the Mg alloy becomes a potential biocompatible material for medical applications, such as cardiovascular and bone stent [3].

In recent years, due to the rapidly rising incidence, cardiovascular disease becomes a widespread concern of public health and accounted for 40% of death rate among human diseases in China [4]. Since a big amount of patients with heart disease were suffering


G. Wang et al. (Eds.): APCMBE 2023, IFMBE Proceedings 103, pp. 381–387, 2024.
https://doi.org/10.1007/978-3-031-51455-5_42

from vascular stenosis, biocompatible implant material is required for making vascular sent. Comparing with degradable polymer material, metal material requires much smaller volume to provide similar supporting force to the blood vessel surrounding the stent. On the other hand, traditional metal stent frequently causes chronic inflammation and thrombosis in clinical applications, which forces the patients to long term use of antiplatelet drugs [5]. As a result, biodegradable magnesium alloy becomes an ideal material for cardiovascular stent. However, studies have shown that the Mg alloy exhibited high corrosion rate when maintained in human body fluid environment [6], which would seriously reduce the stability of the stent, even cause implantation failure. On the other hand, hydrogen is also produced along with the degradation process of the Mg alloy [7], which is known as hydrogen evolution, commonly leads to pH increasing and alkalosis, and causes discomfort [8]. Accumulation of hydrogen in human body can also result in inflammation and tissue necrosis [9]. Accordingly, surface coating is essential for improving resistance to corrosion of the Mg alloy prior to the implantation into human body [10].

Micro-arc oxidation is a commonly used surface coating technique in clinical applications. Ceramic oxide film can be produced on the surface of magnesium alloy by high temperature and high pressure treatment through micro-arc discharge, which distinctly improved the surface hardness of the Mg alloy [11]. The voltage of ceramic oxide film is low, and integrated closely with the coated surface, which decrease corrosion rate by isolating of the inner metal material and the outer body fluid. Moreover, the MAO protocol is simple without requirement of vacuum or reduction of temperature. The produced electrolyte is harmless and can be discharged without treatment. The advantages of MAO technique makes magnesium alloy have great potential in replacing traditional materials in cardiovascular stent development. Although the magnesium alloy stent exhibited good biocompatibility, there are still concerns about the effects of degradation of the material on cell growth after implanting into the human body.

The microfluidic chip-based technology has been applied to construct portable devices with small size, and has received increasing attractions due to the low reagent consumption and short analysis time. Thus, the microfluidic chip can be a favorable platform to perform the research on the Mg alloy' degradation, yet not studied. In this work, MAO-treated and untreated magnesium alloy were tested by co-culturing with vascular endothelial and Schwann cell. Degradation characteristics of the magnesium alloy in the microfluidic chip and their effects to cell growth were analyzed and discussed.

## 2 Experimental Methods

### 2.1 Methods and Materials

ZK60 Magnesium alloy was kindly provided by Institute of Metal Research, Chinese academy of Science. MAO coatings were carried out at a constant voltage of 450 V, 1400 Hz and 30% for 5 min, with based electrolytes consisting of potassium fluoride (8 g/L), hydroxide (0.8 g/L) and sodium hexametaphosphate (3.5 g/L). After the coating, all samples were rinsed using dd$H_2O$, then dried in ambient air. To avoid potential damages to the material, the Mg alloy was cleaned by alcohol then explored to UV light for 30 min, instead of sterilized by a high pressure steam sterilizer before adding into cell culture mixtures. Vascular endothelial cell and Schwann cell were cultured using 1640 and DEMS culture medium, respectively. Regular culture protocols were used for cell culturing.

### 2.2 Effects of Magnesium Alloy on Cell Growth

Cellular morphology and amounts of live cells were recorded using an optical microscope every 24 h for 96 h. Corrosion rates of the Mg alloy were evaluated by recording the pH values. By comparing the pH line chart and cell growth curve, the effects of pH variation on cell growth were analyzed. Cell growth curve was drawn by calculating live cell numbers as following: the live cell numbers were recorded in three microscopic fields that were chosen randomly.

### 2.3 Fabrication of the Microfluidic Chip

The developed microfluidic chip contains two inlets and two outlets. The micro channels on the left side of the chip have a width of approximately 80 um, whereas the bent channels on the right side of the chip have a width of 250 um. Access holes for inputting and outputting reaction mixtures were drilled into the edges of both inlets and outlets with the diameter of 500 um. The standard soft lithography technology was applied to fabricate the microfluidic chip. The SU8-2025 (Microchem, USA) was used to develop the silicon mold with the thickness of approximately 60 um. The polydimethylsiloxane (PDMS) was used to fabricate the chip after baked at 85 °C for 40 min and bonded with the mold. The suspension of the reaction mixtures with cells and with/without the magnesium alloy powder were injected through inlets using a precision syringe. After the micro channels were loaded with the reaction mixtures, the outlets were closed by injecting mineral oil (Sigma) to maintain the reaction system for the degradation characteristics of the Mg alloy.

## 3 Results

In the current study, to determine the effect of the Mg alloy degradation occurring in cell culture medium, the cells were co-cultured with the Mg alloy for 96 h. White precipitation was observed in the cell culture mixture with untreated Mg alloy after 48 h. While, no precipitation was observed for MAO-treated using the same culture conditions. The medium represented series color change appearance: the medium of endothelial cells plus MAO-treated turned from the initial pink to a purple color. While, the medium of endothelial cells plus untreated magnesium alloy turned to transparent. We assumed the pH variation or degradation products resulted in the color change of the medium. PH line chart of 96 h co-culturing was drawn and shown in Fig. 1.

As shown in Fig. 2, massive cell death was observed for both the endothelial cell and Schwann cell after co-culturing with untreated Mg alloy for 2 days. For the cells co-cultured with MAO-treated, massive cell death occurred after co-culturing for 3 days. While, the amount of live cells was larger than those co-cultured with untreated at each time point.

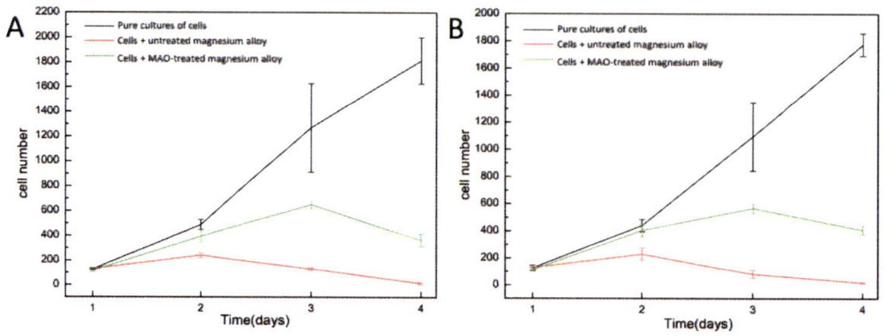


**Fig. 1.** PH line chart of the cell culture medium. **A** Schwann cell. **B** Endothelial cell.

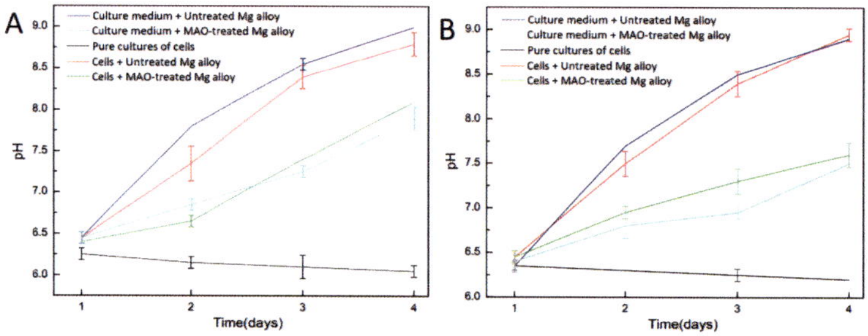


**Fig. 2.** Growth cures of cells culturing with or without magnesium alloy. **A** Growth curve of endothelial cell. **B** Growth curve of Schwann cell.

## 4 Discussion

Magnesium alloy is attracting increased attentions, due to the biodegradable and mechanical characteristics. Besides, the density and elastic modulus of Mg alloy is similar with natural bones, indicating great potential in bone implant applications [12, 13]. A variety of surface coating methods have been applied to the Mg alloy for in vivo application considerations, among which the MAO coating is commonly used since the treatment produce a thick and hard coating with good abrasive resistance [14]. PH values increased distinctly along with the raise culture time extension for the untreated Mg alloy co-cultured with both endothelial cell and Schwann cell. For the two types of cell species, pH values of the culture medium with untreated increased much faster than that with MAO-treated ones. This can be explained considering ceramic oxide film that was created on the surface of the MAO-treated Mg alloy prevented the contact of the Mg alloy with cells and culture medium. On the contrary, there was a decreasing trend for the medium pH of endothelial cell cultured without Mg alloy. We assumed the product reacted with the cells and culture medium component was the main reason caused the pH increasing. Since the survival pH range for normal human cells was 6.0–9.0, the high pH level would cause cell death.

For both endothelial cell and Schwann cell without adding magnesium alloy showed normal growth characteristics. Slight influence on both types of cells was observed in the culture mixture with MAO-treated Mg alloy. Massive cell death was observed after 2 days co-culturing of the two types of cells with untreated Mg alloy. The results were not consistent with our previous study using the MAO coated Mg alloy co-cultured with murine bone marrow stromal cells (BMSCs). The BMSC cells were observed grow well after co-culturing, and showed normal morphology [12]. We assumed the main reason might be the different characteristics of the BMSC cells and Schwann/Endothelia cells. In endothelial cell culture medium with untreated magnesium alloy, spinal precipitation was generated, puncturing the cell bodies, which caused fatal damages to the cells. For Schwann cell, huge rectangular crystal was generated in the culture medium after co-cultured with untreated. The precipitation might be consisted of corrosion products that peeled off the coated surface of Mg alloy, since the porous structure on the coated surface frequently caused degradation [15]. On the other hand, considering more cells would attach on the coated surface than that on the untreated surface of Mg alloy due to the porous structure according to our previous research [12], we assumed the cell bodies might reduce contacts of the Mg alloy and the culture medium, which led to less degradation products. Besides, hydrogen evolution occurred since small amount of air bubbles were observed around the surface of the magnesium alloy. The release of hydrogen upon degradation is a main problem of the Mg alloy, which was still not completely solved till now [12]. However, on obvious precipitation was found in the co-culture system of Schwann cell with MAO-treated Mg alloy. We assumed the ceramic oxide film slowed down the degradation rate of the magnesium alloy in the culture medium, but not fully prevented, since point corrosion was observed on the surface of the MAO-treated after one week co-culturing with cells.

The death rate of endothelial cells was more rapid than that of Schwann cells. We assumed this can be explained by the fact that the generated spinal precipitation in endothelial cell culture medium resulted in physical damages to the cell bodies or affecting on cell attachment. The amount of live cells decreased after 3 days co-culturing with both the MAO-treated and untreated magnesium alloy. Considering the pH values were increasing faster in the cell medium after 3 days co-culturing with MAO-treated (See Fig. 2), we assumed the high pH level was the main reason responsible for the massive cells death.

Previous reports have shown that the Mg ions released by the MAO-coated Mg alloy would promote cell differentiation [16]. While, swelling and rupture of cell membrane might occur if the concentration of the generated Mg ions was too high [17]. On the other, the large pH variation in the cell culture mixture were also the main reason of the massive cell death. Considering the degradation rate of the MAO-treated Mg alloy was apparently slower than the untreated, the ceramic oxidation film generated via MAO treatment was believed to distinctly increasing the corrosion resistance of the Mg alloy, which contributed to extent the service time of the stent. Meanwhile, the reduced hydrogen evolution production would minimize human body responds compared to the fast hydrogen evolution caused by the untreated Mg alloy. While, the MAO treatment still remains to be improved, since after co-culturing with cells for 3 days, degradation occurred, and resulted in high pH levels, indicating the ceramic oxidation film was not completely densified, but exhibiting porous structure. On the other hand, since the MAO coating would be used in vascular stent in our future work, the ceramics coating might peel off due to the big deformation. To solve the problem, we are trying to develop flexible and stretchable coating, which is still in an exploratory stage. Further treatments are necessary to improve the corrosion resistance of the Mg alloy for surgical implantation.

## 5 Conclusions

This study indicated that the MAO-treated magnesium alloy slice was apparently slower than the untreated slice, and the ceramic oxidation film generated via MAO treatment was believed to distinctly increasing the corrosion resistance of the magnesium alloy material. Further treatment is necessary to improve the corrosion resistance of the magnesium alloy materials for surgical implantation applications.

**Acknowledgment.** We thank Prof. Huazhe Yang (China Medical University) for kindly assisting in the study.

## References

1. Chen, Y.H., FritH, J.E., Ali, D.M., et al.: Mechanical properties and biocompatibility of porous titanium scaffolds for bone tissue engineering. J. Mech. Behav. Biomed. **75**, 169–174 (2017)
2. Chu, C.L., Han, X., Jing, B., Feng, X., et al.: Surface modification of biomedical magnesium alloy wires by micro-arc oxidation. Trans. Nonferrous Met. Soc. **24**(4), 1058–1064 (2014)
3. Chang, L., Tian, L.F., Liu, W.: In vitro studies of biomedical magnesium alloys in a simulated physiological environment: a review. Corros. Sci. **72**(3), 118–124 (2013)
4. Xin, Y., Hu, T., Chu, P.K.: Intravenous magnesium in experimental stent thrombosis in swine. Acta Biomater. **7**(4), 1452–1459 (2011)
5. Rukshin, V., Azarbal, B., Shah, P.K.: Arterioscl. Throm. Vas. **21**, 1544 (2001)
6. Peeters, P., Bosiers, M., Verbist, J., et al.: Preliminary results after application of absorbable metal stents in patients with critical limb ischemia. J. Endovasc. Ther. **12**, 1 (2005)
7. Brezina, M., Minda, J., Dolezal, P.: Characterization of powder metallurgy processed pure magnesium materials for biomedical applications. Metals **7**(11), 461 (2017)
8. Song, G.L.: Control of biodegradation of biocompatible magnesium alloys. Corros. Sci. **49**(4), 1696–1701 (2007)
9. Harandi, S.E., Banerjee, P.C., Easton, C.D., et al.: Influence of bovine serum albumin in Hanks' solution on the corrosion and stress corrosion cracking of a magnesium alloy. Mater. Sci. Eng. C-Mater. **80**, 355 (2017)
10. Huang, C., Tang, Y.Z., Zhang, Y.Z.: Microstructure and dry sliding ear behavior of laser clad AlCrNiSiTi multi-principal element alloy coatings. Rare Met. **36**(7), 562–568 (2017)
11. Zhou, M., Xiong, P., Jia, Z.J.: Improved the in vitro cell compatibility and apatite formatioin of porous Ti6A14V alloy with magnesium by plasma immersion ion implantation. Mater. Lett. **202**, 9–12 (2017)
12. Yang, X.M., Li, M., Lin, X., et al.: Enhanced in vitro biocompatibility/bioactivity of biodegradable Mg-Zn-Zr alloy by micro-arc oxidation coating contained $Mg_2SiO_4$. Surf Coat Tech **233**, 65–73 (2013)
13. Witte, F., Fischer, J., Nellesen, J., et al.: In vitro and in vivo corrosion measurements of magnesium alloy. Biomaterials **27**(7), 1013–1018 (2006)
14. Seyfoori, A., Mirdamadi, S., Khavandi, A., et al.: Biodegradation behavior of micro-arc oxidized AZ31 magnesium alloys formed in two different electrolytes. Appl. Surf. Sci. **261**(15), 92–100 (2012)

15. Fischerauer, S.F., Kraus, T., Wu, X., et al.: In vivo degradation performance of micro-arc-oxidized magnesium implants: a micro-CT study in rats. Acta Biomater. **9**(2), 5411–5420 (2013)
16. Park, J.W., Kim, Y.J., Hang, J.H., et al.: Osteoblast response to magnesium ion-incorporated nanoporous titanium oxide surfaces. Clin. Oral Implant Res. **21**(11), 1278–1287 (2010)
17. Wang, D.W., Cao, Y., Qiu, H., et al.: Improved blood compatibility of Mg-1.0Zn-1,0Ca alloy by micro-arc oxidation. J. Biomed. Mater. Res. **99A**, 162–172 (2011)

# Wireless EEG-fNIRS Fusion Signal Acquisition System for Depth of Anesthesia Monitoring

Sanhe Duan[1](✉), Qi Guo[1], Siyuan Lv[1], Ying Liu[2], Hong Tang[2], Dan Liu[1], Jinwei Sun[1], and Qisong Wang[1]

[1] School of Instrumentation Science and Engineering, Harbin Institute of Technology, 92 Xidazhi St., Harbin 150001, China
samduan@hit.edu.cn

[2] Department of Anesthesia, Provincial Hospital of Heilongjiang, Harbin 150001, China

**Abstract.** Depth of anesthesia monitoring has been adopted in clinic in the recent years. However, misjudgments could occur under certain circumstances, which would harm patients mentally or even physically. In this article, we have proposed a novel hybrid EEG-fNIRS signal acquisition system with self-designed EEG and fNIRS acquisition modules. Results show that the EEG module has an indication error between 4 and 14%, the fNIRS module could drive laser sources and acquire signals with a 0.005 V converted signal resolution, and the system could acquire, visualize and save the data with a stable running time of about 1 h. The proposed system has huge potential for DoA monitoring.

**Keywords:** Depth of anesthesia monitoring · EEG · fNIRS · Hybrid-sourced data

## 1 Introduction

Monitoring depth of anesthesia (DoA) plays a vital role in clinical surgery to protect patients, which will be in favor of the administration of anesthetic drugs and others. Monitoring DoA with electroencephalogram (EEG) like bi-spectral index (BIS) [1] and NarcoTrend [2] has been widely used in clinic in the past decades. However, misjudgments could occur under certain circumstances when employing these systems [3, 4]; also, they usually require high purchase and maintenance costs, especially due to their patent protections. To improve the performance of DoA monitoring, new technologies has been gradually applied in this field, such as functional near-infrared spectroscopy (fNIRS). fNIRS assists researchers in understanding functions of different regions of the brain. But it could also be used in DoA monitoring with a high accuracy [5]. It is unaffected by electrical interference like motion artifacts, which makes it superior when the subject is in motion. Combining the advantages of EEG and fNIRS technologies has been studied recently to further improve human signal monitoring. Hybrid EEG-fNIRS systems have been discovered to take advantages in high accuracy and stability in brain-computer interface (BCI) [6, 7]. Because of its collecting more physiological information than standalone systems, we expect the hybrid systems to achieve higher


G. Wang et al. (Eds.): APCMBE 2023, IFMBE Proceedings 103, pp. 388–397, 2024.
https://doi.org/10.1007/978-3-031-51455-5_43

performance in DoA monitoring [8]. In this study, we propose a novel hybrid EEG-fNIRS signal acquisition system, where we have designed EEG and fNIRS acquisition modules. The system can achieve acquiring synchronized signal, visualizing them and saving the data to computers. Experiments have also been conducted to test the system.

## 2 Methodology

The system adopts a fusion of EEG and fNIRS monitoring, which is shown in Fig. 1.

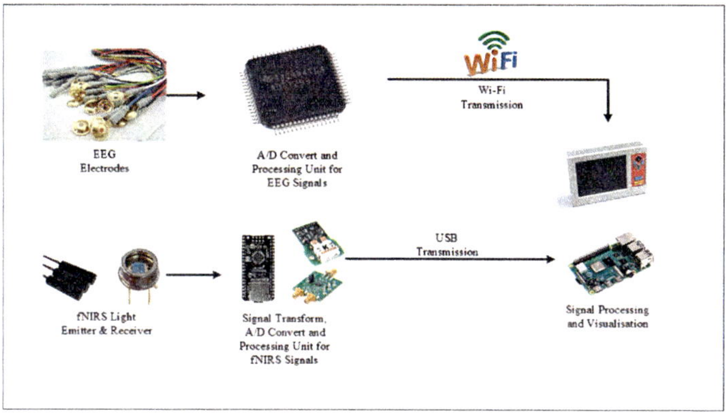


**Fig. 1.** System structure

It comprises vital parts to achieve the acquisition of EEG and fNIRS signals with the ability to generate optical source signals used by fNIRS. Also, it has the function of receiving, processing and visualizing the signals.

### 2.1 Hardware Structure and Process

Acquisition hardware comprises EEG and fNIRS acquisition modules, where they should acquire and process signals respectively. Furthermore, the fNIRS module should be able to drive near-infrared (NIR) light sources. Figure 2 displays the structural processes of these modules.

The A/D converter (ADC) for EEG acquiring typically integrates programmable gain amplifiers and digital filters, which will simplify the design. A photovoltaic cell converts optical signals to current ones. These current signals need to be converted to voltage signals via amplifying circuits for the ADC.

### 2.2 Software Structure

The software employed in the system comprises that managing the acquisition modules from the terminal, and that regulating the individual modules. The software in the modules' microcontrollers (MCU) need to control the ADCs and other peripherals, process the signals and send them. The terminal adopts its software to receive information from the modules, decode and process the signals, visualize and store the signals.

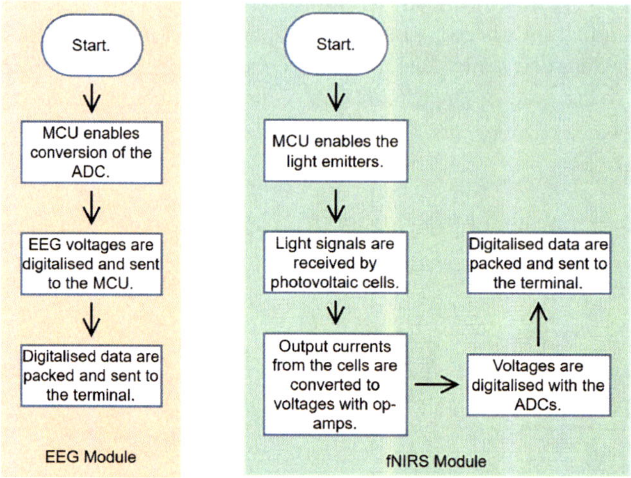


**Fig. 2.** Structural processes of the acquisition modules

# 3 Design

## 3.1 Design of the EEG Acquisition Module

We have designed an EEG acquisition module which comprises parts shown in Fig. 3.

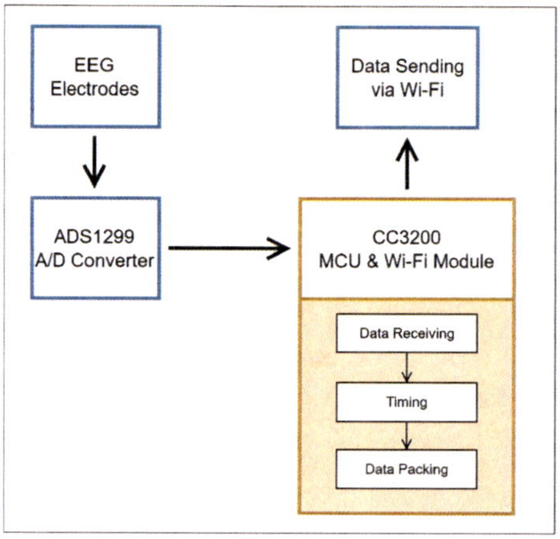


**Fig. 3.** Components of the EEG acquisition module

The ADS1299 ADC is specialized in the acquisition of human electrical signals, and provides differential inputs up to 8 channels. The CC3200 MCU can connect with other devices with Wi-Fi. The acquisition module draws power from a Li-Ion battery. Information sent to the terminal comprises EEG data, battery condition and time the data were acquired.

## 3.2 Design of the fNIRS Acquisition Module

The fNIRS module requires close coordination between the light source and the sensor. Therefore, we have designed a light source driver circuit and an optical signal acquisition circuit.

### 3.2.1 Light Source Driver Sub-module

We have selected infrared laser LED tubes as the fNIRS light source. These tubes run with a voltage between 3 and 5 V and near-infrared wavelengths. We expect the light sources flash at a frequency of 100 kHz, and we have proposed a dedicated driver sub-module circuit as is shown in Fig. 4. The Schmitt trigger is used to convert the voltages generated by the R-C circuit to positive signals, which drive the transistor switch to generate square waves from the DC power. Op-amps in the circuit are implemented using the ADA4891 general amplifier, and the Schmitt trigger is implemented by the 74HC132 chip.

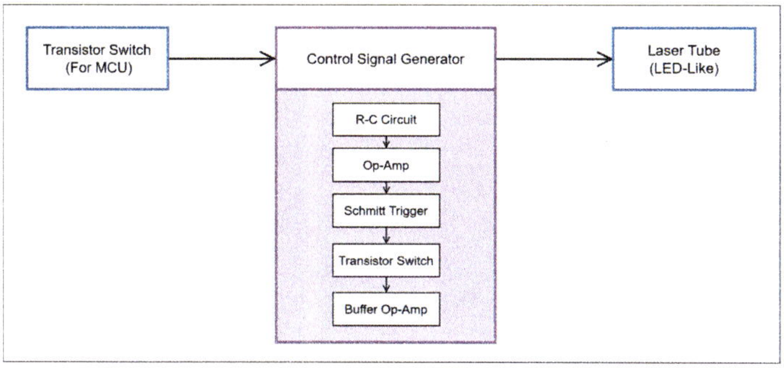


**Fig. 4.** Components of the light driver circuit

### 3.2.2 Optical Signal Acquisition Sub-module

We have used low dark current and wide frequency response photovoltaic cells as light sensors in the signal acquisition sub-module. These cells are most responsive at wavelengths around 800 nm, which are suitable for our tasks. The sub-module circuit is composed of parts shown in Fig. 6. The low-power COS8552 amplifiers are adopted in the circuit. The MS5193T ADC in the circuit has a 24-bit precision, which would provide convenience for further works, such as modeling hemoglobin concentrations and DoA. The GD32F4 MCU has been selected due to its high compatibility with STM32F4 chips.

## 3.3 Design of the Software

As is mentioned above, we need to develop software for the MCUs in the acquisition modules and for the terminal PC. Figure 5 demonstrates the processes of all the software.

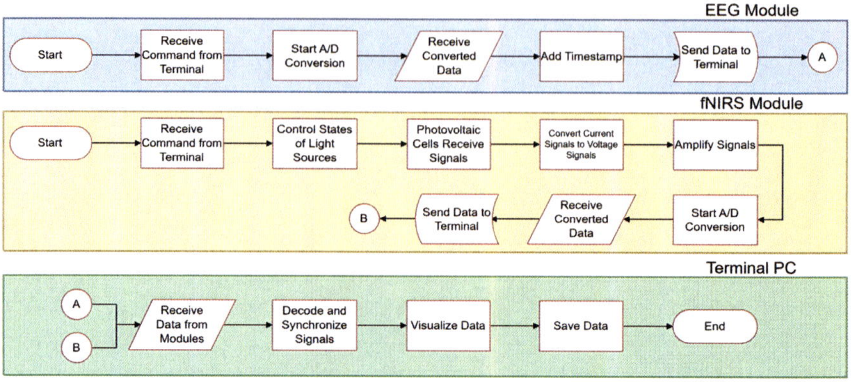


**Fig. 5.** Processes of the software

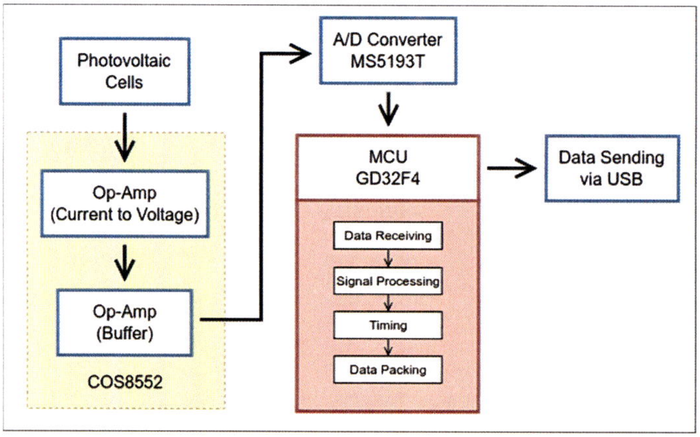


**Fig. 6.** Components of the optical signal acquisition sub-module

The software managing the modules should be able to control the peripherals. Also, the software shall pack the data received and send them to the terminal. Software for the terminal should visualize the data in real time. Data should be saved as common file types after the acquisition process for the convenience of further research.

The software for the EEG acquisition module is written in Energia, an Arduino-based system specialized for the programming of Texas Instruments MCUs. Standard Peripheral Drivers for the STM32 chips are adopted in the software for the fNIRS module. The terminal software is powered by Python and Qt libraries.

# 4 Results

## 4.1 System Prototypes

Figure 7 presents the prototype PCBs for the system. From left to right are the PCBs of the EEG acquisition module (front and back), the fNIRS light source driver sub-module, and the fNIRS signal acquisition sub-module.

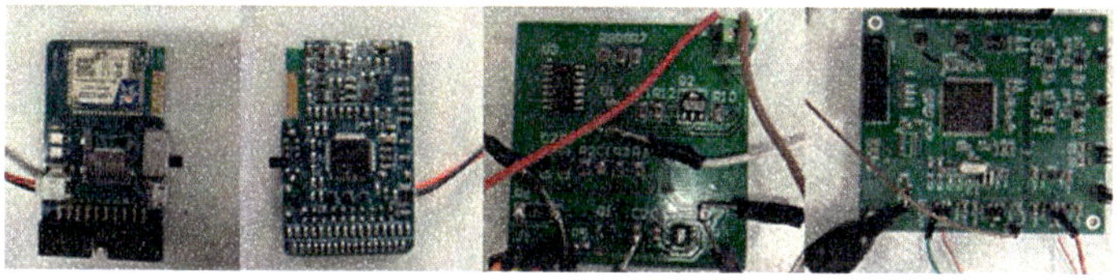

**Fig. 7.** The prototype PCB boards

## 4.2 Testing the Prototypes

We have conducted tests for both the individual modules and the combined system. Individual tests of the modules are to verify their assigned functions, and the combined tests are to verify the components' coordination and the system's stability.

### 4.2.1 Testing the EEG Module

Signal quality tests for the EEG acquisition module have been undertaken to investigate its error characteristics in its operating frequency zone. We have input sine wave and square wave signals with an amplitude of 2 mV and a frequency between 1 and 40 Hz to the module. We monitored output voltages using a digital multimeter. The results are displayed in Fig. 8. Relative indication errors when acquiring sine waves are between 4 and 14%, and tend to decrease on the rise of signal frequency. Square wave acquisition introduces relative indication errors between 4 and 10% with no notable relationships between the errors and signal frequencies. Referring to standards of metrological verification and actual application reports, we consider results above acceptable.

### 4.2.2 Testing the fNIRS Module

Tests for this module consist of those for the light source driver and for the acquisition board. Test results of the driver circuit indicated it could output signals from 2.5 to 3.11 V at a frequency of 170 kHz and powered the laser tube up. Test for the acquisition circuit uses an always-on laser tube (5 mV) to illuminate a photovoltaic cell connected to the circuit. The circuit adopted a 3.3 kΩ resistor to convert current signals to voltage ones. We have moved the laser tube around during the test to simulate lights of different power. The voltages acquired by the ADC are displayed in Fig. 9, in which we found the circuit's display resolution was 0.005 V.

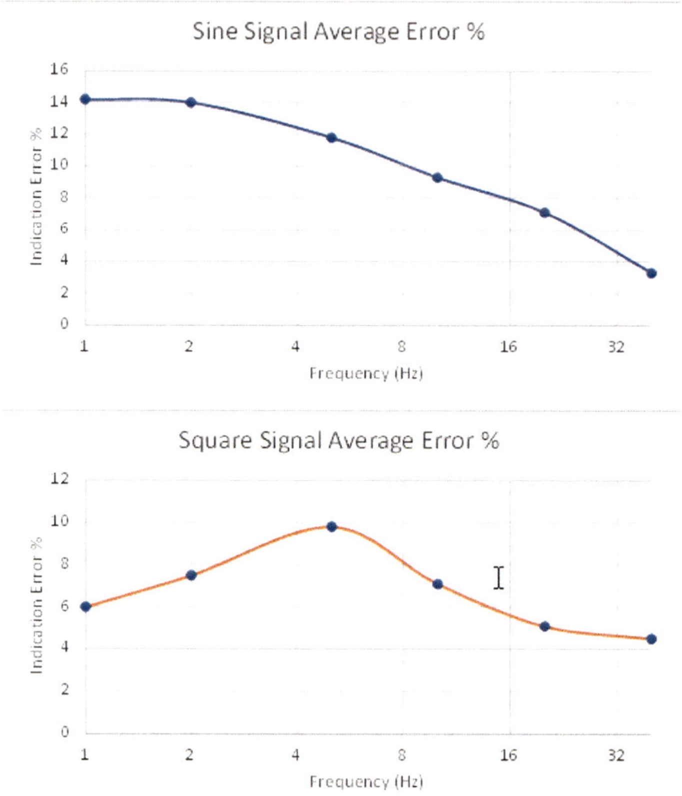


**Fig. 8.** Indication errors of the EEG acquisition module

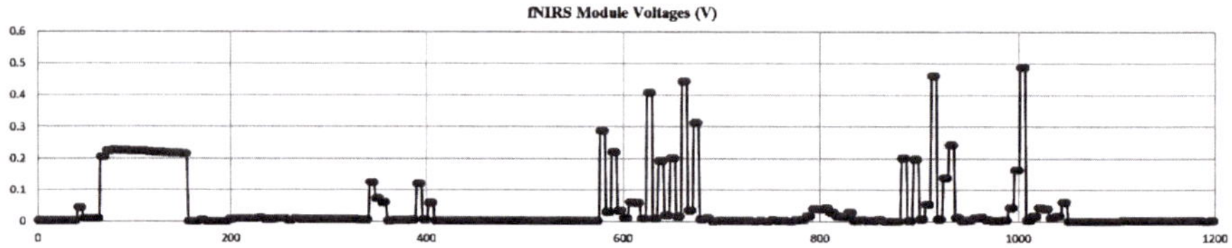


**Fig. 9.** Signals acquired by the fNIRS acquisition module

### 4.3 Combined Tests

We have conducted the tests by connecting a single EEG channel to a square wave signal which had a peak-to-peak voltage of 2 mV and a frequency of 15 Hz. Also, we have used the light source driver circuit to power a low-power laser tube and let the tube illuminate a photovoltaic cell connected to the fNIRS acquisition circuit. Both modules were connected to the terminal PC. The testing system can be seen in Fig. 10.

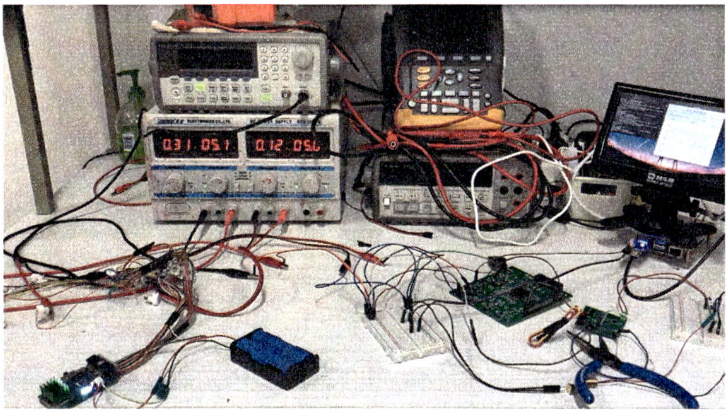

**Fig. 10.** System testing environment

Partial data and visualization of all the data are illustrated in Figs. 11 and 12. These data showed that the system could achieve synchronized acquisition of EEG and NIR signals, visualization and saving of these data. These tests aim to test whether the combined system could achieve such functions: controlling the acquisition modules and receiving data from them, data synchronization, visualization and saving.

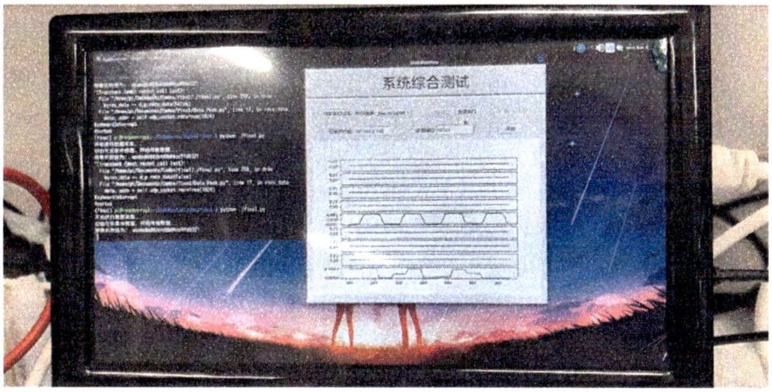


**Fig. 11.** Visualized data in the terminal control software

Furthermore, an endurance test has been conducted to simulate conditions in clinic. Using the same testing system in Fig. 10, we ran the test for 1 h, during which we altered signals and monitored the system's condition every 10 min. Partial data saved after the endurance test could be seen in Fig. 13, where 18,000 groups of data need approximately 1 h to acquire. Results above show the system's stability.

## 5 Discussion

Test results indicate that the system has the ability to ac-quire EEG and fNIRS information and process them in real time. However, the system is still improvable in several aspects:

| | 0 | 1 | 2 | 3 | 4 | 5 | 6 | 7 | 8 | 9 | 10 | 11 | 12 | 13 | 14 | 15 | 16 | 17 | 18 | |
|---|---|---|---|---|---|---|---|---|---|---|---|---|---|---|---|---|---|---|---|---|
| 0 | -0.10706 | -0.02732 | 0.097638 | 0.108546 | 0.108525 | 0.108541 | 0.108553 | 0.108555 | 0.10855 | 0.073074 | -0.07148 | -0.10833 | -0.10831 | -0.10832 | -0.10835 | -0.10835 | -0.10833 | -0.098 | 0.025586 | 0.1 |
| 1 | 0.201667 | 0.201667 | 0.201667 | 0.201667 | 0.201667 | 0.201667 | 0.201667 | 0.201667 | 0.201667 | 0.201667 | 0.201667 | 0.201667 | 0.201667 | 0.201667 | 0.201667 | 0.201667 | 0.201667 | 0.201667 | 0.201667 | 0.2 |
| 2 | 0.201667 | 0.201667 | 0.201667 | 0.201667 | 0.201667 | 0.201667 | 0.201667 | 0.201667 | 0.201667 | 0.201667 | 0.201667 | 0.201667 | 0.201667 | 0.201667 | 0.201667 | 0.201667 | 0.201667 | 0.201667 | 0.201667 | 0.2 |
| 3 | 0.201667 | 0.201667 | 0.201667 | 0.201667 | 0.201667 | 0.201667 | 0.201667 | 0.201667 | 0.201667 | 0.201667 | 0.201667 | 0.201667 | 0.201667 | 0.201667 | 0.201667 | 0.201667 | 0.201667 | 0.201667 | 0.201667 | 0.2 |
| 4 | 0.201667 | 0.201667 | 0.201667 | 0.201667 | 0.201667 | 0.201667 | 0.201667 | 0.201667 | 0.201667 | 0.201667 | 0.201667 | 0.201667 | 0.201667 | 0.201667 | 0.201667 | 0.201667 | 0.201667 | 0.201667 | 0.201667 | 0.2 |
| 5 | 0.201667 | 0.201667 | 0.201667 | 0.201667 | 0.201667 | 0.201667 | 0.201667 | 0.201667 | 0.201667 | 0.201667 | 0.201667 | 0.201667 | 0.201667 | 0.201667 | 0.201667 | 0.201667 | 0.201667 | 0.201667 | 0.201667 | 0.2 |
| 6 | 0.201667 | 0.201667 | 0.201667 | 0.201667 | 0.201667 | 0.201667 | 0.201667 | 0.201667 | 0.201667 | 0.201667 | 0.201667 | 0.201667 | 0.201667 | 0.201667 | 0.201667 | 0.201667 | 0.201667 | 0.201667 | 0.201667 | 0.2 |
| 7 | 0.201667 | 0.201667 | 0.201667 | 0.201667 | 0.201667 | 0.201667 | 0.201667 | 0.201667 | 0.201667 | 0.201667 | 0.201667 | 0.201667 | 0.201667 | 0.201667 | 0.201667 | 0.201667 | 0.201667 | 0.201667 | 0.201667 | 0.2 |
| 8 | 0.001366 | 0.001366 | 0.001366 | 0.001366 | 0.001366 | 0.001366 | 0.001378 | 0.001378 | 0.001378 | 0.001378 | 0.001378 | 0.001378 | 0.001383 | 0.001383 | 0.001383 | 0.001383 | 0.001383 | 0.001383 | 0.001378 | 0.0 |

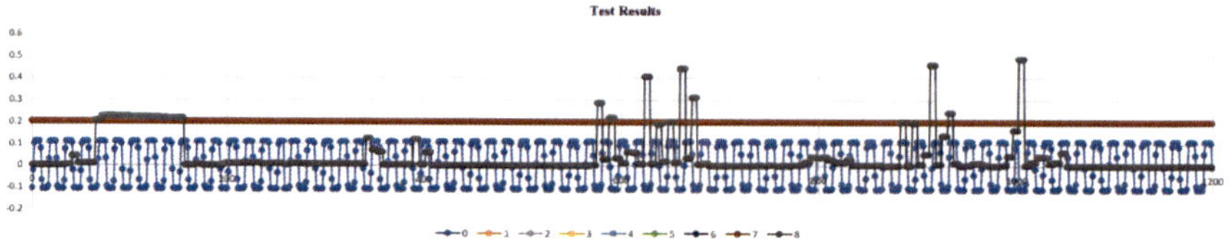


**Fig. 12.** Data saved locally and their visualization

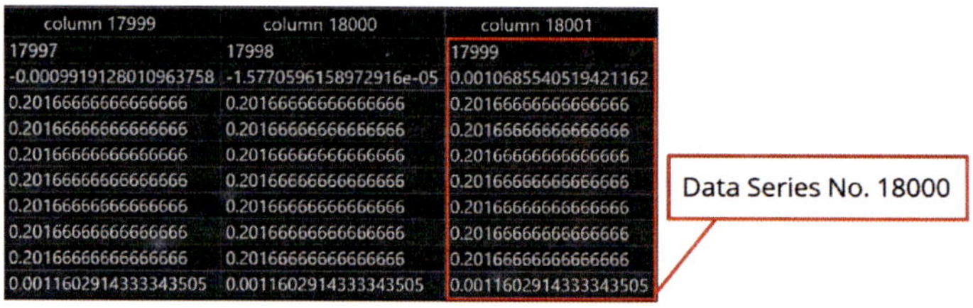

| column 17999 | column 18000 | column 18001 |
|---|---|---|
| 17997 | 17998 | 17999 |
| -0.0009919128010963758 | -1.5770596158972916e-05 | 0.0010685540519421162 |
| 0.20166666666666666 | 0.20166666666666666 | 0.20166666666666666 |
| 0.20166666666666666 | 0.20166666666666666 | 0.20166666666666666 |
| 0.20166666666666666 | 0.20166666666666666 | 0.20166666666666666 |
| 0.20166666666666666 | 0.20166666666666666 | 0.20166666666666666 |
| 0.20166666666666666 | 0.20166666666666666 | 0.20166666666666666 |
| 0.20166666666666666 | 0.20166666666666666 | 0.20166666666666666 |
| 0.20166666666666666 | 0.20166666666666666 | 0.20166666666666666 |
| 0.0011602914333343505 | 0.0011602914333343505 | 0.0011602914333343505 |



**Fig. 13.** Endurance test results of the combined system

*Making the System Fully Wireless*: Current version of the fNIRS acquisition module needs USB connections to communicate with the terminal. Requiring a line would be a nuisance in surgery, where the line could limit operations.

*Alternating the fNIRS Module*: fNIRS based on steady-state spectroscopy doesn't need ahigh-frequency signal. A series of programmable switches would be enough to control the light sources.

*Making the System Smaller and Wearable*: Current system boards are too large to fit on human heads, and a headband needs to be designed to make the system wearable.

*Improving the Stability and Battery Life*: These systems should last for longer time in clinic. So,larger batteries and power optimization of the circuit should be undertaken.

## 6 Conclusion

We have built a hybrid EEG-fNIRS signal acquisition hardware system aiming at monitoring depth of anesthesia in clinic. The system could acquire EEG and NIR signals simultaneously, and achieve visualization and saving of the data, and could run continuously for at least 1 h. But the system still has multiple problems and is not ready for monitoring actual fNIRS signals and DoA levels. A novel proposal of the system has been underway, which includes redesigning the modules and building mathematical models for calculating hemoglobin concentration and DoA.

**Acknowledgment.** This work was sponsored by the Fundamental Research Funds for the Central Universities (Grant No. IR2021222), Future Science and Technology Innovation Team project of HIT(216506).

## References


1. LeBlanc, J.M., Dasta, J.F., Pruchnicki, M.C., Gerlach, A., Cook, C.: Bispectral index values, sedation-agitation scores, and plasma lorazepam concentrations in critically Ill surgical patients. Am. J. Critical Care **21**, 99–104 (2012)
2. Kreuer, S., Wilhelm, W.: The narcotrend monitor best practice and research clinical anaesthesiology **20**, 111–119 (2006)
3. Joshua, L.: Awakening 2013. Section: Health
4. Russell, I.F.: The Narcotrend 'depth of anaesthesia' monitor cannot reliably detect consciousness during general anaesthesia: an investigation using the isolated forearm technique. Br. J. Anaesth. **96** (2006)
5. Hernandez-Meza, G., Izzetoglu, M., Osbakken, M., Green, M., Abubakar, H., Izzetoglu, K.: Investigation of optical neuro-monitoring technique for detection of maintenance and emergence states during general anesthesia. J. Clin. Monitoring Comput. **32**, 147–163 (2018)
6. Yanhua, S.: Research on the Key Technology of EEG-fNIRS Based Few Channel and Bimodel Bain Computer Interface Master's thesis. Southeast University Nanjing, China (2017)
7. Enhui, W.: Research of Emotion Recognition System Based on EEG-fNIRS Master's thesis. Jilin University Changchun, China (2020)
8. Seul-Ki, Y., Dong-Ok, W., Seong, C., et al.: Spatio-temporal dynamics of multimodal EEG-fNIRS signals in the loss and recovery of consciousness under sedation using midazolam and propofol. PLOS ONE **12**, e0187743 (2017). Publisher: Public Library of Science

# The Love Wave Immunosensor for Detecting the Pneumonia Biomarker Procalcitonin (PCT)

X. J. Zhang[1], H. M. Xiong[1], J. Y. Sun[1], Y. J. Hu[2], Y. Zhou[2], H. Wan[1], T. X. Wang[3], and P. Wang[1](✉)

[1] Key Laboratory for Biomedical Engineering of Education Ministry, Department of Biomedical Engineering, Biosensor National Special Laboratory, Zhejiang University, Hangzhou, China
cnpwang@zju.edu.cn

[2] Sir Run Run Shaw Hospital, Zhejiang University, Hangzhou, China

[3] Zhejiang, E-Linkcare Meditech Co., Ltd., No. 30 Baita Tongjiang Road, Taizhou, Zhejiang, China

**Abstract.** Pneumonia refers to infectious inflammation of the pulmonary parenchyma caused by bacterial, viral, and other pathogens. The early screening and identification of the pathogen is essential to the treatment for pneumonia patients. Procalcitonin (PCT) is an acute parameter used to distinguish between bacterial and non-bacterial inflammation. Besides, PCT is clearly correlated with the severity and prognosis of systemic infections such as inflammatory response syndrome, community-acquired pneumonia (CAP), and septic shock (some severe COVID-19 patients will present septic shock symptoms). In this study, we develop an 8-channel automated device based on the Love-type surface acoustic wave sensor to detect PCT, especially in exhaled breath condensates (EBC) of pneumonia patients. This immunosensor is mainly based on SPA self-assembly layer and the sandwich immunoassay. Besides, the signal is amplified by AuNPs and immunogold staining. The initial results show that the Love-SAW immunosensor has a good linear range of PCT detection from 15.62–500 ng/mL (R2 = 0.9703) and the limits of detection (LOD) is 0.85 ng/ml. This high-throughput device based on Love-SAW immunosensor is expected to rapidly detect multiple pneumonia biomarkers including PCT, providing valuable guidance for the diagnosis and prognosis of pneumonia.

**Keywords:** Surface acoustic wave sensor · Biomarker · PCT · Pneumonia · Exhaled breath condensates

## 1 Introduction

Pneumonia refers to infectious inflammation of the pulmonary parenchyma caused bacterial, viral, and other pathogens. Among them, bacterial pneumonia and viral pneumonia are the most common form, the leading cause of death from acute respiratory infections [1]. The early screening and identification of the pathogen is essential to the treatment for pneumonia patients. Currently, it is difficult to identify pathogens by using the clinical imaging methods. Blood tests can detect some biomarkers associated with


G. Wang et al. (Eds.): APCMBE 2023, IFMBE Proceedings 103, pp. 398–406, 2024.
https://doi.org/10.1007/978-3-031-51455-5_44

the disease, but it is invasive. Bacteriological tests requiring days of bacterial cultures are time-consuming. These methods are not conducive to early diagnosis of pneumonia, resulting in delay in the treatment of patients.

Procalcitonin (PCT) is an acute parameter used to distinguish between bacterial and non-bacterial inflammation. A large number of research data have shown that PCT is clearly correlated with the severity and prognosis of systemic infections such as inflammatory response syndrome [2], community-acquired pneumonia (CAP) [3], sepsis [4], and septic shock (some severe COVID-19 patients will present septic shock symptoms [5]). Besides, PCT testing has also received widespread attention in laboratory testing for COVID-19 [5, 6]. In complex clinical situations, PCT with high sensitivity and specificity should be adopted as early as possible to apply antibiotics timely and accurately [7–9].

The level of PCT is very low in healthy people, but it can be significantly increased in patients with bacterial pneumonia, the best cut-off in plasma is 1.09 ng/mL [10]. According to statistics, optical methods [11], electrochemical luminescence (ECL) [12] and electrochemical sensors [13] have been used more often for PCT detection in clinical serum or spiked serum. These methods have high sensitivity and low detection limit, but rely on complex optical and electrochemical systems, which are time-consuming, expensive and invasive.

Exhaled breath condensate (EBC) detection is a promising method for early screening and diagnosis of lung diseases [14, 15]. The non-volatile molecules contained in exhaled breath mainly exist in the form of small droplets [16], which are thought to be produced by the airway lining fluid [17] and condense into EBC when the temperature drops. EBC sampling is noninvasive, rapid and cost-effective. However, due to the extremely low concentration and complex composition of EBC, the detection of biomarkers in EBC remains a challenge. So it is urgent to develop a method to detect potential biomarkers of pneumonia at extremely low concentrations.

The Love wave immunosensor, one of the surface acoustic wave (SAW) sensors, has many advantages such as low attenuation, high sensitivity and corrosion resistance in liquids. The SAW sensor is a piezoelectric mass sensor that can be sensitive to mass loading on the surface, as the loading can influence the propagation of the acoustic wave. Amongst various SAW sensors, Love wave sensor is a favored device for liquid phase applications [18].

In this study, we have developed a system based on the Love wave immunosensor and its 8-channel automated detection instrument to detect PCT in EBC for the diagnosis and prognosis of pneumonia. This high-throughput instrument is expected to be further used to analyze more pneumonia biomarkers including PCT, as well as samples from clinical patients with pneumonia, for a more accurate early diagnosis of pneumonia.

## 2 Materials and Methods

### 2.1 Materials

The Au nanoparticles (AuNPs) solution (d $\approx$ 10–20 nm), staphylococcal protein A (SPA), coating antibody (Ab1) and labeling antibody (Ab2) of PCT as well as PCT antigen were all purchased from Jingqi Biotechnology Co., Ltd. (China). The phosphate buffered solution (PBS) was bought from Hangzhou Chemical Reagent Co., Ltd. (China). The albumin from bovine serum (BSA) was bought from Sigma-Aldrich (USA). EBC collection device was bought from ASCON Tecnologic (Italian).

### 2.2 Love-Saw Sensor

The Love-SAW sensor comprises a piezoelectric material, a cross-finger transducer (IDTs), a waveguide layer, and a top sensitive layer, as shown in Fig. 1a. In this study, ST-Z quartz with balanced properties and pure horizontal shear wave excitation is selected as the piezoelectric substrate for Love wave. IDTs uses a uniform split finger structure and there are 50 pairs on each side of IDTs. The wavelength $\lambda$ is 28 $\mu$m. The cross finger width a of each split finger is $\lambda/8$ and the spacing p is $\lambda/4$. $SiO_2$ is selected as the waveguide layer, and the thickness is 3 $\mu$m. The sensitive layer material is Au with the thickness of 50 nm. The center frequency of the final sensor is about 152.5 MHz.

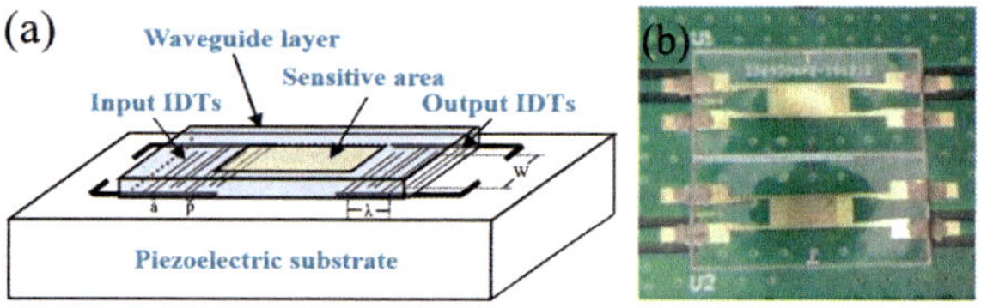


**Fig. 1.** **a** Schematic diagram of Love-SAW sensor structure; **b** Image of dual-channel Love-SAW sensor.

Figure 1b shows the real picture of the two-channel Love-SAW sensor, in which one channel is the sensing channel and the other is the reference channel. By comparing the signals of sensing channel and reference channel, interference of temperature, solution viscoelasticity and other factors can be eliminated.

### 2.3 8-Channels Automated Detection System

The multi-channel automatic detection system is shown in Fig. 2. There are eight Love-SAW sensors on the top of the instrument. A catheter connected to an internal injection pump can deliver samples to the sensor surface through a small hole in the instrument's top cover, enabling portable sampling. The inside of the instrument contains two power modules, a signal generation module, a signal processing module and a main control circuit, which can realize the signal generation and acquisition of the sensor. In addition, there is a sliding table control module, a sliding table sampling module, a sample tank, a injection pump, etc., to realize automatic sampling. Labview software and dual serial ports are used for signal acquisition and human-computer interaction interface where users can adjust the injection pump sampling amount and rate as well as the type of sample to be injected. Meanwhile, users can send and receive signals of 8 channels in real time and efficiently.

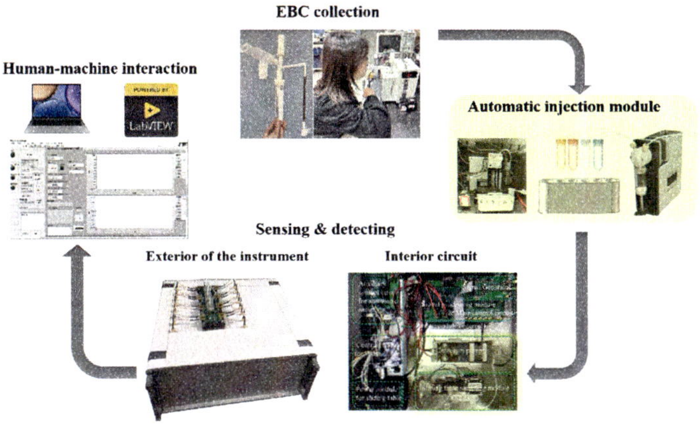


**Fig. 2.** The automated detection system.

### 2.4 Experiment Setup

This immunosensor is mainly based on SPA self-assembly layer and the sandwich immunoassay. The antigen firstly is captured by the coating antibodies (Ab1) which are strongly immobilized on the gold layer of the senor by SPA self-assembly layer. Then labeling antibodies conjugated with gold nanoparticles (AuNP@Ab2) can be captured by antigen which has been on the surface of the immunosensor, and the signal is further amplified by gold staining.

To avoid excessive consumption, we optimized the optimal concentration of PCT labeling antibody (Ab2) binding to Au nanoparticles (AuNP) by enzyme linked immunosorbent assay (ELISA). Firstly, add AuNPs solution into the microplate (200 μL per well) and then add 10 μL Ab2 with different concentrations into each well, blow and mix well. Secondly, add 10 μL 10% NaCl solution into each well, blow and mix well. Finally, measmre OD value and analyze the relative peak values (ΔOD).

After the optimization, the making process of AuNPs@Ab2 was as follows. At first, adjust the pH of AuNPs solution to 8–9 with $K_2CO_3$ solution (pH 9.6). Then, add 50 μL PCT with the most appropriate concentration into 1 mL AuNPs solution with adjusted pH and shake well for 30 min. After that, put the solution into the centrifuge to centrifuge at 4 °C and 14,000 rpm for 30 min. Finally, remove the supernatant and redissolve with 0.2% BSA solution.

Before the experiment, the gold layer of the sensor is washed with 1M NaOH and 1M HCl solution in turn, and then activated by piranha solution, a mixture of 98% sulfuric acid and 30% hydrogen peroxide (7:3). Figure 3, the diagram of PCT detection by Love-SAW sensor, shows the corresponding modification and detection steps.

(a) Self-assembled layer modification: Add 10 μL 1 mg/mL solution of Staphylococcus aureus protein A (SPA) to each sensor surface. The SPA protein has sulfhydryl groups, which can bind to Au on the surface of the sensitive layer to form Au–S bonds. Meanwhile, SPA can still bind to Fc segment of antibody to realize directional fixation of antibody [19]. SPA incubation usually lasts for half an hour.

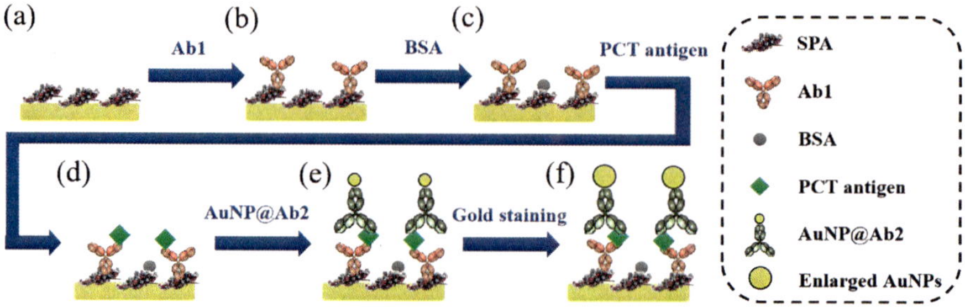


**Fig. 3.** Schematic diagram of immunosensor surface modification and PCT detection process.

(b) Coated with Ab1: After PBS washing and nitrogen gas drying, add 10 μL 100 μg/mL coating antibody (Ab1) of PCT to the surface of the working channel sensor, and 10 μL 10% BSA solution to the surface of the reference channel. Then put the biosensors into the refrigerator to incubate at 4 °C overnight.
(c) Block excess binding sites: After PBS washing and nitrogen gas drying, 10 μL 10% BSA solution is added to both the working channel and the reference channel to block nonspecific binding sites. Half an hour later, the sensor is washed by PBS and dried by nitrogen gas,
(d) Inject PCT samples: After fixing the microfluidic chip made by PDMS, inject PBS into microfluidic chip at a flow rate of 50 μL/min until the sensor signal is stabilized. Then, 40 μL PCT antigen solution with different concentrations is injected into different sensors and static binding lasts for 10 min.
(e) Add AuNP@Ab2: After rinsing with PBS, inject 40 uL AuNP@Ab2 into each sensor and static binding is lasted for about 15 min. The AuNP@Ab2 complex can be specifically captured by the PCT antigen, resulting in an increase of the mass on sensor's surface.
(f) Amplify signal by gold staining: After PBS washing, 100 μL freshly made gold staining solution (10 mM chlorauric acid mixed with 20 mM hydroxylamine hydrochloride in 1:1 equal volume) is injected with the spped of 50 μL/min. At this time, $[AuCl_4]^-$ in the chlorauric acid solution will be catalyzed by AuNPs in the AuNP@Ab2, which will continuously wrap on the surface of AuNPs [20]. The mass amplification is proportional to the number of AuNPs captured on the surface. Finally, clean with PBS until the signals become stable.

## 3 Results and Discussion

### 3.1 Optimization of Labeling Antibody Concentraton

The binding conditions between Ab2 and AuNPs has been optimized. According to the Fig. 4, after adding 10% NaCl, a series of AuNPs solutions combining with different concentrates of Ab2 appeared different degrees of coagulation phenomenon. The lower the concentration of Ab2, the more obvious the coagulation. In the absorption spectrum, the absorbance value of the solution decreased at 520 nm, while the absorbance increased near 700 nm. In addition, the absorption peaks were redshifted due to the increase in particle size of AuNPs complex.

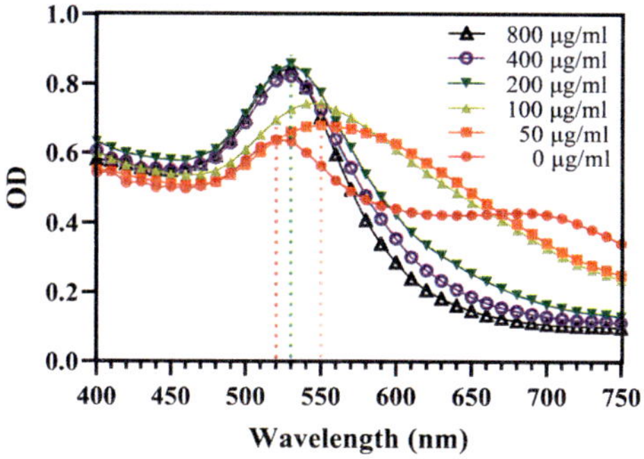


**Fig. 4.** Absorption spectrum of AuNPs solution with different concentrations of PCT Ab2 after adding 10% NaCl

The relative peak absorbance (△OD) between the maximum absorbance at 500–600 nm wavelength and 710 nm wavelength was calculated. Figure 5 shows that △OD increases with the increase of antibody concentration. When the antibody concentration exceedes 200 μg/mL, △OD did not increase significantly. So 200 μg/mL was selected as the minimum antibody concentration to stabilize AuNPs. The most appropriate concentration should be increased by an additional 10% from 200 μg/mL, which is 220 μg/mL.

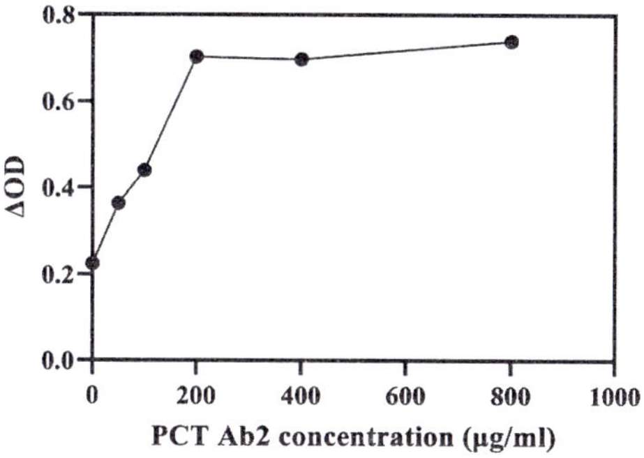


**Fig. 5.** The relative peak absorbance (△OD) of AuNPs with different concentrations of PCT Ab2

## 3.2 Detection of PCT

After each experiment, analyze the phase changes of the working channel and the reference channel over time. After normalization for each channel data, the difference in phase shift change between the working and reference channels was calculated by subtracting the phase change of the reference channel from the phase change of the working channel. Figure 6 shows that the phase shift of Love-SAW sensor will become larger after injecting AuNP@Ab2. Besides, the higher concentration, the greater the phase change. After adding gold staining solution, the phase shift further increased. Similarly, the phase change becomes more obvious with the increase of the concentration.

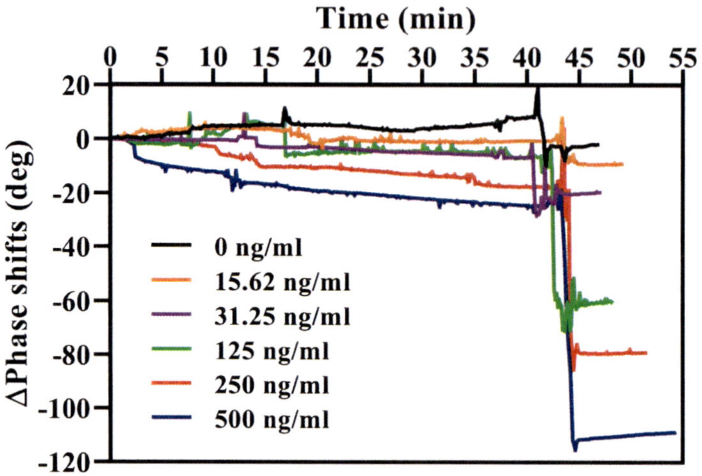


**Fig. 6.** Real-time monitoring of PCT with different concentration based on Love-SAW sensor

The relationship between the concentration of PCT antigen and the final phase shift change is shown in Fig. 7. The results show that in the concentration range of 15.62–500 ng/ml, the Love-SAW biosensor has good linearity in detecting the logarithm base 10 of concentration in standard samples ($R^2 = 0.9703$). Besides, the limits of detection (LOD) for PCT is calculated to be 0.85 ng/ml based on the principle of 3σ, which refers to adding the result of three times the standard deviation and the mean value of the phase shifts of 6 standard blank samples and then substituting the result into the linear equation to calculate the corresponding concentration.

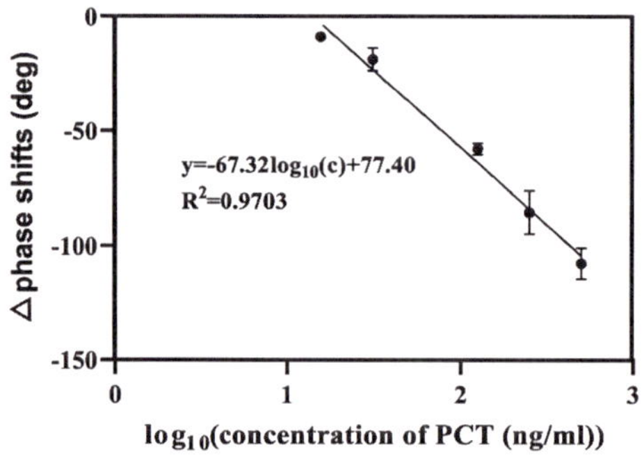


**Fig. 7.** The standard curve of PCT detected by Love-SAW sensor (n = 3)

## 3.3 Discussion

The proposed system based on Love-SAW can realize multi-channel automated detection with detection time less than 1 h. The initial results show that the Love-SAW immunosensor has a good linear range of PCT detection from 15.62 to 500 ng/mL ($R^2 = 0.9703$)

and the limits of detection (LOD) is 0.85 ng/ml. In order to achieve accurate detection of actual EBC samples from patients with pneumonia, the current linear range and detection limit for PCT are not low enough. Therefore, more experiments are needed to detect samples with lower concentrations. Meanwhile, further signal amplification strategies need to be studied such as MOF@Au.

## 4 Conclusions

In this study, we developed a Love type acoustic surface wave immunosensor and designed an automated detection instrument to rapidly detect pneumonia biomarker PCT. The detection principle is based on SPA self-assembly layer and immune sandwich method. In addition, with AuNPs and immunogold staining signal amplification technology, the signal changes caused by the surface antigen quality of the sensor were linearly amplified, thus achieving highly sensitive detection of the pneumonia biomarker PCT. The proposed detection system based on Love-SAW immunosensor is expected to rapidly detect various pneumonia biomarkers including PCT, so as to provide valuable guidance for the diagnosis and prognosis of pneumonia.

**Acknowledgement.** This work was supported by the Funds for International Cooperation and Exchange of the National Natural Science Foundation of China (No. 62120106004), National Key Research and Development Program of China (No. 2021YFB3200801), the Public welfare research program of Zhejiang Provincial Science and Technology Department (No LGF19H010011).

## References

1. Bansal, M., Khatri, M., Taneja, V.: Potential role of periodontal infection in respiratory diseases—a review. J. Med. Life **6**(3) (2013)
2. Feng, X.D., Li, S.S., Sun, Q., et al.: Immune-inflammatory parameters in COVID-19 cases: A Systematic Review and meta-analysis. Front. Med. **7** (2020). ARTN30110.3389/fmed
3. Kim, M.W., Lim, J.Y., Oh, S.H.: Mortality prediction using serum biomarkers and various clinical risk scales in community-acquired pneumonia. Scand. J. Clin. Lab. Inv. **77**(7), 486–492 (2017)
4. Rubio-Diaz, R., Julian-Jimenez, A., del Castillo, J.G., et al.: Ability of lactate, procalcitonin, and criteria defining sepsis to predict 30-day mortality, bacteremia, and microbiologically confirmed infection in patients with infection suspicion treated in emergency departments. Emergencias **34**(3), 181–189 (2022)
5. Li, X., Wang, L., Yan, S., et al.: Clinical characteristics of 25 death cases with COVID-19: A retrospective review of medical records in a single medical center, Wuhan, China. Int. J. Infect. Dis. **94**, 128–132 (2020). https://doi.org/10.1016/j.ijid
6. Hu, R., Han, C.F., Pei, S.Y., et al.: Procalcitonin levels in COVID-19 patients. Int. J. Antimicrob. Agents **56**(2) (2020). 10605110.1016/j.ijantimicag
7. Liu, F., Li, L., Xu, M.D., et al.: Prognostic value of interleukin-6, C-reactive protein, patients with COVID-19 and procalcitonin in. J. Clin. Virol. **127** (2020). ARTN10437010.1016/j.jcv
8. Schuetz, P., Beishuizen, A., Broyles, M., et al.: Procalcitonin (PCT)-guided antibiotic stewardship: an international experts consensus on optimized clinical use. Clin. Chem. Lab. Med. **57**(9), 1308–1318 (2019). https://doi.org/10.1515/cclm

9. Bouadma, L., Luyt, C.E., Tubach, F., et al.: Use of procalcitonin to reduce patients'exposure to antibiotics in intensive care units (PRORATA trial): a muhicentrerandomised controlled trial. Lancet **375**(9713), 463–474 (2010). https://doi.org/10.1016/S0140-6736(09)61879-1
10. Su, W., Ju, L., Hua, Q. et al.: Values of combined C-reactive protein, procalcitonin and serum amyloid A in differential diagnosis of bacterial and non-bacterial community acquired pneumonia in children. Diagn. Microbiol. Infect. Dis. **105**(2) (2023). https://doi.org/10.1016/j.diagmicrobio.2022.115865
11. Hu, X., Wang, Z., Zhu, Z.: Establishment of a quantum-dot cytometric assay for detecting PCT and the value of clinical detection. Chin. J. Gerontol.Gerontol. **33**(8), 1828–1831 (2013)
12. Song, X.Z., Zhao, L., Zhang, N., et al.: Ultrasensitive electrochemiluminescence biosensor with silver nanoclusters as a novel signal probe and Alpha-fe2o3-pt as an efficient co-reaction accelerator for procalcitonin immunoassay. Anal. Chem. (2023). https://doi.org/10.1021/acs.analchem.2c04673
13. Gupta, Y., Pandey, C.M., Ghrera, A.S.: Development of conducting cellulose paper for electrochemical sensing of procalcitonin. Microchim. Acta **190**(1) (2023). https://doi.org/10.1007/s00604-022-05596-9
14. Zou, Y.C., Wang, L., Zhao, C., et al.: CEA, SCC and NSE levels in exhaled breath condensate-possible markers for early detection of lung cancer. J. Breath Res. **7**(4) (2013). Artn04710110.1088/1752-7155/7/4/047101
15. Liang, Y., Yeligar, S.M., Brown, L.A.S.: Exhaled breath condensate: a promising source for biomarkers of lung disease. Sci. World J. (2012). Artn21751810.1100/2012/217518
16. Davis, M.D., Montpetit, A., Hunt, J.: Exhaled breath condensate an overview. Immunol. Allergy. Clin. **32**(3):363−+ (2012). https://doi.org/10.1016/j.iac
17. Effros, R.M., Casaburi, R., Porszasz, J., et al.: Exhaled breath condensates: analyzing the expiratory plume. Am. J. Resp. Crit. Care **185**(8), 803–804 (2012). https://doi.org/10.1164/rccm
18. Li, S.M., Wan, Y., Su, Y., et al.: Gold nanoparticle-based low limit of detection Love wave biosensor for carcinoembryonic antigens. Biosens. Bioelectron.. Bioelectron. **95**, 48–54 (2017)
19. Lee, W., Oh, B.K., Bae, Y.M., et al.: Fabrication of self-assembled protein A monolayer and its application as an immunosensor. Biosens. Bioelectron.. Bioelectron. **19**(3), 185–192 (2003). https://doi.org/10.1016/S0956-5663(03)00195-7
20. Saha, K., Agasti, S.S., Kim, C., et al.: Gold nanoparticles in chemical and biological sensing. Chem. Rev. **12**(5), 2739–2779 (2012). https://doi.org/10.1021/cr2001178

# Active Sensor for Multidimensional Force Detection

Bojing Shi(✉)

School of Biological Science and Medical Engineering, Beihang University, 37 Xueyuan Road, Haidian District, Beijing, China
bjshi@buaa.edu.cn

**Abstract.** The sense of touch is one of the important media for humans and animals to communicate with the environment. It is critical to find a method or device that can detect the multidimensional dynamic micromechanical signals of biological soft tissues such as skin and muscle, quickly and accurately, which is essential for the development of tactile sensing technologies. Here, we demonstrate a triboelectric force sensor (TFS) that can convert the mechanical signals of the living creature's soft tissue into detectable electric signals directly. The TFS contains elastic polymer micro-column and micro-cone structures that can be used to detect normal and tangential dynamic forces quickly, accurately, and synchronously. This work aims to establish an active dynamic microforce sensing model and an overall performance index system of the TFS, which would realize the accurate detection of the mechanical properties of biological soft tissues. It analyses the influencing factors of the sensing performance of the TFS from the aspects of sensitivity, accuracy and stability. This work is intended to explore a new type of active mechanical sensing method and mechanism, and establish a universal connection between electrical outputs and relevant mechanical parameters. It may provide reference ideas and a theoretical basis for the research and development of multi-dimensional biomechanics sensors with simple structure, sensitive signals and fast response, and the exploration of bionic tactile systems.

**Keywords:** Active sensor · Triboelectric effect · Multidimensional force detection

## 1 Introduction

Humans perceive the external world through their skin's sense of touch, such as the perception of temperature, humidity, pressure and vibration, which can identify the size, material, hardness, and other properties of the object in contact [1–3]. For the exploration of tactile mechanism, especially for the study of its biomechanical process, one of the keys lies in whether the dynamic micro-mechanical characteristics of biological soft tissues such as skin and muscle can be obtained quickly and accurately, thus laying the foundation for building a more "realistic" force tactile model. The research work related to tactile sensing published in the journal Science has attracted further attention from researchers in this field (Fig. 1).


G. Wang et al. (Eds.): APCMBE 2023, IFMBE Proceedings 103, pp. 407–414, 2024.
https://doi.org/10.1007/978-3-031-51455-5_45

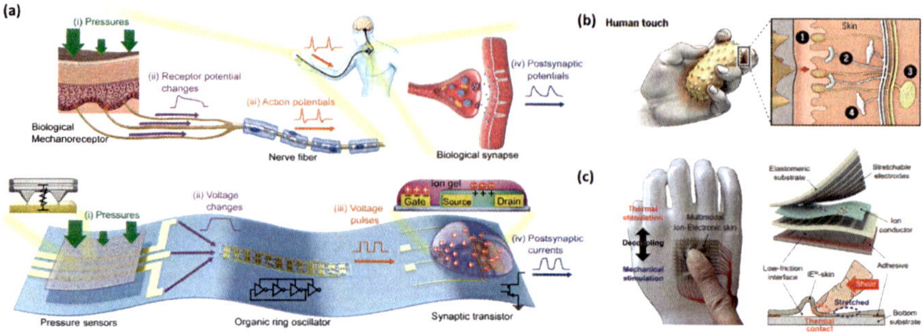

**Fig. 1.** Force sensors used for tactile stimulation. **a** Bionic active tactile sensing [4]; **b** Tactile receptors and perception process [5]; **c** Active tactile sensing based on ionic conductor [6].

The traditional active sensors used for the mechanical detection of biological soft tissue are mostly piezoresistive and capacitive [7–9]. Their dynamic response speed depends too much on the complex signal acquisition and processing system, and some structures need to be made of rigid materials, which increases the difficulty of the flexible preparation of sensors. These bottlenecks will restrict the further development of dynamic micro-force sensing of biological soft tissue. The flexible force sensor based on active sensing technology can solve the above problems. The basic principle of active sensing includes the piezoelectric effect and triboelectric effect, that is, the device can generate piezoelectric potential or friction charge by itself under the action of external force to realize the instantaneous conversion of force signal to electrical signal [10–12]. This active sensing method not only breaks away from the dependence on complex signal sources and processing systems, but also realizes real-time and accurate detection of tactile dynamic micro-forces. At the same time, due to the extensive selection of materials, it is more conducive to its flexible fabrication (Fig. 2).

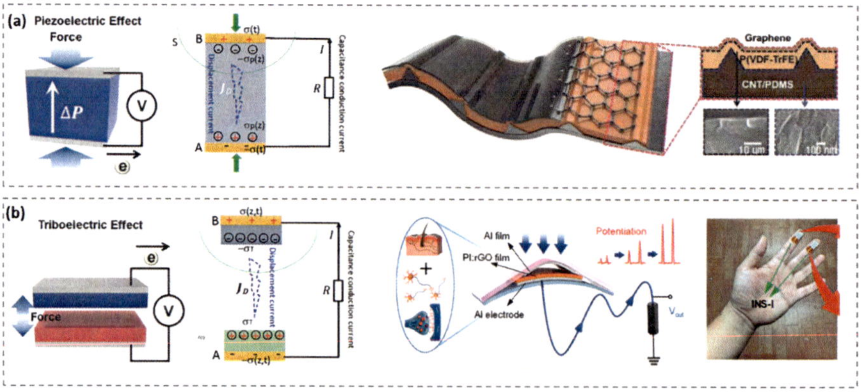

**Fig. 2.** Active force sensors [13–15]. **a** Piezoelectric type; **b** Triboelectric type.

Researchers at home and abroad have made important progress in the field of active mechanical sensing. Professor Zhonglin Wang's team proposed a triboelectric nanogenerator based on friction electrification and electrostatic induction effect, which can be used to collect tiny mechanical energy; Then, combining its principle with Maxwell's displacement current theory, a mechanical-electrical conversion mechanism model of friction nano-generator is constructed [16–18]. Its basic working principle is that when the friction generator nano-motor is deformed due to external force, two kinds of friction layer materials with different electron gain and loss abilities will contact/rub, and generate friction charges at the contact/friction interface. When the external force changes to make the friction layer separate, a potential difference is formed between the two, which will drive the electrons in the back electrode of the friction layer to flow in the external circuit and form a current (Fig. 3).

Researchers of the Chinese Academy of Sciences have developed an intelligent neuro-like tactile sensor that has learning and memory functions based on a triboelectric nanogenerator [14]. Researchers at Peking University have proposed a self-powered smart skin based on contact electricity and planar electrostatic induction, which is used to detect the contact position and speed of objects, which is a typical active mechanical sensor [19]. Researchers from Sungkyunkwan University in South Korea have proposed a graphene friction electronic tactile sensor that is co-coupled with a single-electrode friction nanogenerator and graphene field-effect transistor [20].

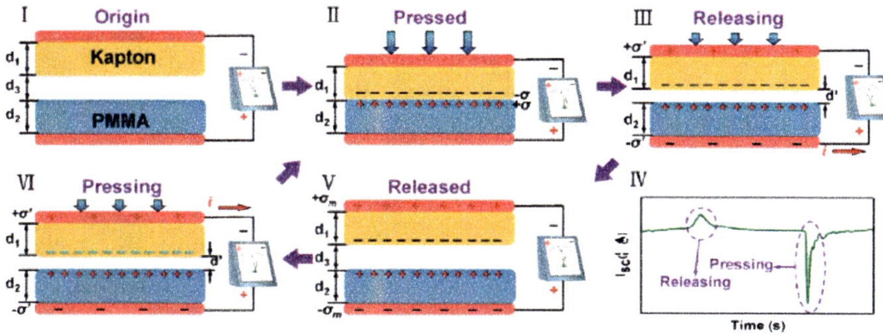


**Fig. 3.** Working principle of triboelectric nanogenerator [21].

Although the active biomechanical sensor has made great progress which has greatly improved the accuracy, rapidity and simplicity of the mechanical properties testing method of biological soft tissue, there are still the following challenges to be solved: how to achieve real-time and accurate detection of tangential force and normal force at the same time? The mechanical process of skin and muscle is fine and complex, with non-linear, anisotropic, viscoelastic and other biomechanical properties [22, 23]. The current active sensing research has not yet proposed a good solution for the multi-dimensional detection of dynamic mechanical behavior of biological soft tissue.

Here, we proposed to combine the friction nano-generator with surface micro-structure (such as micro-cone) with micro-column structure, which not only takes advantage of the sensitivity of the triboelectric effect to force signals, but also realizes the

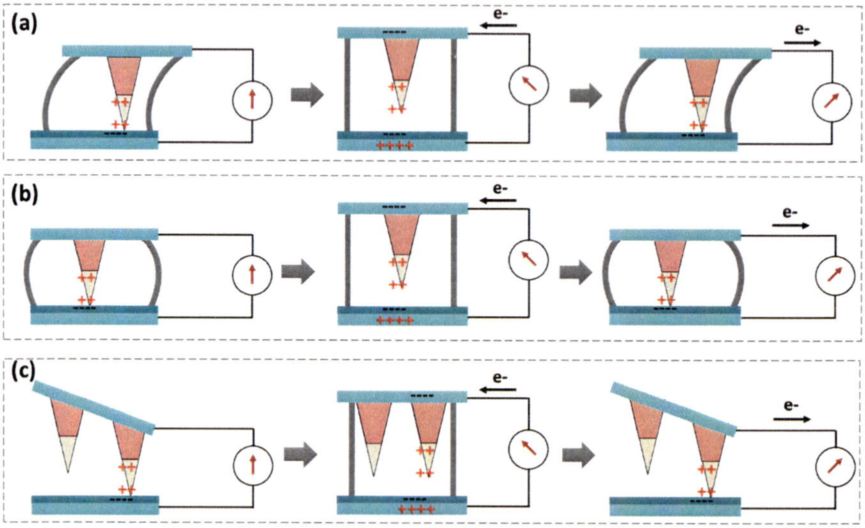


**Fig. 4.** Active multi-dimensional force sensors based on triboelectric effect and its working principle under different forces. **a** Shear force; **b** Pressure; **c** Irregular force.

detection of multi-dimensional force with the help of micro-column. Therefore, the applicant has designed an active multi-dimensional dynamic force sensor TFS based on a triboelectric effect, which can accurately and quickly detect the dynamic micro-force of biological soft tissue in multi-dimension. Compared with the traditional resistance and capacitance sensors, TFS gets rid of the dependence on the signal source, not only simplifies the device structure, but also realizes the instantaneous direct conversion of force signal to the electrical signal. This not only avoids the system error caused by the existence of signal source, improves the sensitivity of force signal acquisition and the integrity of sensing signal, but also realizes the detection of multi-dimensional dynamic force (Fig. 4).

## 2 Results and Discussion

We select the required materials from the polymer materials with good biocompatibility and good flexibility such as silica gel, polydimethylsiloxane (PDMS), polylactic acid (PLA), polytetrafluoroethylene or other synthetic materials, to make the sensor. Materials such as metal or conductive polymer are selected to attach to the flexible substrate to act as the electrode. This sensor will have the characteristics of adapting to the surface and deformation of a variety of complex biological soft tissues. The flexible polymer material with good biocompatibility is used to process the film with a certain thickness (50–200 μm) and microcone/column structure (400–800 μm). The electrode layer (50–200 nm) was prepared by magnetron sputtering, thermal evaporation or ink-jet printing. The different metal or polymer materials were coated on the tip of the cone to study their effect on the friction electrical signal (Fig. 5).

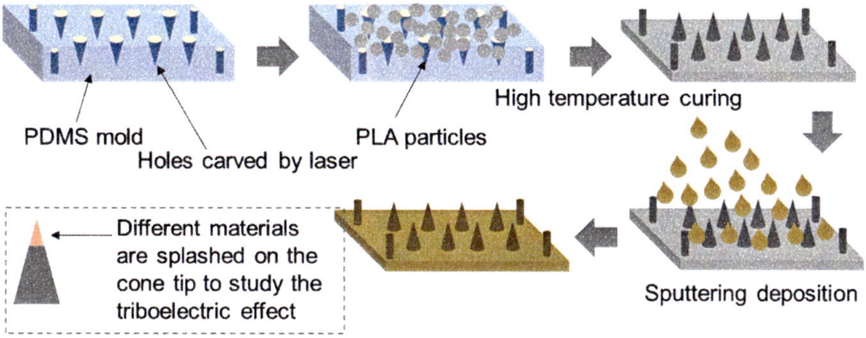


**Fig. 5.** Cone manufacturing process.

To improve the performance of sensors by increasing the amount of electrical charge generated by contact between different materials, friction interface modification technology of the sensors has aroused great interest and become increasingly important in the design of sensor structures. Since various microstructures will lead to different non-uniform stress distribution during the pressure, a variety of microstructures have been investigated according to the needs. Different microstructures will produce different stress distributions under pressure, so we have studied the mechanical properties of various microstructures of the friction layers of the sensor. In this work, we compared the mechanical properties and triboelectric outputs of friction layer surfaces with conical, cylindrical, and rectangular structures through finite element analysis and measured the results. In the simulation, the height of the cylinder, cone, and cuboid is the same, and the bottom radius of the cone and cylinder is consistent with the ground side length of the box.

From the simulation results, the conical structure deforms the most under the same pressure, which means that the smaller the contact surface area at the front end of the microstructure, the greater the deformation under pressure. To verify the simulation results, we made sensors with different microstructures and tested them. The experimental results show that the deformation results of different microstructures have similar trends under the action of the normal force. Although their displacements under lower pressures are almost the same, eventually the deformation of the cone structure is the largest with the increase of the normal force.

At the same time, we have demonstrated the good sensitivity of the sensor and its sensing ability for multi-angle forces to demonstrate its sensing applications in practical scenarios. For example, TFS can be installed on a finger for reagent weighing. In this experiment, TFS is installed on the index finger of a prosthetic hand, which holds the test tube. In the initial state, the surface of the TFS contacts the sidewall of the test tube. Then, we added water to the test tube six times through a pipette to increase weight, with a volume of approximately 2.3 mL of water being added each time. Since the test tube is held with a prosthetic hand, the increased weight of water is equivalent to an increase in the shear force between the TFS and the test tube. Therefore, TFS has been proven to be capable of weighing reagents, providing a more accurate method of weighing reagents or samples during experimental operations.

Meanwhile, we tested the ability of TFS to detect tilt forces. Four conical microstructures are prepared on the friction layer surface of TFS, with the top of each corresponding to an electrode. The four top electrodes of the TFS are sequentially connected to the four data channels of the oscilloscope, which directly records sensing data and displays it on the screen in real-time. The tilt force applied to the sensor is achieved by pressing the sensor with a finger in a directional direction.

The press action in each direction was repeatedly tested to verify its effectiveness and stability. By comparing the output amplitudes of the four channels of the TFS, the direction of the force can be clearly distinguished. For example, when a forward force was applied to the TFS, more force would be concentrated on cones 1 and 2 than on cones 3 and 4, resulting in more deformation and higher voltage output to reflect the characteristics of the external force applied to the sensor. Therefore, by analyzing the output amplitude of each cone, the direction of the force can be distinguished by the TFS.

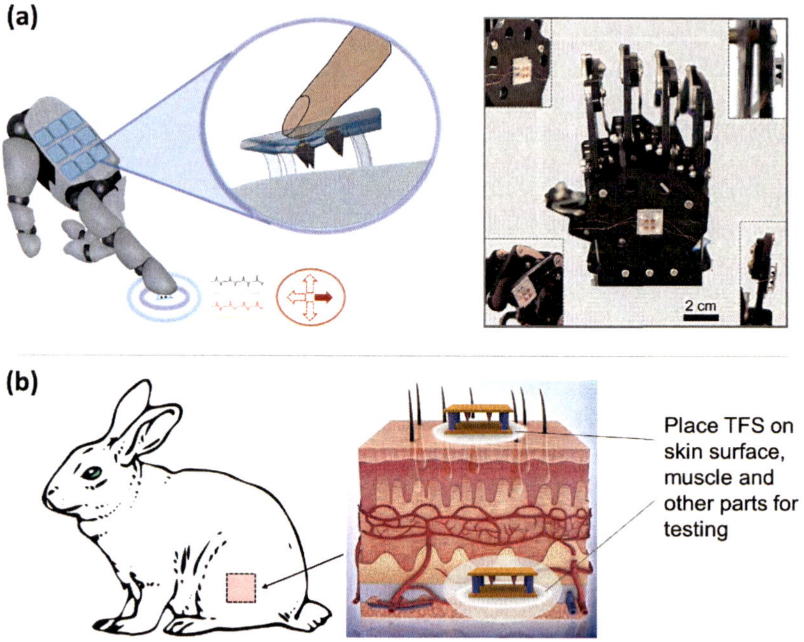


**Fig. 6.** Application scenarios of TFS. **a** Wearable sensor and human-machine interface [24]; **b** Mechanical testing of living biological tissue.

For the mechanical testing of living biological tissue, a flexible TFS with a suitable size and shape is designed and manufactured. Considering the characteristics of the fitting part of a human body (skin) and experimental animal (muscle and tendon), biological glue is used to enhance the fitting of the device and soft tissue. Study the physical and electrical output characteristics of TFS in real-time, and analyze its in-body sensing effect. Combined with the above experimental results, the finite element analysis technology is used to explore the operation law of TFS in vivo, and build a suitable theoretical model, which provides a theoretical basis for further optimizing the structure and output performance, and realizing the effective conversion of biological soft tissue force signal to the electrical signal. In the future, we will improve the construction of TFS from the aspects of material, structure and surface treatment, and realize the differential design and integration of sensor devices for different living soft tissues (Fig. 6).

## 3 Conclusions

In summary, based on the triboelectric sensing architecture of elastic support and surface microstructure, we have developed an active multi-dimensional force sensor that can detect and distinguish between normal and shear forces. We have fabricated and compared different sensor structures and obtained key parameters for improving sensor performance, including the surface structure of the friction layer and the microstructure array layout, to optimize sensor design. At the same time, we also discussed the corresponding sensing mechanism. The results show that the optimized TFS has a good linearity ($R^2 = 0.97$) and a fast response to external forces. The sensitivity of the optimized sensing material and structure for normal force detection is 4.8 times higher than that of a pure PDMS cone configuration. The detection limit of TFS for shear force can reach 255 Pa. Through the response characteristics of multiple microstructures and the output voltage amplitude of different signal paths, real-time detection and determination of the direction of external forces can be achieved. In terms of application verification, we have constructed an intelligent artificial hand for real-time measurement of reagent weight, tactile sensing, and an intelligent multi-dimensional force indication system. In brief, our proposed TFS has great potential as a sensitive force sensor for human-machine interfaces, electronic skins, wearable/implantable electronic devices, and robots in the future.

**Acknowledgment.** This work was supported by the National Natural Science Foundation of China (32101117) and the Fundamental Research Funds for the Central Universities.

## References

1. Lee, W.W., et al.: A neuro-inspired artificial peripheral nervous system for scalable electronic skins. Sci. Robot. **4**(32), eaax2198 (2019)
2. Oh, J.Y., Bao, Z.: Second skin enabled by advanced electronics. Adv. Sci. **6**(11), 1900186 (2019)
3. Chou, H.-H., et al.: A chameleon-inspired stretchable electronic skin with interactive colour changing controlled by tactile sensing. Nat. Commun.Commun. **6**(1), 8011 (2015)
4. Kim, Y., et al.: A bioinspired flexible organic artificial afferent nerve. Science **360**(6392), 998–1003 (2018)
5. Sundaram, S.: How to improve robotic touch. Science **370**(6518), 768–769 (2020)
6. You, I., et al.: Artificial multimodal receptors based on ion relaxation dynamics. Science **370**(6519), 961–965 (2020)

7. Zuk, S., Pietrikova, A., Vehec, I.: Capacitive touch sensor. Microelectron. Int. **35**(3), 153–157 (2018)
8. Chun, S., et al.: A highly sensitive pressure sensor using a double-layered graphene structure for tactile sensing. Nanoscale **7**(27), 11652–11659 (2015)
9. Chen, Z., et al.: Enhancing the sensitivity of percolative graphene films for flexible and transparent pressure sensor arrays. Adv. Func. Mater. **26**(28), 5061–5067 (2016)
10. Hua, Q., et al.: Skin-inspired highly stretchable and conformable matrix networks for multifunctional sensing. Nat. Commun.Commun. **9**(1), 244 (2018)
11. Choi, W., et al.: Enhanced sensitivity of piezoelectric pressure sensor with microstructured polydimethylsiloxane layer. Appl. Phys. Lett. **104**(12), 123701 (2014)
12. Wu, W., Wen, X., Wang, Z.L.: Taxel-addressable matrix of vertical-nanowire piezotronic transistors for active and adaptive tactile imaging. Science **340**(6135), 952–957 (2013)
13. Ryu, H., Yoon, H.-J., Kim, S.-W.: Hybrid energy harvesters: toward sustainable energy harvesting. Adv. Mater. **31**(34), 1802898 (2019)
14. Wu, C., et al.: Self-powered tactile sensor with learning and memory. ACS Nano **14**(2), 1390–1398 (2020)
15. Lee, J.-H., et al.: Highly stretchable piezoelectric-pyroelectric hybrid nanogenerator. Adv. Mater. **26**(5), 765–769 (2014)
16. Fan, F.-R., Tian, Z.-Q., Lin Wang, Z.: Flexible triboelectric generator. Nano Energy **1**(2), 328–334 (2012)
17. Wang, Z.L.: On the first principle theory of nanogenerators from Maxwell's equations. Nano Energy **68**, 104272 (2020)
18. Wang, Z.L.: On Maxwell's displacement current for energy and sensors: the origin of nanogenerators. Mater. Today **20**(2), 74–82 (2017)
19. Shi, M., et al.: Self-powered analogue smart skin. ACS Nano **10**(4), 4083–4091 (2016)
20. Khan, U., et al.: Graphene tribotronics for electronic skin and touch screen applications. Adv. Mater. **29**(1), 1603544 (2017)
21. Wang, Z.L.: Triboelectric nanogenerators as new energy technology for self-powered systems and as active mechanical and chemical sensors. ACS Nano **7**(11), 9533–9557 (2013)
22. Nardinocchi, P., Teresi, L.: On the active response of soft living tissues. J. Elast.Elast. **88**(1), 27–39 (2007)
23. Yem, V., Kajimoto, H.: Comparative evaluation of tactile sensation by electrical and mechanical stimulation. IEEE Trans. Haptics **10**(1), 130–134 (2017)
24. Zhang, W., et al.: Self-powered force sensors for multidimensional tactile sensing. ACS Appl. Mater. Interfaces **14**, 20122–20131 (2022)

# Quantitative Hematocrit Measurement on a Pressure-Actuated Microfluidic Chip

Haonan Li[1], Muyang Zhang[1], Zejingqiu Chen[2], Zhiqing Xiao[3], Zitao Feng[3], Eric S. Hald[3], and Weijin Guo[3](✉)

[1] Department of Electronic Engineering, Shantou University, Shantou, China
[2] Department of Biology, Shantou University, Shantou, China
[3] Department of Biomedical Engineering, Shantou University, 243 Daxue Road, Shantou, China
guoweijin@stu.edu.cn

**Abstract.** In point-of-care diagnostics, hematocrit (HCT), which is the volume percentage of red blood cells in the whole blood sample, is closely related to human health status. Here, we developed a pressure-actuated, polydimethylsiloxane (PDMS) microfluidic chip for quantitative measurement of HCT. The narrowest part of its flow channel is 8 μm and acts as a constriction for blood cells, which can lead to retardance of blood flow in the chip. The amount of red blood cells has an influence on the transport time of passing through the constriction for the blood samples, so we can use the transport time to infer the HCT value. We found a linear calibration curve between blood transport time and HCT value, which showed a correlation coefficient ($R^2$) of 0.9506 for blood samples with HCT ranging from 0.35 to 0.55. This microfluidic chip can provide the results of HCT measurement within 1 min, making it well-suited for point-of-care diagnostics.

**Keywords:** Hematocrit measurement · Microfluidic · PDMS · Point-of-care diagnostics · Pressure-actuated

## 1 Introduction

Blood is made up of blood cells and plasma and is very important for human body function. It stores a lot of information about overall health status, and diagnostics of many diseases require whole blood tests. HCT is the volume percentage of red blood cells in the whole blood sample. For healthy adults, the hematocrit can range from 35 to 47% for women and 41–54% for men [1]. HCT measurement is widely used to evaluate human health in clinical practice [2]. It is often used as an indicator for the diagnosis and classification of anemia [3]. HCT can also be used to determine whether the patients need fluid replenishment. It is a significant index of some diseases.

At present, the commonly used clinical methods for HCT measurement include centrifugal method, blood analyzer method and radionuclide method. These methods are very accurate, but generally time-consuming and inefficient. Moreover, most of clinical methods require specialized instrumentation and are not suitable for applications in point-of-care diagnostics. Many microfluidic chips have been developed to measure


G. Wang et al. (Eds.): APCMBE 2023, IFMBE Proceedings 103, pp. 415–420, 2024.
https://doi.org/10.1007/978-3-031-51455-5_46

HCT quantitatively, aiming for HCT measurements at home or clinics in resource-limited regions [2, 4–9]. Lee et al. developed an electrochemical method to measure the HCT on a microfluidic chip by checking the current response of blood in a fluidic channel under DC voltage [4]. Petersson et al. used an acoustic microfluidic chip for the separation of blood cells and plasma, followed by optical detection for the measurement of HCT [5]. Browne et al. used a microfluidic chip with spiral fluidic channels for plasma separation and quantification of HCT [6]. Berry et al. used a multi-layer paper microfluidic chip to measure the HCT according to the flow distance of blood samples [2]. Frantz et al. developed a flow tracking app on smartphone for characterizing the blood flow on a lateral flow test strip and used it for HCT measurement [7]. Laha et al. developed a smartphone based method to screen the pattern of a blood drop on a paper strip pre-soaked by glycerol and related the topological features of the pattern to HCT value [8]. However, the majority of these methods need external electrical or fluidic power, which is not suitable for point-of-care diagnostics; take a long time to perform HCT measurement, which can cause the problems such as stagnancy of blood flow or drying of blood samples (such problems can introduce errors for the measurement); or need to develop some specific computer program or algorithm for image process.

In this study, we develop a PDMS microfluidic chip for quantitative measurement of HCT. The design of the chip was inspired by previous work [10]. This chip is actuated by pressure from finger through a pen tip and does not need external power supply. Only 6 μL whole blood sample is needed for one test, and the test can be done in less than 1 min. The fluidic channel for blood sample has a constriction of 8 μm. Since most of blood cells are red blood cells and the shape of red blood cells is similar to a pancake, of which the diameter is 6–8 μm, blood cells passing through the constriction will experience some retardance. The amount of blood cells will have an influence on the total retardance caused by the constriction. By recording the transport time of blood samples through the constriction, we can use it to reflect the HCT value. The timer function of smartphone can be used to record the transport time. In this way, HCT is measured by recording the blood transport time of an unknown blood sample.

## 2 Experiment

The blood samples for the experiment are taken from pigs, which is provided by a local food supplier. Blood samples from the pigs were directly put into the test tubes with anticoagulant EDTA coating (BD Vacutainer®, K2 EDTA 10.8 mg, 6 mL, REF: 367863, Franklin Lakes, NJ, USA) and stored at 4 °C before use.

For the preparation of SU-8 mold of the microfluidic chips, it follows a standard protocol. Briefly, SU-8 2015 (Yilan Micro Electronics, Suzhou, China) was spin-coated on a 4-inch silicon wafer. Next, the silicon wafer was baked at 95 °C for 4 min. Then, we performed photolithography on the silicon wafer with a patterned plastic film mask (Jixian Opto-electronic, Shenzhen, China) using a lithography machine (URE-2000/35AL, Institute of Optics and Electronics, Chinese Academy of Sciences, China). After that, the silicon wafer was baked at 95 °C for 5 min. Then, the silicon wafer was developed in propylene glycol methyl ether acetate (PGMEA) and washed by isopropanol. Lastly, the silicon wafer was hard baked at 150 °C for 20 min before it was ready for use. In addition, the silicon wafer was treated with trichloro (1H, 1H, 2H, 2H-perfluorooctyl) silane before it was used for replica molding of PDMS.

We pasted a PDMS block of 7 × 7 × 2 mm on the SU-8 mold, and used it for molding the air pocket (Fig. 1, top). This PDMS block was also treated with trichloro (1H, 1H, 2H, 2H-perfluorooctyl) silane.

For the chips used in the experiment, we used PDMS (Sylgard 184, Dow Corning Corporation, USA) with a 10:1 ratio of base to curing agent. We stirred the PDMS and used a vacuum chamber to remove the bubbles. Then, we poured the PDMS onto the mold, and again removed the bubbles using a vacuum chamber. After confirming that there were no bubbles in the PDMS, we placed them in an oven (80 °C) for more than 50 min to cure the PDMS. Then, we cut and peeled PDMS from the SU-8 mold. We did plasma hydrophilic treatment of PDMS pieces and glass slides by a plasma cleaner (PDC-002, Harrick Plasma, Ithaca, NY, USA) and bonded them together. Then, we put them in the oven (80 °C) for 24 h before storing at room temperature in preparation for experimental use.

We used a profiler (Dektak XT, Bruker, Billerica, MA, USA) for the characterization of SU-8 mold and PDMS microfluidic chips. The height of fluidic channel is 25 ± 2 μm, and the width of the constriction is 8 ± 1 μm. The diameter of the sample loading well on the chip is 2 mm. After the blood samples pass through the constriction, it will reach an area of pillars. The shape of the pillar is a rectangle slot with length as 120 μm and radius as 30 μm. The schematic and real pictures of the chip are shown in Figs. 1 and 2.

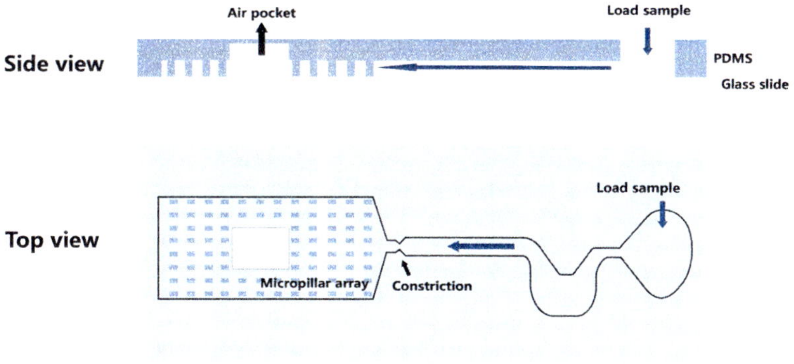


**Fig. 1.** The schematic of the microfluidic chip. It is formed by bonding a PDMS chip to a glass slide. It mainly consists of four parts: a sample loading well, a fluidic channel with a constriction, a chamber of micropillar arrays, and an air pocket.

For the preparation of blood samples, we filled blood samples in capillary tubes and centrifuged them to separate the blood cells and plasma. Then we used the software ImageJ (https://imagej.nih.gov/ij/) to analyze and calculate the volume proportion of plasma and RBC in the capillary tubes, and obtained the HCT values of the blood samples. After that, we adjusted the HCT of blood samples by extracting or adding plasma. We prepared blood samples with HCT of 35, 40, 45, 50 and 55%. In order to reduce the surface energy of the blood samples, avoid gas bubbles in the fluidic channel, and avoid blockage caused by aggregated blood cells, we then added phosphate buffered saline mixed with 0.2% Tween-20 (PBST; Tween 20, Macklin, Shanghai, China) to the blood with a volume ratio of blood to PBST of 4:1.

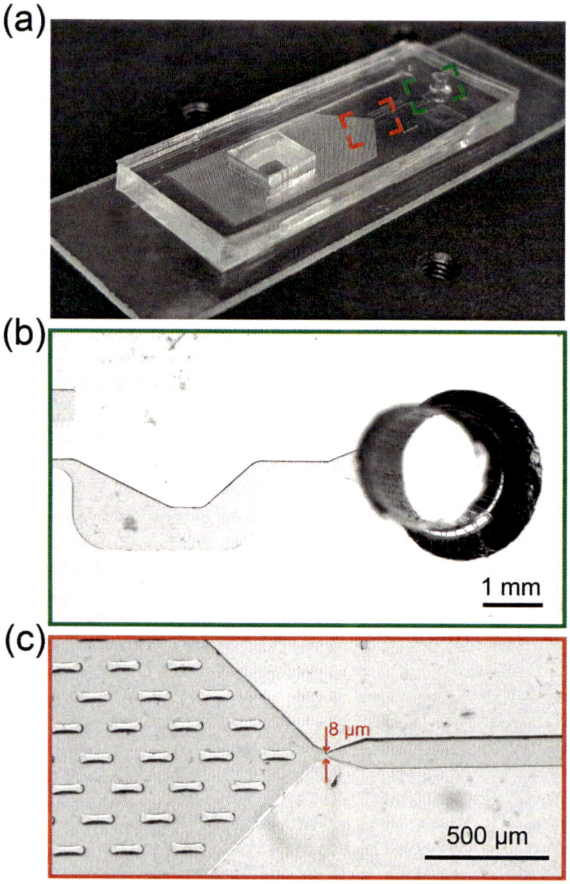


**Fig. 2.** Pictures of the microfluidic chip **a**: The loading well of the samples **b**: the enlarged view of green bracket in (**a**) and the constriction point of the fluidic channel **c**: the enlarged view of red bracket in (**a**). The narrowest point of the constriction has a width of 8 μm.

For the experiment, at first, we pressed the air pocket on the chip using a pen tip, then used a pipette to add a drop of 6 μL blood sample into the chip's loading well. Before sample addition, we gently shook it to prevent the sedimentation of blood cells. When the blood sample fully filled the loading well, we released the pressure on the air pocket. Then, the top roof of the air pocket began to restore and caused a low pressure inside the fluidic channel, causing blood to be drawn into the fluidic channel. We started timing when the blood samples started flowing and ended timing when the blood samples had passed through the 8 μm constriction completely. Each experiment was repeated at least three times. A timer was used to record the transport time of blood samples.

## 3 Results

According to the experimental data shown in Fig. 3, blood transport time shows an obvious increasing trend with the increase of HCT from 35 to 55%, the fitting equation is $Time = 50.3 \times HCT - 7.50$ with a linear fitting coefficient $R^2$ greater than 95%. Considering the low cost of the microfluidic chip and low requirement on the instrument for time recording, this chip is quite promising for HCT measurement in the scenario of point-of-care diagnostics.

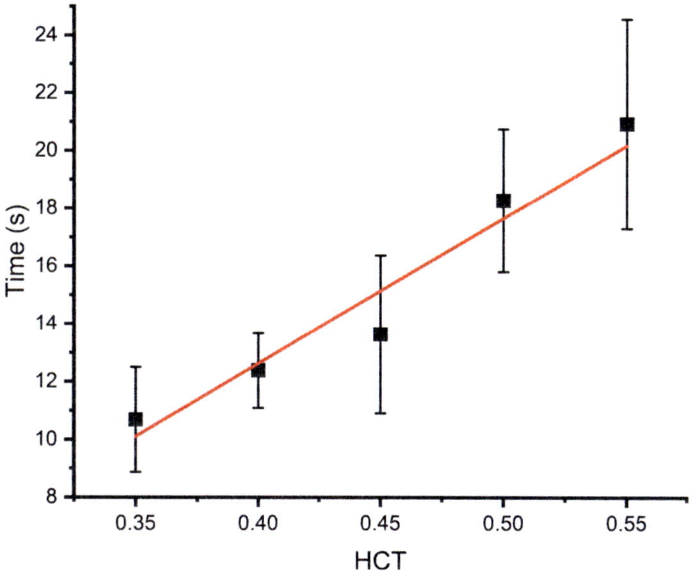


**Fig. 3.** The average transport time data (black) and linear fitting curve (red solid line) of time versus hematocrit values. The equation of fitting curve: $Time = 50.3 \times HCT - 7.50$, fitting coefficient: $R^2 = 0.9506$.

## 4 Discussion

The error bars in Fig. 3 seem to be high, and we suspected variations from chip to chip are the main reasons. There may be some defects in the chip bonding. In addition, since the operation of this device needs two persons, one for handling the device and one for recording the time, there exists some variations in the pressure applied on the air pocket and acuity of time recording. For the next steps, we plan to further test blood samples with HCT as 30 and 60% to check if it still works or not. Testing real blood samples with unknown HCT will be another experiment in the near future.

In the experiment, we found that when the HCT was high, such as 50 and 55%, the chance of chip blockage (blood samples pause or stop flowing during experiment due to cell blockage at the constriction) was higher than that for low HCT samples. We suspect that this is due to the non-Newtonian fluid nature of blood [11], and we need further experiments to test this hypothesis by diluting the blood samples more, trying to transfer them into Newtonian fluids and improving the accuracy of the test.

## 5 Conclusion

We developed a HCT measurement method based on blood flow velocity difference in a microfluidic chip. We configured blood samples with different HCT values and diluted the blood samples with PBST to optimize blood flow in our chip. We recorded the transport time of different blood samples and performed fitting of experimental data. Our experimental results showed that the transport time of blood samples with different HCT is indeed related to the HCT value, with a linear fitting coefficient greater than 0.95. Our method can perform an estimate of HCT in less than 1 min without the need for external power supply or fluidic pumping. With the possibility of further lowering the cost of chip fabrication by injection molding or hot embossing, we envision our method can be used to measure HCT at home or clinics in resource-limited regions.

**Acknowledgment.** This research was funded by Shantou University (STU Scientific Research Foundation for Talents: NTF20034), Department of Education of Guangdong Province (Scientific Research Project: 2022KQNCX019), and Guangdong Basic and Applied Basic Research Foundation (2022A1515110855).

## References

1. Giorno, R., Clifford, J.H., Beverly, S., et al.: Hematology reference values analysis by different statistical technics and variations with age and sex. Am. J. Clin. Pathol. **74**(6), 765–770 (1980)
2. Berry, S.B., Fernandes, S.C., Rajaratnam, A., et al.: Measurement of the hematocrit using paper-based microfluidic devices. Lab Chip **16**(19), 3689–3694 (2016)
3. Kosiborod, M., Smith, G.L., Radford, M.J., et al.: The prognostic importance of anemia in patients with heart failure. Am. J. Med. **114**(2), 112–119 (2003)
4. Lee, H.Y., Barber, C., Rogers, J.A., et al.: Electrochemical hematocrit determination in a direct current microfluidic device. Electrophoresis **36**(7–8), 978–985 (2015)
5. Petersson, K., Jakobsson, O., Ohlsson, P., et al.: Acoustofluidic hematocrit determination. Anal. Chim. Acta **1000**, 199–204 (2018)
6. Browne, A.W., Ramasamy, L., Cripe, T.P., et al.: A lab-on-a-chip for rapid blood separation and quantification of hematocrit and serum analytes. Lab Chip **11**(14), 2440–2446 (2011)
7. Frantz, E., Li, H., Steckl, A.J.: Quantitative hematocrit measurement of whole blood in a point-of-care lateral flow device using a smartphone flow tracking app. Biosens. Bioelectron.. Bioelectron. **163**, 112300 (2020)
8. Laha, S., Bandopadhyay, A., Chakraborty, S.: Smartphone-integrated label-free rapid screening of anemia from the pattern formed by one drop of blood on a wet paper strip. ACS sensors **7**(7), 2028–2036 (2022)
9. Xiao, Z., Feng, Z., Yang, Y., et al.: Quantitative hematocrit measurement on a paper microfluidic chip pretreated by sodium chloride. In: IEEE 17th International Conference on Nano/Micro Engineered and Molecular Systems, pp. 59–62 (2022)
10. Wang, G., Chu, L.T., Hartanto, H., et al.: Microfluidic particle dam for visual and quantitative detection of lead ions. ACS Sens. **5**(1), 19–23 (2019)
11. Zeng, H., Zhao, Y.: Rheological analysis of non-Newtonian blood flow using a microfluidic device. Sens. Actuators, A **166**(2), 207–213 (2011)

# A Novel Glutamate Three-Electrode System Based on Microelectrode Sensing Technology

Lu Yang[1], Zexuan Meng[1], Jiajia Chen[1], Jian Wang[1], Qiang Zhou[1,4], Guixue Wang[2,3], and Guangchao Zang[1,3,4](✉)

[1] Institute of Life Science, and Laboratory of Tissue and Cell Biology Lab Teaching & Management Center, Chongqing Medical University, University City Middle Road 61#, Chongqing 400016, People's Republic of China
zangguangchao@cqmu.edu.cn

[2] Key Laboratory for Biorheological Science and Technology of Ministry of Education State and Local Joint Engineering Laboratory for Vascular Implants, Bioengineering College of Chongqing University, Chongqing 400030, People's Republic of China
wanggx@cqu.edu.cn

[3] Jinfeng Laboratory, Chongqing 401329, People's Republic of China

[4] Department of Pathophysiology, Chongqing Medical University, Chongqing 400016, People's Republic of China

**Abstract.** Glutamate(Glu) plays an important role in brain function. The analysis of variations in Glu in physiological or pathological situations can be done using neuroelectrochemical sensing technology. Since the electrode is susceptible to interference in vivo and $H_2O_2$ is difficult to oxidize on carbon materials, it is necessary to improve the stability and sensitivity of the electrode when modifying the electrode. In this work, we first modified Pt nanoparticles and 3-thiopheneacetic acid(3-TAA) on the surface of carbon fiber microelectrode(CFME) in sequence, and finally fixed glutamate oxidase (GLOD) covalently on the surface of 3-TAA. So we successfully built the CFME/Pt-PTAA-GLOD sensor which is utilized to detect glutamate, providing a foundation for future neuroscience research.

**Keywords:** Glutamate · 3-Thiopheneacetic acid · Glutamate oxidase · Electrochemical sensor · Carbon fiber microelectrode

## 1 Introduction

Glutamate(Glu) is the main excitatory neurotransmitter with the highest concentration in the central nervous system [1]. It is involved in the majority of excitatory synaptic activities and is crucial for neurodevelopment, synaptic plasticity, learning, memory, sensation, movement, and other essential processes [2, 3]. Glu exhibits a paradoxical property. On the one hand, glutamate-induced excitation can regulate brain activity under normal stimulation. On the other side, the constant stimulation brought on by Glu can cause the occurrence of pathological circumstances of the nervous system, which can result in neuro-related diseases such as cerebral ischemia, epilepsy, and hypoxic-ischemic encephalopathy. Under normal physiological conditions, the concentration of


G. Wang et al. (Eds.): APCMBE 2023, IFMBE Proceedings 103, pp. 421–427, 2024.
https://doi.org/10.1007/978-3-031-51455-5_47

Glu in nerve cells is 10 mM while in the intercellular space only has 50–350 μM [4]. And the amount of Glu in cerebral fluid is even less, only 0.5–2 μM [5]. The content of Glu in cerebral fluid can reach 350 μM in pathological conditions [6]. In conclusion, the study of Glu alterations in physiological and pathological states plays a significant part in the nervous system and the pathways that are connected to it.

Carbon fiber microelectrode (CFME), one of the most widely used flexible microelectrodes, is used due to the characteristics of high conductivity, superior biocompatibility and easy miniaturization. Enzyme sensors with excellent sensitivity and selectivity have been employed extensively in the production of Glu biosensors due to the complexity of brain neurotransmitters. Glu oxidizes to α-ketoglutaric acid and generates hydrogen peroxide when subjected to glutamate oxidase (GLOD) action. The reaction formula is as follows. The generated $H_2O_2$ was detected by electrochemical means to detect glutamate.

$$L - glutamate + O_2 + H_2O \overset{GLOD}{\rightarrow} 2 - oxoglutarate + NH_3 + H_2O_2$$

As is common knowledge, electrooxidizing of $H_2O_2$ on carbon materials is challenging and time-consuming. Due to its good electrochemical performance, Pt nanoparticles are frequently modified on CFME to meet the goal of detecting Glu at low concentrations [7–9]. A crucial step is the modification of glutamate oxidase on the Pt layer. The existing methods of enzyme fixation include crosslinking, adsorption, covalent fixation, and embedding. Due to the problems such as leakage and instability of bioactive molecules in adsorption and embedding method, intensive cross-linking reaction and a poor recovery of the immobilized enzyme activity in cross-linking. The covalent fixation method is chosen due to its benefits, including firm combination, high stability, and long-term continuous use. 3-thiopheneacetic acid (3-TAA), as an intrinsically conducting polymers (ICPs) replaced by carboxy, has attracted much attention due to its significant environmental stability, excellent electrochemical stability, and –COOH functionality. Glutamate oxidase(GLOD) was covalently fixed on the surface of 3-TAA, which enhanced the electrode stability. Therefore, we created CFME/Pt-PTAA-GLOD to prepare Glu biosensors.

## 2 Materials and Methods

### 2.1 Preparation of CFME

A glass capillary tube (i.d. 1.5 mm, length 100 mm) was drawn into two sections of similar length using a micropipette puller (MP-500, RWD, Shenzhen, China), with the diameter of each tip between 40 and 70 μm. On a copper wire that was just a little bit longer than the glass tube, a carbon fiber (7 μm in diameter, Shenzhen Tony Electronics Co., Ltd., Shenzhen, China) was applied using conductive silver paste and allowed to cure. Threaded into the ready capillary glass tube is the copper wire connected to the carbon fiber. The carbon fiber is threaded out at the tip and the copper wire is exposed at the end. Finally, carbon fiber was lengthened to 300–500 μm under a microscope and sealed with paraffin wax from the end of the glass capillary.

### 2.2 Preparation of CFME/Pt-PTAA-GLOD

First, CFME was immersed in a mixture of 0.2M $Na_2SO_4$ and 1 mM $H_2PtCl_6$. Pt was electrodeposited on the electrode surface for 1200 s on the electrode surface at 100 mV/s sweep speed and −0.6V constant potential. Following that, 14 segment was deposited using cyclic voltammetry (CV) in an acetonitrile solution containing 50 mM tetrabutylammonium hexafluorophosphate (TBAHFP) and 0.1M 3-TAA in the potential range of -1.0–2.5 V, with a sweep rate of 100 $mV{\cdot}s^{-1}$. Finally, to activate the carboxyl group on PTAA, CFME/Pt-PTAA was placed to a solution containing 30mM N-hydroxysuccinimide(NHS), 15 mM 1-Ethyl-3-(3-dimethylaminopropyl)carbodiimide hydrochloride(EDC·HCl). Following that, it was immediately dissolved in a solution containing 5U/mL GLOD for 6 h, and when not in use, it was kept in 0.1M PBS at 4 °C.

### 2.3 Preparation of Ag/AgCl Reference Microelectrode

CFME was scanned for 10 cycles of electrodeposition silver at a scanning rate of 0.1 $V{\cdot}s^{-1}$ using CV from −0.9 V to 0.9 V while immersed in a solution containing 5 mM $AgNO_3$ and 1 M $KNO_3$. They were then moved to an electrolyte with 0.1 M KCl and 0.01 M HCl. By performing 2 cycles of CV scanning from −0.15 V to 1.05 V at 0.05 $V{\cdot}s^{-1}$, the Ag/AgCl reference microelectrode was created. Then the Ag/AgCl reference microelectrode was prepared by coating Nafion solution polymer film on the surface of the prepared reference electrode, which was dried at room temperature for further use.

### 2.4 Preparation of Pt Microelectrode

CFME was immersed in a mixture of $H_2PtCl_6$ and $Na_2SO_4$, and Pt was electrodeposited on the electrode surface for 3600 s at a sweep speed of 100 $mV{\cdot}s^{-1}$ and a constant potential of −0.6V. Then the prepared electrode surface was coated with Nafion solution polymer film.

## 3 Results

### 3.1 Electrode Performance of Self-made Ag/AgCl Reference Microelectrode and Pt Microelectrode

By using CV, the successfully constructed flexible Ag/AgCl reference microelectrode and Pt microelectrode were compared to the commercial Ag/AgCl reference electrode and Pt electrode. The outcomes demonstrated that the performance of the self-made Ag/AgCl reference microelectrode and Pt microelectrode matched that of the commercial electrode (Fig. 1), providing a crucial tool for future in vivo research (Commercial electrodes and homemade electrodes were both treated equally.).

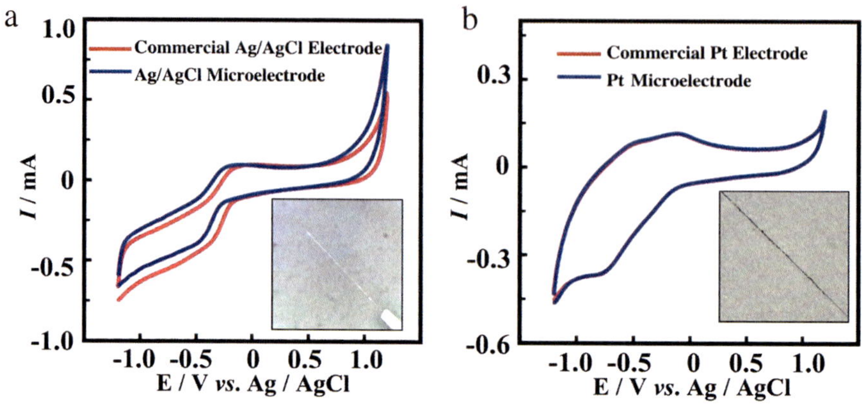


**Fig. 1.** Performance comparison between self-made electrodes and commercial electrodes. **a** reference electrodes (inset: Macro picture of a home-made Ag/AgCl reference microelectrode); **b** Pt electrodes (inset: Macro view of home-made Pt microelectrode). Background electrolyte is 0.1 M PBS (pH 7.4).

### 3.2 CFME/Pt-PTAA-GLOD Electrode Optimization

After the successful preparation of CFME, we initially modified carbon fiber and treated it with acid [10]. Then the electrical activity of CFMEs was raised, which was advantageous to the efficient deposition of Pt. On the surface of carbon fiber, the –COOH was increased. Since the charge used during hydrogen adsorption/desorption affected the electrochemically active surface area of Pt nanoparticles, the loading of Pt nanoparticles on CFME was tuned (Fig. 2a), and the ideal deposition time was chosen as 1200 s. After that, we deposited 3-TAA via CV. After numerous tries, it was found that stable CV curve was obtained when the deposition of 3-TAA was the most effective (Fig. 2b). Considering that a high load of glutamate oxidase would lead to poor substrate response, and a low load would lead to poor sensitivity, we initially soaked CFME/Pt-PTAA in 6U/ml GLOD solution for 6 h to support glutamate oxidase. The produced CFME/ Pt-PTAA-GLOD was kept in 0.1M PBS at 4 °C since low temperature and less air exposure can improve the stability of nanomaterials on electrode surface.

### 3.3 CFME/Pt-PTAA-GLOD Electrode Performance

Figure 3 shows the excellent electrochemical performance of the prepared CFME/Pt-PTAA-GLOD for Glu detection. The CV of CFME/Pt-PTAA-GLOD was recorded in glutamate-free and glutamate-containing artificial cerebral spinal fluid (aCSF, pH 7.4). Figure 3a depicted the cyclic voltammetry curve. Upon the addition of Glu, a significant reduction current was visible on the electrode. Maximum response was observed at −0.2 V, so subsequent amperage studies were conducted at this voltage.

The potential of CFME/Pt-PTAA-GLOD was held at −0.2 V and aliquots of glutamate was injected into aCSF(pH = 7.4) at a regular intervals (Fig. 4b). The electrode can successfully detect $H_2O_2$ catalyzed by glutamate oxidase. And the illustration in Fig. 3b also shows that the electrode has a certain linearity.

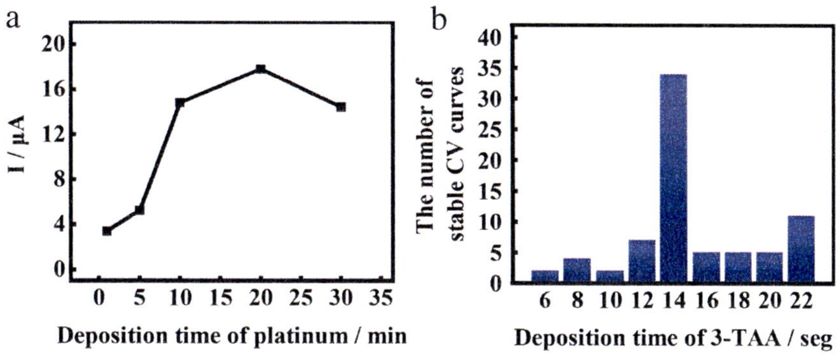


**Fig. 2.** Optimization diagram of CFME/Pt-PTAA-GLOD electrode. **a** Optimal deposition time diagram of Pt (4mM ferricyanide solution, 0.1V/s); **b** Optimal deposition time diagram of 3-TAA.

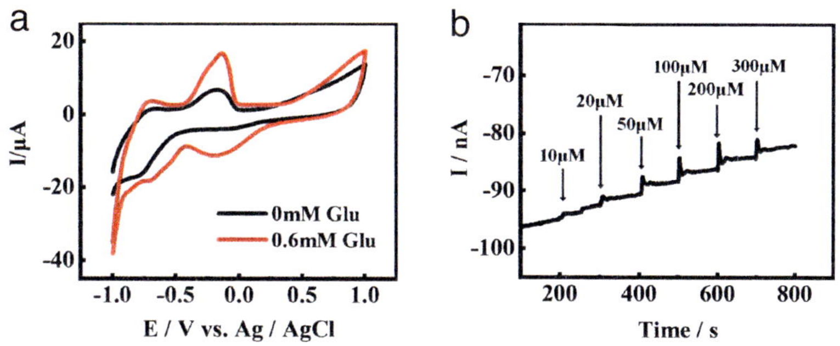


**Fig. 3.** Performance diagram of CFME/Pt-PTAA-GLOD. **a** CFME/Pt-PTAA-GLOD's CV curve; **b** CFME/Pt-PTAA-GLOD i–t graph.

## 4 Discussion

The mammalian brain is the most complex and superlative part of the nervous system. One of the main strategies to study the physiological and pathological changes of the brain is to study the qualitative and quantitative changes of neurotransmitters occurring in the process of brain nerve phenomena. Compared with non-invasive imaging techniques, neuroelectrochemical sensing technology has become a research hotspot with the advantages of high spatial and temporal resolution and in situ study. Commercial Ag/AgCl electrode and Pt electrode cannot be applied to in vivo studies due to their large size and poor biocompatibility. Therefore, we successfully constructed Ag/AgCl reference microelectrode and Pt microelectrode for follow-up in vivo experimental studies (Fig. 1).

Studies have shown that the extracellular content of Glu is very low under physiological conditions, while the extracellular content of Glu can be increased by several hundred times under pathological conditions. So it requires that the Glu sensor we constructed has a low detection limit and a wide linear range. Later, we successfully constructed CF/Pt-PTAA-GLOD for Glu detection (Fig. 3), which can realize the detection of Glu.

In the system, glutamate can be specifically recognized and bound by glutamate oxidase molecules covalently fixed on the surface of CF/Pt-PTAA-GLOD. These molecules then carry out intricate enzymatic reactions to produce α-ketoglutaric acid, ammonia, and $H_2O_2$, which in turn produce a variety of biochemical signals. These biochemical signals are converted into electrical signals under the action of an electric current, which are then captured by PTAA film and transmitted to the Pt layer, and finally detected and recorded by a computer-controlled CHI 630e electrochemical analyzer (Fig. 4).

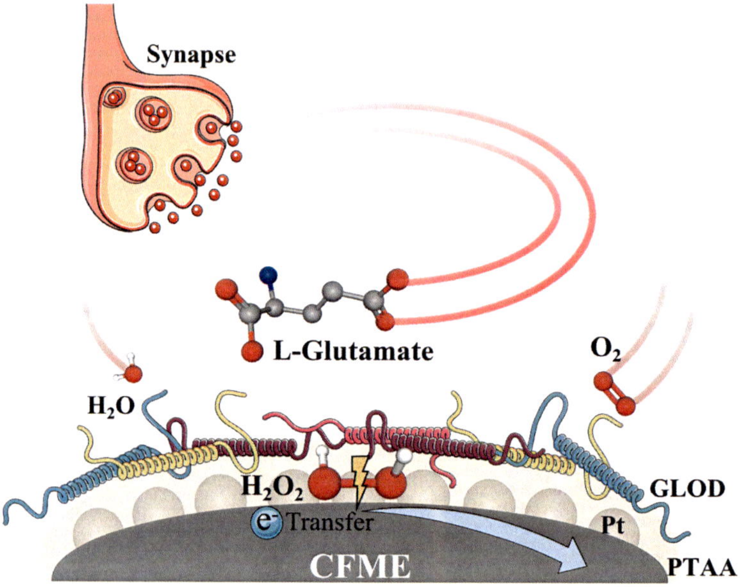


**Fig. 4.** Schematic diagram of CFME/Pt-PTAA-GLOD detection.

Glu is a potential biomarker that can be used to detect and monitor abnormal conditions in the brain. Glu is synthesized in the nerve terminal region of the neuron, which is then stored in glutamate vesicles and released in the synaptic space between the nerve terminal and the postsynaptic neuron membrane. When diffused into the postsynaptic membrane, L-glutamate interacts with various types of receptors (e.g., NMDA, AMPA receptors), ions (e.g., calcium ions, sodium ions), causing postsynaptic membrane depolarization. This activity lasts until Glu is reabsorbed into the neuron that releases it, or until adjacent neurons cease. Under pathological conditions, the increased release or decreased reuptake of Glu leads to calcium overload and apoptosis of neurons, resulting in excitotoxicity and nerve injury. By using neuroelectrochemical sensing technology, glutamic acid sensors are ready to monitor changes in intracellular, intercellular, and cerebrospinal fluid under physiological and pathological conditions, investigate the interactions between Glu and related nerve small molecules (such as NMDA receptors, ascorbic acid, and dopamine) in the neural pathway, and examine associated physiological and pathological mechanisms.

## 5 Conclusion

The advantages of high sensitivity, high selectivity, high spatial and temporal resolution of neurosensing technology over conventional brain tissue imaging technology have made it a research hotspot in the interdisciplinary fields of analytical science, materials science, neuromedicine, and physical science. In this study, we successfully created CFME/Pt-PTAA-GLOD that made it possible to detect Glu. Further characterization and electrode performance measurement of the electrode, as a tool, it is expected to achieve real-time detection of glutamate in cells, brain slices and in vivo SD rats. So it can support the investigation of the pathological alterations of associated neurological illnesses to advance research on neurotransmitters.

**Acknowledgment.** This work was supported by grants the Natural Science Foundation of Chongqing (cstc2020jcyj-msxmX0330); the JinFeng Laboratory Foundation, Chongqing, China (jfkyjf202203001).

## References

1. Salt, T.E., Eaton, S.A.: Functions of ionotropic and metabotropic glutamate receptors in sensory transmission in the mammalian thalamus. Prog. Neurobiol.Neurobiol. **48**(1), 55–72 (1996)
2. Dagani, F., D'Angelo, E.: Glutamate metabolism, release, and quantal transmission at central excitatory synapses: implications for neural plasticity. Funct. Neurol.. Neurol. **7**(4), 315–336 (1992)
3. Jamain, S., et al.: Linkage and association of the glutamate receptor 6 gene with autism. Mol. Psychiatry **7**(3), 302–310 (2002)
4. Jamal, M., Xu, J., Razeeb, K.M.: Disposable biosensor based on immobilisation of glutamate oxidase on Pt nanoparticles modified Au nanowire array electrode. Biosens. Bioelectron.. Bioelectron. **26**(4), 1420–1424 (2010)
5. Hawkins, R.A.: The blood-brain barrier and glutamate. Am. J. Clin. Nutri. **90**(3, Suppl. S), 867S–874S (2009)
6. Hu, Y., et al.: Direct measurement of glutamate release in the brain using a dual enzyme-based electrochemical sensor. Brain Res. **659**(1–2), 117–125 (1994)
7. Chen, J., et al.: A highly sensitive amperometric glutamate oxidase microbiosensor based on a reduced graphene oxide/prussian blue nanocube/gold nanoparticle composite film-modified pt electrode. Sensors **20**(10) (2020)
8. Batra, B., Pundir, C.S.: An amperometric glutamate biosensor based on immobilization of glutamate oxidase onto carboxylated multiwalled carbon nanotubes/gold nanoparticles/chitosan composite film modified Au electrode. Biosens. Bioelectron.. Bioelectron. **47**, 496–501 (2013)
9. Schuvailo, O.M., et al.: Ultramicrobiosensor for the selective detection of glutamate. Electroanalysis **19**(1), 71–78 (2007)
10. Wu, Z., et al.: Platinum nanoparticle-modified carbon fiber ultramicroelectrodes for mediator-free biosensing. Sens. Actuat. B-Chem. **119**(1), 295–301 (2006)

# Fast Sample Entropy Atrial Fibrillation Analysis Towards Wearable Device

Chao Chen[1], Bruno da Silva[2(✉)], Caiyun Ma[1], Jianqing Li[1], and Chengyu Liu[1(✉)]

[1] School of Instrument Science and Engineering, Southeast University, Sipailou2, Nanjing, China
chengyu@seu.edu.cn

[2] Department of Electronics and Informatic/Vrije Universiteit Brussel, Plaine 2, Brussels, Belgium
bdasilva@etrovub.be

**Abstract.** Atrial Fibrillation (AF) is a common and often debilitating heart rhythm disorder characterized by an irregular, rapid, and sometimes chaotic heart rate. This paper proposes to use fast entropy estimation algorithm to analyze AF on wearable processors for ECG R wave interval. The suggested fast entropy method requires less computation time to detect AF. Information entropy, typical as Sample Entropy (SampEn), is a popularly used complexity measurement metric for AF detection. However, the quadratic time complexity of conventional SampEn restricts its analysis ability. The fast entropy estimation map original signals by Merge Sort (MS) and use a lightweight (LW) similarity-checking method to avoid unnecessary operations on entropy analysis. The proposed algorithm is verified on the long-term recordings from MIT-BIH AF database. This fast entropy measurement, MS-LW, has the same complexity measurement result as SampEn but is three times faster, which is convenient for long-term data. Altogether, this lightweight SampEn is suitable for wearable applications.

**Keywords:** Sample entropy · Complexity analysis · Fast sample entropy · Atrial fibrillation

## 1 Introduction

Atrial fibrillation (AF) is a common heart rhythm disorder characterized by an irregular and often rapid heart rate [1]. It is one of the most important and common arrhythmias and is associated with an increased risk of stroke, heart failure, and premature death [2]. The accurate diagnosis and effective management of AF are essential to reduce the associated morbidity and mortality. As such, there is a need for reliable and effective methods of AF analysis.

AF usually has an irregular heartbeat, leading to high complexity and entropy measurement values. Sample Entropy (SampEn) is a popular information complexity measurement metric. Estimating complexity for heart rate or RR intervals could aid in AF detection, making SampEn a promising no-liner analysis for AF [3].


G. Wang et al. (Eds.): APCMBE 2023, IFMBE Proceedings 103, pp. 428–434, 2024.
https://doi.org/10.1007/978-3-031-51455-5_48

However, conventional SampEn requires traversing each mode in sequence and checking similarity with all other modes. This process is a quadratic time complexity dual-loop process. The computation for long-term data will be unacceptable and will have an impact on the online AF monitor.

To obtain a quick result, some research reduces time complexity through approximate analysis; however, this introduces bias from complexity analysis [4]. Some researchers believe that not all similarity checking is required for SampEn computation; some modes differ significantly from others and avoiding similarity checking is acceptable for these modes. Manis conducts thorough research on this topic and discovers lightweight work well by avoiding unnecessary similarity checking in biomedical signal analysis. The lightweight (LW) method only checks for similarity when two modes match in at least one dimension on a sorted space. Otherwise, no further similarity checking is required because they do not match within the similarity threshold [5].

Previous work compared the time performance of serval known fast entropy methods on different platforms, such as Central Processing Unit (CPU) and Field Programmable Field Array (FPGA), using three multi-source biomedical signals [6]. The lightweight method demonstrated promising speed and stability with the Merge Sort (MS) algorithm. Because MS is a fast and stable Sorting method integrated into many official computation packages in modern languages for its time performance, this study evaluates MS based LW entropy measurement (MS-LW) in terms of speedup and computation resources. This study confirms that MS-LW has the same entropy estimation value as standard SampEn but with a faster computation time. The contributions of this study are:

- Evaluation of MS-LW fast entropy estimation algorithm for AF detection based on R-wave intervals.
- Comparison of the MS-LW with conventional SampEn entropy measurement in terms of computational efficiency.

# 2 Method

## 2.1 Algorithm Description

SampEn is a widely used nonlinear method for analyzing time series data. It was developed in the early 2000 s and is based on self-similarity. SampEn measures the uncertainty in a series of data points and is used to detect patterns in data that may not be detectable using linear methods. It is also helpful for quantifying a signal's complexity and determining a system's predictability.

On the other hand, SampEn must traverse all inner modes and compare them to all other modes. A double traverse of all the data in order is necessary for SampEn. Due to the excessive similarity checking, this dual-loop process cannot perform online entropy analysis.

The recently proposed MS-LW is an optimization of the original SampEn algorithm. MS-LW SampEn provides a faster assessment of time series complexity and has been measured by various signals, including electrocardiogram (ECG), electroencephalogram (EEG), and photoplethysmogram (PPG) [7]. MS-LW is a helpful tool for diagnosing and treating arrhythmias like AF because it is efficient at measuring the complexity and predictability of a signal. To avoid performing extraneous similarity checks, MS-LW only performs similarity checks in the neighbor part of the sorted series, as shown in Fig. 1.

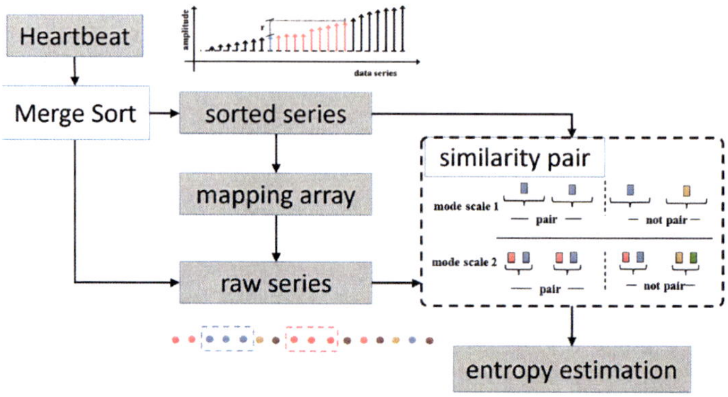


**Fig. 1.** The commutating architecture for MS-LW.

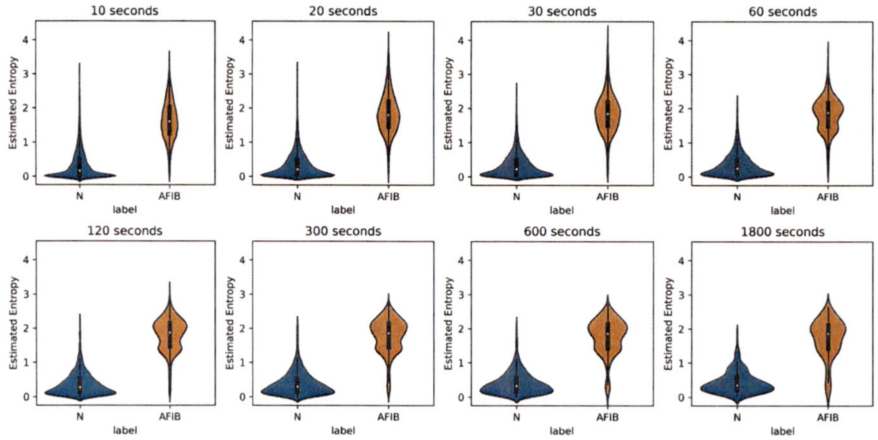


**Fig. 2.** Entropy measurement for AF and N-labeled data as a iolin graph.

## 2.2 Dataset

The MIT-BIH Atrial Fibrillation Database (AFDB) is a publicly available dataset [8]. It consists of 25 long-term (10 h) ECG recordings, most of which have paroxysmal AF. The ECG signals are sampled at a frequency of 250 Hz. This dataset contains 25 records of ten hours of RR interval beat annotation files and corresponding rhythm annotation files for arrhythmia detection and analysis researchers and engineers. Almost all rhythms are labeled atrial fibrillation (AFIB) and other not included rhythms (N), with only a few atrial flutter (AFL) and AV junctional rhythm (J) labels.

### 2.3 Experiment Setup

The beat and arrhythmia annotation files are transferred and saved as an array for the C/C++ performance test. The SampEn and MS-LW entropy estimation algorithms are tested on the same wearable CPU to evaluate their timing and classification ability for AF detection. The low-end CPU is a dual-core ARM Cortex-A9 with a working frequency of 666 MHz.

Input test data for the entropy analysis in this study are segments of 10, 20, 30, 60, 120, 180, 300, 600, and 1800 s.

Segment length, segment location within particular dataset records, segment entropy estimation value, and computation time are all measured and recorded. The segment length, corresponding entropy estimation value, and computation time are used in this study for analysis.

## 3 Result

### 3.1 Measured Entropy Value Compared with SampEn

SampEn is widely acceptable in biomedical signal analysis for complexity measurement. SampEn traverse all inner modes and counts their probability. The similarity checking for all inner modes makes SampEn stable for entropy estimation.

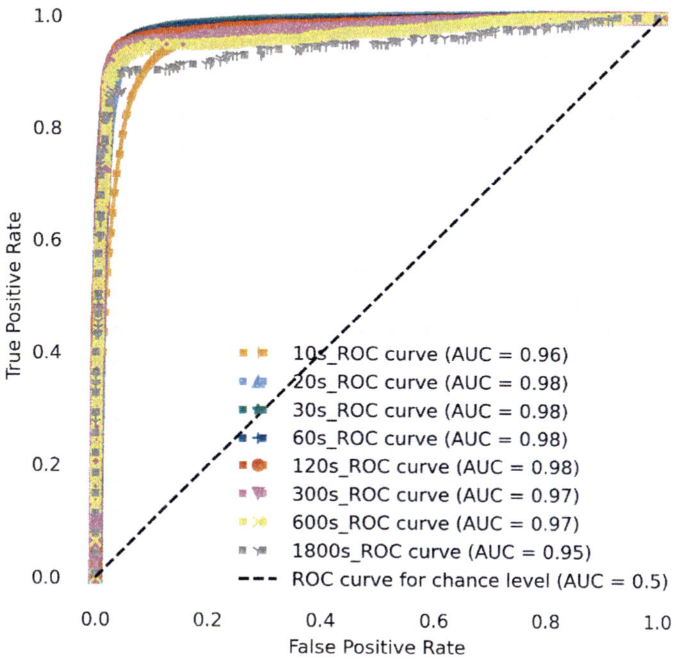


**Fig. 3.** ROC curve for entropy measurement in AF analysis.

This study compares the value of MS-LW with SampEn for each segment, using SampEn as the gold standard for conditional entropy estimation. Both entropy algorithms have the same estimated value distribution as shown in Fig. 2, and MS-LW has exactly the same entropy estimation as SampEn with zero error, making it a valid alternative to SampEn.

## 3.2 Description Ability for AF

Our previous research employs the 10 s segment to reduce computation time, which is widely used in AF analysis. Some researchers, however, claim that long-term segments have superior classification ability. As illustrated by the violin Fig. 2, entropy estimation calculated by SampEn or MS-LW has a good discriminatory ability for AFIB and N in both short-term and long-term segments.

As expected in Fig. 2, AFIB-labeled data with an irregular heartbeat has a higher complexity value than N-labeled data. The long segment generally has a more stable complexity estimation value than the short segment. Even for N-labeled segments with low complexity, some extremely high value exceeds three in short-term segments such as 10 and 20 s. However, the long-term segment usually has a lower value close to zero because it is more prone to irregularity.

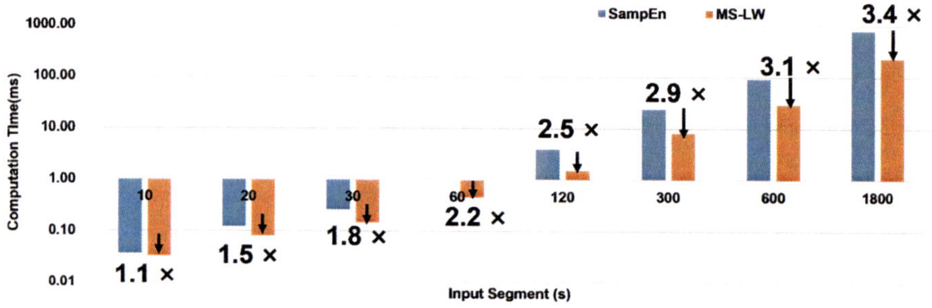


**Fig. 4.** Execution time comparison with MS-LW and conventional SampEn.

In Fig. 2, AFIB-labeled long segments, like the 1800 s segment, have a few slight peaks with low entropy values, whereas N-labeled segments have a high entropy value. It might originate from the test system's rhythm annotation approach. The long-term segment of paroxysmal AF may contain both AFIB and N segments. The AFIB segments in N labeled 1800 s will increase the complexity and have a high entropy estimation. While N segments in AFIB labeled data will reduce complexity with a low entropy value.

The estimated entropy from SampEn and MS-LW has good classification ability for AF, as shown in the Receiver Operating Characteristics curve (ROC) graph Fig. 3. However, a segment that is either too short (10 s) or too long (1800 s) will decrease the Area under the ROC Curve (AUC). The best AUC value is 0.98 for segment lengths ranging from 20 to 120 s. This phenomenon is because long-term segments may have mixed rhythm and are difficult to categorize as AFIB or N, whereas random factors more easily influence short-term segments.

### 3.3 Speedup Comparison on Wearable Processors

MS-LW outperforms SampEn in terms of real-time AF detection capability. The SampEn computation time increases rapidly with input data length, as shown in Fig. 4 with a logarithmic axis. It is due to the SampEn complexity estimation algorithm's quadratic time complexity. In this study, MS-LW improved execution time for avoiding massive unnecessary similarity checking in long-term data by about three times. Furthermore, as shown in the Fig. 4, the speedup increases with input length. Because of this, MS-LW will be a better alternative for complexity analysis on detecting online AF, especially for wearable processors, which has quick response with limited resources.

## 4 Discussion

A fast complexity analysis algorithm could quickly and accurately assess the degree of complexity in a given data system, making it ideal for use in real-time applications, such as in the case of wearable low-end CPUs.

This study employs a fast complexity analysis algorithm to classify AF, characterized by an irregular heartbeat and a high level of complexity in the heart rate or RR interval sequence.

Long-term signal analysis requires a quick and accurate complexity metric; the time complexity of traditional Sample Entropy limits its online analysis for long-term signals; MS-LW should be a better alternative.

A quick and accurate complexity measurement is always vital for biomedical signal analysis research and engineering. The method highlighted here may bring something different to the no-linear information complexity research topic.

Furthermore, it may enable the development of improved algorithms, models, and tools for biomedical signal analysis. Finally, it may provide valuable insights that may help further advance the biomedical signal analysis field.

## 5 Conclusions

The irregular heartbeat of AF atrial fibrillation (AF) makes complexity analysis an excellent tool for AF analysis. This study uses a fast complexity analysis method to estimate entropy quickly, based on Merge Sort (MS) and lightweight similarity checking (LW). The MS-LW entropy estimation technique was found to have the same absolute complexity estimated result as the commonly used Sample Entropy method. Additionally, the MS-LW approach is suitable for wearable devices with low-end processors, making it applicable to wearable applications.

**Acknowledgment.** This research was funded by the National Natural Science Foundation of China (62171123, 62071241, 62201144 and 62211530112), China Scholarship Council (202106090175).

## References

1. McManus, D.D., Lee, et al.: A novel application for the detection of an irregular pulse using an iPhone 4S in patients with atrial fibrillation. Heart Rhythm **10**(3), 315–319 (2013)
2. Marini, C., Santis, De., et al.: Contribution of atrial fibrillation to incidence and outcome of ischemic stroke: results from a population-based study. Stroke **36**(6), 1115–1119 (2005)
3. Alcaraz, R., Rieta, J.J.: A review on sample entropy applications for the non-invasive analysis of atrial fibrillation electrocardiograms. Biomed. Signal Process. Control **5**(1), 1–14 (2010)
4. Tomčala, J.: New fast ApEn and SampEn entropy algorithms implementation and their application to supercomputer power consumption. Entropy **22**(8), 863 (2020)
5. Manis, G., Aktaruzzaman, M., Sassi, R.: Low computational cost for sample entropy. Entropy **20**(1), 61 (2018)
6. Chen, C., da Silva, B., Chen, R., Li, S., Li, J., Liu, C.: Evaluation of fast sample entropy algorithms on FPGAs: from performance to energy efficiency. Entropy **24**(9), 1177 (2022)
7. Chen, C., da Silva, B., Li, J., Liu, C.: Acceleration of fast sample entropy towards biomedical applications on FPGAs. In: 2022 International Conference on Field-Programmable Technology (ICFPT), pp. 1–4. IEEE (2022)
8. PhysioBank, P.: Physionet: components of a new research resource for complex physiologic signals. Circulation **101**(23), e215–e220 (2000)

# A Novel Electrophoresis Devices Combined with Immunosensor for the Rapid Detection of Carcinoembryonic Antigen

Xiaoting Wu[1], Qing Lu[1], Yusha Li[1], Yuchan Zhang[1], Yuansheng Lan[1], Xiaoqing Ming[1], Wei Jiang[1], Guixue Wang[2,3](✉), and Guangchao Zang[1,3,4](✉)

[1] Institute of Life Science, Laboratory of Tissue and Cell Biology Lab Teaching and Management Center, Chongqing Medical University, Chongqing 400016, People's Republic of China
zangguangchao@cqmu.edu.cn

[2] Key Laboratory for Biorheological Science and Technology of Ministry of Education State and Local Joint Engineering Laboratory for Vascular Implants, Bioengineering College of Chongqing University, Chongqing 400030, People's Republic of China
wanggx@cqu.edu.cn

[3] Jinfeng Laboratory, Chongqing 401329, People's Republic of China

[4] Department of Pathophysiology, Chongqing Medical University, Chongqing 400016, People's Republic of China

**Abstract.** Carcinoembryonic antigen (CEA) is a broad-spectrum cancer marker, that is significantly more highly expressed in cancer patients than in healthy individuals. The short time, high sensitivity and specificity detection of CEA can greatly help in the early clinical detection and screening of cancer. Now, the concentration monitoring of CEA is also widely used in the postoperative detection of cancer to judge its prognosis and recurrence. Electrochemical immunoassay is an ideal technique for detecting tumor markers, it has attracted much attention due to its special advantages such as high sensitivity, low cost and convenient handling. Still, traditional immunosensors generally have the problems of long detection time and high detection limit. In this work, we have constructed an electric field enhanced electrochemical immunosensor based on the electrophoresis principle for detecting CEA rapidly and sensitively. Upon incubation with CEA, the proposed electrophoresis device imparts the electric field force on CEA, allowing CEA to swim up quickly in the system. It greatly shortens the incubation time of CEA to 5 min and enables to achieve the rapid detection of CEA, which has a good application prospect in the rapid and accurate diagnosis of clinical cancer and biological analysis in the future.

**Keywords:** Electrophoresis device · Glassy carbon electrode · Electrochemical immunosensor · Carcinoembryonic antigen


G. Wang et al. (Eds.): APCMBE 2023, IFMBE Proceedings 103, pp. 435–442, 2024.
https://doi.org/10.1007/978-3-031-51455-5_49

# 1 Introduction

Cancer disease poses an increasingly serious threat to human health, and early evaluation and diagnosis are crucial to improve the rate of cancer treatment and improve the lifestyle of patients. The rapid and sensitive detection of tumor markers is one of the ways to early diagnosis of cancer. Carcinoembryonic antigen (CEA) as a high-precision analytical cancer biomarker, is often used for early screening, diagnosis and prognostic evaluation of colorectal cancer, gastric cancer, lung cancer and other cancers [1, 2]. The rapid and accurate detection of CEA plays a very important role in clinical diagnosis. One of the outstanding challenges in early cancer diagnosis are the development of rapid and highly sensitive biomarker detection technologies [3]. Many methods have been developed for detecting CEA, and electrochemical immunosensors have attracted significant attention due to their fast response speed and strong specificity [4]. The label-free electrochemical immunosensor uses the antibody fixed to the surface of the base material as the recognition molecule, which aims to specifically bind the antigen and finally output the electrical signal for the immunoassay of the assay.

At present, there are many problems in clincal antigen detection, such as system interference and long time consuming. Therefore, exploring the rapid and accurate detection method of antigen is indispensable. Yan et al. prepared a sandwich electrochemical immunosensor based on supramolecular labeling strategy, and the incubation time of CEA was 1 h [5]. Wang et al. constructed a labeled free electrochemical immunosensor based on pattern-shaped Ag/MoS2/rGO nanocomposites to detect CEA with ultrasensitivity, and the incubation time of CEA was also 1 h [6]. Most immune sensors can now achieve high sensitivity detection of CEA, but the operation is generally complicated and does not solve the problem of long time consuming in clinical detection.

To this end, we developed a sensing device with an electrophoresis system coupled with label-free electrochemical immunosensors for rapid incubation detection of CEA. CEA is an acidic glycoprotein with a human embryonic antigen-determining cluster negatively charged in a specific buffer solution system. Through electrochemical signals, CEA is subjected to an upward electric field force in the electrophoretic system, which then quickly swims to the surface of the glassy carbon electrode (GCE) to bind to the antibody (Ab). The combination of CEA and Ab can be completed in 5 min, which greatly reduces the detection time. In addition, in the previous work, our team members successfully applied the electrophoresis device in electrochemical molecular imprinting sensing [7]. It indicates that the electrophoretic device has excellent practical application potential and development space in biosensing and clinical diagnosis.

# 2 Materials and Methods

## 2.1 Design of the Novel Electrophoresis Device

The UTP1306S series is an economical DC stable power supply instrument to provide DC power supply for the electrophoresis device. The 5 ml particular beaker with platinum wire (Pt) at the bottom is fixed on the fixing frame, the solution system in the beaker device is 5 ml PBS (0.1M, pH $=$ 8.0). And the working electrode is placed 1mm from the upper liquid level, and kept parallel to the Pt plate at the bottom, as shown in Fig. 1. In the device, the working electrode is the anode, and the platinum disk electrode at the bottom is the cathode. After providing the DC voltage, a vertical electric field is generated between the two. The DC power supply is turned on to provide a voltage of 300 mV for the electrophoretic device. After running for 5 min, the power supply is turned off and the electrophoresis device completes the rapid incubation of CEA.

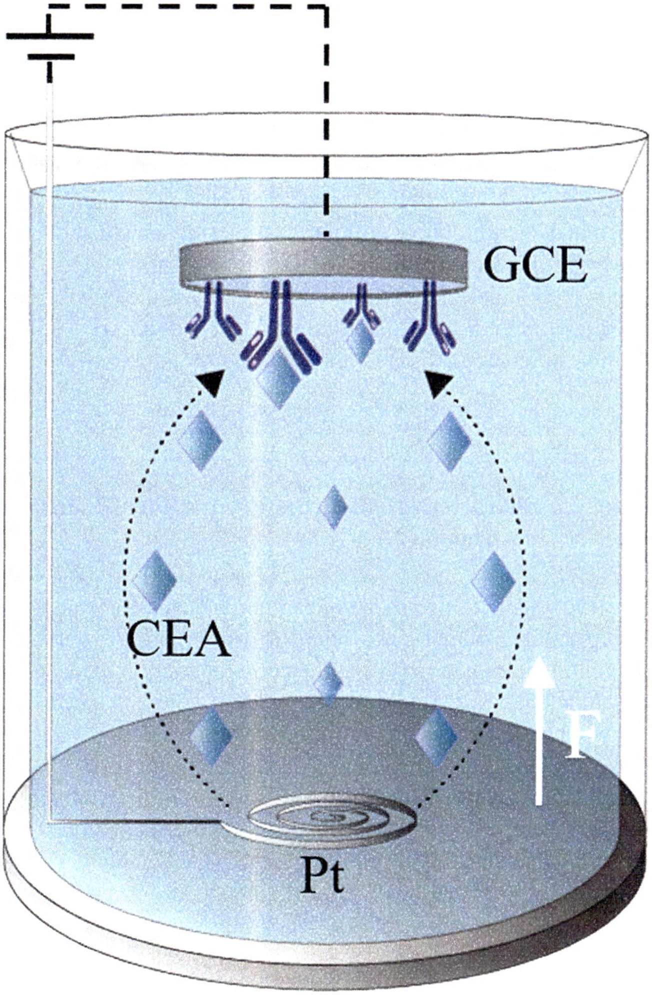


**Fig. 1.** Schematic diagram of the electrophoresis device.

### 2.2 Preparation of an Electric-Field-Enhanced Immunosensor

The bare GCE was polished with 0.3 μm and 0.05 μm alumina powder, ultrasonically cleaned by ultrapure water (18.2 MΩ), absolute ethanol and ultrapure water, respectively, and dried at room temperature. Electrodeposition in 10 ml of diamino terephthalic acid (ATA, 10 mM ATA dissolved in 0.01 M PBS) solution at 50 mV/s. Electroactivation was scanned for four cycles from 0 to 1.6 V in 100 mM $K_2S_2O_8$ and 60 mM $H_2O_2$ of PBS to reduce GCE/ATA impedance. Further incubated with 10 μL 10 μg/mL Ab for 1h and blocked with PBS solution containing 2.0 wt% BSA for 30 min to block nonspecific binding sites. The Ab and BSA incubation procedures were performed in a 37 °C environment. After natural drying and the next step, each modification was eluted with 0.1 M PBS. Incubation of the target protein CEA was performed in an electrophoresis device, 10 ul of detection concentration of CEA was added to the electrophoresis device system for 5 min to obtain GCE/ATA-Ab-Ag. The current response after incubation with CEA at different detection concentrations was determined with the differential pulse voltammetry (DPV) at the electrochemical workstation. The three-electrode system used is a glassy carbon electrode as the working electrode, Pt as the opposite electrode, and silver chloride as the reference electrode. The scan rate was all set at 0.1 V/s. The final obtained sensor was stored at 4 °C when not in use.

## 3 Results

### 3.1 Electrochemical Characterization of the Electric-Field-Enhanced Immunosensor Construction

To verify the construction of the electrochemical immunosensor and the successful application of the electrophoresis device, we selected two effective electrochemical methods, including cyclic voltammetry (CV) and electrochemical impedance spectroscopy (EIS). Electrochemical characterization of the electric field enhanced immunosensors was described by monitoring the changes on the electrode surface.

CV method records the current response of the electrode surface by CV scanning to analyze the conductive performance of the material. We determined the CV of the bare GCE, modified electrode with Ab, BSA sealing and incubating CEA with electrophoresis. According to the CV result (Fig. 2a), ATA conductivity was extremely poor, after further fixing Ab, it seriously affected the electron transfer rate, and the CV peak current decreased. After the sealing of free site with BSA and incubating CEA with electrophoresis device. Protein molecules limited the electron conversion between the electrode surface and the redox probe, and the peak current continued to decrease, indicating that the binding process at each step was effective.

In addition, EIS was used to monitor the manufacturing process of the immunosensor, where the semicircle diameter (SD) was positively correlated with the electron transfer resistance (Ret) at the electrode interface in Nyquist's diagram. In Fig. 2b, When the ATA/Ab was fixed on the GCE surface, its SD was much larger than the bare GCE due to its low conductivity. After the sequential assembly of BSA and CEA, Ret increased sequentially because of biomolecules hindering electron transfer. The results of EIS and CV agree well, both demonstrating the successful application of the electrophoresis device and the successful preparation of the electric field-enhanced immunosensor.

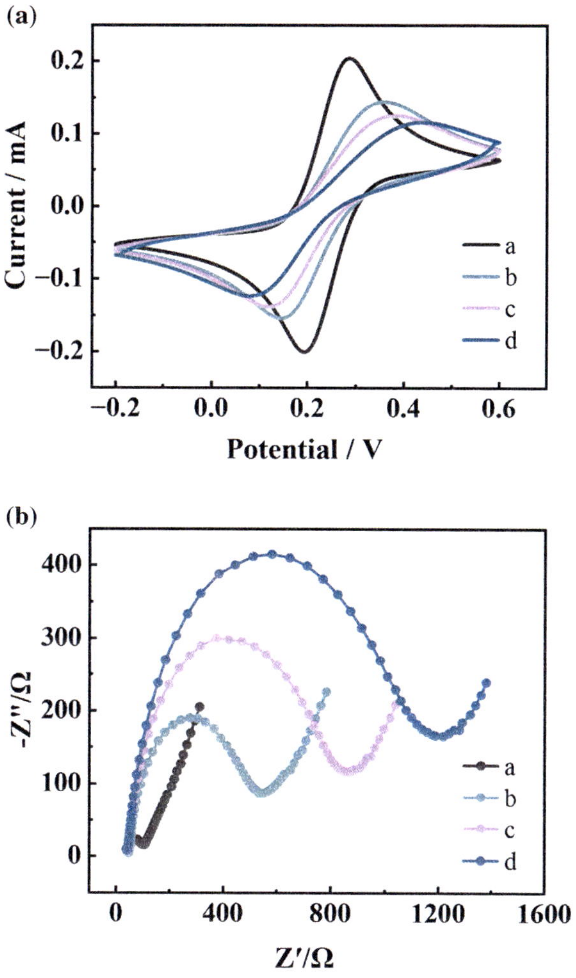


**Fig. 2.** CV (**a**) and EIS (**b**) were respectively performed in $Fe(CN)_6{}^{3-/4-}$ (5 mM) containing KCl (1 M) and 5 mM $K_3Fe(CN)_6/K_4Fe(CN)_6$ (1:1) with 0.1 M PBS solution. **a** Bare GCE, **b** GCE/ATA/Ab, **c** GCE/ATA/Ab/BSA, **d** GCE/ATA/Ab/BSA/CEA. The CEA concentration in electrophoresis incubation was 0.1 ng/ml.

### 3.2 Analysis of Differential Pulse Voltammetry (DPV) Measurement

After incubation of CEA in the electrophoresis device, CEA concentration was determined by DPV and analyzed by the current response of DPV. We focus on exploring the successful application of electrophoretic devices in electrochemical immunosensors. According to the current response (Fig. 3) before and after electrophoresis, the CEA rapid incubation was successfully achieved for 5 min, which significantly shortened the CEA detection time.

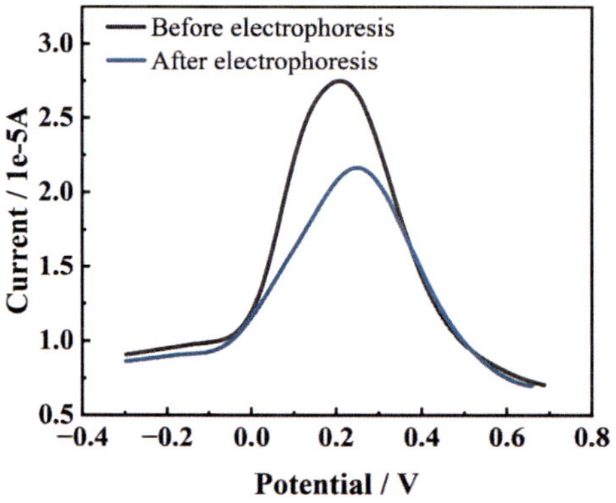


**Fig. 3.** For the DPV determination, the black curve represents the current response on the electrode surface before electrophoresis, and the blue curve indicates the current response after incubation of CEA with the electrophoresis device. The electrolyte solution used was 0.1 M PBS containing 5 mM $[Fe(CN)_6]^{3-/4-}$ and 1 M KCl. The CEA concentration was 0.1 ng/ml.

## 4 Discussion

At present, various kinds of sensors are developing rapidly in the fields of biological detection and clinical diagnosis, but the rapid and accurate detection of analytes still faces enormous challenges. The Electrophoresis method can effectively realize the rapid enrichment of charged substances and reduce background interference. The most common is the protein blotting method that Western blotting. The detection principle for denaturing polyacrylamide gel electrophoresis for protein concentration and separation, transfers it to the NC membrane or PVDF membrane, using antigen-antibody reaction for specific signal detection, the technology has been widely used in protein level expression research, antibody activity detection and disease early diagnosis, but cumbersome steps and long operation time [8–10]. Based on the principle of directional protein swimming by electrophoresis. We are considering applying electrophoresis in biosensors and designing a new electrophoresis device for the rapid enrichment detection of analytes.

Our team constructs the principle and device of electrophoresis. In the previous work, o-phenylenediamine (o-PD) is the template molecule, and BSA is the target detection material. The experimental results proved the traditional molecular imprinting sensor BSA detection time from 15 min to 5 min, the detection of a lower detection limit, and good clinical applicability to real fetal calf serum samples, showing the successful construction of the electrophoresis device.

In this work, we explored the effect of the electrophoretic system in the immunoassay. CEA is a broad-spectrum tumor marker that can be present in adult serum and can be used as an auxiliary diagnostic marker for various cancers, rapid and sensitive detection of markers is very important in clinical diagnosis. By analyzing the current response results of DPV, we demonstrated that the constructed electric field-enhanced electrochemical immunosensor can achieve rapid incubation of CEA within 5 min, while the traditional immunosensor basically requires 1 h incubation time, and the electrophoresis device we applied shortened the antigen detection time by at least 12 times. According to the isoelectric point and molecular weight properties of different substances, the electrophoretic system also provides a new possibility for the anti-interference strategy. In conclusion, the electrophoresis device was successfully used in label-free electrochemical immunosensors.

The proposed electrophoretic system showed remarkable potential for the rapid detection of cancer markers. In addition, we are studying to further expand its ability in the future practical application of cancer detection, as follows: (1) Optimize the electrophoresis device, imagine that electrophoresis incubation system and detection system are integrated. Electrochemical detection of CEA will be performed simultaneously during the incubation, which can be more intuitive observation concentration change, build convenient sensing system, and realize low cost, fast, general function, etc. (2) The electrophoresis system will be applied to the field of electrochemiluminescence immune sensing, so as to realize higher precision detection while rapidly detecting CEA, and promote the practical application in clinical samples.

## 5 Conclusions

In conclusion, we constructed an electrifield enhanced electrochemical immunosensor combined with an electrochemical immunosensor, which can incubate the antigen in a very short time, enabling rapid and accurate detection of CEA. With excellent electrochemical analysis performance and low cost, the electrophoresis device has good applications in CEA biological detection and clinical cancer diagnosis. In the future, we will try the application of electrophoresis devices in biosensing such as small molecules and aptamer sensors, further improve the overall detection performance of traditional electrochemical sensors, and constantly explore the huge application potential of the electrophoretic system.

**Acknowledgments.** This work was supported by grants the Natural Science Foundation of Chongqing (cstc2020jcyj-msxmX0330); the JinFeng Laboratory Foundation, Chongqing, China (jfkyjf202203001).

## References

1. Hong, W., et al.: A reusable electrochemical immunosensor fabricated using a temperature-responsive polymer for cancer biomarker proteins. Biosens. Bioelectron. **78**, 181–186 (2016)
2. Miksad, R.A., Meropol, N.J.: Carcinoembryonic antigen-still more to learn from the real world. JAMA Oncol. **4**(3), 315–316 (2018)

3. Li, J., et al.: A highly specific and sensitive fluorescence quenching probe for carcinoembryonic antigen detection based on tetrapod Au nanostars with Ag coating. Mater. Today Commun. **25**, 101373 (2020)
4. Yang, Z., et al.: Efficient streptavidin-functionalized nitrogen-doped graphene for the development of highly sensitive electrochemical immunosensor. Biosens. Bioelectron. **89**, 312–318 (2017)
5. Yan, Z., et al.: An ultrasensitive sandwich-type electrochemical immunosensor for carcino embryonie antigen based on supermolecular labeling strategy. J. Electroanal. Chem. **781**, 289–295 (2016)
6. Wang, Y., et al.: Label-free electrochemical immunosensor based on flower-like Ag/MoS2/rGO nanocomposites for ultrasensitive detection of carcinoembryonic antigen. Sens. Actuators, B Chem. **255**, 125–132 (2018)
7. Lu, Q., et al.: Novel electrophoresis device with a molecularly imprinted polymer sensor for high-performance detection. Electrochem. Commun. **141**, 107355 (2022)
8. Kongsuphol, P., et al.: Melatonin attenuates methamphetamine-induced deactivation of the mammalian target of rapamycin signaling to induce autophagy in SK-N-SH cells. J. Pineal Res. **46**(2), 199–206 (2009)
9. Minsker, K., et al.: Characterization of rVSVDeltaG-ZEBOV-GP glycoproteins using automated capillary western blotting. Vaccine **38**(45), 7166–7174 (2020)
10. Li, C., Arakawa, T.: Application of native polyacrylamide gel electrophoresis for protein analysis: bovine serum albumin as a model protein. Int. J. Biol. Macromol. **125**, 566–571 (2019)

# Design of a Soft Exoskeleton with Motion Perception Network for Hand Function Rehabilitation

Xiaodong Li[1,2,3], Dehao Duanmu[2,3], Junlin Wang[2,3], and Yong Hu[1,2,3](✉)

[1] Orthopedic Center, The University of Hong Kong-Shenzhen Hospital, Shenzhen, China
yhud@hku.hk

[2] Department of Orthopaedics and Traumatology, The University of Hong Kong, Hong Kong, SAR, China
cnlixd@163.com

[3] The University of Hong Kong-Shenzhen Institute of Research and Innovation, Shenzhen, China

**Abstract.** Hand dysfunction seriously affects patients' activities of daily life. Rehabilitation exoskeleton can effectively improve the hand function of patients and reduce the burden of their families. However, most of the existing exoskeletons lack the ability to detect the state of hands during rehabilitation, which is a potential safety risk for rehabilitation. In order to improve the safety of hand function rehabilitation training, we proposed a soft wearable exoskeleton equipped with motion perception network. The soft exoskeleton is composed of guided bending bellows actuators, and has good mechanical properties. Besides, the soft bending sensor used to build the perception network has high measurement accuracy. The results showed that the soft exoskeleton with motion perception network not only realizes the full range of finger motion, but also measures the angle of each joint during the movement process. Therefore, this device can improve the rehabilitation effect, avoid secondary injury during rehabilitation training, and meet the rehabilitation needs of patients with hand dysfunction.

**Keywords:** Soft exoskeleton · Motion perception network · Soft actuator · Bending sensor · Hand function rehabilitation

## 1 Introduction

Whether at work or in daily life, hands participate in various activities, such as perception, movement, holding, manipulation, etc. Almost all survival activities are inseparable from hand function, so hands play a vital role in human life [1]. However, many neurological diseases or injuries cause hand dysfunctions, such as stroke, cerebral palsy, spinal cord injury, hand trauma, and central nervous system injury [2]. The traditional approach to hand functional rehabilitation relies heavily on the experience of therapists and requires their significant physical effort and strength to perform manual interventions [3]. As a result, the traditional treatment is difficult to cope with the surge of patients and the strict


G. Wang et al. (Eds.): APCMBE 2023, IFMBE Proceedings 103, pp. 443–450, 2024.
https://doi.org/10.1007/978-3-031-51455-5_50

requirements of rehabilitation training on intensity, duration and consistency. In order to solve these problems, with the development of soft robotic technology in recent years [2, 4], the field of rehabilitation medicine has embraced wearable robots as a common practice. Wearable exoskeleton, for instance, are frequently employed in hand functional rehabilitation to encourage the re-establishment of connections between damaged central nervous system and patients' hand.

In the past few decades, the development of soft robotics technology has provided a solid guarantee for the safety requirements of wearable exoskeleton rehabilitation robots [5, 6]. In terms of structures, the trend is from the traditional series link hinge mechanism of rigid robots to innovative mechanisms by utilizing advancements in power transmission technology and exploring new materials, such as cable-driven exoskeleton gloves and pneumatic artificial muscle exoskeleton gloves. In a previous study, we designed a pneumatically guided binding bellows actuators, and developed the wearable rehabilitation gloves, which not only meet the mechanical needs of rehabilitation training, but also ensure safety during the rehabilitation process [7].

In robot-assisted hand function rehabilitation, the reliability and safety of the devices are crucial to avoid causing secondary harm to patients [8, 9]. Even though the soft robot has the natural characteristics of high safety, it would be better to monitor the training process in order to further enhance the safety of rehabilitation [10, 11]. For the existing soft exoskeletons, most of them lack the ability to monitor the motion state, due to no sensors embedded [12]. Therefore, the integration of sensing technology into the soft exoskeleton to achieve motion monitoring has important application value for clinical rehabilitation.

This study aims to develop a soft exoskeleton with motion perception network to monitor the hand motion and enhance safety during hand function rehabilitation process. We used the flexible bending sensors to establish a motion perception network, and then combine it with the rehabilitation glove based on guided binding bellows actuators to design a soft exoskeleton with perceptive function. The actuators and sensors in the exoskeleton were measured to evaluate the performance of the exoskeleton for hand function rehabilitation.

## 2 Methodology

### 2.1 Mechanical Structures

The design of the execution mechanism for hand function rehabilitation is inseparable from the rehabilitation requirements, including passive techniques like muscle and joint relaxation in the initial phase, followed by active training in the intermediate phase, and additional training in daily activities during the later phase [5, 13]. In size, the hand joints are small with high motion complexity, it is not suitable to use rigid active exoskeleton structures as the hand function rehabilitation exoskeleton robots. In addition, the power and transmission of rigid mechanical structures require large space, and it is difficult to accomplish wearing comfort and fit, which will increase the burden on the hands, and even cause secondary injuries [14]. In conclusion, the soft wearable hand function rehabilitation device is a more appropriate choice. Considering that the rehabilitation training requires bi-directional force for the joints, we choose fluidic driving instead of cable. Because the weight of the rehabilitation exoskeleton should be borne by the participants in training, the pneumatic driving is finally selected in order to reduce the weight of exoskeleton as much as possible comparing to the hydraulic driving mode.

In this study, we used a kind of pneumatic actuator called guided bending bellows actuators (GBBAs) as the driving mechanism of the rehabilitation glove [7], which can obviously provide bidirectional mechanical output and reduce the weight of the patient's hand compared to other flexible actuators. As shown in Fig. 1, at each finger joint, an independent actuator is configured to provide the force to make the finger joint bend. Connected to the glove through two fixed plates, the output force of the pneumatic actuator can be transmitted to the joints on both sides. When the internal output of the actuator is positive pressure, the output force at both ends acts as thrust, driving the finger to flexion, while the internal output of the actuator is negative pressure, the output force at both ends acts as pulling force, driving the finger to extension.

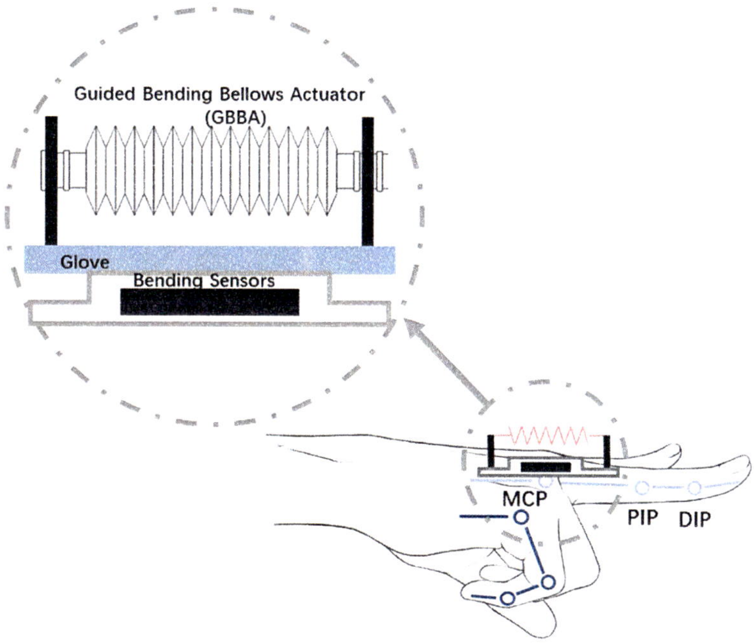


**Fig. 1.** Schematic diagram of the working principle of the soft exoskeleton with bending sensors.

In order to establish a motion perception network, we placed the bending sensors on the finger joints, including the interphalangeal (IP) and metacarpophalangeal (MCP) joints of thumb and the distal interphalangeal (DIP), proximal interphalangeal (PIP) and MCP joints of the other four fingers, as shown in Fig. 1. These sensors are constructed with a novel material that functions as an electrical semiconducting tape. This material is made of soft and flexible ethylene propylene rubber (Scotch Electrical Semi-Conducting Tape 13, 3M), and its impedance changes in response to bending. The effectiveness of this material as a bending sensor has been evaluated in our previous works [15, 16].

During hand function rehabilitation training, the pneumatic actuator provides pushing or pulling force at both ends according to the change of internal pressure. These output forces are transmitted to the fingers on both sides of the knuckle through the fixed plate to drive the joint to rotate. The flexible film bending sensor embedded in the glove follows the finger motion to generate corresponding bending changes, thus obtaining real-time data on the knuckle bending.

## 2.2 Working Principles of Control System

The control system of the soft rehabilitation glove can perform both open-loop control by setting the rehabilitation intensity, and closed-loop control based on the feedback provided by the sensor network in the system. The entire control system can be categorized into three distinct routes, including the information route, the electric circuit route and the gas route. These routes correspond to the transmission of control signals, electric energy and gas flow direction in the system, respectively. Figure 2 depicts the physical diagram of the lower controller and gas drive system based on the three schematic routes.

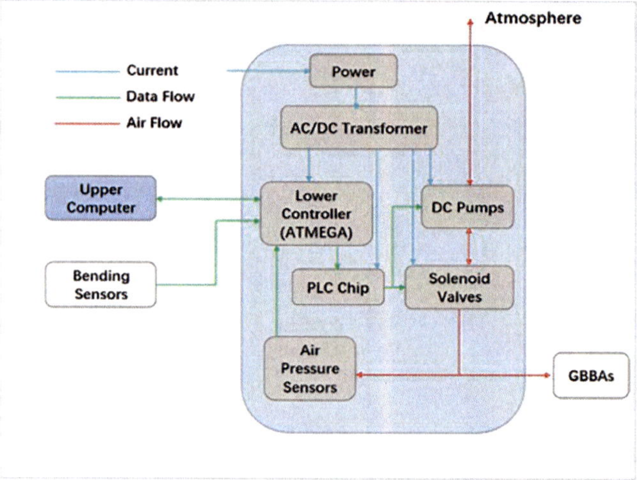


**Fig. 2.** Schematic diagram of control system.

The open-loop control system functions by transmitting control signals from the upper computer to the lower controller (AT-MEGA328P-AU) via the serial port. The lower controller then sends the processed analog signals to the PLC drive chip (Macrowis, 4 WAYs), which activates the pneumatic components, including drive pumps (Chaofei, ES-3910, DC24V) and solenoid valves (OST Solenoid 2/2 NC, 24V). The system's air pressure sensors and bending sensors directly send signals to the lower controller for collection. To power the system, the AC power supply (JC Power, 24V 72W) converts electrical energy into 24V DC power, which is used by the PLC chip module, DC pumps and solenoid valves. The compressed or vacuum gas is transferred from the compression and vacuum pump to the main gas route via two parallel solenoid valves. A manual flow valve is located after the solenoid valves to maintain stable flow rates in the gas circuit. Ultimately, the control instructions issued by the upper computer are carried out by passing compressed or vacuum gas through GBBAs with the cooperation of the control system's modules.

In the closed-loop system, the self-developed soft bending sensor network mentioned above mainly provides rehabilitation state awareness. By detecting the real-time angle of the corresponding knuckles through the bending sensor, the angle change trend of each knuckle can be calculated [17, 18], and compared with the input command of the pneumatic system, the patient's motion trend can be obtained. The input signal of the pneumatic generating system (input air pressure, duration, etc.) will be passively adjusted according to the patient's motion trend [4, 19], which not only prevents secondary damage to the patient's knuckles by the rehabilitation equipment, but also improves the recovery efficiency.

## 3 Results

In order to test the performance of a single GBBA, we measured its displacement changes during inflation and extraction. The results are shown in Fig. 3. Considering the original length of GBBA, it is clear that its elongation ratio exceeds 200%. This elongation ratio ensures that the fingers can move in a large range driven by the soft exoskeleton. Then we evaluated the measurement characteristics of a single bending sensor. As shown in Fig. 4, bending sensor has high measurement accuracy, with mean absolute error (MAE) of 2.99°. It is acceptable for the measurement of hand motion.

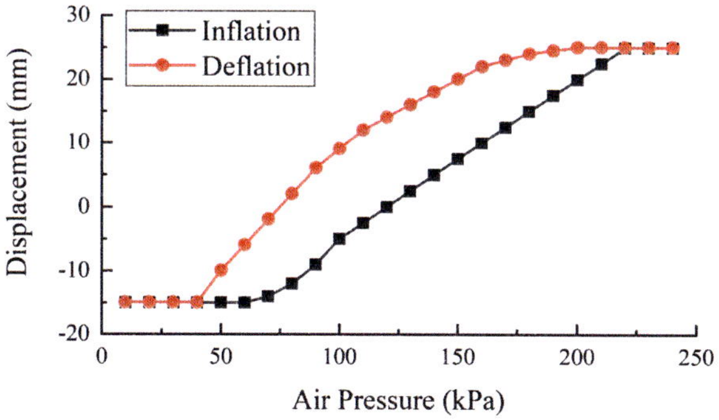


**Fig. 3.** The displacement change of GBBA during inflation and deflation.

Through the measurement of a single actuator and sensor, it is believed that the soft exoskeleton made up of these components would have good performance. In order to evaluate the performance of the soft exoskeleton, we designed a bionic finger model with three joints [7], and its total range of motion is 270°. We use soft exoskeleton to drive the finger model, and record the air pressure and motion amplitude. The result is shown in Fig. 5. It is obvious that the soft exoskeleton can achieve full range of motion. Due to the measurement error of the bending sensors, there may be an obvious error on

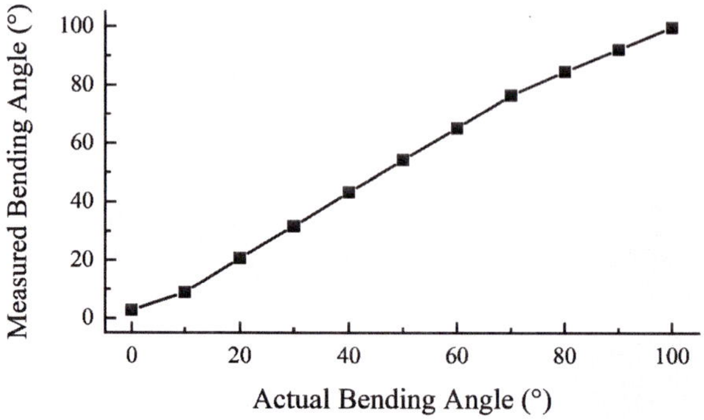


**Fig. 4.** Performance test of bending sensor.

angle measurement when the movement amplitude is large. However, there is no doubt that with motion perception network, the motion angle of each joint can be measured in real time, so as to estimate the motion state of the hand.

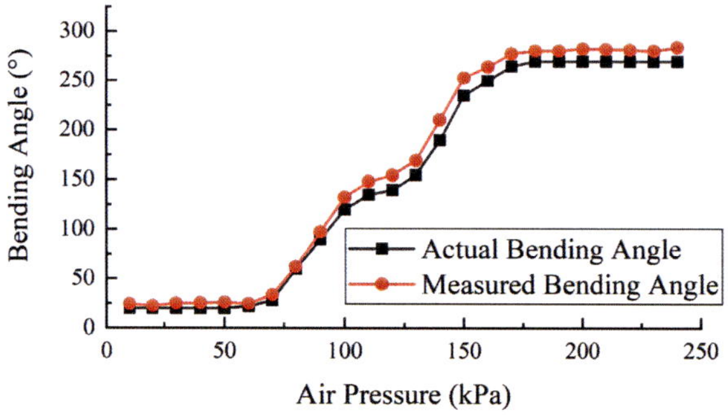


**Fig. 5.** Flexion of a finger model under soft exoskeleton.

## 4 Conclusions

In this study, we proposed a soft exoskeleton integrating bending sensor array as a perception network. At each knuckle, the exoskeleton is equipped with a pneumatic guided bending bellows actuator as the driving mechanism and a soft membrane bending sensor to collect motion information. As a novel wearable hand functional rehabilitation device with motion perception system, our exoskeleton not only provides patients with active rehabilitation training, but also obtains the motion trend during the training process and adjust the input signals of the pneumatic control system in time. The real-time detection of motion state and trends during rehabilitation training can both effectively avoid secondary injuries to patients and greatly improve rehabilitation efficiency.

**Acknowledgment.** This work was supported in part by the National Key Research and Development Program of China (2021YFF0501600); Shenzhen-Hong Kong-Macau Technology Research Programme (Type C. SGDX20190816232011196); Shenzhen Local Science and Technology Development Fund guided by the Chinese Central Government (2021Szvup130).

## References

1. Aftabi, H., Nasiri, R., Ahmadabadi, M.N.: Simulation-based biomechanical assessment of unpowered exoskeletons for running. Sci. Rep. **11**(1), 11846 (2021). https://doi.org/10.1038/s41598-021-89640-3
2. Ambrosini, E., Ferrante, S., Rossini, M., et al.: Functional and usability assessment of a robotic exoskeleton arm to support activities of daily life. Robotica **32**(8), 1213–1224 (2014). https://doi.org/10.1017/S0263574714001891
3. Wang, W., Zhang, J., Kong, D., et al.: Research on control method of upper limb exoskeleton based on mixed perception model. Robotica **40**(10), 3669–3685 (2022). https://doi.org/10.1017/S0263574722000480
4. Daratany, C., Taveira, A.: Quasi-experimental study of exertion, recovery, and worker perceptions related to passive upper-body exoskeleton use during overhead, low force work, pp. 369–373. Springer International Publishing (2020). https://doi.org/10.1007/978-3-030-44267-5_55
5. Proietti, T., O'Neill, C., Hohimer, C.J., et al.: Sensing and control of a multi-joint soft wearable robot for upper-limb assistance and rehabilitation. IEEE Robot. Autom. Lett. **6**(2), 2381–2388 (2021). https://doi.org/10.1109/LRA.2021.3061061
6. Moyon, A., Poirson, E., Petiot, J.-F.: Experimental study of the physical impact of a passive exoskeleton on manual sanding operations. Procedia CIRP **70**, 284–289 (2018). https://doi.org/10.1016/j.procir.2018.04.028(28thCIRPDesignConference23-25May2018Nantes)
7. Duanmu, D., Wang, X., Li, X., et al.: Design of guided bending bellows actuators for soft hand function rehabilitation gloves. Actuators (2022)
8. Peng, X., Acosta-Sojo, Y., Wu, M.I., et al.: Actuation timing perception of a powered ankle exoskeleton and its associated ankle angle changes during walking. IEEE Trans. Neural Syst. Rehabil. Eng. **30**, 869–877 (2022). https://doi.org/10.1109/TNSRE.2022.3162213
9. Graser, J.V., Prospero, L., Liesch, M., et al.: Test-retest reliability of upper limb robotic exoskeleton assessments in children and youths with brain lesions. Sci. Rep. **12**(1), 16685 (2022). https://doi.org/10.1038/s41598-022-20588-8
10. Fanti, V., Sanguineti, V., Caldwell, D.G., et al.: Assessment methodology for human-exoskeleton interactions: kinetic analysis based on muscle activation. Front. Neurorobot. **16**, 982950 (2022). https://doi.org/10.3389/fnbot.2022.982950
11. Mochizuki, G., Centen, A., Resnick, M., et al.: Movement kinematics and proprioception in post-stroke spasticity: assessment using the Kinarm robotic exoskeleton. J. Neuroeng. Rehabil. **16**(1), 146 (2019). https://doi.org/10.1186/s12984-019-0618-5
12. Louie, D.R., Mortenson, W.B., Lui, M., et al: Patients' and therapists' experience and perception of exoskeleton-based physiotherapy during subacute stroke rehabilitation: a qualitative analysis. Disab. Rehab. 1–9 (2021). ahead-of-print. https://doi.org/10.1080/09638288.2021.1989503
13. Bortole, M., Venkatakrishnan, A., Zhu, F., et al.: The H2 robotic exoskeleton for gait rehabilitation after stroke: early findings from a clinical study. J. Neuroeng. Rehabil. **12**(1), 54 (2015). https://doi.org/10.1186/s12984-015-0048-y

14. Guo, N., Wang, X., Duanmu, D., et al.: SSVEP-based brain computer interface controlled soft robotic glove for post-stroke hand function rehabilitation. IEEE Trans. Neural Syst. Rehabil. Eng. **30**, 1 (2022). https://doi.org/10.1109/TNSRE.2022.3185262
15. Shen, Z., Yi, J., Li, X., et al.: A soft stretchable bending sensor and data glove applications. Robot. Biomimetics **3**(1), 22 (2016)
16. Li, X., Wen, R., Shen, Z., et al.: A wearable detector for simultaneous finger joint motion measurement. IEEE Tran. Biomed. Circ. Syst. **12**(3), 644–654 (2018)
17. Delgado, P., Alekhya, S., Majidirad, A., et al.: Shoulder kinematics assessment towards exoskeleton development. Appl. Sci. **10**(18), 6336 (2020). https://doi.org/10.3390/app10186336
18. Muijzer-Witteveen, H., Sibum, N., van Dijsseldonk, R., et al.: Questionnaire results of user experiences with wearable exoskeletons and their preferences for sensory feedback. J. Neuroeng. Rehabil. **15**(1), 1–8 (2018). https://doi.org/10.1186/s12984-018-0445-0
19. Galofaro, E., D'Antonio, E., Patané, F., et al.: Three-dimensional assessment of upper limb proprioception via a wearable exoskeleton. Appl. Sci. **11**(6), 2615 (2021). https://doi.org/10.3390/app11062615

# In Silico Investigation of the Effect of Atrial Fibrosis on High-Frequency Electrocardiogram

Hanyu Wang, Na Zhao(✉), Jianqing Li, and Chengyu Liu(✉)

School of Instrument Science and Engineering, Southeast University, Nanjing, China
{zhaona,chengyu}@seu.edu.cn

**Abstract.** Atrial fibrosis plays an important role in the occurrence and maintenance of atrial fibrillation (AF). The assessment of atrial fibrosis is of great significance in the prediction, evaluation and treatment of AF. Currently, the development of high-frequency electrocardiogram (ECG) suggests that it may become a new and potential method to assess atrial fibrosis, which is relatively convenient and non-invasive. However, there is little relevant research on this issue. In this study, we investigated the effect of atrial fibrosis on high-frequency ECG using a two-dimensional (2D) atrial electrophysiological model. The effects of diffusion coefficient, fibrosis density and ion channel remodeling on high-frequency ECG were simulated. Simulation results demonstrated that the degree of atrial fibrosis (changes in diffusion coefficient and fibrosis density) would lead to a decrease in the maximum amplitude of about 30–63% on high-frequency ECG, while the ion channel remodeling would limitedly affect the maximum amplitude. The more severe the fibrosis density or the smaller the diffusion coefficient, the lower the maximum amplitude on high-frequency ECG. These findings may provide new insights into the assessment of atrial fibrosis by high-frequency ECG.

**Keywords:** High frequency electrocardiogram signal · Atrial fibrosis · Atrial electrophysiology modeling

## 1 Introduction

Atrial fibrosis is an important factor in the substrate of atrium, which is involved in the occurrence and maintenance of atrial fibrillation (AF) [1, 2]. If we can detect the degree of atrial fibrosis in advance, we can intervene and prevent it in advance, effectively reduce the incidence and severity of AF. In addition, atrial fibrosis assessment can assist physicians in selecting patients who can undergo catheter ablation for AF, because if atrial fibrosis is more severe, the prognosis is poor even after catheter ablation. Therefore, accurate assessment of the severity of atrial fibrosis in patients with AF is an important basis for guiding the treatment of AF, which is of great significance in clinical practice. At present, there are two main methods to assess fibrosis: late gadolinium enhancement by cardiac MR (LGE-CMR) and three-dimensional mapping of cardiac electrophysiology [2, 3]. The former requires specialized equipment that is not available in every hospital, while the latter is a method of invasive surgery. They both have their own limitations.


G. Wang et al. (Eds.): APCMBE 2023, IFMBE Proceedings 103, pp. 451–458, 2024.
https://doi.org/10.1007/978-3-031-51455-5_51

Therefore, the highly available and non-invasive method for the assessment of atrial fibrosis is needed. Recently, in view of the superior performance of high-frequency electrocardiogram (ECG) in detection of myocardial ischemia, we propose to use high-frequency ECG as an entry point to assess atrial fibrosis. However, there is little relevant research on this issue, thus this study focuses on it.

The purpose of this study is to investigate the effect of atrial fibrosis on high-frequency ECG and to help to develop a high-frequency ECG-based method for assessing atrial fibrosis which can be used in physical examinations and in medical settings lacking specialized equipment.

## 2 Methods

### 2.1 Two-Dimensional Atrial Tissue Model

In this study, the Courtemanche-Ramirez-Nattel model was used to represent action potentials of human atrial myocytes [4]. The updated fibroblast model developed by Zhao et al. [5] was implemented to couple to atrial myocytes. Then, a two-dimensional (2D) atrial tissue that consisted of 300 $\times$ 300 cells with a size of 4.5 $\times$ 4.5 cm$^2$ was constructed to investigate the effect of atrial fibrosis on high-frequency ECG. In the 2D atrial tissue model, as shown in Fig. 1, adjacent atrial myocytes were coupled by gap junctions. Gap junctions allowed ions to pass through when the potential difference occurred between the coupled neighboring cells, thus enabling action potentials propagation between the adjacent atrial myocytes. Fibroblasts in the atria were much smaller in volume than atrial myocytes, thus a single atrial myocyte could couple with multiple fibroblasts. The gap junction conductance between each fibroblast and the atrial cell is $G_{gap}$. In this study, atrial myocytes in the area of fibroblast proliferation were randomly coupled with 0 or 4 fibroblasts. In addition, the simulation of a one-dimensional model with 300 cells was performed to determine the conduction velocity of 60 cm/s from the 100th cell to the 200th cell under normal conditions, which was within the scope of physiological experiments [6]. Pacing stimuli with a cycle length of 750 ms for 20 beats were applied to the corner of the 2D atrial tissue to evoke action potentials to propagate throughout the whole tissue.

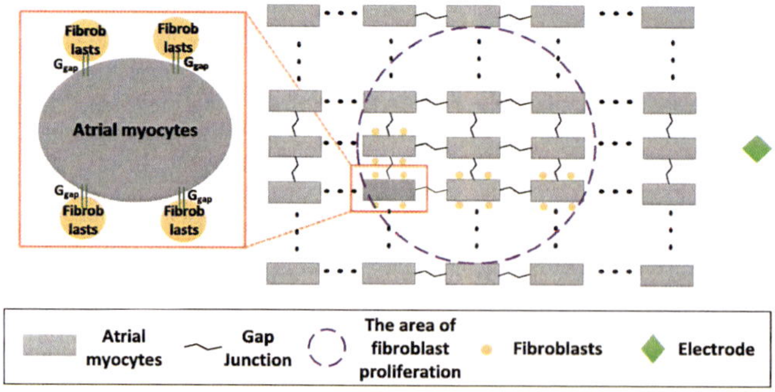


**Fig. 1.** 2D atrial tissue model

Grey rectangles indicate atrial myocytes; yellow circles indicate fibroblasts; green diamond indicates the location of the electrode; the purple dotted line indicates the area of fibroblast proliferation; and black broken lines indicate gap junctions.

### 2.2 Simulation of Atrial Fibrosis

The simulation of atrial fibrosis contained two parts: fibrosis density and diffusion coefficient. To investigate the effects of high-density and low-density atrial fibrosis on high-frequency ECG, the study by Ashihara et al. [7] was referenced. As shown in Fig. 1, the area of fibroblast proliferation is represented by a circle with a diameter of 3.0 cm in the central area. Within the area, the proportion of atrial myocytes coupled with four fibroblasts reached 50% and 12.5% of the area, representing high-density and low-density atrial fibrosis, respectively. In addition, to investigate the effect of diffusion coefficient on high-frequency ECG, the diffusion coefficient was reduced by 25% and 50%, respectively.

### 2.3 Simulation of Ion Channel Remodeling

During the process of AF, the degree of atrial fibrosis will change, so will ion channel remodeling, which may also affect the changes of high-frequency ECG. In this study, ion channel remodeling in paroxysmal AF and persistent AF was selected as two representatives to investigate the effect of ion channel remodeling on high-frequency ECG. To represent ion channel remodeling in different types of AF, the different modifications in ion channel conductance were incorporated in the atrial myocyte model. For persistent AF, the maximum conductance of the transient potassium current ($I_{to}$), the delayed rectifier potassium current ($I_{Kur}$), the L-type calcium current ($I_{CaL}$) and the inward rectifier potassium current ($I_{K1}$) were assumed to be 50%, 50%, 30% and 200% of the initial values, respectively [8]. For paroxysmal AF, the maximum conductance of $I_{to}$, $I_{Kur}$, $I_{CaL}$ and $I_{K1}$ were assumed to be 75%, 75%, 65% and 200% of the initial values, respectively [9].

### 2.4 Simulation of High-Frequency ECG

Electrocardiogram show the potential accumulation of the heart tissue at the electrode, and the potential is relatively small at points within the heart tissue far from the electrode. The ECG calculation is given by the following formula [10]:

$$ECG = \int \frac{\boldsymbol{D}\nabla V_m \cdot \vec{r}}{r^3} dV \tag{1}$$

where $V$ is the integral domain to be calculated, and in this study it is the 2D atrial tissue; $D$ is the diffusion tensor; $\vec{r}$ is the directional vector pointing from each point within the tissue to the electrode, and in this study the electrode was placed 2 cm to the right of the 2D atrial tissue [11], as shown in Fig. 1; r is the length of the directional vector.

In order to obtain high-frequency ECG, fast Fourier transform and bandpass filtering were performed on the obtained ordinary ECG. The ordinary ECG signals in the normal model with a 1000 Hz sampling rate is shown in Fig. 2a, the high-frequency ECG with 150–250 Hz signal component preserved is shown in Fig. 2b, and its spectrogram is shown in 2C.

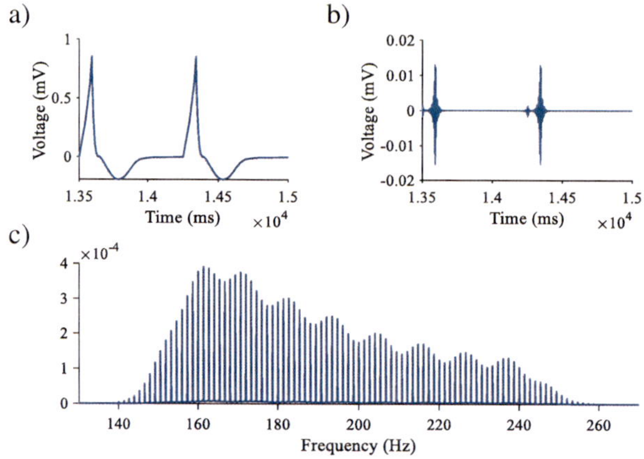


**Fig. 2.** Simulation results of ECG in the normal model. **a** ordinary ECG signal in the normal model, **b** signal after 150–250 Hz filtering, **c** spectrogram

## 3 Retsults

Firstly, to investigate the effect of the diffusion coefficient on high-frequency ECG, the ion channel remodeling and the fibrosis density were set to the same, and the diffusion coefficient was reduced by 25% and 50%, respectively. As showed in Fig. 3a, the blue solid line represents the normal model, the red dotted line represents a 25% decrease in the diffusion coefficient, and the purple dashed line represents a 50% decrease in the diffusion coefficient. In Fig. 3a, their maximum amplitudes were reduced by about 30% and 41%, respectively, compared with the normal model. The more the diffusion coefficient decreased, the greater the proportion of the components biased to 250 Hz in the spectrogram, and the lower the maximum amplitude on high-frequency ECG. The spectrograms in Fig. 3b are both different from the normal model.

Secondly, the effect of the fibrosis density on high-frequency ECG was investigated under the condition of the same diffusion coefficient and ion channel remodeling. As shown in Fig. 4a, the blue solid line represents the normal model, the red dotted line represents low-density fibrosis, and the purple dashed line represents high-density fibrosis. The maximum amplitude of the high-density fibrosis model was reduced by about 63%, while that of the low-density fibrosis model was reduced by about 41%. The spectrogram in Fig. 4b showed that the high-frequency components of the low-density fibrosis model

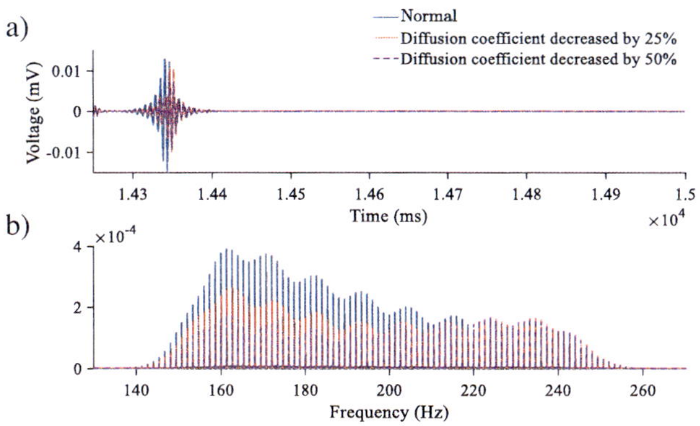


**Fig. 3.** Effect of the diffusion coefficient on high-frequency ECG. **a** Signal after 150–250 Hz filtering, **b** spectrogram

were quite different from those of the high-density fibrosis model. Compared with the low-density fibrosis model, the high-density fibrosis model had a larger proportion of the spectrogram biased towards 250 Hz.

Thirdly, the effect of ion channel remodeling on high-frequency ECG was investigated under the same diffusion coefficient and the same fibrosis density. Paroxysmal AF model and persistent AF model were simulated by ion channel remodeling. After filtering, the 150–250 Hz high frequency component of the signal was preserved, as shown in Fig. 5a. The maximum amplitude of the high-frequency ECG signals in the paroxysmal and persistent AF models decreased by almost the same degree, and it was difficult to distinguish paroxysmal and persistent AF by high-frequency ECG. In addition, compared with the normal model, the influence of ion channel remodeling on the spectrum was very limited, as shown in Fig. 5b.

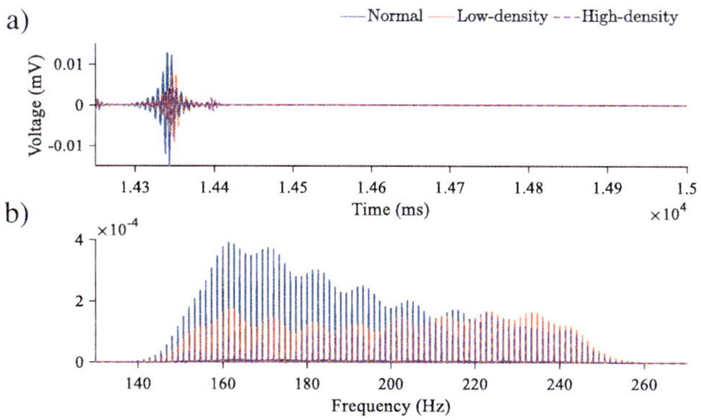


**Fig. 4.** Effect of the fibrosis density on high-frequency ECG. **a** Signal after 150–250 Hz filtering, **b** spectrogram

Furthermore, the different decrease of diffusion coefficient was combined with different fibrosis density to investigate how the degree of fibrosis had effects on high-frequency ECG. As shown in Fig. 6a, the blue solid line represents the normal model, the red dotted line represents the low fibrosis model with low-density fibrosis and a decline of 25% in the diffusion coefficient, and the purple dashed line represents the high fibrosis model with high-density fibrosis and a decline of 50% in the diffusion coefficient. Compared with the normal model, the maximum amplitude of the low fibrosis model decreased by about 30%, while the maximum amplitude of the high fibrosis model decreased by about 63%. With the degree of fibrosis increasing, the compositions of the spectrum were more biased towards 250Hz in Fig. 6b.

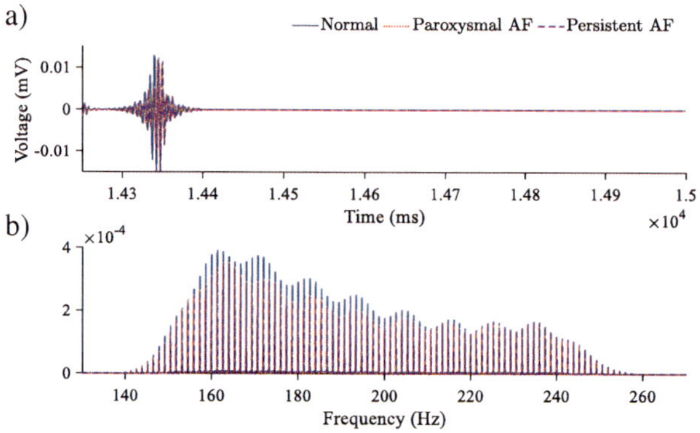


**Fig. 5.** Effect of ion channel remodeling on high-frequency ECG. **a** Signal after 150 Hz-250 Hz filtering, **b** spectrogram

In addition, the cause of high-frequency ECG changes was explored in the context of atrial fibrosis. Figure 6c shows the electrical conduction schematics of the normal model and the fibrosis models at different times. The top row is the normal model, the middle row is the low fibrosis model, and the bottom row is the high fibrosis model. The different color represents the different voltage. The results showed that the conduction process in the fibrosis models was slower and less uniform than that in the normal model at the same time. Because atrial myocytes randomly coupling with fibroblasts caused a decrease in their own action potentials and impeded the electrical conduction process between adjacent cells. Therefore, the potential accumulation in Formula (1) was declined in high-frequency ECG under fibrosis conditions.

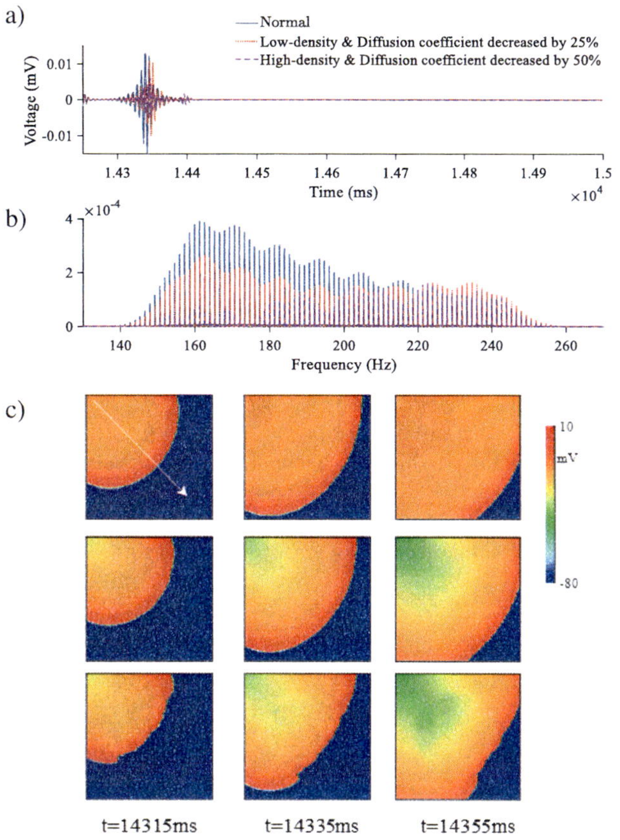


**Fig. 6.** Effect of the diffusion coefficient and the degree of atrial fibrosis on high-frequency ECG. **a** Signal after 150–250 Hz filtering, **b** spectrogram, **c** electrical conduction schematics

## 4 Conclusion

In this study, the effects of diffusion coefficient, fibrosis density and ion channel remodeling on high-frequency ECG were simulated in the 2D atrial tissue model. The simulation results demonstrated that fibrosis would lead to the decrease of the maximum amplitude on high-frequency ECG, but the effect of ion channel remodeling on high-frequency ECG was not significant. These findings may provide new insights into the assessment of atrial fibrosis by high-frequency ECG.

**Acknowledgment.** This work was supported by the National Natural Science Foundation of China (62171123, 62071241, 62201144 and 62211530112), the Project funded by China Postdoctoral Science Foundation (2022M720725), and the Fundamental Research Funds for the Central Universities (2242022R20065).

## References


1. Goldberger, J.J., Arora, R., Green, D., et al.: Evaluating the atrial myopathy underlying atrial fibrillation: identifying the arrhythmogenic and thrombogenic substrate. Circulation **132**(4), 278–291 (2015). https://doi.org/10.1161/CIRCULATIONAHA.115.016795
2. Lee, D.K., Shim, J., Choi, J.I., et al.: Left atrial fibrosis assessed with cardiac MRI in patients with paroxysmal and those with persistent atrial fibrillation radiology. Radiology **00**(0), 1–8: 575–582 (2019). https://doi.org/10.1148/radiol.2019182629
3. Harrison, J.L., Jensen, H.K., Peel, S.A., et al.: Cardiac magnetic resonance and electroanatomical mapping of acute and chronic atrial ablation injury: a histological validation study. Eur. Heart J. **35**(22), 1486–1495 (2014). https://doi.org/10.1093/eurheartj/eht560
4. Courtemanche, M., Ramirez, R.J., Nattel, S.: Ionic mechanisms underlying human atrial action potential properties: insights from a mathematical model. Am. J. Physiol. **275**(1), H301-321 (1998). https://doi.org/10.1152/ajpheart.1998.275.1.H301
5. Zhao, N.: Study on mechanism of atrial fibrillation induced by heart failure based on multiscale atrial computational model. Harbin Inst. Technol. (2020). https://doi.org/10.27061/d.cnki.ghgdu.2020.004745
6. Dössel, O., Krueger, M.W., Weber, F., et al.: Computational modeling of the human atrial anatomy and electrophysiology. Med. Biol. Eng. Comput. **50**(8), 773–799 (2012). https://doi.org/10.1007/s11517-012-0924-6
7. Ashihara, T., Haraguchi, R., Nakazawa, K., et al.: The role of fibroblasts in complex fractionated electrograms during persistent/permanent atrial fibrillation implications for electrogram-based catheter ablation. Circ. Res. **110**(2), 275–284 (2012). https://doi.org/10.1161/circresaha.111.255026
8. Tobon, C., Palacio, L.C., Chidipi, B., et al.: The antimalarial chloroquine reduces the burden of persistent atrial fibrillation. Front. Pharmacol. **10**, 1–12 (2019). https://doi.org/10.3389/fphar.2019.01392
9. Palacio, L.C., Ugarte, J.P., Tobón, C.: In-silico study of the ionic current gradients determining left-to-right atrial frequencies during paroxysmal atrial fibrillation. In: International Conference on Advances in System Simulation. SAGE Publications Sage UK: London, England (2019)
10. Keldermann, R.H., Tusscher, K., Nash, M.P., et al.: A computational study of mother rotor VF in the human ventricles. AJP Heart Circul. Physiol. **296**(2), H370-379 (2009). https://doi.org/10.1152/ajpheart.00952.2008
11. Li, Y., Wan, R., Liu, J., et al.: In silico mechanisms of arsenic trioxide-induced cardiotoxicity. Comput. Physiol. Med. **13**, 1–17 (2022). https://doi.org/10.3389/fphys.2022.1004605

# GCN-ResNet: A Multi-label Classifier for ECG Arrhythmia

Jing Wu[1], Shuo Zhang[2], Xingyao Wang[2], and Chengyu Liu[2](✉)

[1] The School of Software, Southeast University, Suzhou, China
[2] The School of Instrument Science and Engineering, Southeast University, Nanjing, China
chengyu@seu.edu.cn

**Abstract.** Automatic ECG classification using artificial intelligence technology is of great significance for the early prevention and diagnosis of cardiovascular diseases. Over the past few years, there have been many studies having demonstrated impressive performance in the area of single label ECG classification. Nonetheless, in real-world clinical scenarios, a single ECG recording may exhibit multiple types of arrhythmia concurrently, thus highlighting the significance of investigating multi-label ECG classification. This paper proposes a multi-label ECG classification model based on GCN-CNN framework, named GCN-ResNet, which can complete the task of multi-label ECG classification by using GCN to extract label information and CNN to extract ECG information. At the same time, two loss function improvement strategies are proposed to address the imbalance problem. Experiments show that our method can achieve F1 score of 0.832 in classifying 55 kinds of arrhythmias, which can help doctors to conduct early rapid ECG diagnosis.

**Keywords:** ECG · Multi-label classification · Arrythmia · GCN

## 1 Introduction

Cardiovascular disease is the number one health killer in the world, and electrocardiogram is the simplest and most effective method to diagnose cardiovascular disease. How to make good use of the advantages of artificial intelligence technology which developed rapidly in recent years, to realize the early detection and treatment of cardiovascular diseases has become the key of cardiovascular disease prevention and treatment.

In clinical practice, a patient with cardiovascular diseases may correspond to multiple arrhythmia types simultaneously. Compared with the single-label abnormal ECG classification task, the multi-label abnormal ECG classification task is more in line with the clinical practice.

Deep learning, particularly convolutional neural network (CNN), are capable of automatically extracting essential features from ECG signals. In the task of single-label ECG classification, some studies have achieved very high classification accuracy by using deep learning technology. There is also some tentative work in the field of multi-label ECG classification.


G. Wang et al. (Eds.): APCMBE 2023, IFMBE Proceedings 103, pp. 459–465, 2024.
https://doi.org/10.1007/978-3-031-51455-5_52

In order to realize efficient and high-precision multi-label ECG classification and effectively use the related information between ECG labels, this paper proposes a multi-label classification model named GCN-ResNet which based on GCN-CNN framework. A one-dimensional convolution ResNet model is used to extract the characteristics of ECG signals, and a 3-layer GCN model is used to mine the related information of labels. In this paper, the dataset used contains 55 kinds of arrhythmia. The algorithm's evaluation criterion is based on the F1 score.

This paper makes the following significant contributions:

(1) Combining the advantages of GCN and ResNet, an algorithm model GCN-ResNet for multi-label ECG classification is proposed, which can detect 55 arrhythmia symptoms at the same time.
(2) This paper designs a loss function to address the issue of highly unbalanced distribution of 55 sample types in the dataset.

The rest of this paper is structured as follows: Sect. 2 introduces the progress of multi-label classification task and ECG classification task in recent years. Section 3 outlines the proposed classification model. Section 4 details the implementation process. Section 5 provides an overview of the results. Section 6 summarizes this paper and discusses the future work.

## 2 Related Work

### 2.1 Multi-label Classification Task

At present, the models used for multi-label classification tasks can be divided into three distinct categories [1], problem transformation method, algorithm transformation method and neural network modeling method. The problem transformation method ignores the correlation between labels and transforms them into multiple single-label classification tasks [2–4]. Algorithm transformation extends specific machine learning algorithms and is directly applied to multi-label classification tasks. Neural network makes the model have better generalization ability by capturing the correlation between labels.

Most of the multi-label classification work using neural network uses CNN to extract features, and the second network to extract the correlation between labels. References [5, 6] used RNN/LSTM to extract semantic relations between labels. Durand et al. [7] use GCN to do the same work. Yan et al. [8] regarded the multilabel classification task as a sequence generation problem to consider the label correlation.

### 2.2 Electrocardiogram Classification Task

Deep learning technology has made some progress in the field of ECG classification [9]. An end-to-end DNN model was proposed to classify 12 types of single-lead ECG signals, resulting in an F1 score of 0.837. Kamaleswaran et al. [10] designed a 13-layer CNN model to classify four kinds of ECG signals, and the F1 score reached 0.83.

The application of deep learning in the study of single-label ECG classification tasks has achieved high accuracy. Some researchers have also explored the problem of multi-label ECG classification [11]. Multi-ECGNet was developed to simultaneously identify 55 types of abnormal heart rates, achieving an F1 score of 0.863. Li et al. [12] proposed a model combining GRU and attention mechanism, and nine kinds of multi-label classification are realized on private data sets, with an accuracy rate of 92.8%. Although the methods discussed realize multi-label ECG classification, they do not make effective use of ECG data label information and do not address the issue of imbalanced data set distribution. Therefore, it is still a challenge to apply deep learning to multi-label ECG classification.

## 3 Methods

To complete the task of multi-label ECG classification, the key factor is to construct an efficient algorithm for classifying multi-label ECG signals and use the relevant information of labels. To address this problem, this paper proposes a GCN-ResNet architecture based on GCN and CNN, which can extract effective information from multi-lead ECG for multi-label ECG classification.

### 3.1 Model Structure

The GCN-ResNet model's overall architecture consists of two components: an ECG feature learning module based on CNN and a classifier learning module based on GCN. The network is mainly designed according to ML-GCN [13] and ResNet [14]. Figure 1 illustrates the model structure.

The ECG feature learning module is a one-dimensional ResNet18. The feature of ECG signal is obtained by applying the global maximum pooling after the last convolution layer. The input signal is an ECG signal.

The GCN classifier module contains 3-layer GCN, which learns label features. At each GCN layer, the previous layer's node feature is used as input, and a new node feature is produced as output. The input signal of GCN part is the word embedding vector of 55 class labels, and the last layer produces 55 classifiers as output.

The classifier learned by GCN module was applied to the ECG features learned by ResNet18 module, and the prediction scores for 55 categories were obtained.

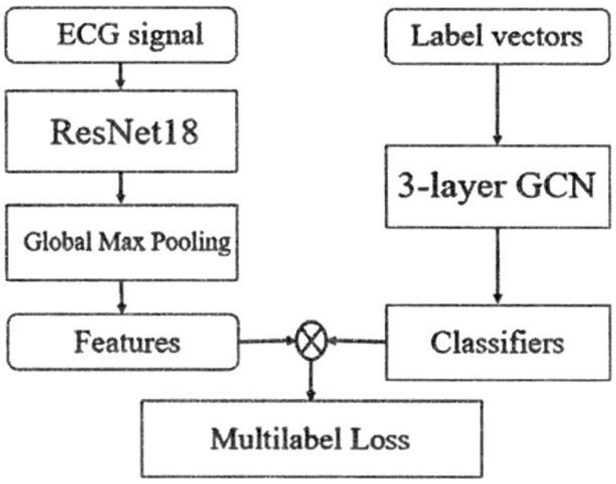


**Fig. 1.** The model structure

### 3.2 Adjacency Matrix

GCN transmits information between nodes based on adjacency matrix. This paper defines co-occurrence mode between labels as adjacency matrix. The number of label pairs in the training set is counted to get the matrix $M \in R^{C \times C}$ . Based on , the conditional probability matrix $P_i = M_i/N_i$ is obtained. Where $N_i$ is the total number of times that label $i$ appears. The label co-occurrence mode may appear as a long tail distribution, binary processing is carried out to obtain the final co-occurrence matrix.

### 3.3 Optimization Strategy of Loss Function

The multi-label classification problem is to select K target categories from N candidate categories. The simplest way is to activate them with sigmoid function, sum the cross entropy of each two categories as loss, as formula 1.

$$L = \sum_{c=1}^{C} y^c log(\sigma(\hat{y}^c)) + (1 - y^c) log(1 - \sigma(\hat{y}^c)) \tag{1}$$

where $\sigma(x)$ is sigmoid function, $1/(1+e^{-x})$, $y^c$ and $\hat{y}^c$ are vectors, representing the real label and the network output without any activation.

However, when $n>>k$, this approach will face a serious category imbalance problem, which usually requires some balancing strategies. In this paper, two strategies are used to improve the loss function. The first is weighted sigmoid cross entropy loss, as formula 2.

$$L = mean\left(\sum_{c=1}^{C} w^c (y^c log(\sigma(\hat{y}^c)) + (1 - y^c) log(1 - \sigma(\hat{y}^c)))\right) \tag{2}$$

where $w^c$ is the weight of each category, $w^c = 1/logn^c$ , and $n^c$ is the number of labels of each category. Weighting the loss function makes the model pay more attention to categories with a small number of samples, so it can alleviate the imbalance of data distribution.

The second strategy is softmax cross-entropy scheme, with the advantage of self-adaptability[15].

Cross entropy loss is equivalent to comparing all non-target class scores $s_{1,2,\ldots,t.t+1,\ldots,n}$ with the target class score $s_t$, and making the maximum difference less than 0 as far as possible. Formula 3 can be used to express the loss function.

$$L = log\left(1 + \sum_{i \in neg, j \in pos}^{C} e^{s_i - s_j}\right) \tag{3}$$

By introducing an additional 0 class, our objective is for the target classes to have scores greater than $s_0$, and for the non-target classes to have scores less than $s_0$, in this paper, suppose $s_0 = 0$. Formula 4 can be used to express the loss function.

$$L = log\left(1 + \sum_{i \in n, j \in p}^{C} e^{s_i - s_j}\right) + log\left(1 + \sum_{i \in n}^{C} e^{s_i - s_0}\right) + log\left(1 + \sum_{j \in p}^{C} e^{s_0 - s_j}\right) \tag{4}$$

In which neg and pos represent positive and negative sample sets respectively.

# 4 Implementation

## 4.1 Dataset

This paper utilizes a dataset from the "Hefei Hi-tech Cup" ECG intelligence competition, which contains 32,142 ECG records. Each sample has 8 leads, namely I, II, V1, V2, V3, V4, V5 and V6, with a sampling frequency of 500 Hz and a duration of 10 s. The data set contains 55 arrhythmia categories, and each record contains one or more labels. Through $III = II - I$, $aVR = -(II + I)/2$, $aVL = I - II/2$ and $aVF = II - I/2$ to obtain 12-lead ECG signal.

## 4.2 Data Preprocessing

The ECG records were augmented by size transformation, vertical flipping and other data enhancement operations, and resampled to 2048 points.

Cleaning the label data of the training set. Delete ECG records with mutually exclusive labels, such as ECG records with sinus rhythm and sinus arrhythmia.

## 4.3 Label Word Vector Embedding

This paper uses Chinese medical word segmentation toolkit pkuseg [16] to segment clinical ECG documents and establish a clinical ECG corpus. Glove model [17] is used to train ECG corpus. The word vectors corresponding to the 55 categories are obtained.

# 5 Results

## 5.1 Loss Function Optimization

Loss function is an important factor that affects the performance of deep learning. Therefore, this paper sets up a comparative experiment of different multi-label classification loss functions, namely sigmoid cross-entropy loss function (GRes18-SL), weighted sigmoid cross-entropy loss function (GRes18-WSL), and softmax cross-entropy loss function (GRes18-SML). The model structure and other parameters are fixed. The result is shown in Table 1.

**Table 1.** Results of different loss function

| | GRes18-SL | GRse18-WSL | GRse18-SML |
|---|---|---|---|
| Rec | 0.839 | 0.836 | 0.835 |
| Pre | 0.810 | 0.827 | 0.825 |
| F1 | 0.824 | 0.832 | 0.830 |

The highest F1 score of GRse18-WSL is 0.832, and the highest F1 score of GRes18-SML is 0.830, both of which are higher than GRes18-SLwith the original loss function, so the optimization of the loss function can improve the performance of the model. The F1 scores of each category are also calculated. Taking GRes18-SML model as an example, the F1 scores of categories with large number of samples, like complete right bundle branch block, sinus bradycardia and sinus rhythm are all above 0.95. However, in categories with small number of samples, like atrioventricular conduction and ST segment changes, the F1 score is about 0.5, which means the model does not perform well in these categories. On the whole, the model can achieve a high level of performance in most categories, but further research is needed for categories with small number of samples.

### 5.2 Comparison with Previous Studies

This paper also makes a comparative experiment with other models on the same data set. The contrast models used in the experiment include the original one-dimensional ResNet18 and ECGNet. The results are illustrated in Table 2.

**Table 2.** The results of different models

| | GCN-ResNet18 | ResNet18 | ECGNet |
|---|---|---|---|
| Rec | 0.836 | 0.839 | 0.838 |
| Pre | 0.827 | 0.817 | 0.827 |
| F1 | 0.832 | 0.828 | 0.833 |

Finally, the GCN-Res18 model proposed in this paper improves the F1 score to 0.832 compared to ResNet18.

The results of the above experiments prove that the GCN-ResNet model proposed in this paper can achieve the current high-performance level of multi-label ECG classification, and assist doctors in detecting patients during clinical diagnosis and treatment.

## 6 Conclusions

In this paper, a classification model GCN-ResNet based on GCN and CNN is proposed for ECG multi-label classification. By preprocessing the data and labels, improving the loss function and model, the method was able to achieve the highest F1 score of 0.832 on a 12-lead ECG dataset, thus demonstrating its ability to achieve high performance in multi-label ECG classification tasks.

There are still some limitations. The CNN used to extract ECG features in this paper is simple. It may be better to use the updated network model combined with attention mechanism. Furthermore, the model is unable to fully learn the characteristics of certain categories due to the insufficient number of samples. In addition, the model of this paper has not been verified on other data sets, and additional research is necessary to expand on the results of this study.

**Acknowledgment.** The study was partly supported by the National Natural Science Foundation of China (62171123, 62071241 and 62211530112).

## References

1. Zhang, M., Zhou, Z.: A review on multi-label learning algorithms. IEEE Trans. Knowl. Data Eng. **26**(8), 1819–1837 (2014)
2. Boutell, M.R., Luo, J., Shen, X., et al.: Learning multi-label scene classification. Pattern Recogn. **37**(9), 1757–1771 (2004)
3. Johannes, F., Eyke, H., et al.: Multilabel classification via calibrated label ranking. Mach. Learn. **73**(2), 133–153 (2008)
4. Read, J., Pfahringer, B., Holmes, G., et al.: Classifier chains for multi-label classification. Mach. Learn. **85**(3), 333–359 (2011)
5. Wang, J., Yang, Y., Mao, J., et al.: CNN-RNN: a unified framework for multi-label Image classification, In: 2016 IEEE Conference on Computer Vision and Pattern Recognition (CVPR), 2016, pp. 2285–2294. https://doi.org/10.1109/CVPR.2016.251
6. Yang, Y.Y., Lin, Y.A., Chu, H.M., et al.: Deep learning with a rethinking structure for multi-label classification. Proceedings of Machine Learning Research **101**, 1–16 (2019)
7. Durand, T., Mehrasa, N., Mori, G.: Learning a deep ConvNet for multi-label classification with partial labels. In: 2019 IEEE/CVF Conference on Computer Vision and Pattern Recognition (CVPR), Long Beach, CA, USA, 2019, pp. 647–657. https://doi.org/10.1109/CVPR.2019.00074
8. Yang, P., Sun, X., et al.: SGM: sequence generation model for multi-label classification. In: Proceedings of the 27th International Conference on Computational Linguistics (COLING), 2018, pp.3915–3926. arxiv.org/abs/1806.04822
9. Hannun, A.Y. et al.: Cardiologist-level arrhythmia detection and classification in ambulatory electrocardiograms using a deep neural network. Nat. Med. **25**(1), 65–69 (2019)
10. Kamaleswaran, R., Mahajan, R., Akbilgic, O.: A robust deep convolutional neural network for the classification of abnormal cardiac rhythm using varying length single lead electrocardiogram. Physiol. Meas. Akbilgic **39**(3), 035006 (2018)
11. Cai, J., Sun, W., Guan, J., You, I.: Multi-ECGNet for ECG arrhythmia multi-label classification. IEEE Access **8**, 110848–110858 (2020). https://doi.org/10.1109/ACCESS.2020.3001284
12. Li, D., Wu, H., et al.: Automatic classification system of arrhythmias using 12-lead ECGs with a deep neural network based on an attention mechanism. Symmetry **12**(11), 1827 (2020). https://doi.org/10.3390/sym12111827
13. Chen, Z.M., Wei, X.S., Wang, P., Guo, Y.: Multi-label image recognition with graph convolutional networks. In: 2019 IEEE/CVF Conference on Computer Vision and Pattern Recognition (CVPR), Long Beach, CA, USA, 2019, pp. 5172–5181
14. He, K., Zhang, X., Ren, S., Sun, J.: Deep residual learning for image recognition. In: 2016 IEEE Conference on Computer Vision and Pattern Recognition (CVPR), Las Vegas, NV, USA, 2016, pp. 770–778. https://doi.org/10.1109/CVPR.2016.90
15. Github: bert4keras [Source code] (2022). https://github.com/bojone/bert4keras
16. Luo, R., Xu, J., Zhang, Y., Zhang, Z., Ren, X., Sun, X.: PKUSEG: a toolkit for multi-domain Chinese word segmentation (2019)
17. Pennington, J., Socher, R., Manning, C.: GloVe: global vectors for word representation. In: Proceedings of the 2014 Conference on Empirical Methods in Natural Language Processing (EMNLP), 2014, pp. 1532–1543

# Automatic Analyzer for Urinary Stone Detection in Urine

Xianyou Sun[1,2], Yanchi Zhang[1], Chiyu Ma[1], Tianxing Wang[3], Hao Wan[1,2], and Ping Wang[1](✉)

[1] Key Laboratory for Biomedical Engineering of Ministry of Education, Department of Biomedical Engineering, Biosensor National Special Laboratory, Zhejiang University, Hangzhou 310027, China
12015014@zju.edu.cn
[2] Binjiang Institute of Zhejiang University, Hangzhou 310053, China
[3] Zhejiang, E-Linkcare Meditech Co., LTD, Baita Tongjiang Road, Taizhou, NoZhejiang, China

**Abstract.** Currently, the world's population is aging and sub-healthy, but due to the stressful life of people or medical pressure, most people are unable to go to the hospital in time for medical checkups to screen for hidden problems. Therefore, we developed an automated analyzer based on the principle of optical detection sensors for home or community use to help people screen for diseases. The analyzer uses non-invasive body fluids, such as urine and saliva, as the detection target, and it can automate the extraction and detection of disease markers in body fluids. The analyzer is also equipped with a unique upper computer operating system, which facilitates human-computer interaction. In this study, a detection protocol and sensing system were developed for urinary stone markers (citric acid and oxalic acid) in urine. The concentration of the target is converted into absorbance at a specific wavelength by nano-sensitive materials, and then the absorbance is quantitatively converted into an electrical signal by a photodiode and transmitted to the upper computer of the analyzer, and a detection report is generated. This study has completed the verification of the experimental principle and the optimization of the detection conditions. The analyzer can complete the extraction and detection of citric acid and oxalic acid in urine within 20 min, and the recovery rate in actual samples can reach more than 90%, which has the value of promotion and application.

**Keywords:** Biomedical sensors and instrument · Urinary stone detection · Urine pretreatment · Nano-sensitive materials

## 1 Introduction

With the accelerated pace of life, more and more young people are in a state of sub-health, and failure to go for medical check-ups may lead to the deterioration of diseases when minor symptoms appear in the body. In addition, due to aging, the elderly population is increasing, and the need for health care or early screening of diseases is even greater [1]. Therefore, there is an urgent need for timely medical checkups to avoid disease


G. Wang et al. (Eds.): APCMBE 2023, IFMBE Proceedings 103, pp. 466–474, 2024.
https://doi.org/10.1007/978-3-031-51455-5_53

progression. However, the reality has contradicted this need. On the one hand, people do not go to hospitals frequently for medical checkups due to the stressful life, and on the other hand, the rampant viral infectious diseases has aggravated the global medical resource constraint, and frequent hospital checkups increase the risk of contracting virus. Therefore, there is an urgent need for some medical detection instruments for home or community use to meet people's needs for early screening of diseases.

Popular medical instruments for home use include blood glucose meters, electrocardiographs and blood pressure monitors. Although these instruments serve the purpose of health monitoring, they can only provide some common physiological indicators, such as blood pressure or blood sugar, and cannot accurately determine people's diseases. Test strips are another type of medical testing product. Although they offer the advantage of low cost, they also fail to provide reliable screening results for diseases because their readings are easily affected by light or vision (especially in the elderly) and they do not provide quantitative results [3]. For this situation, we developed a portable analyzer that can automate the extraction and detection of disease markers using body fluids accessible non-invasively as the detection target (Fig. 2a). This analyzer integrates filtration, extraction, sample preparation, detection and self-cleaning functions for home use.

Urinary stones are a prevalent disorder that obstructs the urinary tract, harms local organs, and can potentially lead to kidney failure [4, 5]. The most common type of urinary calculus is calcium oxalate calculus, so the level of oxalate in urine can be one of the markers of urinary calculus [6, 7]. However, citrate inhibits crystal formation, so a low concentration of citric acid (CA) in the urine is also a cause of urolithiasis [8]. Measurement of citrate and oxalate levels in urine is important for the early prevention of urolithiasis in patients. [9, 10] We have developed a method to detect oxalic acid (OA) and CA in urine using this analyzer, which can provide early screening for patients with urolithiasis. More importantly, the analyzer is expected to become a universal analyzer for the detection of multiple disease markers, and any protocol that fits the same pre-treatment and detection process can be completed using it.

## 2 Materials and Methods

### 2.1 Detection Principle

CA was detected using citrate lyase. CA is broken down into oxaloacetate and acetate by the catalytic action of citrate lyase, and oxaloacetate is reduced to L-type malate by reduced nicotinamide adenine dinucleotide (NADH) in the presence of L-type malate dehydrogenase. The concentration of oxidized $NAD^+$ is linearly correlated with the concentration of CA in the sample. And due to the optical properties of NADH, which absorbs light at 340 nm, the concentration of CA can be quantified by measuring the decrease in the absorbance of NADH at 340 nm.

OA was detected using oxalate oxidase, which oxidizes OA to produce carbon dioxide and hydrogen peroxide. In this study, copper nanoclusters modified with dithiothreitol and bovine serum proteins (BSA-DTT-CuNCs) were used as a bionanocatalytic enzyme for catalyzing hydrogen peroxide, which maintains better activity over a wider pH range and temperature range compared to horseradish peroxidase. Hydrogen peroxide reacts with phenol and 4-aminoantipyrine (AAP) as chromogenic agents catalyzed by

BSA-DTT-CuNCs to form quinone dyes, which produce an absorption peak at 500 nm. Therefore, the amount of OA in urine can be measured by spectroscopic detection of an increase in absorbance at 500 nm. The principles of detection of CA and OA are shown in Fig. 1.

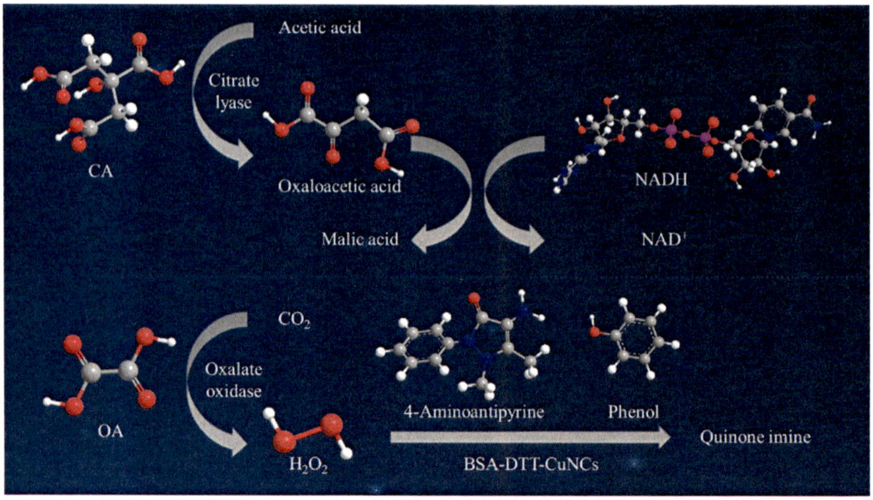


**Fig. 1.** Principle of citric acid and oxalic acid detection

## 2.2 Hardware

The analyzer consists of three parts: pre-processing module, detection module and control module (Fig. 2c). The function of the pre-treatment module is to complete the extraction and enrichment of OAs and CAs in urine. The pre-treatment module consists of a filtration unit, an extraction unit, a sample pool, a multichannel switching valve, two peristaltic pumps, two micro syringe pumps and three 2-position 3-way solenoid valves.

The detection module allows for the detection of 8 samples in one pass (Fig. 2b). A commercial microplate is mounted in a bracket with 8 light-transmitting holes at the bottom. The bracket is mounted on a screw nut, and the rotation of the screw stepper motor drives the displacement of the microplate. Its core components are two light sources emitting at 340 and 500 nm and two photodiodes that are sensitive to light at 340 and 500 nm, respectively, located directly above the light sources.

The control module consists of an Arduino mega2560 as the core controller with a sufficient number of I/O interfaces and some driver chips for driving various appliances. In addition, the analyzer is equipped with an LCD display and a built-in host computer containing Win10 system for human-computer interaction. The analyzer can also establish interaction with external computers through the USB interface.

### 2.3 Software

The design of software is divided into upper part and lower part. The upper part is programmed using Labview-2017, which is divided into editing command unit, displaying result unit and data post-processing unit. The editing command unit allows setting the operating mode and operating parameters of the analyzer and displays the connection status of the serial port. The displaying result unit shows the working process of the analyzer and the real-time data during the inspection. The data post-processing unit allows saving of the original experimental data and processing of the data such as generating calibration curves or generating test reports. The lower part is programmed with the Arduino IDE and interacts with the upper part through the serial port. The lower part program adopts modular design and can be divided into decoding subroutine, pre-processing subroutine and detection subroutine. After the lower part receives the command string containing the working parameters and working modes from the upper part, it first executes the decoding subroutine, assigns the decoded working parameters to each subroutine, and then executes the corresponding subroutine according to the decoded working modes.

### 2.4 Operating Principle

The pretreatment is divided into filtration, enrichment and extraction steps. The filtration unit contains three filters with progressively smaller screens, which can filter out impurity particles above 0.22 um from the urine. The multi-channel switching valve and peristaltic pumps will then pass the methanol solution and deionized water through the extraction unit to activate the filler. Next, the filtered urine will be passed through the extraction unit at a slow speed to enrich the OAs and CAs in the urine, while other impurities flow to the waste pool. Finally, dilute sulfuric acid solution will be passed through the extraction unit to dissolve OAs and CAs and then flow to the sample pool.

The micro syringe pumps with high precision drops the sample from the sample pool into the microplate through the droppers. The reaction of OAs and CAs in urine with the reaction substrate in the microplate will produce changes in absorbance at 500 nm and 340 nm, respectively. The screw will drive the microplate successively through the middle of the two light sources and the two photodiodes. The light emitted by the source passes through the bracket, the sample, and ultimately reaching the photodiode. Here, the real-time light intensity values are measured and then transmitted to the host computer. In addition, this analyzer has a calibration function where two miniature syringe pumps will drop standard samples and dilutions into specific wells, respectively, to formulate the concentration gradient specified in the upper unit.

## 3 Analysis of Results

### 3.1 Pre-processing Performance

The recovery of the pretreatment is a significant indicator to assess the performance of the analyzer pretreatment. A 10 mL artificial urine sample spiked with 1.5 mM OA was divided into two equal portions, one of which was pre-treated automatically by the analyzer and the other was left untreated. The two samples were analyzed separately for

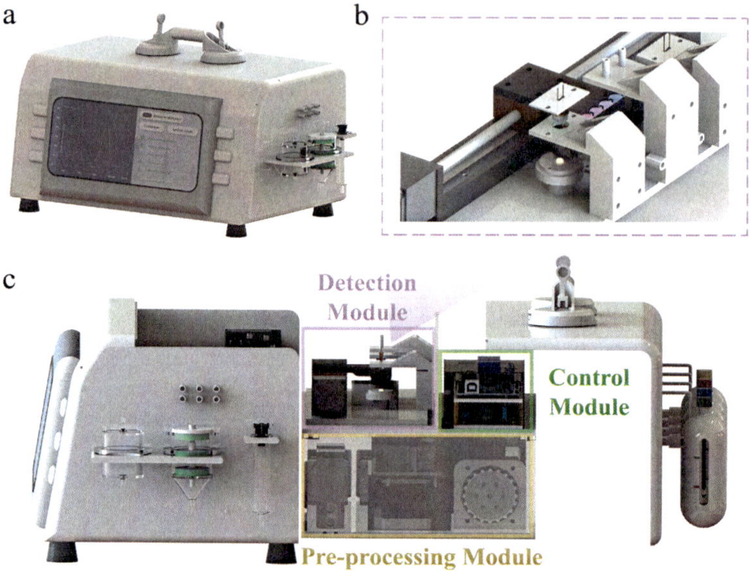


**Fig. 2.** Structure of the automatic analyzer. **a** The appearance of the automatic analyzer, its length, width and height are 440 mm, 300 mm, 250 mm; **b** Structure of the detection module; **c** Exploded view of the automatic analyzer.

OA using high performance liquid chromatography (HPLC) and the results are shown in Fig. 3a. The peak value of the OA sample (OA-P) pretreated by the analyzer was divided by the peak value of the original OA sample (OA-O) without pretreatment to obtain a recovery of 93.3% for OA. Similarly, 10 mL of the artificial urine sample spiked with 1.5 mM CA was treated identically, and the peak value of the CA sample (CA-P) pretreated by the analyzer was divided by the peak value of the original CA sample without pretreatment (CA-O) to obtain a recovery of 95.9% for CA. The analyzer pretreatment causes a small loss of OA and CA in the urine due to traces of OA and CA remaining in the analyzer pipeline and extraction column after the pretreatment.

## 3.2 Detection Performance

To verify the sensitivity and linearity of the analyzer detection module, OA solutions ranging from 1mM-10mM and CA solutions ranging from 0.2 mM to 10 mM were prepared. The reaction substrate was added to the microplate and the different concentrations of OA solution were then added dropwise to the 6 wells in turn. The absorbance of the solution at 500 nm was tested by the microplate reader and the analyzer, and two standard curve sets were generated. (Fig. 3b). The linear fitting equation is $y = 0.0427x + 0.1109$ with an $R^2$ coefficient of 0.9978 and $y = 0.0346x + 0.0848$ with an $R^2$ coefficient of 0.9998, respectively, achieved by the microplate reader and the analyzer.

Subsequently, different concentrations of CA solutions were added dropwise to the 6 wells of the microplate containing the reaction substrate, and the absorbance of the solutions at 340 nm was tested by the microplate reader and the analyzer, and two standard curve sets were generated. (Fig. 3c). The linear fitting equation is y = – 0.0945x + 1.3949 with an $R^2$ coefficient of 0.9982 and y = – 0.0653x + 0.8381 with an $R^2$ coefficient of 0.9941, respectively, achieved by the microplate reader and the analyzer. The results show that the analyzer has comparable sensitivity and linearity to the enzyme marker in the linear range. Therefore, it is suitable for the detection of OA and CA.

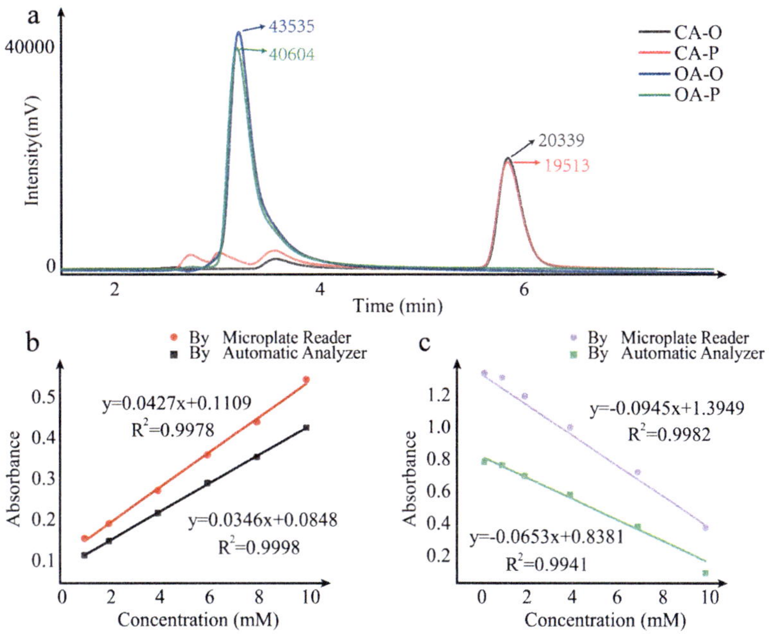


**Fig. 3.** Results of performance verification of the analyzer. **a** Verification of the analyzer pretreatment performance, where CA-O and CA-P represent CA samples without the analyzer pretreatment and CA samples with the analyzer pretreatment, respectively, and OA-O and OA-P represent OA samples without the analyzer pretreatment and OA samples with the analyzer pretreatment, respectively; **b** Verification of the detection performance of OA; **c** Verification of the detection performance of CA.

### 3.3 Detection of Real Samples

Real urine spiked with different concentrations of OA and CA was pre-treated and detected automatically by the analyzer. The experiment was repeated three times for each concentration, and the results are shown in Tables 1 and 2. The results showed that the recovery of OA in the real sample by the analyzer ranged from 91% to 94% with a coefficient of variation of less than 7.97%, while the recovery of CA in the real sample ranged from 92% to 95% with a coefficient of variation of less than 6.41%. It indicates that the analyzer has good recovery and stability for the real samples.

**Table 1.** The detection results of OA in real samples

| Spiked concentration | Detection concentration | Coefficient of variation (%) | Recovery (%) |
|---|---|---|---|
| 2 mM | 1.848 ± 0.095 | 5.150 | 92.405 |
| 4 mM | 3.672 ± 0.047 | 1.293 | 91.793 |
| 6 mM | 5.617 ± 0.415 | 7.396 | 93.609 |
| 8 mM | 7.464 ± 0.058 | 0.775 | 93.300 |

**Table 2.** The detection results of CA in real samples

| Spiked concentration | Detection concentration | Coefficient of variation (%) | Recovery (%) |
|---|---|---|---|
| 2 mM | 1.841 ± 0.107 | 5.816 | 92.056 |
| 4 mM | 3.746 ± 0.068 | 1.816 | 93.661 |
| 6 mM | 5.712 ± 0.005 | 0.089 | 95.206 |
| 8 mM | 7.441 ± 0.477 | 6.409 | 93.007 |

## 4 Discussion

We have successfully developed a detection method for OA and CA and demonstrated its feasibility through experimental results. CuNCs were innovatively utilized as the catalyst, and the traditional HRP and TMB colorimetric system was replaced with a phenol-APP colorimetric system. The stability of CuNCs enhanced the method's anti-interference ability, making it more suitable for complex on-site detection environments.

The success of our detection method also confirms the excellent performance of the automatic analyzer. It is important to note that on-site biochemical detection instruments must possess the capability to pre-treat biological samples; otherwise, the complexity of the samples can lead to significant interference during detection. Our instrument exhibits exceptional pre-treatment performance, as validated through HPLC. The automatic pre-processing scheme based on solid-phase extraction that we designed can serve as a reference for the extraction of other biomarkers. Although there is room for improvement in the pre-processing module of our instrument, such as enhancing the recovery rate, sample loss is inevitable even with careful manual pre-processing. Fortunately, the recovery rate of the analyzer's pre-processing is stable within a small range. Therefore, establishing an algorithm model to compensate for sample loss may be a suitable approach. In addition, the detection module of our analyzer cleverly miniaturizes the microplate reader, maintaining the same detection performance and 8 channels while reducing the volume.

In urinary stone screening applications, while hyperoxaluria and hypocitraturia are the most common types of urinary stones [6–8], accounting for approximately 80% of cases, uric acid concentration and pH are also important reference factors. [11, 12]

Therefore, further research should be conducted to expand the instrument's detection capabilities to include uric acid and pH, achieving a more comprehensive evaluation of urinary stones. On the other hand, it is also worth exploring how to integrate screening protocols for other diseases into the instrument, making it a multi-disease screening device for use in households or communities.

## 5 Conclusions

In summary, an automatic analyzer that can automate the extraction and detection of OAs and CAs in urine was established. After experimental validation, the automatic analyzer pre-treatment module can achieve 93.3% and 95.9% recovery of OA and CA in urine, while the detection module has comparable sensitivity and linearity to the microplate reader for the detection of OA and CA standard solutions. Finally, the results of the detection of real samples showed that the automatic analyzer could automate the extraction and detection of CA and OA in urine within 20 min with good recovery and stability. In addition, the analyzer has great potential to be used for the detection of other biomarkers. Due to its ease of operation, it can be used at home or in the community, and has the value of promotion.

**Acknowledgment.** This work was supported by National Key Research and Development Program of China (No. 2021YFB3200801), Key International Cooperation Project of NSFC (No. 62120106004) and the Research Program of Zhejiang Provincial Science and Technology Department (No. 2023C03104).

## References

1. Chang, A.Y., Skirbekk, V.F., Tyrovolas, S., et al.: Measuring population ageing: an analysis of the Global Burden of Disease Study 2017. In: The Lancet Public Health, pp. e159-e167 (2017)
2. Jaul, E., Barron, J.: Age-related diseases and clinical and public health implications for the 85 years old and over population. In: Frontiers in Public Health, Mini Review, vol. 5 (2017). Accessed 11 Dec 2017
3. Sajid, M., Kawde, A.N, Daud, M.: Designs, formats and applications of lateral flow assay: a literature review. J. Saudi Chem. Soc. 689–705 (2015)
4. Türk, C. et al.: EAU guidelines on diagnosis and conservative management of urolithiasis. In: European Urology, pp. 468–474 (2016)
5. Scales, C.D., Smith, A.C., Hanley, J.M., et al.: Prevalence of kidney stones in the United States. In: European Urology, pp. 160–165 (2012)
6. Cochat, P., Rumsby, G.: Primary hyperoxaluria. N. Engl. J. Med. 649–658 (2013)
7. Garrelfs, S.F., et al.: Lumasiran, an RNAi therapeutic for primary hyperoxaluria type 1. N. Engl. J. Med. 1216–1226 (2021)
8. Wu, J., Zhao, J., Zhao, Z., et al.: Significance of TRPV5 and OPN biomarker levels in clinical diagnosis of patients with early urinary calculi. Am. J. Transl. Res. 6778–6783 (2021)
9. Spradling, K., Vernez, S.L., Khoyliar, C., et al.: Prevalence of hyperoxaluria in urinary stone formers: chronological and geographical trends and a literature review. J. Endourol. **30**(4), 469–475 (2016)

10. Zuckerman, J.M., Assimos, D.G.: Hypocitraturia: pathophysiology and medical management. Rev. Urol. **11**(3), 134 (2009)
11. López, M., Hoppe, B.: History, epidemiology and regional diversities of urolithiasis. Pediatr. Nephrol. **25**, 49–59 (2010)
12. Türk, C., Knoll, T., Petrik, A., et al.: Guidelines on urolithiasis. Eur. Assoc. Urol. (2011)

# A U-Sleep Model for Sleep Staging Using Electrocardiography and Respiration Signals

Kaiyue Si[1], Kejun Dong[1,2], Jingyi Lu[1], Lina Zhao[1], Wentao Xiang[3], Jianqing Li[3], and Chengyu Liu[1(✉)]

[1] School of Instrument Science and Engineering, Southeast University, Nanjing, China
chengyu@seu.edu.cn

[2] School of Information Science and Engineering, Southeast University, Nanjing, China

[3] School of Biomedical Engineering and Informatics, Nanjing Medical University, Nanjing, China

**Abstract.** Recognizing sleep stages has significant clinical relevance for assessing the physical and mental health of people and for treating sleep-related illnesses. Since manual sleep stage requires experienced clinician to carry out and the process is time-consuming and laborious, the automatic methods for sleep staging have been widely investigated. To perform a five-class (wake, N1, N2, N3 and rapid eye movement) sleep staging task, 255 subjects with polysomnography signals including a single-lead electrocardiography (ECG) signal and single-channel respiration signal from the DCSM dataset is utilized. Notably, ECG and respiration signals are reflecting in heart rate and respiratory rhythm, respectively. The sleep stages are scored in standard 30s-length epochs. This work describes an automatic sleep staging method based on the U-Sleep network, a typical U-Net architecture, which includes three sub-modules: the encoder, the decoder, and the segment classifier. The subject-independent experiment shows an overall accuracy of 0.641 and F1-score of 0.45 for the five sleep stages on test set by the applied U-sleep network. Our findings confirm to some extent that ECG and respiratory signals contain comprehensive information for sleep staging.

**Keywords:** ECG · Respiration · U-Sleep model · Sleep staging

## 1 Introduction

Sleep is a basic human physiological process and important for maintaining health. A series of physiological and biochemical changes can be occurred in the different sleep stages, which helps restore physical strength, boost immunity, overcome diseases and physical recovery [1]. Moreover, adequate sleep helps promote optimal learning, memory, concentration, mood, and decision-making processes for brain cognition [2]. Normally, the sleep cycle of people can be divided into three phases: wakefulness (W), rapid eye movement (REM), and non-rapid eye movement (NREM) phases, where NREM is

This Work Was Supported in Part By the National Natural Science Foundation of China (62171123, 62211530112, 62201144, 62001240 and 62071241).


G. Wang et al. (Eds.): APCMBE 2023, IFMBE Proceedings 103, pp. 475–482, 2024.
https://doi.org/10.1007/978-3-031-51455-5_54

can be further divided into progressive depth stages (e.g. N1, N2, and N3 stages). Besides, The phases and cycles of sleep, which display the underlying neurophysiological processes, are valuable resource for identifying the diagnostic indicators of a variety of sleep disorders, such as sleep apnea, insomnia, depression, Alzheimer's disease and cardiovascular diseases [3, 4]. So, sleep staging has significant clinical relevance for assessing the physical and mental health of people and for treating sleep-related illnesses.

Polysomnography (PSG) technique is viewed as international recognized gold standard for objective physiological quantification of human sleep stages by monitoring continuous breathing, arterial oxygen saturation, electroencephalogram (EEG), electrocardiogram (ECG), heart rate, and other indicators at night. However, this technique needs to be fixed in the designated parts of the body of the person being monitored, suffering discomfort with multiple-channel EEG, multiple-lead ECG recordings and it is not convenient for long-term monitoring. So many studies prefer to monitor sleep from single-lead ECG signal. For example, Radha et al. used the single-lead ECG signal to extract RR intervals, heart rate variability features, and finally completed the classification of sleep stages [5]. But this method can only characterize small information about the state of the heart. Later, Thomas et al. developed an automated measurement method for cardiopulmonary coupling (CPC) using respiration signals during sleep, which verified that CPC and ECG are consistent [6] and provided more accurately sleep staging [7].

In recent years, with the development of machine learning and deep learning techniques, some automatic sleep staging algorithms using ECG signal and respiration signals have emerged [8]. Sun et al. achieved the best performance for staging all five sleep stages with a Cohen's kappa of 0.585 by developing deep neural networks to stage sleep from ECG and respiratory signals, validating that ECG and respiratory effort provide substantial information about sleep stages [9]. Recently, fully convolutional networks have achieved great success in medical image analysis, where U-net is widely utilized in the field of medical image segmentation. Notably, the typical U-net for image domain can be viewed as the encoder-decoder structure, where encoder is used as feature extraction and decoder structure is up-sampling to further feature reconstruction [10]. To deal with the temporal sequences, U-Time network, a fully convolutional encoder-decoder network, was proposed by mapping continuous inputs of arbitrary length to sequences of class labels on freely selected timescales [11]. Recently, the U-Sleep network was established using PSG recordings for sleep staging with only two-lead ECG signals from 15,660 participants of 16 clinical studies, with a mean F1-score being 0.79 for healthy adults and 0.76 for patients with sleep apnea [12]. The U-Sleep network extends the U-Time model by building on the repository. Individual instances of the model can be trained, accurate and resilient sleep staging can be performed in a wide range of clinical populations and polysomnography (PSG) acquisition protocols. Inspired the excellent performance of U-Sleep network [7, 12], we propose an automatic sleep staging method based on the U-Sleep network with the ECG and respiratory signals by considering the comprehensive information.

The rest of this work is structured as follows. Materials and methods are described in Sect. 2. Sections 3 and 4 present results and conclusions, respectively.

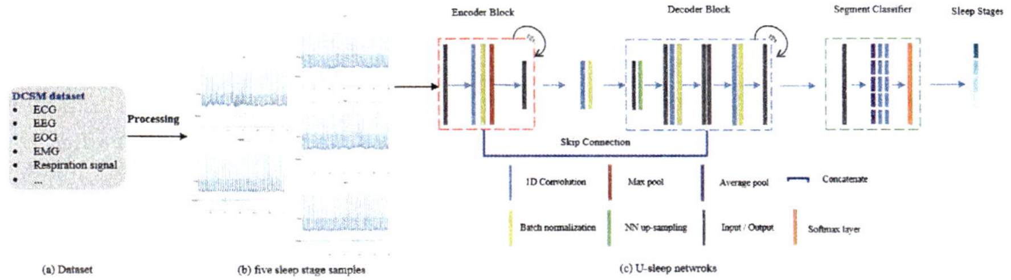


**Fig. 1.** The overview of the proposed U-sleep framework with **a** dataset, **b** typical fives samples contain 30s-length of signals, **c** the U-Sleep networks for classification, respectively

## 2 Materials and Methods

### 2.1 Dataset

As shown in Fig. 1a, the DCSM dataset originates from the Danish Center for Sleep Medicine (DCSM), which consists of 255 randomly selected subjects visiting the DCSM for the diagnosis of non-specific sleep-related disorders with a fully anonymized overnight lab-based PSG recordings [12]. The DCSM dataset represents a diverse cohort of Danish patients for demographic characteristics, diagnostic background, and sleep/non-sleep-related medication usage. The PSG recordings were collected from 2015 to 2018. Each PSG includes ECG signal, respiratory signals recorded from the chest and abdominal bands, EOG signal and EMG signal. Note that all signals for PSG recordings were sampled at 256 Hz and acquired from subjects about 20 h.

### 2.2 Pre-processing

A band pass filter (0.3–70 Hz with 3 dB limits) was applied to eliminate high-frequency noise, the intended purpose of the DCSM dataset is the development and benchmarking of clinically applicable sleep staging. In our work, we only used a single-lead ECG signal (ECG-II) and single-channel respiration signal (NASAL) from the individuals as the input signals. The ECG and respiratory signals are resampled to 128 Hz using polyphasic filtering. The sleep scoring is accomplished by dividing the night of PSG recording into standard 30-s epochs and sleep staging labels are annotated by experts according to AASM criteria. Typical fives epochs contain 30 s-length of ECG and respiration signals with respect to W, REM, N1, N2 and N3 stages, as shown in Fig. 1b. Note that, after the pre-processing, the dataset includes 187076, 6593, 8049, 55982, 10021 epochs of all 255 subjects for W, REM, N1, N2 and N3 stages, respectively.

### 2.3 The U-Sleep Model

As also shown in Fig. 1c, the U-Sleep model consists of three sub-modules: encoder, decoder, and segment classifier. The encoder takes the original two channels physiological signals (ECG-II and NASAL) as the input and represents it with a deep stack of feature maps, where the input signal is sampled multiple times. The decoder learns the mapping from the feature stack back to the input signal domain, providing dense point-by-point segmentation. The segmentation classifier applies tight representations at selected temporal resolution to predict the final sleep stages.

*Encoder:* this module consists of 12 encoder blocks, each of them includes a 1D convolutional layer and a layer of exponential linear unit (ELU) activation functions, batch normalization, and max-pooling. The size of convolutional kernel is 9 with a stride of 1, a kernelless expansion is expanded following a batch normalization and max-pooling operation. Notably, the length of input to the encoder are two channels physiological signals in this work.

*Decoder:* it also consists of 12 decoder blocks, where each of them performs nearest neighbour (NN) up-sampling on its input signal and applies 1D convolution layer (with convolution kernel size of 2 and a stride of 1), the ELU activation function, and batch normalization. Here, the length of the feature mapping along the time axis can be doubled after the NN up-sampling operation. Note that, the up-scaled input is combined with the output of the corresponding encoder block's batch parametric operation, then it is subjected to convolution, non-linearity, and batch normalization. Finally, the output of the decoder module has the same temporal resolution as the initial input signal.

*Segment classifier:* it aggregates sample scores into longer time segments. For a given $i$-th length of window, the segment classifier performs the channel dimensional averaging pooling with width $i$ and stride $i$, , followed by two point-by-point convolutions (with a convolution kernel width of 1 and a stride of 1). The output of the segment classifier is $T \times K$ right random matrix, where T is the number of segments and $K = 5$ is the number of sleep stages. The scores are converted to probabilistic predictions using the softmax operation.

The main parameters of the U-Sleep model include epochs, batch size, learning rate, maximum step during model training, given Table 1.

**Table 1.** Some main parameters settings using for U-Sleep model.

| Parameter | Value |
|---|---|
| Epochs | 641 |
| Batch size | 16 |
| Learning rate | 0.000005 |
| Maximum step | 2000 |

# 3 Results and Discussion

## 3.1 Evaluation Metrics

To evaluate the performance of the classification, we focus on the precision, recall, and F1-score metrics. The precision and recall are defined as follows:

$$Precision = \frac{TP}{TP + FP} \tag{1}$$

$$Recall = \frac{TP}{TP + FN} \tag{2}$$

where $TP$, $FP$, and $FN$ are the numbers of true positives, false positives, and false negatives for a given sleep stages. Note that precision represents the proportion of true examples returned. The recall represents the proportion of true cases returned to all positive cases. The above two metrics are contradictory, to balances both precision and recall, another widely used metric F1-score, defined as:

$$F_1 = \frac{2TP}{2TP + FN + FP} \tag{3}$$

### 3.2 Subject-independent Experiment

To evaluate the performance of our proposed U-sleep model, we conducted the subject-independence classification, the individual differences physiology signals patterns across subjects leads to inferior accuracy as expected, but this is very useful for clinical application in practical. Specifically, the DCSM dataset includes 255 subjects, which is divided into training set (resp. 74.5%), validation set (resp. 10.2%), and test set (resp. 15.4%), each accounting for 190, 26, and 39 subjects. All records from subjects in the training set are used to train the U-Sleep model. The records in the validation set are utilized to do fine-tuning parameters to improve the performance of U-Sleep model. Records from the test set are provided for evaluation.

### 3.3 Performance

The classification performance of individual sleep stages with respect to five-class task are tested. Table 2 presents the confusion matrix for all samples over 39 subjects in test set. The diagonal elements represent the number of samples (TP) that are correctly classified by the U-Sleep model, whereas the off-diagonal elements show the number of samples that are mislabeled to other classes. From this table, we have unbalance dataset where the numbers of samples for W, R, N1, N2 and N3 are 30501 (resp. 47.74%), 6805 (resp. 10.65%), 3821 (resp. 5.98%), 16580 (resp. 25.95%) and 6188 (resp. 9.68%), respectively. The overall accuracy of our proposed U-Sleep model for five-class sleep stages from this confusion matrix is obtained 0.641. Compared to other machine learning technologies to monitor sleep using ECG and respiratory singals has attracted increasing attention.

According to the confusion matrix in Table 2, the corresponding precision, recall, and F1-score metrics for each sleep stages are calculated and presented in Table 3. From this table, we can obtain that the W stage performed well on all three indicators (>0.7), R stage has a high precision (*e.g.* 0.79) while the other two indicators have low values. The precisions of N1 and N2 sleep stages are very low, only 0.23 and 0.55. The W sleep stage has the highest overall recall at approximately 0.94. Besides, the N1 sleep stage shows a lower overall recall of only 0.322. This result is consistent with this sleep stage often showing very low agreement across human sleep scorers (<45%) [15]. Regarding the F1-score metric, the performance of the five stages is along with the samples proportion. Finally, the overall mean F1-score of 5 stages is equal to 0.45.

**Table 2.** The confusion matrix for all 39 subjects in test set.

| | Predicted | | | | | |
|---|---|---|---|---|---|---|
| True | | W | REM | N1 | N2 | N3 |
| | W | 28611 | 85 | 778 | 1023 | 4 |
| | REM | 3047 | 1008 | 553 | 2152 | 45 |
| | N1 | 1485 | 25 | 1232 | 1045 | 34 |
| | N2 | 5130 | 138 | 2428 | 8556 | 328 |
| | N3 | 1659 | 19 | 306 | 2668 | 1536 |
| TP = 40943, Total = 63895, ACC = 0.641 | | | | | | |

**Table 3.** The classification metrics with respect to precision, recall, and F1-score for all 39 subjects in test set.

| | $F_1$ | Precision | Recall |
|---|---|---|---|
| W | 0.81 | 0.72 | 0.94 |
| REM | 0.25 | 0.79 | 0.15 |
| N1 | 0.27 | 0.23 | 0.32 |
| N2 | 0.53 | 0.55 | 0.52 |
| N3 | 0.38 | 0.79 | 0.25 |
| Mean | 0.45 | 0.62 | 0.43 |

Finally, we also investigate the classification performance for each subject with respect to the five stages in the test set in the context of F1-score metric. The mean, standard deviation, the maximum and minimum values for F1-score related to the 39 subjects are presented in Table 4. The mean, minimum and maximum values of the F1-score are equal to 0.878, 0.558 and 0.976, which are presented the best performance in W stage. Regarding the N2 stage, we can obtain that it has a larger range of F1-score from 0.205 to 0.700 where presents the highest standard deviation among the five stages. These results reflect the large difference for subjects in N2 stage.

**Table 4.** Some statistical distributions about F1-score values of five sleep stages among all the 39 subjects.

| | mean | std | min | max |
|---|---|---|---|---|
| W | 0.878 | 0.085 | 0.558 | 0.976 |
| REM | 0.399 | 0.077 | 0.280 | 0.599 |
| N1 | 0.325 | 0.076 | 0.205 | 0.445 |
| N2 | 0.512 | 0.132 | 0.205 | 0.700 |
| N3 | 0.371 | 0.079 | 0.247 | 0.571 |

Some previous studies and our work with similar input signals are summarized in Table 5. Compared to the two studies, our work uses a larger sample size of training and testing sets, which can provide more robust study. Moreover, our propsed U-Sleep model for the five-class sleep stages shows similar results with respect to the two studies.

**Table 5.** Related work in the literature

| Study | Year | Dataset size | Type of signal | Performance |
|---|---|---|---|---|
| [13] | 2006 | 37 subjects | ECG, ribcage respiratory effort and EEG | 3 stages (W, REM, and non-REM sleep); accuracy = 67% |
| [14] | 2015 | 48 subjects | ECG and respiratory inductance plethysmography | 4 stages (W, light sleep, deep sleep, REM); accuracy = 69% |
| Our work | 2023 | 255 subjects | ECG and respiration signal (NASAL) | 5 stages (W, REM, N1, N2, N3); accuracy = 64% |

## 4 Conclusions

In this work, we applied U-Sleep network to perform the five-stage sleep staging (W, REM, N1, N2, N3) using single-lead ECG signal and single-channel respiratory signal from a public open dataset, named DCSM. This method enables sleep monitoring with only two physiological signals, making a small step towards application in actual situations. However, this work has some limitations, such as the discrepancy of physiological signals for different subjects and unbalance samples problems. In our future work, we try to apply domain adaptation methods and some data augmentation strategies to overcome these limitations. Moreover, the optimal combination of ECG and respiratory signals should become the directions that need to be explored in depth.

## References

1. Besedovsky, L., Lange, T., Haack, M.: The sleep-immune crosstalk in health and disease. Physiol. Rev. **99**(3), 1325–1380 (2019)
2. Simon, E.B., Vallat, R., Barnes, C.M., Walker, M.P.: Sleep loss and the socio-emotional brain. Trends Cogn. Sci. **24**(6), 435–450 (2020)
3. Leary, E.B., Watson, K.T., Ancoli-Israel, S., Redline, S., Stone, K.L.: Association of rapid eye movement sleep with mortality in middle-aged and older adults. JAMA Neurology, **77**(10), 1241–1251
4. Lucey, B.P., Mccullough, A., Landsness, E.C., Toedebusch, C.D., Holtzman, D.M.: Reduced non-rapid eye movement sleep is associated with tau pathology in early Alzheimer's disease. Sci. Transl. Med., **11**(474), (2019)
5. Radha, M., Fonseca, P., Moreau, A., Ross, M., Aarts, R.M.: Sleep stage classification from heart-rate variability using long short-term memory neural networks. Sci. Rep. **9**(1), 14149 (2019)
6. Thomas, R.J., Mietus, J.E., Peng, C.K., Goldberger, A.L.: An electrocardiogram-based technique to assess cardiopulmonary coupling during sleep. Sleep (9), 28,1151–1161 (2005)
7. Ji, H.C., et al.: Sleep quality change after upper airway surgery in obstructive sleep apnea: Electrocardiogram-Based Cardiopulmonary Coupling Analysis. Laryngoscope **125**(7), 1737–1742 (2015)
8. Fiorillo, L., Puiatti, A., Papandrea, M., Ratti, P.L., Faraci, F.D. : Automated sleep scoring: A review of the latest approaches. Sleep Med. Rev., **48**, (2019)
9. Sun, H., Ganglberger, W., Panneerselvam, E., Leone, M.J., Quadri, S.A., Goparaju, B., Westover, M.B.: Sleep staging from electrocardiography and respiration with deep learning. Sleep, **43**(7), (2020)
10. Ronneberger, O., Fischer, P., Brox, T.: U-Net: convolutional networks for biomedical image segmentation. MICCAI, 234–241 (2015)
11. Perslev, M., Jensen, M. H., Darkner, S., Jennum, P.J., Igel, C.: U-Time: a fully convolutional network for time series segmentation applied to sleep staging. (2019)
12. Perslev, M., Darkner, S., Kempfner, L., Nikolic, M., Jennum, P.J., Igel, C.: U-Sleep: resilient high-frequency sleep staging. NPJ Digit Med **4**(1), 72 (2021)
13. Redmond, S.J., Heneghan, C.: Cardiorespiratory-based sleep staging in subjects with obstructive sleep apnea. IEEE Trans. Biomed. Eng. **53**(3), 485–496 (2006)
14. Fonseca, P., Long, X., Radha, M., Haakma, R., Aarts, R.M., Rolink, J.M.: Sleep stage classification with ECG and respiratory effort. Physiol. Meas., **36**(10), (2015)
15. Atul, M., Magdy, Y., Kuna, S. T., Ruth, B., Kushida, C. A., James, W., Pien, G.W.: Performance of an automated polysomnography scoring system versus computer-assisted manual scoring. Sleep (4), 573–582

# Author Index





G. Wang et al. (Eds.): APCMBE 2023, IFMBE Proceedings 103, pp. 483–486, 2024.
https://doi.org/10.1007/978-3-031-51455-5

**Z**